MW01701285

12

AMERICAN ACADEMY™
OF OPHTHALMOLOGY

Retina and Vitreous

Last major revision 2015–2016

2016–2017
BCSC
Basic and Clinical Science Course™

Funded in part by the Educational Trust Fund/Retina Research Foundation

Protecting Sight. Empowering Lives.™

EB
Published after collaborative review with the European Board of Ophthalmology subcommittee

The American Academy of Ophthalmology is accredited by the Accreditation Council for Continuing Medical Education to provide continuing medical education for physicians.

The American Academy of Ophthalmology designates this enduring material for a maximum of 15 *AMA PRA Category 1 Credits*™. Physicians should claim only the credit commensurate with the extent of their participation in the activity.

CME expiration date: June 1, 2018. *AMA PRA Category 1 Credits*™ may be claimed only once between June 1, 2015, and the expiration date.

BCSC® volumes are designed to increase the physician's ophthalmic knowledge through study and review. Users of this activity are encouraged to read the text and then answer the study questions provided at the back of the book.

To claim *AMA PRA Category 1 Credits*™ upon completion of this activity, learners must demonstrate appropriate knowledge and participation in the activity by taking the posttest for Section 12 and achieving a score of 80% or higher. For further details, please see the instructions for requesting CME credit at the back of the book.

The Academy provides this material for educational purposes only. It is not intended to represent the only or best method or procedure in every case, nor to replace a physician's own judgment or give specific advice for case management. Including all indications, contraindications, side effects, and alternative agents for each drug or treatment is beyond the scope of this material. All information and recommendations should be verified, prior to use, with current information included in the manufacturers' package inserts or other independent sources, and considered in light of the patient's condition and history. Reference to certain drugs, instruments, and other products in this course is made for illustrative purposes only and is not intended to constitute an endorsement of such. Some material may include information on applications that are not considered community standard, that reflect indications not included in approved FDA labeling, or that are approved for use only in restricted research settings. **The FDA has stated that it is the responsibility of the physician to determine the FDA status of each drug or device he or she wishes to use, and to use them with appropriate, informed patient consent in compliance with applicable law.** The Academy specifically disclaims any and all liability for injury or other damages of any kind, from negligence or otherwise, for any and all claims that may arise from the use of any recommendations or other information contained herein.

AAO, AAOE, American Academy of Ophthalmology, Basic and Clinical Science Course, BCSC, EyeCare America, EyeNet, EyeSmart, EyeWiki, Focal Points, IRIS, ISRS, OKAP, ONE, Ophthalmic Technology Assessments, *Ophthalmology,* Preferred Practice Pattern, ProVision, SmartSight, The Ophthalmic News & Education Network, and the AAO logo (shown on cover) and tagline (Protecting Sight. Empowering Lives) are, among other marks, the registered trademarks and trademarks of the American Academy of Ophthalmology.

Cover image: From BCSC Section 10, *Glaucoma.* Typical gonioscopic appearance of angle recession. *Courtesy of Steven T. Simmons, MD.*

MIX
Paper from responsible sources
FSC
www.fsc.org
FSC® C103061

Copyright © 2016
American Academy of Ophthalmology
All rights reserved
Printed in the United States of America

Basic and Clinical Science Course

Louis B. Cantor, MD, Indianapolis, Indiana, *Senior Secretary for Clinical Education*
Christopher J. Rapuano, MD, Philadelphia, Pennsylvania, *Secretary for Ophthalmic Knowledge*
George A. Cioffi, MD, New York, New York, *BCSC Course Chair*

Section 12

Faculty

Colin A. McCannel, MD, *Chair,* Los Angeles, California
Neal H. Atebara, MD, Honolulu, Hawaii
Stephen Jae Kim, MD, Nashville, Tennessee
Brian C. Leonard, MD, Ottawa, Canada
Richard B. Rosen, MD, New York, New York
David Sarraf, MD, Los Angeles, California
Emmett Cunningham, Jr, MD, PhD, MPH, *Consultant,* Hillsborough, California
Graham E. Holder, PhD, *Consultant,* London, England

The Academy wishes to acknowledge the American Society of Retina Specialists (ASRS), the Macula Society, and the Retina Society for recommending faculty members to the BCSC Section 12 committee.

The Academy also wishes to acknowledge the following committees for review of this edition:

Committee on Aging: Helen Ka-Fun Li, MD, Houston, Texas

Vision Rehabilitation Committee: Joseph L. Fontenot, Daphne, Texas

Practicing Ophthalmologists Advisory Committee for Education: David J. Browning, MD, PhD, *Primary Reviewer,* Charlotte, North Carolina; Edward K. Isbey III, MD, *Chair,* Asheville, North Carolina; Alice L. Bashinsky, MD, Asheville, North Carolina; Robert G. Fante, MD, Denver, Colorado; Bradley D. Fouraker, MD, Tampa, Florida; Dasa V. Gangadhar, MD, Wichita, Kansas; Steven J. Grosser, MD, Golden Valley, Minnesota; James A. Savage, MD, Memphis, Tennessee

EBO

European Board of Ophthalmology: Alain Gaudric, MD, *Chair,* Paris, France; Catherine Creuzot-Garcher, MD, PhD, FEBO, *Liaison,* Dijon, France; Bahram Bodaghi, MD, PhD, Paris, France; Giovanni Staurenghi, MD, Milan, Italy; Adnan Tufail, MBBS, MD, London, United Kingdom

The EBO wishes to acknowledge EURETINA for recommending reviewers to the EBO committee.

Financial Disclosures

Academy staff members who contributed to the development of this product state that within the past 12 months, they have had no financial interest in or other relationship with any entity discussed in this course that produces, markets, resells, or distributes ophthalmic health care goods or services consumed by or used in patients, or with any competing commercial product or service.

The authors and reviewers state that within the past 12 months, they have had the following financial relationships:*

Dr Bodaghi: Abbott Medical Optics (C), Allergan (C, S), Bausch + Lomb Surgical (C), Novartis Pharmaceuticals (S), Santen (C), Xoma (C)

Dr Browning: Aerpio Therapeutics (S), Alimera Sciences (C), Diabetic Retinopathy Clinical Research Network (S), Genentech (S), Novartis Pharmaceuticals (S), Pfizer (S), Regeneron Pharmaceuticals (S)

Dr Creuzot-Garcher: Alcon Laboratories (C, S), Bausch + Lomb (C), Laboratoires Thea (C), Novartis Pharmaceuticals (C, L, S)

Dr Fante: Ophthalmic Mutual Insurance Company (C)

Dr Fouraker: Addition Technology (C), Alcon Laboratories (C), KeraVision (C), Ophthalmic Mutual Insurance Company (C)

Dr Gaudric: Alcon Laboratories (C), Alimera Sciences (C), Bayer (C), Novartis Pharmaceuticals (C, S), ThromboGenics (C)

Dr Grosser: Ivantis (O)

Dr Holder: Servier (C), Isis Pharmaceuticals (C)

Dr Leonard: Annidis (O), Bayer Healthcare Pharmaceuticals (C), Merck & Co (C), Novartis Pharmaceuticals (C), Orbis International (C), Pfizer (S), Regeneron Pharmaceuticals (C)

Dr McCannel: DORC Dutch Ophthalmic Research Center (International)/Dutch Ophthalmic USA (C)

Dr Rosen: Allergan (S), Clarity Medical Systems (C), Genentech (S), OD-OS (L), Optovue (C)

Dr Sarraf: Alcon Laboratories (S), Allergan (S), DORC Dutch Ophthalmic Research Center (International)/Dutch Ophthalmic USA (S), Genentech (S), Heidelberg Engineering (L), Regeneron Pharmaceuticals (S), ThromboGenics (S)

Dr Savage: Allergan (L)

Dr Staurenghi: Alcon Laboratories (C, L), Allergan (C), Bayer (C, L), Canon (C), GlaxoSmithKline (C), Heidelberg Engineering (C, L), Kowa (S), Novartis Pharmaceuticals (C, L, S), Ocular Instruments (P), OD-OS (C), Optos (C), Optovue (C), QLT Phototherapeutics (C), Roche (C), Zeiss (S)

Dr Tufail: Alcon Laboratories (C), Allergan (C, L), Bayer Healthcare Pharmaceuticals (C), Genentech (C), Heidelberg Engineering (C), Notal Vision (S), Novartis Pharmaceuticals (C, L, S)

The other authors and reviewers state that within the past 12 months, they have had no financial interest in or other relationship with any entity discussed in this course that produces, markets, resells, or distributes ophthalmic health care goods or services consumed by or used in patients, or with any competing commercial product or service.

*C = consultant fees, paid advisory boards, or fees for attending a meeting; L = lecture fees (honoraria), travel fees, or reimbursements when speaking at the invitation of a commercial sponsor; O = equity ownership/stock options of publicly or privately traded firms (excluding mutual funds) with manufacturers of commercial ophthalmic products or commercial ophthalmic services; P = patents and/or royalties that might be viewed as creating a potential conflict of interest; S = grant support for the past year (all sources) and all sources used for a specific talk or manuscript with no time limitation

Recent Past Faculty

Richard S. Kaiser, MD
Adam A. Martidis, MD
Hermann D. Schubert, MD
David N. Zacks, MD, PhD

In addition, the Academy gratefully acknowledges the contributions of numerous past faculty and advisory committee members who have played an important role in the development of previous editions of the Basic and Clinical Science Course.

American Academy of Ophthalmology Staff

Dale E. Fajardo, *Vice President, Education*
Beth Wilson, *Director, Continuing Professional Development*
Ann McGuire, *Acquisitions and Development Manager*
Stephanie Tanaka, *Publications Manager*
D. Jean Ray, *Production Manager*
Beth Collins, *Medical Editor*
Naomi Ruiz, *Editorial Assistant*

American Academy of Ophthalmology
655 Beach Street
Box 7424
San Francisco, CA 94120-7424

Contents

General Introduction

The Basic and Clinical Science Course (BCSC) is designed to meet the needs of residents and practitioners for a comprehensive yet concise curriculum of the field of ophthalmology. The BCSC has developed from its original brief outline format, which relied heavily on outside readings, to a more convenient and educationally useful self-contained text. The Academy updates and revises the course annually, with the goals of integrating the basic science and clinical practice of ophthalmology and of keeping ophthalmologists current with new developments in the various subspecialties.

The BCSC incorporates the effort and expertise of more than 80 ophthalmologists, organized into 13 Section faculties, working with Academy editorial staff. In addition, the course continues to benefit from many lasting contributions made by the faculties of previous editions. Members of the Academy's Practicing Ophthalmologists Advisory Committee for Education, Committee on Aging, and Vision Rehabilitation Committee review every volume before major revisions. Members of the European Board of Ophthalmology, organized into Section faculties, also review each volume before major revisions, focusing primarily on differences between American and European ophthalmology practice.

Organization of the Course

The Basic and Clinical Science Course comprises 13 volumes, incorporating fundamental ophthalmic knowledge, subspecialty areas, and special topics:

1 Update on General Medicine
2 Fundamentals and Principles of Ophthalmology
3 Clinical Optics
4 Ophthalmic Pathology and Intraocular Tumors
5 Neuro-Ophthalmology
6 Pediatric Ophthalmology and Strabismus
7 Orbit, Eyelids, and Lacrimal System
8 External Disease and Cornea
9 Intraocular Inflammation and Uveitis
10 Glaucoma
11 Lens and Cataract
12 Retina and Vitreous
13 Refractive Surgery

In addition, a comprehensive Master Index allows the reader to easily locate subjects throughout the entire series.

References

Readers who wish to explore specific topics in greater detail may consult the references cited within each chapter and listed in the Basic Texts section at the back of the book.

These references are intended to be selective rather than exhaustive, chosen by the BCSC faculty as being important, current, and readily available to residents and practitioners.

Videos

This edition of Section 12, *Retina and Vitreous,* includes videos related to topics covered in the book. The videos were selected by members of the BCSC faculty and are available to readers of the print and electronic versions of Section 12 (www.aao.org/bcscvideo_section12). Mobile-device users can scan the QR code below (a QR-code reader must already be installed on the device) to access the video content.

Study Questions and CME Credit

Each volume of the BCSC is designed as an independent study activity for ophthalmology residents and practitioners. The learning objectives for this volume are given on page 1. The text, illustrations, and references provide the information necessary to achieve the objectives; the study questions allow readers to test their understanding of the material and their mastery of the objectives. Physicians who wish to claim CME credit for this educational activity may do so by following the instructions given at the end of the book.

Conclusion

The Basic and Clinical Science Course has expanded greatly over the years, with the addition of much new text and numerous illustrations. Recent editions have sought to place a greater emphasis on clinical applicability while maintaining a solid foundation in basic science. As with any educational program, it reflects the experience of its authors. As its faculties change and as medicine progresses, new viewpoints are always emerging on controversial subjects and techniques. Not all alternate approaches can be included in this series; as with any educational endeavor, the learner should seek additional sources, including such carefully balanced opinions as the Academy's Preferred Practice Patterns.

The BCSC faculty and staff are continually striving to improve the educational usefulness of the course; you, the reader, can contribute to this ongoing process. If you have any suggestions or questions about the series, please do not hesitate to contact the faculty or the editors.

The authors, editors, and reviewers hope that your study of the BCSC will be of lasting value and that each Section will serve as a practical resource for quality patient care.

Objectives

Upon completion of BCSC Section 12, *Retina and Vitreous,* the learner should be able to

- describe the basic structure and function of the retina and its relationship to the pigment epithelium, choroid, and vitreous
- select appropriate methods of examination and ancillary studies for the diagnosis of vitreoretinal disorders
- identify specific pathologic processes that affect the choroid, retina, or vitreous
- describe the principles of medical and surgical treatment of vitreoretinal disorders
- incorporate data from major prospective clinical trials in the management of vitreoretinal disorders whenever possible

Introduction

The retina is the delicate neuroepithelium that lines the posterior aspect of the eye, adhering firmly to the optic nerve head posteriorly and to the ora serrata anteriorly. Divided into central and extra-areal periphery, this layer of modified sensory cilia serves important aspects of visual function:

- detail discrimination
- color perception
- vision in dim illumination
- peripheral vision

The vitreous is the transparent structure that fills the posterior segment eye cavity and is composed of connective tissue, predominantly type II collagen, glycosaminoglycans, and hyaluronic acid. It plays an important role in many diseases of the posterior segment. Understanding its structure and the changes it can undergo with aging is key to understanding many vitreoretinal disorders.

BCSC Section 12, *Retina and Vitreous,* is arranged into 3 parts. Part I, Fundamentals and Diagnostic Approaches, covers retinal anatomy, imaging, and functional evaluation in 3 chapters. Chapter 1 provides an overview of the anatomy of the posterior segment. Chapter 2 discusses techniques of examination, including dilated slit-lamp biomicroscopy in combination with precorneal non–contact or contact lenses, and indirect ophthalmoscopy, often aided by scleral indentation to facilitate viewing the anterior retina.

Documenting clinical findings, either descriptively or by illustration, remains an essential element of a complete posterior segment examination. In addition, ancillary tests, such as fundus autofluorescence, fluorescein angiography, indocyanine green angiography, optical coherence tomography (OCT), scanning laser ophthalmoscopy, microperimetry, and electrophysiology, may provide additional diagnostic information. Optical coherence tomography in its various incarnations (time-domain, spectral-domain, and swept-source OCT) deserves special mention, as it has become perhaps the most commonly ordered ancillary ophthalmic test and is revolutionizing the understanding of many vitreoretinal conditions.

Chapter 3 reviews electrophysiologic tests and their significance in diagnosis and follow-up of retinal disease. Ultrasonography, or echography, employing both A- and B-scan techniques, is useful for patients with opaque media, can aid in the diagnosis of retinal or choroidal lesions, and can be used to monitor a lesion's size.

Depending on their location, developmental or acquired alterations in the posterior segment may or may not be symptomatic. Many vitreoretinal diseases, such as diabetic retinopathy or age-related macular degeneration, may be asymptomatic until the more advanced stages are reached. Vitreoretinal disease symptoms, when they occur, may include the following:

- transient or persistent reduction in visual acuity
- dyschromatopsias (alterations in color vision or perception)
- delayed photostress recovery (delayed adaptation to reduced lighting)
- photophobia
- metamorphopsia (wavy or distorted vision)
- floaters
- photopsia (flashes)
- scotomata (blind spots/areas)
- loss of visual field
- nyctalopia (night blindness)

Part II, Disorders of the Retina and Vitreous, discusses specific diseases of and trauma to the posterior segment in Chapters 4 through 17. Appropriate diagnostic techniques are indicated throughout these discussions. By necessity, the illustrative findings associated with the described vitreoretinal disorders are presented as highlights—using schematics as well as the different imaging technologies—rather than as a comprehensive collection. Narratives describing the management of, and therapy for, the retinal disorders covered in Part II are complemented by descriptions of many important clinical trials that have helped establish appropriate evidence-based practices.

Part III, Selected Therapeutic Topics, offers more detailed information in Chapters 18 and 19 on the 3 most important posterior segment treatment approaches: vitreoretinal surgery, laser surgery, and intravitreal injection of effective pharmacologic agents, especially anti–vascular endothelial growth factor treatments. The emergence of each of these treatment approaches has been associated with dramatic improvements in the outcomes retina specialists can accomplish in terms of preserving or restoring vision for our patients.

Increasingly, when treating patients with vitreoretinal disorders, clinicians are basing treatment decisions on evidence from clinical trials. Readers should familiarize themselves with topics important for interpreting the scientific literature, such as study design, levels of evidence, results interpretation, and clinical practice applications of trial results (see BCSC Section 1, *Update on General Medicine,* Chapter 1).

This book is not meant as a thorough review of the field but rather serves as what a group of experts considers the most important highlights of the specialty. Thus, readers interested in more comprehensive information can obtain additional detail from the selected references as well as from references that appear at the end of the book under Basic Texts. Lastly, a new feature with this edition is the inclusion of videos to better illustrate specific topics; these edited clips are accessible through the print and electronic forms of this volume.

PART I

Fundamentals and Diagnostic Approaches

CHAPTER 1

Basic Anatomy

The Vitreous

The vitreous is a transparent gel composed of water, collagen, and hyaluronic acid; it occupies 80% of the volume of the eye. The vitreous body is divided into 2 main topographic areas: the central, or core, and the peripheral, or cortical, vitreous. The vitreous gel is composed of collagen fibrils separated by hydrated hyaluronic acid molecules, which act as fillers and separators between adjacent collagen fibrils.

The anterior surface of the vitreous body is called the anterior cortical gel, a condensation of collagenous fibers that attach to the posterior lens capsule, forming the ligament of Wieger (Fig 1-1). The retrolental indentation of the anterior vitreous is called the patellar fossa. The potential space between lens and anterior cortical gel bordered by the Wieger ligament is called the Berger space. In the vitreous base, the collagen fibers are especially dense; they insert firmly into a ringlike area that extends 2 mm anterior and 3–4 mm

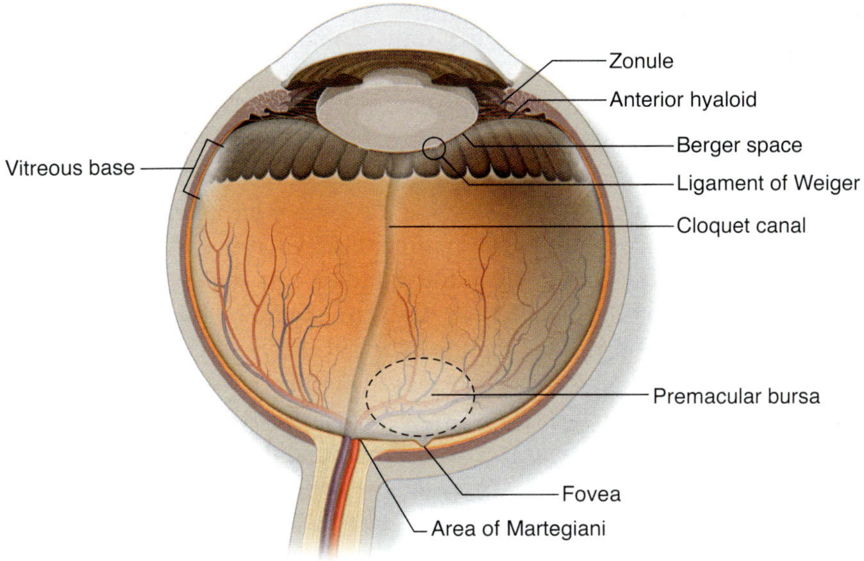

Figure 1-1 The vitreous is most firmly attached to the retina at the vitreous base, and it also has adhesions at the optic nerve, along vessels, at the fovea, and to the posterior lens capsule. A prominent area of liquefaction of the premacular vitreous gel is called the *premacular bursa,* or *precortical vitreous pocket.* *(Illustration by Mark M. Miller.)*

posterior to the ora serrata. The vitreous is not only attached at its base; it is also firmly attached to the lens capsule, retinal vessels, optic nerve, and macula. The collagen fibrils in the cortical vitreous are densely packed, forming the cortical gel. Posteriorly, fibers course in a direction roughly parallel to the inner surface of the retina, forming the preretinal tract. Thus, the vitreous may be regarded as transparent connective tissue surrounded by a basal laminar bag provided by the lens and retina. There is no basement membrane between the vitreous base and lens, an area called the annular gap, which is a ringlike zone important for diffusion between the aqueous and vitreous compartments. The posterior attachment of the vitreous to the macula forms a space known as the premacular bursa, or the precortical vitreous pocket (see Fig 1-1). Attachment of the collagenous vitreous to the disc is at the area of Martegiani. The anatomy of the vitreous is difficult to delineate in vivo, but the vitreous appears to contain interconnected cisterns and canals, most notably the ciliobursal canal connecting the ciliary body and macula and possibly mediating some forms of cystoid macular edema.

Neurosensory Retina

The central area, or macula, measures 5.5 mm in diameter and is centered between the disc and the temporal vascular arcades. Histologically, it is an area featuring 2 or more layers of ganglion cells, totaling half of all the ganglion cells in the retina. Oxygenated carotenoids, in particular lutein and zeaxanthin, accumulate within the central macula and contribute to its yellow color.

The central 1.5 mm of the macula is called the *fovea* (or *fovea centralis*), which is specialized for high spatial acuity and for color vision. The fovea has a margin, declivity, and floor known as the *foveola,* a 0.35-mm-diameter region where cones are slender, elongated, and densely packed. The very center of the foveola is a small depression, 150–200 μm in diameter, known as the *umbo.* Within the fovea is a region devoid of retinal vessels known as the *foveal avascular zone* (FAZ). The geometric center of the FAZ is often taken to be the center of the macula and thus the point of fixation; it is an important landmark in fluorescein angiography. Surrounding the fovea is a ring 0.5 mm in width called the *parafovea,* where the ganglion cell layer, inner nuclear layer, and outer plexiform layer (also known as *Henle layer*) are thickest. Surrounding this zone is a ring approximately 1.5 mm wide termed the *perifovea* (Table 1-1). Thus, the umbo forms the center, and the periphery of the perifovea forms the margin, of the area centralis, or macula (Fig 1-2).

The retina outside the macula, the extra-arcal periphery, is commonly divided into a few concentric regions, starting with a 1.5-mm ring peripheral to the temporal major vascular arcades called the *near periphery.* The retina around the equator is called the *equatorial retina,* and the region anterior to it is called the *peripheral retina.* In the far periphery, the border between the retina and the pars plana is called the *ora serrata.* The posterior border of the vitreous base is located between the ora serrata and the equator of the eye. This region is where most retinal tears occur. Jetties of retinal tissue, called *dentate processes,* extend anteriorly into the pars plana. These processes are more prominent nasally. *Ora bays* are posterior extensions of the pars plana toward the retinal side. On occasion, dentate processes may wrap around a portion of ora bay to form an enclosed ora bay. A

Table 1-1 Anatomical Terminology of the Macula (Area Centralis)

Term	Synonym	Histologic Definition	Clinical Observation and Size
Macula	Posterior pole Area centralis	Contains 2 or more ganglion cell layers	Area between vascular arcades 5.5 mm in diameter centered 3.0 mm temporal and 0.8 mm inferior to the center of the optic disc
Perifovea		From the outermost limit of the parafovea to the outer limit of the macula	Ring 1.5 mm in width surrounding the parafovea
Parafovea		Margin, where the ganglion cell layer, inner nuclear layer, and Henle layer are thickest (ie, the retina is thickest)	Ring 0.5 mm in width surrounding the fovea
Fovea	Fovea centralis	A depression in the inner retina; has a margin, slope, and floor, the photoreceptor layer of which is entirely cones	A concave central retinal depression seen on slit-lamp examination 1.5 mm in diameter (about 1 disc diameter, or 5°)
Foveola		The floor of the fovea features cones only, arranged in the shape of a cake (gâteau nucléaire), where the inner nuclear layer and ganglion cell layer are laterally displaced	0.35 mm in diameter, usually smaller than the foveal avascular zone
Umbo	Fixation Light reflex	Small (150–200 μm) center of the floor of the foveola; features elongated cones forming a bouquet of cones	Observed point corresponding to the normal light reflex but not solely responsible for this light reflex

meridional fold is a radially oriented, prominent thickening of retinal tissue extending into the pars plana. When aligned with a ciliary process, such folds are known as a *meridional complex* (Fig 1-3).

The layers of the retina can be seen in cross-sectional histologic preparations. They are listed here in order from the inner to outer retina (Fig 1-4):

- internal limiting membrane (ILM)
- nerve fiber layer (NFL; the axons of the ganglion cell layer)
- ganglion cell layer (GCL)
- inner plexiform layer (IPL)
- inner nuclear layer (INL)
- middle limiting membrane (MLM)
- outer plexiform layer (OPL)
- Henle fiber layer (HFL)
- outer nuclear layer (ONL; the nuclei of the photoreceptors)
- external limiting membrane (XLM)
- rod and cone inner and outer segments (IS/OS)

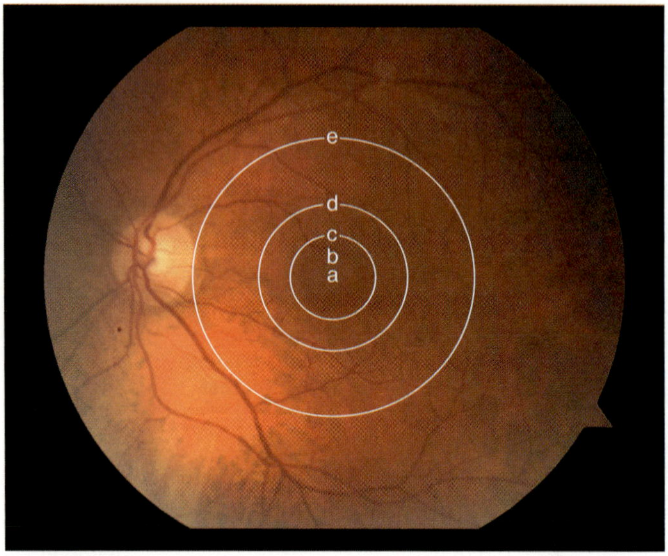

Figure 1-2 Anatomical macula, also called *area centralis* or *posterior pole*. The anatomical fovea and foveola are contained within the center of the anatomical macula. Letters indicate borders of: a = umbo; b = foveola; c = fovea; c to d = parafoveal macula; d to e = perifoveal macula; e = macula. *(Courtesy of Hermann D. Schubert, MD.)*

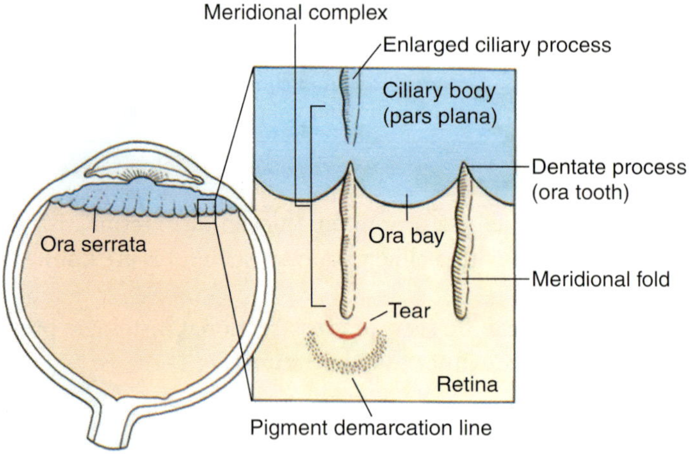

Figure 1-3 Schematic of the ora serrata, showing an ora bay and dentate process. Meridional folds are pleats of redundant retina. Tears may occur at the posterior end of such folds. *(Used with permission from Federman JL, Gouras P, Schubert H, et al. Retina and vitreous. In: Podos SM, Yanoff M, eds.* Textbook of Ophthalmology. *Vol 9. London: Mosby; 1988.)*

Light must travel through the full thickness of the retina to reach the photoreceptors. The density and distribution of photoreceptors vary with topographic location. In the fovea, densely packed cones are predominantly red- and green-sensitive, with a density exceeding 140,000 cones/mm^2. The fovea has no rods; it contains only cones and processes of Müller cells. The number of cone photoreceptors decreases rapidly away from

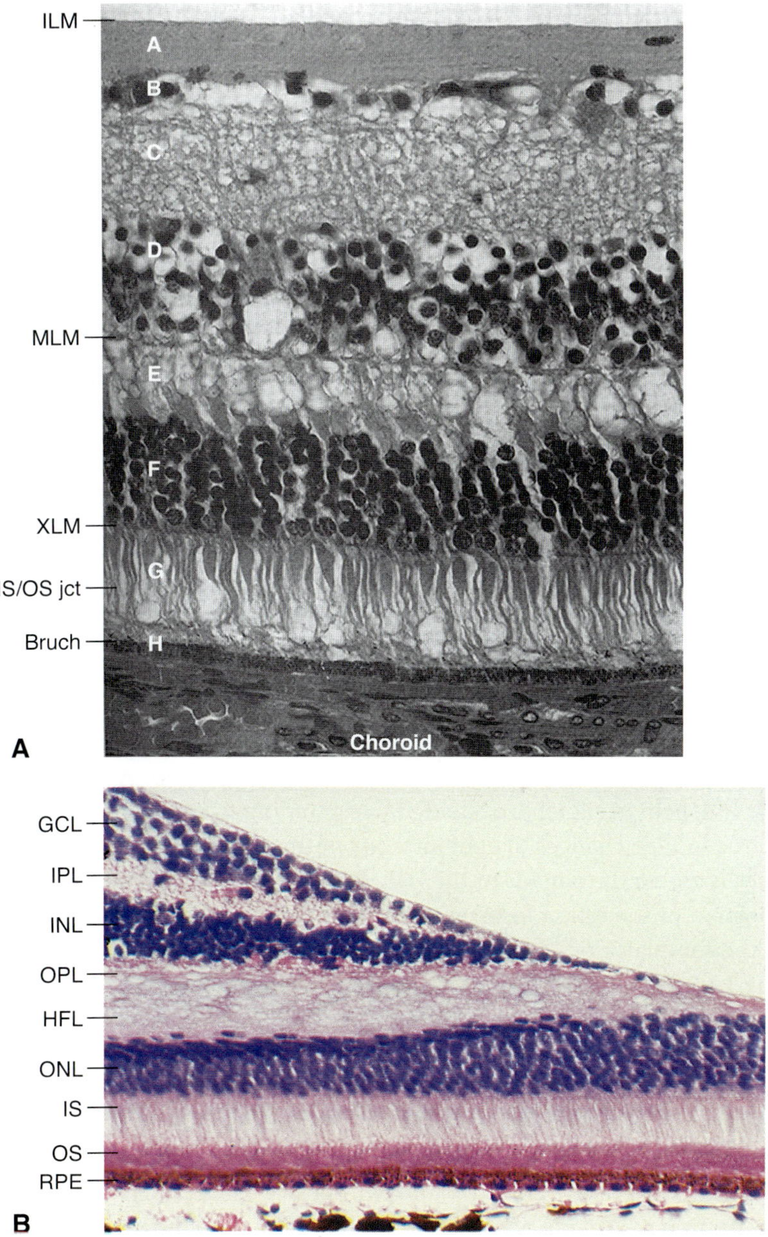

Figure 1-4 **A,** Cross section of the retina and choroid, showing the nerve fiber layer (A), ganglion cell layer (B), inner plexiform layer (C), inner nuclear layer (D), outer plexiform layer (E), outer nuclear layer (F), photoreceptor outer segments (G), and retinal pigment epithelium (H). **B,** In the fovea, the inner cellular layers are laterally displaced, and there is an increased density of pigment in the retinal pigment epithelium (RPE). The incident light falls directly on the photoreceptor outer segments, reducing the potential for scattering of light by overlying tissue elements. Bruch = Bruch membrane; IS/OS jct = inner-outer segment junction; GCL = ganglion cell layer; HFL = Henle fiber layer; ILM = internal limiting membrane; INL = inner nuclear layer; IPL = inner plexiform layer; IS = inner segment of photoreceptors; MLM = middle limiting membrane; ONL = outer nuclear layer; OPL = outer plexiform layer; OS = outer segment of photoreceptors; XLM = external limiting membrane. *(Part A used with permission from Spaide RF, Miller-Rivera NE. Anatomy. In: Spaide RF, ed.* Diseases of the Retina and Vitreous. *Philadelphia: Saunders; 1999; part B courtesy of David J. Wilson, MD.)*

the center, even though 90% of cones overall reside outside the foveal region. The rods have their greatest density in a zone lying approximately 20° from fixation, where they reach a peak density of about 160,000 rods/mm^2. The density of rods also decreases toward the periphery.

The light-sensitive molecules in rods and cones are derived from vitamin A and are contained in the disc membranes of the photoreceptor outer segments. The discs are attached to a cilium, which is rooted through neurotubules in the ellipsoid and myoid of the inner segment. The ellipsoid, which is adjacent to the cilium, contains mitochondria and is responsible for the cone shape. The myoid, which is closer to the photoreceptor nucleus, contains endoplasmic reticulum. The mitochondria, cilia, and inner discs together form the *inner-outer segment junction,* which is apparent with optical coherence tomography (OCT) as the ellipsoid zone and provides evidence of the origin of the photoreceptor as a modified sensory cilium prone to the full range of ciliopathies. Rod outer segments may contain up to 1000 discs stacked like coins. These discs are renewed in and shed from the outer retina and are phagocytosed by the retinal pigment epithelium (RPE) for processing and recycling of components (Fig 1-5).

Cone photoreceptors have a 1-to-1 synapse with a type of bipolar cell known as a *midget bipolar cell.* Other types of bipolar cells also synapse with each cone. Conversely, more than 1 rod—and sometimes more than 100 rods—converge on each bipolar cell. Bipolar cells, the first neurons of the visual pathway, synapse with ganglion cells, the second neurons of the visual pathway in the IPL. The ganglion cells summate responses from bipolar and amacrine cells and develop action potentials that are conducted to the dorsolateral geniculate nucleus and the third neuron in the brain. Amacrine cells on the inside of the INL help in signal processing by responding to specific alterations in retinal stimuli, such as sudden changes in light intensity or the presence of certain sizes of stimuli. Horizontal cells are on the outside of the INL. In the NFL, axons of the GCL course along the inner portion of the retina to form the optic nerve, a brain tract. The ILM, which is formed by the footplates of Müller cells, is attached to the posterior cortical gel of the vitreous (Fig 1-6).

Two additional intraretinal "membranes," the XLM and MLM, were identified by histologists but in actuality are not true membranes but junctional systems. At the outer extent of the Müller cells, zonular attachments between photoreceptors and Müller cells create the XLM, a structure visible with both light microscopy and OCT. Thus, the Müller cells whose nuclei reside in the INL course through almost the entire thickness of the retina. The inner third of the OPL has a linear density where synaptic and desmosomal connections occur between the photoreceptor inner fibers and the processes of the bipolar cells. This linear density, which is also apparent with OCT, is the junctional system that has been called the MLM.

The central retinal artery (a branch of the ophthalmic artery) enters the eye and divides into 4 branches, each supplying blood to a quadrant of the retina. These branches are located in the inner retina. Occasionally, a cilioretinal artery, derived from the ciliary circulation, will supply a portion of the inner retina between the optic nerve and the center of the macula (Fig 1-7). On a tissue level, the retina is supplied by up to 4 layers of capillaries, 1 superficial in the NFL (the radial peripapillary network) and 2 on either

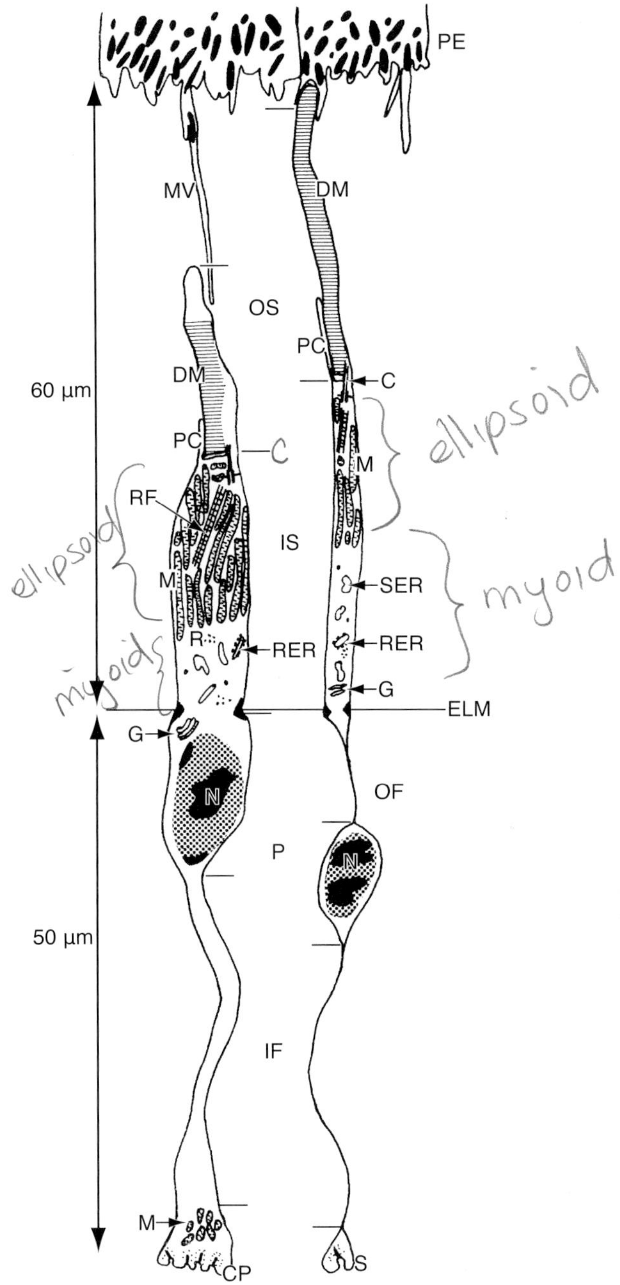

Figure 1-5 Schematic of a cone cell *(left)* and a rod cell *(right)* in the peripheral retina. C = cilium; CP = cone cell pedicle; DM = membranous discs; ELM = external limiting membrane; G = Golgi apparatus; IF = inner fiber; IS = inner segment; M = mitochondria; MV = microvilli of pigment epithelial cells; N = nucleus; OF= outer fiber; OS = outer segment; P = perikaryon; PC = processus calycoides; PE = pigment epithelium; R = free ribosomes; RER = rough endoplasmic reticulum; RF = rootlet fiber; S = rod cell spherule; SER = smooth endoplasmic reticulum. *(Used with permission from Krebs W, Krebs I.* Primate Retina and Choroid. Atlas of Fine Structure in Man and Monkey. *New York: Springer Verlag; 1991.)*

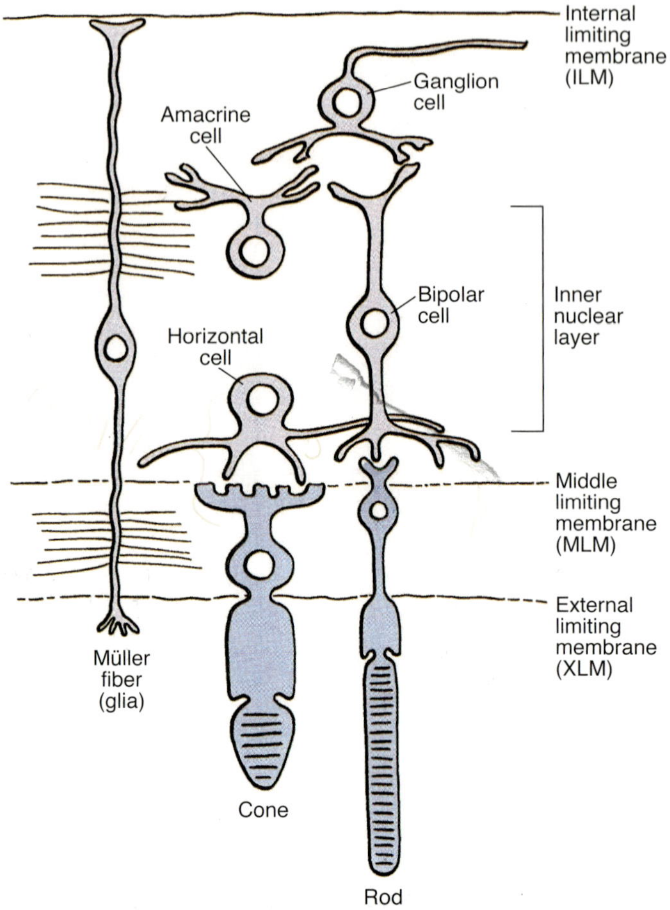

Figure 1-6 Schematic of the neuronal connections in the retina and participating cells. *(Used with permission from Federman JL, Gouras P, Schubert H, et al. Retina and vitreous. In: Podos SM, Yanoff M, eds.* Textbook of Ophthalmology. *Vol 9. London: Mosby; 1988.)*

side of the INL as a superficial and a deep capillary plexus. The metabolic needs of the outer retina are met by the choriocapillaris, a capillary system of the choroidal arteries supplied by the short posterior ciliary arteries. The boundary between the retinal vascular supply and the diffusion from the choriocapillaris varies according to the topographic location, retinal thickness, and amount of light present. The retinal vasculature, including its capillaries, retains the blood–brain barrier with tight junctions between capillary endothelial cells. Blood collected from the capillaries accumulates within a branch retinal vein, which in turn forms the central retinal vein. The retinal vascular system is thought to supply a portion of the oxygen used in the fundus; the choroid supplies the majority. See also Part I, Anatomy, of BCSC Section 2, *Fundamentals and Principles of Ophthalmology.*

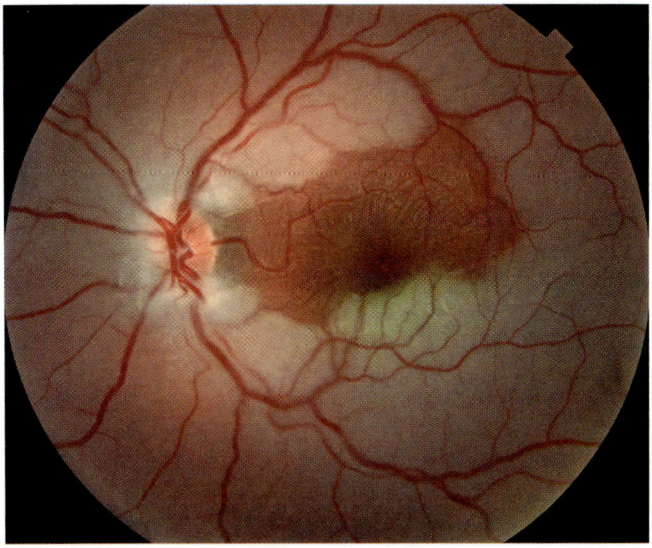

Figure 1-7 A central retinal artery occlusion in a young patient with a previously unknown patent foramen ovale. Fortunately, the patient had a patent cilioretinal artery. Note the inner retinal ischemic whitening in the distribution of the central retinal artery but preservation of the normal retinal transparency in the zone supplied by the cilioretinal artery. *(Used with permission from Ho IV, Spaide RF. Central retinal artery occlusion associated with a patent foramen ovale.* Retina. *2007;27(2):259–260.)*

Retinal Pigment Epithelium

The RPE is a monolayer of pigmented cells derived from the outer layer of the optic cup and thus maintains the apex-to-apex arrangement with müllerian glia (Fig 1-8). This layer is continuous with the pigment epithelium of the ciliary body and iris. Each RPE cell has an apex and base; the apical portion envelopes the outer segments of the photoreceptor cells with villous processes. RPE cells are hexagonal, cuboidal cells approximately 16 μm in diameter. In the macula, however, the cells are taller and denser than in the periphery. The lateral surfaces of adjacent cells are closely apposed and joined by tight junctional complexes (zonulae occludentes) near the apices, forming apical girdles and the outer blood–ocular barrier. The basal surface of the cells shows a rich infolding of the plasma membrane. The basement membrane does not follow these infoldings. The RPE contributes to retinal function in several ways; it

- absorbs light
- phagocytoses rod and cone outer segments
- participates in retinal and polyunsaturated fatty acid metabolism
- forms the outer blood–ocular barrier
- maintains the subretinal space
- heals and forms scar tissue

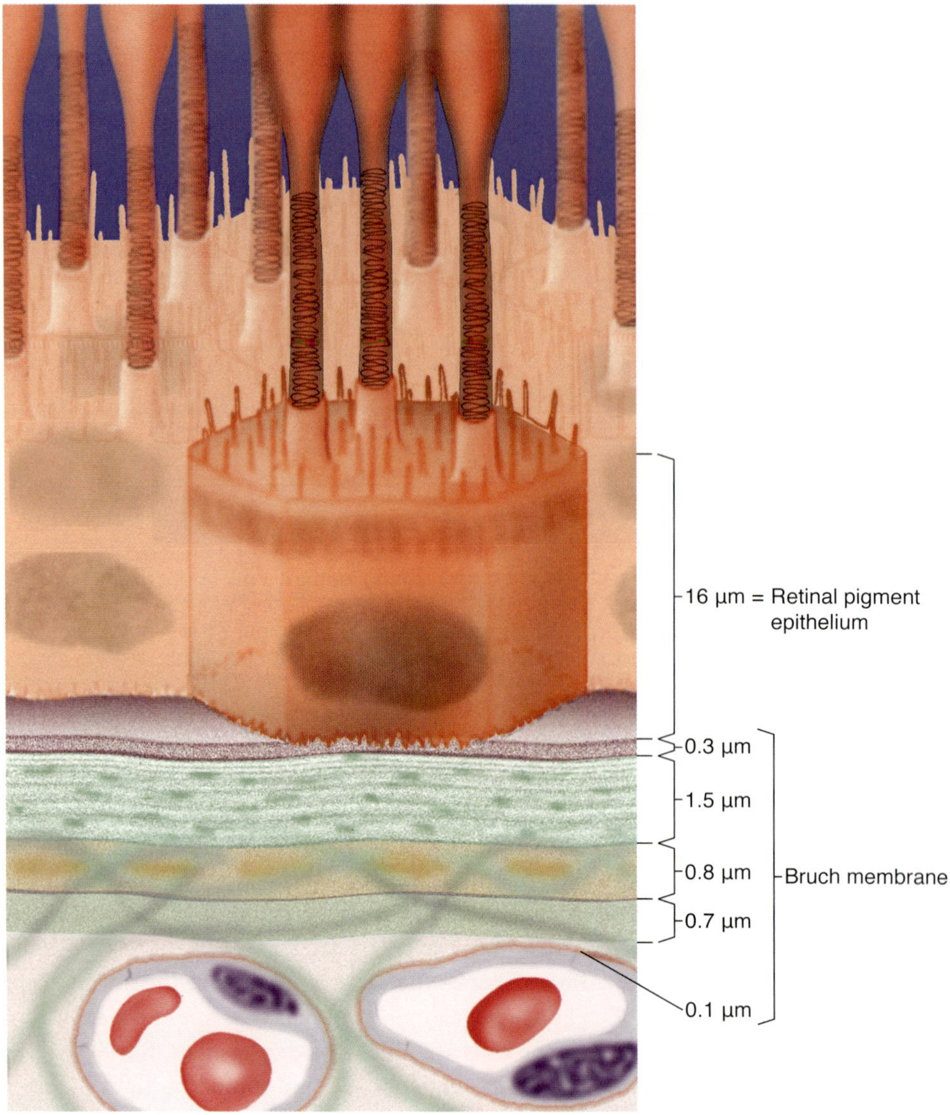

Figure 1-8 Retinal pigment epithelium (RPE) and Bruch membrane. The folded plasmalemma of the RPE rests on its smooth basement membrane (0.3 μm thick) bordering the inner collagenous layer (1.5 μm thick). The outer collagenous layer (0.7 μm thick) borders the elastic layer (0.8 μm thick) and is continuous with intercapillary bridges and the subcapillary fibrous tissue. *(Illustration by Daniel Casper, MD, PhD.)*

The typical RPE cell has a number of melanosomes, each designed to be a biological light absorber. Melanosomes are spheroidal, with their melanin distributed on protein fibers.

RPE cells serve a phagocytic function, continually ingesting the membranes, or discs, shed by the outer segments of the photoreceptor cells. Over the course of a lifetime, each RPE cell is thought to phagocytose billions of outer segments. This process of shedding, phagocytosis, and photoreceptor renewal follows a daily (circadian) rhythm. Rods shed discs at dawn, and cones shed them at dusk. The ingested outer segments are digested gradually through the action of enzymes within cytoplasmic organelles known as *lysosomes.*

Visual pigments contain 11-*cis*-retinaldehyde that is converted to 11-*trans*-retinaldehyde. Most of the steps of regeneration of the 11-*cis* configuration occur in the RPE. A variety of pathologic changes—caused by such factors as genetic defects, drugs, dietary insufficiency (of vitamin A), or senescence—can impair this process of phagocytosis and renewal. Physical separation of the retina from the RPE, such as occurs when subretinal fluid or blood is present, also disrupts the important exchange of metabolites. The biochemical cycle of visual pigments is discussed further in BCSC Section 2, *Fundamentals and Principles of Ophthalmology.*

The barrier function of the RPE prevents diffusion of metabolites between the choroid and the subretinal space. Because of this barrier, the environment of the photoreceptors is largely regulated by the selective transport properties of the RPE. The RPE has a high capacity for water transport, so fluid does not accumulate in the subretinal space under normal circumstances. This RPE-mediated dehydration of the subretinal space also modulates the bonding properties of the interphotoreceptor matrix, which bridges between the RPE and photoreceptors and helps bond the neurosensory retina to the RPE. With deterioration or loss of the RPE, there is corresponding atrophy of the overlying photoreceptors and underlying choriocapillaris.

Bruch Membrane

The basal portion of the RPE is attached to the Bruch membrane, which has 4–5 layers. Starting with the innermost, these layers (see Fig 1-8) are the

- basement membrane of the RPE
- inner collagenous zone
- middle layer of elastic fibers
- outer collagenous zone
- basement membrane of the endothelium of the choriocapillaris

Throughout life, lipids and oxidatively damaged materials build up within the Bruch membrane. Some disease states, such as pseudoxanthoma elasticum, are associated with increased fragility of the Bruch membrane, presumably caused by abnormalities within the membrane's collagen or elastic portions.

Choroid

Blood enters the choroid through the posterior ciliary arteries (Fig 1-9). The outer layer of large-caliber choroidal vessels, known as the Haller layer, is relatively thick. The choroidal vessels in this layer divide into smaller-diameter vessels and precapillary arterioles in a layer known as the Sattler layer. These vessels distribute the blood over the extent of

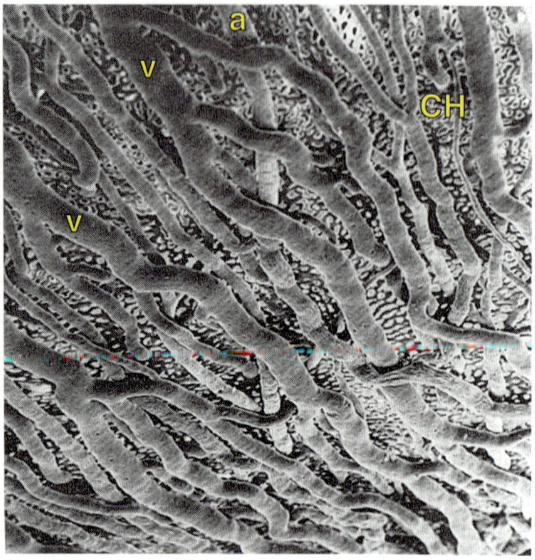

Figure 1-9 Scanning electron micrograph of the choroid. Vascular cast of the choroid from the posterior pole of a 62-year-old man, demonstrating arteries (a), veins (v), and the choriocapillaris (CH). (70×) *(Courtesy of A. Fryczkowski, MD.)*

the choroid, reducing arterial pressure to the relatively low pressure found in the choriocapillaris. The choroid has a maximal thickness posteriorly, where it is 0.22 mm thick, and becomes progressively thinner anteriorly; at the ora serrata, it is 0.1 mm thick. In the posterior pole, the choriocapillaris forms a plexus of capillaries that functionally act as endarterioles, even though the capillaries themselves are not arranged strictly into lobules. The capillary arrangement becomes more irregular toward the periphery, where the capillaries are arranged more radially.

After passing through the choriocapillaris, the blood is collected in venules, which coalesce into collecting channels, or ampullae, of the vortex veins. Most eyes have 4 or 5 vortex veins, which exit the eye at or posterior to the equator. The vortex veins drain into the superior and inferior ophthalmic veins. The retina has one of the highest metabolic rates per gram of tissue in the body; it is served by the choroid, which has the highest blood flow of any tissue. The venous blood exiting the choroid still has a very high oxygen tension. The RPE cells, which are based on the choriocapillaris, are exposed to the highest oxygen tensions of any perfused tissue, increasing the risk of oxidative damage. The rapid flow in the choroid acts as a heat sink to remove thermal energy from light absorption. Interspersed between the vessels of the choroid are loose connective tissue, fibroblasts, and melanocytes.

Sclera

The sclera is composed of collagen and a few elastic fibers embedded in a matrix of proteoglycans. Compared with the cornea, the sclera has less hydration and a more irregular arrangement of fibers. It terminates at the histologists' limbus. The sclera does not have uniform thickness; it is thinnest immediately behind the muscle insertion, whereas it is thicker just posterior to the limbus.

The sclera is normally permeable to the passage of molecules in both directions. Fluid is thought to leave the eye through the sclera. Scleral permeability allows drugs to be delivered to the eye by means of injection into the Tenon space. The sclera is a hydrophilic tissue and is therefore only variably permeable to hydrophobic or amphiphilic substances or medications. This characteristic is an important consideration for periocular injection of pharmacologic agents.

Hogan MJ, Alvarado JA, Weddell JE. *Histology of the Human Eye.* Philadelphia: Saunders; 1971:chaps 5, 8, 9, 11.

Polyak SL. *The Retina.* Chicago: University of Chicago Press; 1941.

Rochon-Duvigneaud A. Recherches sur la fovea de la rétine humaine et particulièrement sur le bouquet des cônes centraux. *Arch Anat Microsc.* 1907(IX):315–342.

Worst JGF, Los LI. *Cisternal Anatomy of the Vitreous.* Amsterdam: Kugler; 1995.

CHAPTER 2

Diagnostic Approach to Retinal Disease

Techniques of Examination

Diagnosing retinal disease requires a combination of careful clinical examination and specialized imaging techniques. The macula can be examined without pupillary dilation, but performance of a complete retinal examination requires a fully dilated pupil. Pupil dilation is accomplished through a variety of pharmacologic agents, including tropicamide, 1%, phenylephrine, 2.5%, and cyclopentolate, 1%. In general, longer-acting dilating drugs are not required.

Ophthalmoscopy

The simplest examination technique is to use the direct ophthalmoscope, which provides an upright, monocular, high-magnification (15×) image of the retina. However, the instrument's lack of stereopsis, small field of view (~6°), and poor view of the retinal periphery limit its use. The binocular indirect ophthalmoscope (BIO), in combination with a handheld magnifying lens, overcomes these limitations, providing an increased field of view (~30°) with lower magnification (2–5×). This combination yields an inverted binocular image capable of revealing most of the retina; for a view of the entire retinal periphery to the ora serrata, the BIO examination must be combined with scleral depression. Typically, 20, 28, and 30 D hand lenses are employed. Magnification is inversely proportional—and the field of view is directly proportional—to the power of the lens; for example, the 30 D lens has the lowest magnification and the widest field. Clinicians can easily learn to correct for the image reversal by turning the retinal drawing sheet upside down to draw the retina and the pathology as seen through the lens.

Magnification of even the lowest-power BIO lens is insufficient to evaluate subtle retinal changes or abnormalities of the vitreous body. Evaluation of these structures requires slit-lamp biomicroscopy. A variety of lenses are available for viewing the retina with the slit lamp. Historically, the 3-mirror contact lens was considered the gold standard. Contact lenses offer the advantage of image stability, better stereopsis, and higher resolution. They are placed directly on the cornea to eliminate its power and the cornea–air interface; their use generally requires topical corneal anesthesia. Cushioning fluids used to protect the cornea range from contact lens wetting solutions to viscous clear gels. The more viscous the solution, however, the more its residual presence interferes with the quality of any subsequent photography or angiography performed following the examination. Non–contact lenses are generally more convenient, allowing rapid evaluation of the retina. Non–contact lenses use the power of the lens in combination with that of the cornea to produce an inverted image with a wider field of view. Because the biconvex indirect lenses used with the slit lamp do not touch the cornea, they circumvent the need for topical anesthesia and avoid potential disturbance to the ocular surface. Typically, high-plus-power lenses ranging from 60 to 90 D are used. Whereas lower-dioptric-power lenses offer more axial resolution and better stereopsis, higher-power lenses offer easier viewing in smaller pupils. The Hruby lens, the original non–contact lens option for fundus biomicroscopy, is a high-negative optical power planoconcave lens attached to the slit-lamp frame. Although it uniquely provides an upright image, its less-versatile smaller field and single-power option have resulted in its decline in use.

The detection of diffuse retinal thickening and cystic spaces in cystoid macular edema or the presence of subretinal fluid over choroidal neovascularization (CNV) is facilitated by using a thin slit beam, at a 45° angle, with a high-magnification lens. The inner aspect of the beam is directed at the surface of the retina and retinal vessels, the outer aspect at the retinal pigment epithelium (RPE). The distance between the inner and outer aspects reveals the thickness of the retina. Once the examiner has a sense of the normal retinal thickness for a given location within the macula, comparisons with other areas can suggest regions of abnormal thickness. The same technique is useful for determining the level of a hemorrhage—preretinal, intraretinal, or subretinal. Careful examination of the beam as it intersects with the retina can differentiate between elevation and depression of a retinal lesion.

Transillumination is another technique that may help highlight cystic changes of the neurosensory retina or help detect pigment epithelial detachments, where the edge of the beam appears to glow. Red-free (green) light may also be useful to help detect small microaneurysms, dots of hemorrhage, or vessels (such as intraretinal microvascular abnormalities or retinal neovascularization) that are difficult to distinguish against the orange background with the normal slit beam. Under red-free light, fluid, fibrin, or fibrous tissue associated with CNV may give a lighter color to the retina, whereas the xanthophyll macular pigment will appear darker, highlighting the foveal avascular zone.

Friberg TR. Examination of the retina: ophthalmoscopy and fundus biomicroscopy. In: Albert DM, Miller JW, Azar DT, Blodi BA, eds. *Albert & Jakobiec's Principles and Practice of Ophthalmology.* 3rd ed. Philadelphia: Saunders; 2008:chap 127.

Imaging Technologies

Scanning Laser Ophthalmoscopy

The confocal scanning laser ophthalmoscope (SLO) generates retinal images that are analogous to those of fundus photography, yet the technology offers greater versatility than fundus photography. It uses a laser beam in the near-infrared (NIR) range (675, 790, or 810–890 nm) that rapidly sweeps back and forth across the retina, building an image line by line from individual point reflections. The reflected light is captured by a confocal photodiode detector that is conjugate to the retinal plane and reconstructed to form a digital image. The confocal optics ensures that only light reflected from the narrow spot illuminated by the laser is recorded.

High-resolution images can be produced either with contrast agents such as fluorescein or indocyanine green (ICG) or without contrast agents to reveal autofluorescence patterns. The SLO is capable of imaging structures at very high magnification and high frame rate, which allows delineation of fine retinal structures that are poorly defined by ordinary fundus cameras, such as those causing autofluorescence. Thus, SLO has the ability to capture transient phenomena such as feeder vessels. Its improved contrast is achieved using low levels of light exposure, enhancing patient comfort. Ultra-high-resolution images to the level of retinal cellular structures (eg, photoreceptors, capillaries, and nerve fibers) can also be obtained using SLO instruments outfitted with adaptive optics, wavefront-flattening systems.

The SLO, with its multiple light sources and tracking capability, enabled the development of multimodal, localized functional testing of the retina in the form of fundus-based perimetry or microperimetry. Threshold-sensitivity determination, focal acuity testing, and even integrated optical coherence tomography (OCT) imaging allow the clinician to correlate anatomical features with visual performance.

SLO-NIR reflectance imaging is especially useful for detecting abnormalities of the outer retina, RPE, and Bruch membrane, as well as the presence of subretinal fluid. Lesions of acute macular neuroretinopathy, reticular pseudodrusen (subretinal drusenoid debris), and subretinal fluid in central serous chorioretinopathy are more easily seen with NIR imaging than with the visible light of the fundus camera.

Recently, the availability of high-quality, ultra-wide-angle SLO systems has facilitated color, fluorescein, and autofluorescent imaging of the peripheral retina. Expanded-field imaging has revealed areas of nonperfusion, neovascularization, and autofluorescent disturbances beyond the view of conventional fundus camera systems.

Freeman WR, Bartsch DU, Mueller AJ, Banker AS, Weinreb RN. Simultaneous indocyanine green and fluorescein angiography using a confocal scanning laser ophthalmoscope. *Arch Ophthalmol.* 1998;116(4):455–463.

Scripsema NK, Rosen RB. Scanning laser ophthalmoscope in the management of age-related macular degeneration. *US Ophthalmic Rev.* 2012;5(2):111–118.

Optical Coherence Tomography

OCT is a noninvasive, noncontact imaging modality that produces micrometer-resolution, cross-sectional images of ocular tissue. OCT is based on imaging reflected light. The technique produces a 2-dimensional image of the backscattered light from different layers in the retina, analogous to B-scan ultrasound (Fig 2-1). OCT, however, uses the principle of low-coherence interferometry, which allows measurement of optical rather than acoustic reflectivity. The use of light instead of sound enhances the resolution through light's inherent speed. Current commercial OCT scanners offer a resolution of 5–10 μm, which is at least 10 times that of ultrasound.

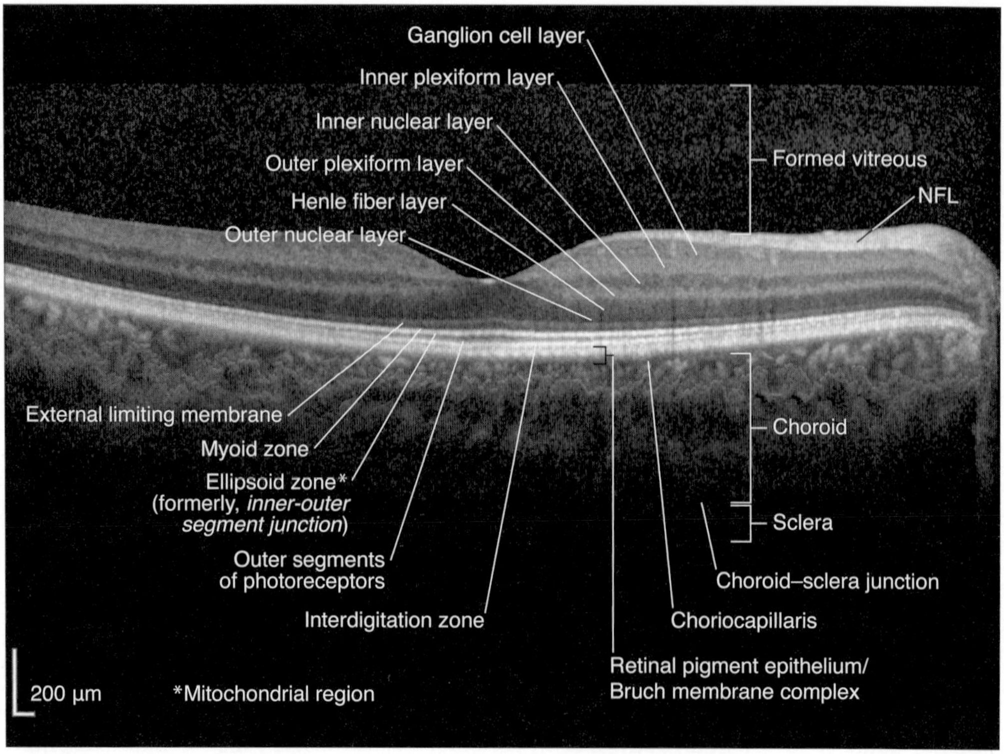

Figure 2-1 Spectral-domain optical coherence tomography (SD-OCT) image, showing a cross section of the retina and choroid. Nomenclature is based on the International Nomenclature for OCT Meeting Consensus for Normal OCT Terminology. Not shown are posterior cortical vitreous, preretinal space, and internal limiting membrane. NFL = nerve fiber layer. *(Courtesy of Colin A. McCannel, MD.)*

Spectral-domain OCT (SD-OCT) technology, delivers a 100-fold improvement in speed over previous-generation, time-domain OCT scanners. With SD-OCT images, the axial resolution is typically less than 7 μm, represented by 2048 pixels per A-scan, and the scan velocity is 18,000–70,000 A-scans per second. SD-OCT images are captured faster and with less motion artifact and higher resolution than time-domain OCT images, enabling 3-dimensional reconstruction and point-to-point registration for reproducible follow-up scans. The density of scans over a given area is also greater, reducing imaging gaps that can result in missing subtle tissue defects.

OCT single-scan, cross-sectional views (tomograms) of the retina appear similar to histologic specimens and have been termed "optical biopsies" (Fig 2-2). Tissues with higher reflectivity, such as the RPE or nerve fiber layer (NFL), appear brighter on gray-scaled images; minimally reflective structures, such as the vitreous and subretinal fluid, appear darker; and intermediately reflective retinal layers or edema appear as shades of gray. OCT systems that employ pseudocolor-scaled images typically represent high reflectivity as white-red, intermediate reflectivity with mixed colors, and low reflectivity as blue-black.

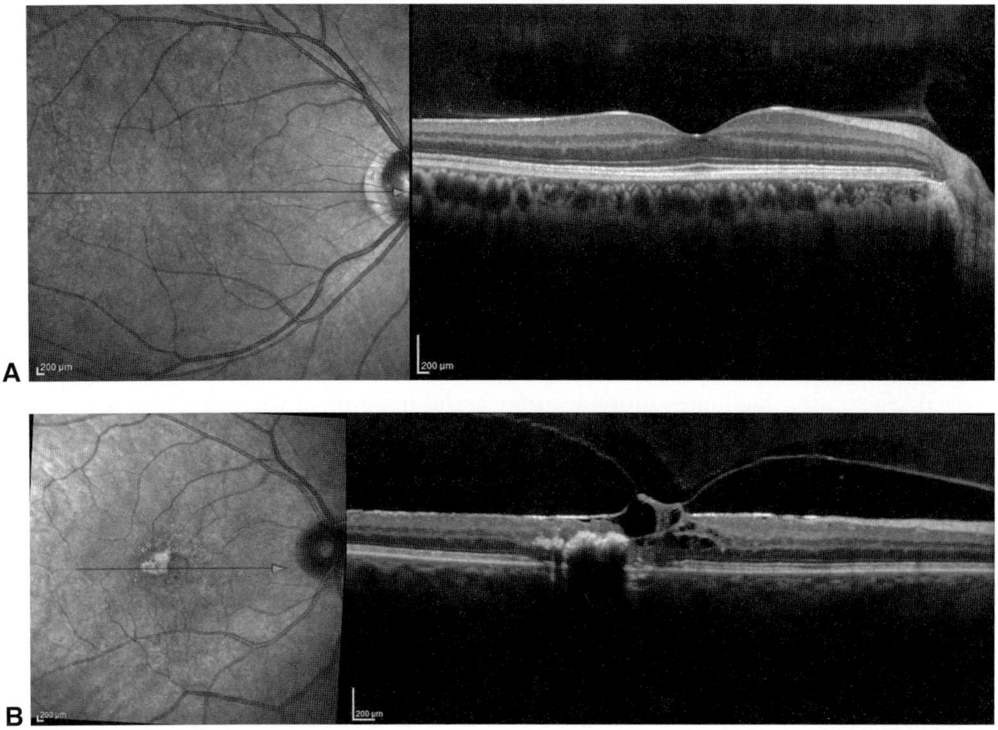

Figure 2-2 SD-OCT and near-infrared reflectance imaging. **A,** SD-OCT scan showing normal foveal depression and retinal thickness with normal near-infrared scanning laser ophthalmoscope (SLO) fundus image. **B,** SD-OCT scan from a patient with macular telangiectasia and vitreous traction. Note the posterior hyaloid pulling on the retina and distorting the foveal contour. The telangiectasia complex appears as a highly reflective lesion in the deeper retina and can also be seen as a bright-appearing lesion in the accompanying SLO fundus image. *(Courtesy of Richard B. Rosen, MD, and Patricia MT Garcia, MD.)*

OCT is useful for revealing epiretinal membranes or cystoid macular edema, differentiating lamellar from pseudo- and full-thickness macular holes, diagnosing vitreomacular traction, differentiating forms of diabetic macular edema, monitoring the course of central serous chorioretinopathy (Fig 2-3), making treatment decisions in the management of age-related macular degeneration (AMD) and macular edema, and detecting subtle subretinal fluid or structural anomalies that are often not revealed by angiography. A benefit of higher-resolution systems includes better delineation of the finest retinal layers, including the internal and external limiting membranes and the outermost retinal layers such as the ellipsoid zone (previously referred to as the *inner-outer segment junction,* or *IS/OS junction*), the cone outer segment line, the interdigitation zone, and the RPE.

OCT can be used to generate a macular thickness map. The OCT software automatically detects the inner and outer retinal boundaries and produces a pseudocolor-scaled topographic map delineating areas of increased thickening in brighter colors and thinner areas in darker colors. A volumetric assessment of regions of the macula can also be determined from the same map. By evaluating changes in retinal volume or macular thickness

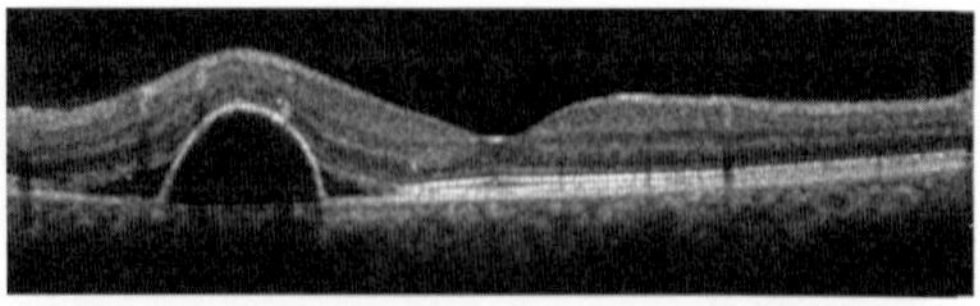

Figure 2-3 OCT image of central serous chorioretinopathy showing subretinal fluid and a small pigment epithelial detachment within the area of serous detachment. *(Courtesy of Gennady Landa, MD, and Patricia MT Garcia, MD.)*

over time, the clinician can judge the efficacy of therapy. Time-domain OCT produces macular thickness maps using 6 radial scans, 6 mm in length, centered on the fovea by interpolation of the thicknesses between the scan lines. In contrast, SD-OCT, taking advantage of its increased speed, can scan the entire macula using tightly spaced sequential horizontal lines to improve the accuracy of thickness and volume measurements; its improved registration facilitates more accurate serial imaging at the same location during follow-up visits. Next-generation devices, such as swept-source (SS) OCT and megahertz SD-OCT, should offer real-time monitoring for surgical applications and more revealing 3-dimensional video renderings.

Dillworth B, Kagemann L, Wollstein G, et al. From the operator's perspective. In: Schuman JS, Puliafito CA, Fujimoto JG, eds. *Everyday OCT.* Thorofare, NJ: Slack; 2006:1–3.

Khurana RN, Bhisitkul RB, Foster BS. Retinal optical coherence tomography. *Focal Points: Clinical Modules for Ophthalmologists.* San Francisco: American Academy of Ophthalmology; 2014, module 5.

Kiernan DF, Mieler WF, Hariprasad SM. Spectral-domain optical coherence tomography: a comparison of modern high-resolution retinal imaging systems. *Am J Ophthalmol.* 2010; 149(1):18–31.

Lumbroso B, Rispoli M. *Guide to Interpreting Spectral Domain Optical Coherence Tomography.* 2nd ed. New Delhi, India: Jaypee Brothers Medical; 2011.

Fundus Autofluorescence

Fundus autofluorescence (AF) is a rapid, noncontact, noninvasive way to evaluate RPE function. Autofluorescence is the intrinsic fluorescence emitted by a substance after being stimulated by excitation energy. Ocular structures that normally autofluoresce include the corneal epithelium and endothelium and lens, macular, and RPE pigments. Some pathologic conditions that autofluoresce are optic nerve drusen and subretinal deposits from photoreceptor outer segments, as seen in Best disease (Fig 2-4). The clinical use of fundus AF relies on the fact that the predominant source of autofluorescence in the macula is lipofuscin. When the RPE phagocytoses photoreceptor outer segments, oxidative by-products of the digested retinoids, fatty acids, and proteins form lipofuscin, which accumulates within the RPE cells. One pigment within lipofuscin that autofluoresces is A2E, a component derived from 2 molecules of vitamin A aldehyde and 1 molecule of ethanolamine. As RPE cells die within a specific area, the normal autofluorescence for that location disappears.

Fundus AF is typically imaged with (1) an SLO that employs blue laser excitation (488 nm) with a 500-nm barrier filter, (2) an SLO that uses green laser excitation (530 nm) and a 600-nm barrier filter, or (3) a fundus camera using a green 550-nm excitation filter with a 660-nm barrier filter. Fundus AF images allow clinicians to evaluate the status

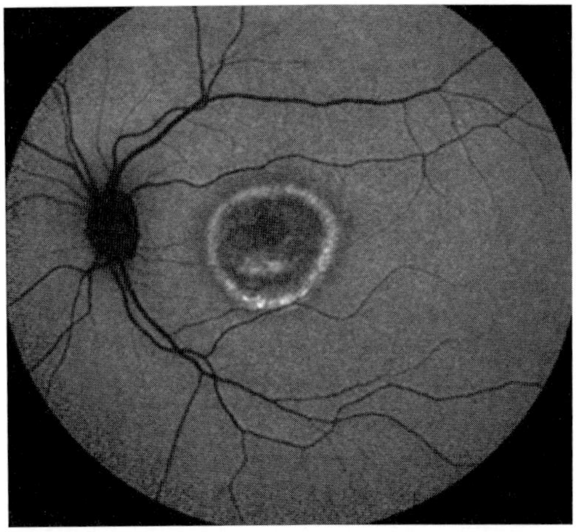

Figure 2-4 Fundus autofluorescence (AF) image from a patient with Best vitelliform dystrophy. The hyperautofluorescent ring visible around the fovea represents lipofuscin accumulation. The central stippled hypoautofluorescent area represents a region of serous elevation with a background of focal lipofuscin deposits and atrophy. *(Courtesy of Hamid Ahmadieh, MD.)*

of the RPE based on lipofuscin levels. Areas of geographic atrophy are devoid of normal autofluorescence and appear dark because of the loss of lipofuscin-containing RPE. Increased autofluorescence at the leading edge of these dark areas is thought to reflect pathologic lipofuscin accumulation, which may predict the direction of future expansion of the atrophy. Autofluorescence has become an important tool for evaluating hereditary retinal disease, largely replacing fluorescein angiography. It has also been helpful in revealing RPE alterations indicative of chronic or recurrent central serous retinopathy, as well as delineating serous pigment epithelial detachments. Although its value in monitoring expansion of geographic atrophy is established, the relationship of various AF patterns to progression of disease needs further exploration.

Near-infrared fundus autofluorescence (NIA) imaging using 787-nm excitation and greater than 800-nm emission reveals fluorescence emitted by melanin and melanofuscin from the RPE and deeper layers of the choroid. NIA images appear somewhat different from images recording the shorter-wavelength fundus AF. Subretinal fluid causes much greater signal attenuation in NIA than in shortwave fundus AF, possibly due to more pronounced scattering and absorption of NIR light by the subretinal fluid. Although less commonly used than shortwave AF imaging, NIA appears to reveal some pathologic changes more precisely and reproducibly than clinical examinations or standard fundus photographs and may find value in the longitudinal monitoring of disease progression.

Kellner U, Kellner S, Weinitz S. Fundus autofluorescence (488 NM) and near-infrared autofluorescence (787 NM) visualize different retinal pigment epithelium alterations in patients with age-related macular degeneration. *Retina.* 2010;30(1):6–15.

Oishi A, Ogino K, Makiyama Y, Nakagawa S, Kurimoto M, Yoshimura N. Wide-field fundus autofluorescence imaging of retinitis pigmentosa. *Ophthalmology.* 2013;120(9):1827–1834.

Oishi M, Oishi A, Ogino K, et al. Wide-field fundus autofluorescence abnormalities and visual function in patients with cone and cone–rod dystrophies. *Invest Ophthalmol Vis Sci.* 2014; 55(6):3572–3577.

Schmitz-Valckenberg S, Holz FG, Bird AC, Spaide RF. Fundus autofluorescence imaging: review and perspectives. *Retina.* 2008;28(3):385–409.

Retinal Angiographic Techniques

Fluorescein angiography

Fluorescein is an orange-red crystalline hydrocarbon with a molecular weight of 376; it transits through the vasculature and diffuses most rapidly into other body fluids where blood–tissue barriers are disturbed. Eighty percent of the fluorescein is protein-bound, primarily to plasma albumin, and therefore does not fluoresce; the remaining 20% circulates unbound within the vasculature and diffuses into tissues of the retina and choroid, where it can be visualized. Fluorescein fluoresces at 520–530 nm (green) when a molecule is excited by light of 465–490 nm (blue).

Fluorescein angiography (FA) allows study of the circulation of the retina and choroid in normal and diseased states. Photographs of the retina are taken following intravenous injection of sodium fluorescein. Typically, 2–3 mL of a 25% solution or 5 mL of a 10% sterile aqueous solution is used. To image the dye's fluorescence, special combinations of excitation and barrier filters are required. The white light from the camera flash passes through a blue excitation filter illuminating the inside of the eye with blue light; in an SLO, a blue laser is swept over the retina. The blue light excites the unbound fluorescein molecules, stimulating them to emit a longer-wavelength green light (520–530 nm). A yellow-green (barrier) filter on the camera lens blocks the reflected blue light, permitting only the yellow-green light emitted by the fluorescein molecules to be imaged. Wide-field SLO systems have also gained increasing favor because of their versatility and simplified ability to image peripheral retina.

Interpreting a fluorescein angiogram requires an understanding of retinal vasculature. The retina has a dual blood supply. The central retinal artery and derived retinal capillary plexus serve the inner half of the retina, and the endothelial cell tight junctions provide the inner blood–retina barrier. Normally, neither bound nor unbound fluorescein can pass this barrier. The choroidal circulation serves the outer half of the retina, and the tight junctional girdles of the RPE provide the outer blood–retina barrier. Fluorescein particles that are not bound to protein can pass through the fenestrated walls of the choriocapillaris but do not normally pass through the RPE cells or through the zonulae occludentes joining RPE cells to gain access to the subretinal space. Thus, fluorescein from the choroid does not enter the neurosensory retina unless the RPE is defective. The fluorescence in the choroid is normally contained by the pigment of the RPE but appears as deep, diffuse background fluorescence.

Fluorescein is injected into a peripheral vein and enters the ocular circulation via the ophthalmic artery 8–12 seconds later, depending on the site, the rate of injection, and the patient's age and cardiovascular health. The retinal and choroidal vessels progressively fill during the transit phase, which generally spans 10–15 seconds. Choroidal filling appears as a deep patchy flush, which often reveals choriocapillary lobular structure. The flow rate in the choroid is higher than that of the retinal vessels. The arterial phase of the transit follows the choroidal phase as dye enters the retinal arteries. The arteriovenous phase begins as the retinal arteries and capillaries completely fill and the retinal veins show evidence of laminar filling. This phase, which usually occurs within 1 minute of dye injection, is considered the peak phase of fluorescence, the point in time when the most capillary detail is shown in the fovea. Following complete venous filling, the dye recirculates and fluorescence gradually declines. In the late phases of the study, the choroid, Bruch membrane, and sclera stain. The larger choroidal vessels frequently appear as a hypofluorescent pattern against the brighter choroidal interstitium.

Fluorescein leaks out of retinal capillaries into the retina only where the capillary endothelium is damaged, as occurs in diabetic retinopathy or vasculitis. Similarly, fluorescein can pass from the choriocapillaris through pigment epithelial cells into the subretinal space and the retinal interstitium only when the pigment epithelial cells or intercellular junctions are abnormal, as in central serous chorioretinopathy or exudative macular degeneration. Patterns of hyperfluorescence combined with stereoscopic images can yield valuable information regarding the depth of leakage from retinal vessels or from abnormal pigment epithelium.

Abnormalities observed with FA can be grouped into 3 categories, each associated with one of the following types of fluorescence:

- autofluorescence
- hypofluorescence
- hyperfluorescence

*Auto*fluorescence is fluorescence that appears with the excitation and barrier filters in place before the fluorescein dye is injected; it is caused by endogenously fluorescent constituents of tissue such as lipofuscin or optic nerve drusen. *Hypo*fluorescence occurs when normal fluorescence is reduced or absent; it is present in 2 major patterns:

1. vascular filling defects
2. blocked fluorescence

Vascular filling defects are defects in which retinal or choroidal vessels fail to fill because of an intravascular obstruction that results in nonperfusion of an artery, vein, or capillary. These defects appear as either a delay in or complete absence of filling of the involved vessels. *Blocked fluorescence* occurs when the stimulation or visualization of the fluorescein is obstructed by fibrous tissue, pigment, or blood blocking normal retinal or choroidal fluorescence in the area.

Blocked fluorescence is easily differentiated from a filling defect by comparing the angiographic and ophthalmoscopic appearances of the area in question. Lack of correspondence in appearances suggests that the problem is more likely a vascular filling defect rather than blocked fluorescence. The depth of a lesion is easily determined by relating the level of the blocked fluorescence to details of the retinal circulation. For example, if lesions block the choroidal circulation but retinal vessels are present on top of this blocking defect, then the lesions are located above the choroid and below the retinal vessels.

*Hyper*fluorescence occurs when there is abnormally excessive fluorescence, typically extending beyond the borders of recognized structures; it manifests in a few major patterns:

- leakage
- staining

- pooling
- transmission, or window, defect
- autofluorescence

Leakage refers to a gradual, marked increase in fluorescence over the course of the study; it results from seepage of fluorescein molecules across the blood–retina barrier. When the outer blood–retina barrier is incompetent, the dye traverses across the pigment epithelium into the subretinal space or neurosensory retina. When the inner blood–retina barrier is incompetent, the dye leaks through vascular walls, into the retinal interstitium, and/or into the vitreous cavity. This leakage can occur secondary to the normal retinal vasculature becoming incompetent or from inherently leaky retinal neovascularization. In the late phases of the study, the borders of hyperfluorescence become increasingly blurred and intense as the fluorescein dye escapes into the extravascular space. Examples of disorders involving leakage include CNV (Fig 2-5), diabetic macular edema (via microaneurysms or intraretinal microvascular abnormalities [IRMAs]), and neovascularization of the disc.

Staining refers to a pattern of hyperfluorescence in which the fluorescence increases in intensity through transit views and persists in late views but in which the borders remain intact throughout the study. Staining results from fluorescein entry into a solid tissue or material that retains the fluorescein, such as a scar, drusen, optic nerve tissue, or sclera (see Fig 2-5B).

Pooling refers to the accumulation of fluorescein in a fluid-filled space in the retina or choroid. At the beginning of the study, the fluid in the space contains no fluorescein

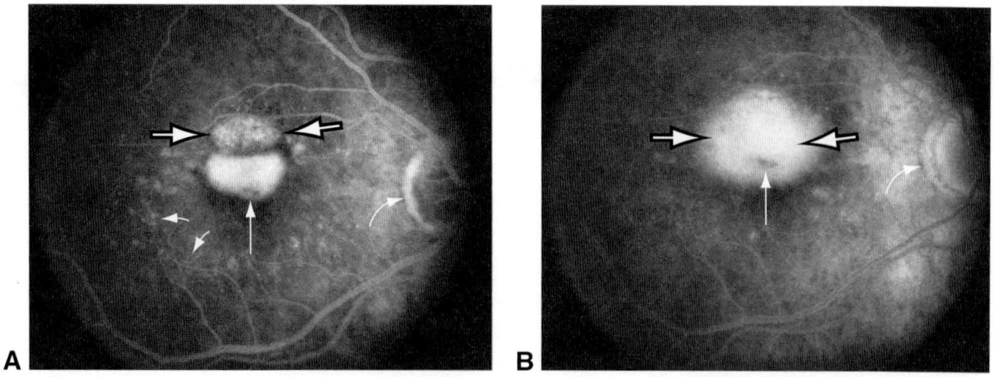

Figure 2-5 Classic and occult CNV in age-related macular degeneration. **A,** Early-phase fluorescein angiogram demonstrates classic CNV *(solid straight arrow)* and the boundaries of occult CNV *(open arrows). Small curved arrows* indicate a slight transmission of fluorescence (window defect) from drusen. The *large curved arrow* shows transmission resulting from retinal pigment epithelium (RPE) atrophy around the optic nerve. **B,** Late-phase angiogram demonstrates leakage of dye from classic CNV *(solid straight arrow)* and occult CNV *(open arrows)*. The transmission of fluorescence from drusen (see the *small curved arrows* in **A**) has faded. The *large curved arrow* shows staining of the sclera around the optic nerve. *(Used with permission from Bressler SB. Management of a small area of choroidal neovascularization in an eye with age-related macular degeneration [AMD] and relatively good visual acuity.* The Wilmer Retina Update. *1995;1:3–7.)*

and is invisible. As fluorescein leaks into the space, the margins of the space trap the fluorescein and appear distinct, as seen, for example, in an RPE detachment in central serous chorioretinopathy (Fig 2-6). As more fluorescein enters the space, the entire area fluoresces.

A *transmission defect,* or *window defect,* refers to a view of the normal choroidal fluorescence through a defect in the pigment of the RPE, such as that shown in Figures 2-5A and 2-5B. In a transmission defect, the hyperfluorescence occurs early, corresponding to filling of the choroidal circulation, and reaches its greatest intensity with the peak of choroidal filling. The fluorescence does not increase in intensity or shape and usually fades in the late phases as the choroidal fluorescence becomes diluted by blood that does not contain fluorescein. The fluorescein remains in the choroid and does not enter the retina.

Adverse effects of fluorescein angiography All patients injected with fluorescein incur a temporary yellowing of the skin and conjunctiva that lasts 6–12 hours and an orange-yellow

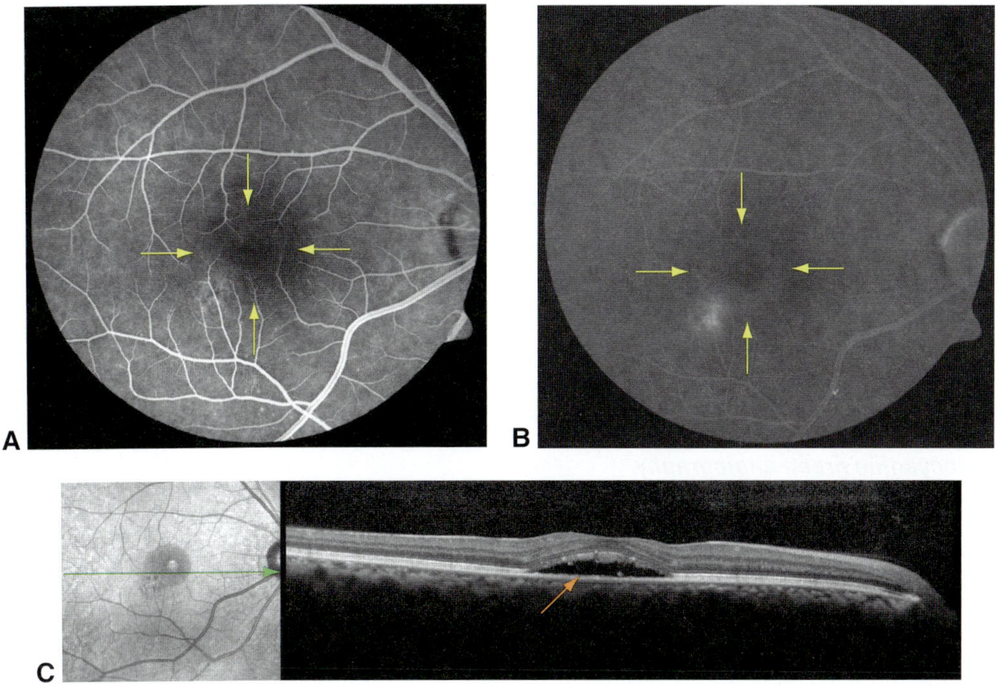

Figure 2-6 Fluorescein angiography (FA) images and OCT scan of central serous chorioretinopathy. **A,** Early-phase FA image of a patient with central serous chorioretinopathy. The *yellow arrows* outline the area of serous retinal detachment. In the inferotemporal aspect of the serous retinal detachment, there is early minimal hyperfluorescence, with diffuse leakage in late views **(B). C,** Corresponding OCT image illustrating the subretinal fluid accumulation *(orange arrow).* Accumulation of deposits on the outer surface of the photoreceptors can be seen. This material is thought to represent shed photoreceptor outer segments or fibrin. The *green arrow and line* on the infrared reflectance imaging shows the scan location of the OCT image. *(Courtesy of Colin A. McCannel, MD.)*

discoloration of the urine that lasts 24–36 hours. Although fluorescein is a relatively safe, injectable drug, adverse effects may include

- nausea, vomiting, or vasovagal reactions following approximately 10% of injections; more severe vasovagal reactions, including bradycardia, hypotension, shock, and syncope, are rare
- extravasation with subcutaneous granuloma, toxic neuritis, or local tissue necrosis—these are extremely rare
- urticarial *(anaphylactoid)* reactions in less than 1% of cases
- *anaphylactic* reactions (cardiovascular shock) at a rate of probably less than 1 in 100,000 injections

Prior urticarial reactions increase a patient's risk of having a similar reaction after subsequent injections; however, premedicating the individual with antihistamines, corticosteroids, or both decreases the risk. Nausea with the risk of subsequent vomiting can often be relieved by rapid application of a cold compress to the neck at the base of the skull at the first sign of distress.

Extravasation of the dye into the skin during injection can be painful, requiring application of ice-cold compresses to the affected area for 5–10 minutes. Close follow-up of the patient over hours or days until the edema, pain, and redness resolve is advised. Although teratogenic effects have not been identified, many ophthalmologists avoid using FA in pregnant women in the first trimester unless absolutely necessary. Also of note, fluorescein is transmitted to breast milk in lactating women.

Berkow JW, Flower RW, Orth DH, Kelley JS. *Fluorescein and Indocyanine Green Angiography: Technique and Interpretation.* 2nd ed. Ophthalmology Monograph 5. San Francisco: American Academy of Ophthalmology; 1997.

Kwiterovich KA, Maguire MG, Murphy RP, et al. Frequency of adverse systemic reactions after fluorescein angiography. Results of a prospective study. *Ophthalmology.* 1991;98(7): 1139–1142.

Indocyanine green angiography

Indocyanine green (ICG) is a water-soluble, tricarbocyanine dye that is almost completely protein bound (98%) after intravenous injection. Because the dye is protein bound, diffusion through the small fenestrations of the choriocapillaris is limited. The intravascular retention of ICG, coupled with low permeability, makes ICG angiography ideal for imaging choroidal vessels. ICG is metabolized in the liver and excreted into the bile. It fluoresces in the near-infrared range (790–805 nm). Because its fluorescence efficacy is only 4% that of fluorescein dye, ICG can be detected only with specialized infrared angiography systems.

The 2 principal technologies used for imaging ICG angiographic studies are standard fundus camera–based systems and SLO-based systems. The fundus camera–based systems use an excitation filter in the range of 805 nm and a barrier filter at 835 nm. ICG angiography performed using an SLO device uses a diode laser illumination system with an output of 805 nm and barrier filters at 500 and 810 nm. High-speed ICG angiography can produce up to 30 frames per second in a continuous recording of the angiogram. This process has allowed visualization of structures that appear only briefly during the study, such as feeder vessels of CNV. The longer wavelength of ICG fluorescence allows for the dye's detection through pigment, fluid, lipid, and hemorrhage, thereby allowing for imaging of abnormalities such as CNV that lie beneath RPE or a thin, subretinal hemorrhage.

The fundus camera–based imaging systems result in ICG angiographic images that do not consistently produce patterns of fluorescence resembling the traditional FA patterns. For example, unlike the traditional CNV FA pattern, CNV imaged with a fundus camera–based system appears as a plaque, a focal hot spot, or a combination of both. Plaques are formed by late-staining vessels and usually correspond to occult CNV. Focal hot spots are well-delineated fluorescent spots that are less than 1 disc diameter in size; their presence often suggests retinal angiomatous proliferations (RAP) or polypoidal vasculopathy (a variant of CNV).

With confocal SLO, it is possible to observe the anatomy of vascular lesions in detail on early frames of the angiography. For example, visible structures and findings include the intraretinal network of RAP; abnormal aneurysmal outpouchings of the inner choroidal vascular network, as found in idiopathic polypoidal choroidal vasculopathy; and focal areas of choroidal hyperpermeability, as occur in central serous chorioretinopathy. Confocal SLO angiography may also differentiate abnormal vasculature in intraocular tumors and reveal the abnormal fluorescence patterns of choroidal inflammatory conditions such as serpiginous-like choroiditis (also called *multifocal serpiginoid choroiditis*), acute multifocal placoid pigment epitheliopathy (AMPPE), multiple evanescent white dot syndrome (MEWDS) (Fig 2-7), birdshot uveitis, and multifocal choroiditis.

A 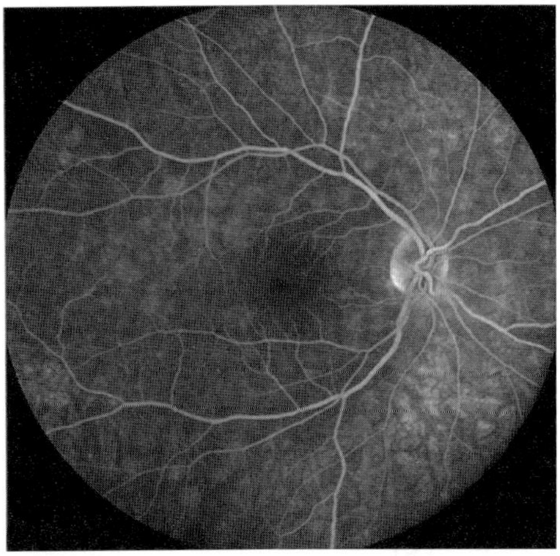

B 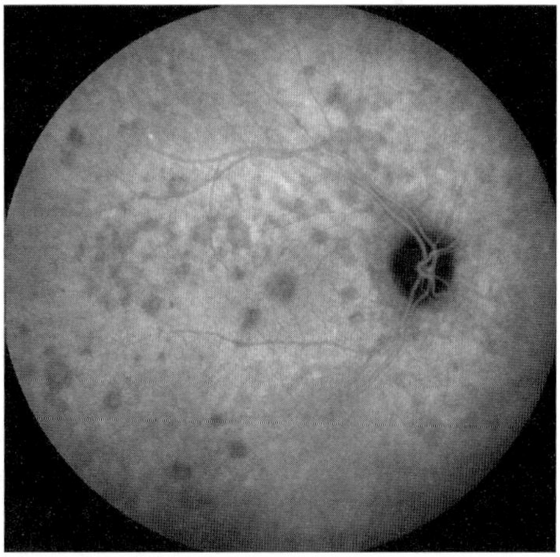

Figure 2-7 Angiographic images from a patient with multiple evanescent white dot syndrome (MEWDS) using fluorescein **(A)** and indocyanine green **(B)** contrast agents. Note the different response of the lesions to the 2 agents. The spots that appear bright on the FA image appear dark on the ICG image. *(Courtesy of Richard B. Rosen, MD, and Patricia MT Garcia, MD.)*

Indications for ICG angiography may include the following:

- CNV
- pigment epithelial detachment
- polypoidal choroidal vasculopathy
- RAP
- central serous chorioretinopathy
- intraocular tumors
- choroidal inflammatory conditions

Adverse effects of indocyanine green angiography Mild adverse events occur in fewer than 1% of patients. Allergic reactions may occur in individuals with a history of allergy to iodides or shellfish because ICG contains 5% iodide. Angiographic facilities should have emergency plans and establish protocols to manage complications associated with either fluorescein or ICG administration, including anaphylaxis. Contraindications to ICG may include liver disease, renal disease, sulfa or penicillin allergy, or use of the drug metformin to control type 2 diabetes mellitus.

American Academy of Ophthalmology. Indocyanine green angiography. *Ophthalmology.* 1998;105(8):1564–1569.

Cheung CM, Lai TY, Chen SJ, et al. Understanding indocyanine green angiography in polypoidal choroidal vasculopathy: The Group Experience With Digital Fundus Photography and Confocal Scanning Laser Ophthalmoscopy. *Retina.* 2014;34(12):2397–2406.

Hope-Ross M, Yannuzzi LA, Gragoudas ES, et al. Adverse reactions due to indocyanine green. *Ophthalmology.* 1994;101(3):529–533.

B-Scan Ultrasonography

B-scan (brightness scan) ultrasonography is an important technique for evaluating intraocular structures when direct visualization is difficult or not possible because of eyelid problems, corneal opacities, anterior segment opacities (eg, hyphema, hypopyon, miosis, pupillary membranes, dense cataracts), vitreous opacities (eg, hemorrhage, inflammatory debris), or extraocular/orbital lesions (Fig 2-8). It utilizes high-frequency sound (10–20 Mhz) from a piezoelectric crystal emitter/receiver that penetrates the tissue and bounces back. The echo that returns to the detector provides a reflection of the different acoustic impedances of the structures in its path. B-scan images are composed of multiple A-scans (axial scans), which emanate in a fan-shaped cone from the probe as the internal emitter is rapidly swept back and forth. Examination involves moving the probe around the globe to acquire different perspectives, which can be reconstructed in the examiner's mind to produce a 3-dimensional impression of the intraocular contents.

B-scan ultrasonography can provide valuable information on alterations of internal ocular structures, and in many instances, it is used even though pathology is clinically visible. For example, the technique may be helpful in differentiating iris masses, ciliary body lesions, or intraocular tumors; ruling out ciliary body, choroidal, or retinal detachments; confirming vitreous detachment; looking for foreign bodies following globe trauma;

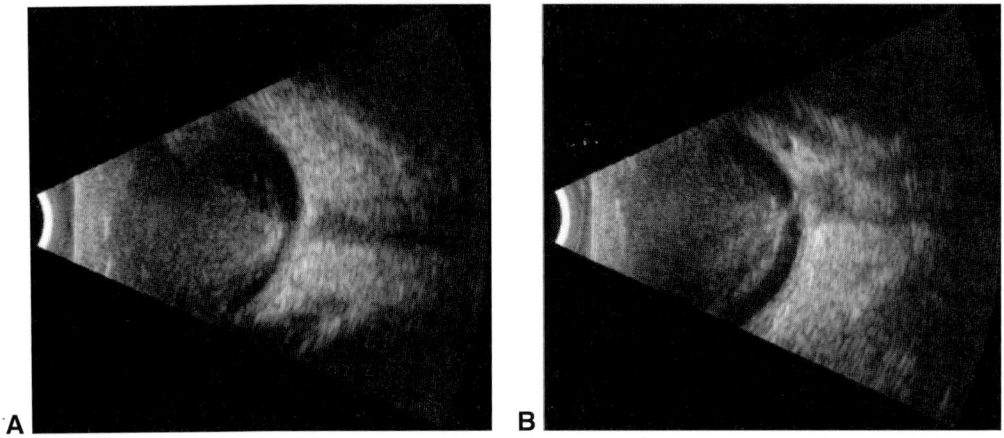

Figure 2-8 B-scan ultrasound images from a patient with vitreous opacities and vitreous separation except for attachment at the optic nerve. Image obtained from the probe scanning horizontally **(A)**; image taken from the probe scanning vertically **(B)**. The retina appears attached, there is no shadowing or appearance of masses, and the optic nerve appears normal. *(Courtesy of Alfonso Ponce, MD, and Julian Garcia, MD.)*

characterizing choroidal and retinal detachments; or identifying disc drusen in suspected papilledema.

Coleman DJ, Silverman RH, Lizzi FL et al. *Ultrasonography of the Eye and Orbit.* 2nd ed. Philadelphia: Lippincott Williams & Wilkins; 2006.

DiBernardo CW, Greenberg EF. *Ophthalmic Ultrasound: A Diagnostic Atlas.* 2nd ed. New York: Thieme; 2006.

Fisher Y. *Essential lectures in ophthalmic ultrasound.* Available at www.ophthalmicedge.org. Accessed July 1, 2014.

Garcia Jr, JP, Finger PT, Rosen RB. *Dynamic Ophthalmic Ultrasonography: A Video Atlas for Ophthalmologists and Imaging Technicians (The Advanced Retinal Imaging Center Collection of The New York Eye and Ear Infirmary).* Baltimore: Lippincott Williams & Wilkins; 2010.

CHAPTER 3

Retinal Physiology and Psychophysics

Clinical electrophysiologic and psychophysical testing allows assessment of much of the visual pathway. Most electrophysiologic tests are types of evoked potential whereby a controlled stimulus is used to evoke an electrophysiologic response. By adjusting stimulus and recording parameters, the examiner can measure the functions of the visual system; these measurements extend from changes in the retinal pigment epithelium (RPE) to the occipital cortical potentials. It is, however, important always to place the test results in clinical context and to consider that dysfunction at one level will usually give abnormalities further along the visual pathway. For example, an abnormal pattern visual evoked cortical potential could reflect an uncorrected refractive error, maculopathy, optic neuropathy, dysfunction of the posterior visual pathways, or other conditions.

A careful history and ophthalmic examination will help the clinician determine the most appropriate tests; it is then important to ensure that all tests are performed to standardized protocols. The International Society for Clinical Electrophysiology of Vision (ISCEV) publishes minimum standards for performing the routine tests, thus enabling meaningful interlaboratory comparison and literature searches. Many laboratories, particularly if they have a strong research interest, use far more complex test protocols but always include the standard responses. The International Federation for Clinical Neurophysiology has also published guidelines for visual system testing, which incorporate suggested test protocols based on symptoms.

Fishman GA, Birch DG, Holder GE, Brigell MG. *Electrophysiologic Testing in Disorders of the Retina, Optic Nerve, and Visual Pathway.* 2nd ed. Ophthalmology Monograph 2. San Francisco: American Academy of Ophthalmology; 2001.

Holder GE, Celesia GG, Miyake Y, Tobimatsu S, Weleber RG; International Federation of Clinical Neurophysiology. International Federation of Clinical Neurophysiology: recommendations for visual system testing. *Clin Neurophysiol.* 2010;121(9):1393–1409.

International Society for Clinical Electrophysiology of Vision. *Standards, recommendations and guidelines.* www.iscev.org/standards/index.html. Accessed July 2, 2014.

Electroretinography

The clinical electroretinogram (ERG) is a measurement of a mass electrical response from the retina, usually evoked by a brief flash of light. ERGs are recorded using active electrodes that contact the bulbar conjunctiva, with reference electrodes at the outer canthi. The active electrodes can be contact lens electrodes, although gold foil electrodes, H-K loop electrodes, and DTL fiber electrodes are also in common use. There are 3 main types of electroretinogram: the full-field (Ganzfeld) ERG, the multifocal ERG (mfERG), and the pattern ERG (PERG).

Full-Field (Ganzfeld) ERG

In the full-field ERG, a Ganzfeld bowl is used to illuminate the entire retina uniformly with a full-field luminance for photopic adaptation or a stimulus for photopic recording. Regular calibration of flash strength is required for clinical accuracy. Figure 3-1 shows typical response amplitudes and timings, but normal values will vary with recording technique, and each laboratory should establish its own normative data. Even with standardized recordings, variations in the type of electrode and specific equipment will affect the test results.

The procedure in most laboratories is to dark adapt the patient while the pupils are dilating, position the corneal electrodes under dim red light, and then commence stimulation using an interstimulus interval sufficient to allow the retina to recover. Many

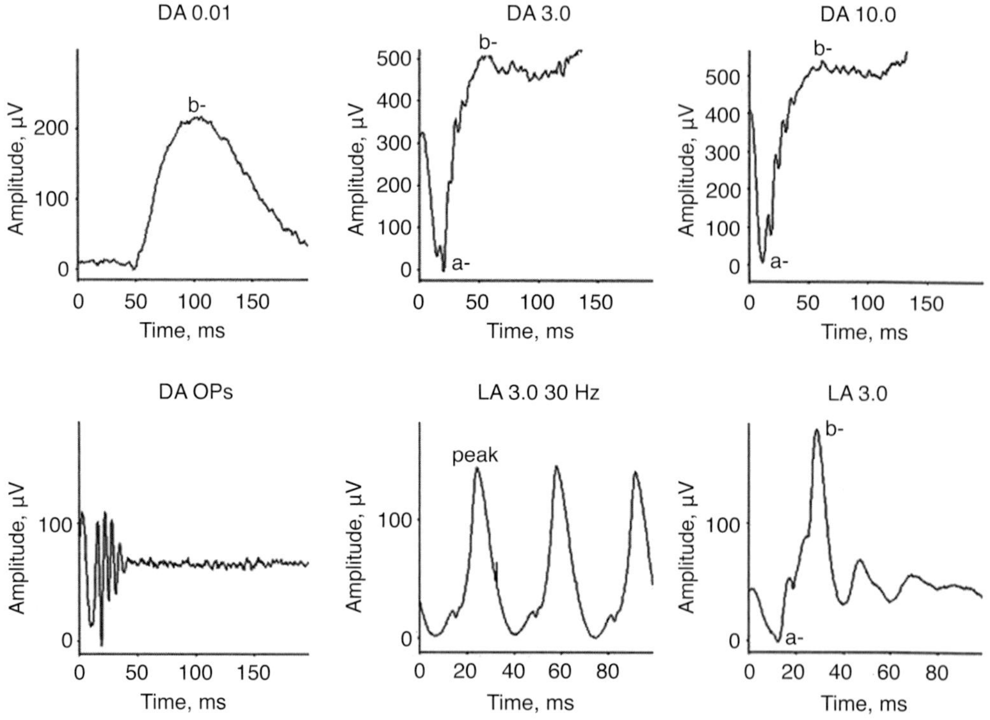

Figure 3-1 Basic electroretinogram (ERG) responses as defined by the International Society for Clinical Electrophysiology of Vision, including the additional "recommended" brighter-flash ERG (DA 10.0). The amplitude and peak times are typical, but normal values must be established for each laboratory using local techniques. See text for further details. a- = a-wave; b- = b-wave; DA = dark-adapted; LA = light-adapted; OPs = oscillatory potentials; numbers following abbreviations denote stimulus intensity (in candela-seconds per meter squared). *(Courtesy of Graham E. Holder, PhD.)*

laboratories perform an intensity series. The patient is then light adapted (using standard background intensity and time of adaptation), and photopic stimuli are delivered.

The ISCEV standard full-field ERG consists of 5 different responses with a suggested sixth (see Fig 3-1). Nomenclature is based on the flash strength as measured in cd (candelas) · s/m^2 and the adaptive state of the eye (ie, dark adapted [DA] or light adapted [LA]). Older terms are given in parentheses. ERG measurement is that of the size and timing of the major components as indicated in Figure 3-1.

1. *DA 0.01 (rod-specific):* This response consists of a b-wave but almost no detectable a-wave. The response arises in the on-bipolar cells (BPCs) (inner nuclear layer) of the rod system. A reduction in this response therefore identifies dysfunction within the rod system, but as the response arises at an inner retinal level, it cannot differentiate between dysfunction at the level of the photoreceptor and inner retinal dysfunction. It therefore acts as a measure of rod system sensitivity.
2. *DA 3.0 (mixed rod–cone):* This response consists of an a-wave and a b-wave. The a-wave at this flash strength usually has 2 peaks between approximately 15 and 21 ms, either of which may be prominent. As only approximately the first 8 ms or so of the DA a-wave reflects photoreceptor hyperpolarization, ISCEV suggests additional DA 10.0/30.0 testing for better diagnostic specificity.
3. *DA 10.0/30.0:* At either of these flash strengths, the a-wave has an easily measurable peak, and most of the a-wave reflects photoreceptor function. It is this response that gives anatomical specificity by localizing the dysfunction either to photoreceptor or inner-retinal level. Thus, a reduced DA 0.01 response accompanied by marked reduction in the a-wave of the DA 10.0/30.0 response indicates photoreceptor dysfunction, but if the a-wave is normal or near normal and the b-wave is of lower amplitude than the a-wave—a so-called negative ERG—then dysfunction is occurring post-phototransduction, that is, at an inner-retinal level.
4. *Oscillatory potentials:* These small oscillations on the ascending limb of the b-wave probably arise largely in the amacrine cells and can be made more visible by filtering. They are reduced in retinal ischemic states and in most cases of congenital stationary night blindness but overall have limited diagnostic value.
5. *LA 3.0 (photopic single-flash):* This ERG is obtained by stimulating with a flash superimposed upon a rod-suppressing background. The a-wave relates to function in the cone photoreceptors and off-bipolar cells. The b-wave is a synchronized component arising in on- and off-BPCs, enabling some localization of dysfunction.
6. *LA 3.0 30 Hz (photopic flicker):* The temporal resolution of the rod system is poor, and this response arises in the cone system. It is the more sensitive measure of cone-system dysfunction but allows no anatomical specificity. Both timing and amplitude are important parameters; delay in the flicker ERG response is a sensitive measure of generalized retinal cone system dysfunction, whereas reduced amplitude but normal peak time is indicative of restricted loss of function.

A number of factors influence the size and timing of the normal ERG, including pupil size; thus, pupil diameter should always be measured. ERG amplitude declines with age, so age-related normal controls are needed. Newborns have small signals, resulting in blunted-waveform ERGs. The response matures rapidly to reach adult values in the first year of life. The ERG is relatively insensitive to refractive error; however, highly myopic eyes will have lower amplitude signals but do not show the peak-time delay usually associated with hereditary retinal degeneration.

As a biological signal, there is inherent noise in ERGs. If amplitudes remain within the normal range, a reduction over time of more than 25% is usually considered significant. For peak-time measures, a change of greater than 3 ms is regarded as significant for cone-derived response a- or b-waves and brighter-flash dark-adapted a-waves, and a change greater than 6 ms is significant for dark-adapted b-waves.

In general, ERG peak-time shift suggests generalized dysfunction, whereas simple amplitude reduction suggests restricted loss of function such as may occur in branch vascular occlusion, regional uveitic damage, or restricted ("sector") forms of retinitis pigmentosa (RP). Timing is often best assessed using the 30-Hz flicker ERG peak time. Generalized inflammatory disease may be associated with delay but preservation of amplitude.

Examples of ERG patterns in specific disorders appear in Figure 3-2. The full-field ERG is a mass response from the whole retina, and dysfunction confined to the macula is therefore accompanied by a normal ERG. Even though the central macula is cone dense, the vast majority of retinal cones lie outside the macula; thus, the macula contributes little to a full-field ERG. Because abnormal photopic ERGs indicate cone dysfunction outside the macula, ERG testing therefore facilitates the distinction between a macular dystrophy (normal ERG) and a cone or cone–rod dystrophy with more serious visual implications for the patient.

Figure 3-2 *Opposite:* ERG findings in various disorders. **A,** Typical normal, control waveforms. **B,** Macular dystrophy: full-field ERGs are all normal, but the pattern ERG (PERG) is undetectable. **C,** Cone dystrophy: DA 0.10 (rod-specific) and DA 10.0 ERG responses are normal; photopic flicker and single-flash ERGs are reduced and delayed; PERG is subnormal, indicating macular involvement. **D,** Rod–cone dystrophy (retinitis pigmentosa [RP]) with macular involvement: all ERGs are markedly subnormal, with rod ERGs more affected than cone ERGs, severe reduction of the DA 10.0 a-wave, indicating photoreceptor disease, and delayed 30-Hz and single-flash cone ERGs, indicating generalized cone system dysfunction. Abnormal PERG shows macular involvement. **E,** Rod–cone dystrophy (RP) with macular sparing: full-field ERGs show a rod–cone pattern of abnormality similar to that shown in **D,** but normal PERG shows macular sparing. **F,** "Complete" congenital stationary night blindness (CSNB): findings show loss of on-pathway function at a postreceptoral level. DA 0.01 response is undetectable; DA 10.0 response is profoundly electronegative, with the normal a-wave reflecting normal photoreceptor function and the marked relative b-wave reduction showing inner retinal disease; 30-Hz flicker ERG shows only minor changes in waveform and mild delay; LA 3.0 ERG shows changes diagnostic of loss of cone on-pathway function but sparing of the off-pathway. The a-wave commences normally but then shows a broadened trough. The b-wave is sharply rising, with loss of the photopic oscillatory potentials, and marked reduction in the b:a ratio. PERG is markedly subnormal. **G,** "Incomplete" CSNB: DA 0.01 response is subnormal but detectable; DA 10.0 response is markedly electronegative; 30-Hz flicker ERG is markedly subnormal, showing delay and a characteristic triphasic waveform; LA 3.0 single-flash photopic ERG shows a subnormal a-wave and a markedly subnormal b-wave, reflecting involvement of both on- and off-cone pathways; PERG is subnormal. **H,** X-linked retinoschisis: DA 0.01 response is severely reduced; DA 10.0 response is profoundly electronegative; 30-Hz flicker ERG shows delay; LA 3.0 ERG shows delay and marked reduction in the b:a ratio; PERG is markedly subnormal. **I,** S-cone monochromatism: DA 0.01 and DA 10.0 ERGs are normal; 30-Hz flicker ERG is virtually undetectable; LA 3.0 response shows only a small b-wave at approximately 50 ms consistent with an S-cone origin; PERG is undetectable. *(Courtesy of Graham E. Holder, PhD.)*

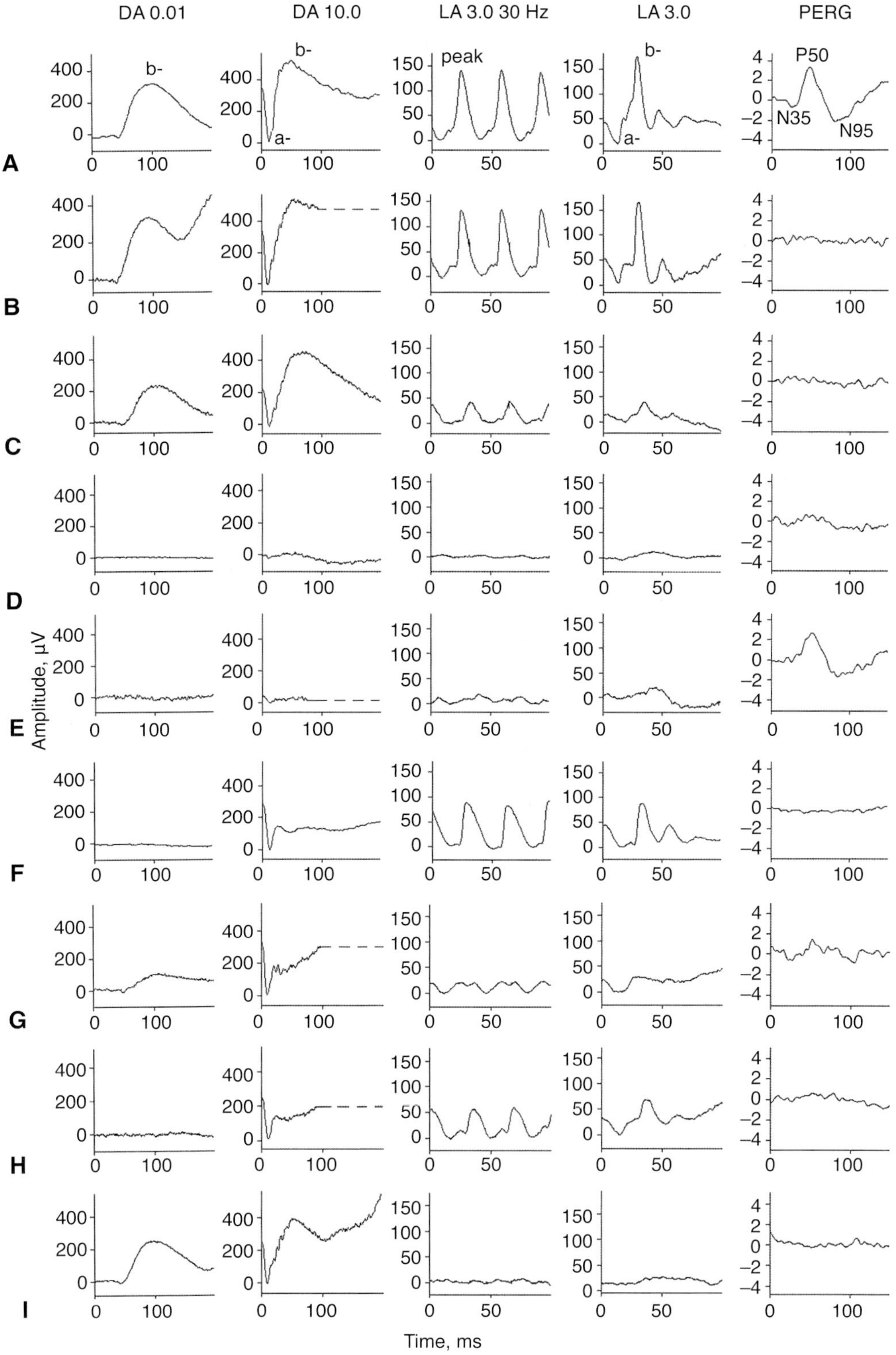
DA 0.01
DA 10.0
LA 3.0 30 Hz
LA 3.0
PERG
b-
a-
peak
P50
N35
N95
A
B
C
D
E
F
G
H
I
Amplitude, μV
Time, ms

Multifocal ERG

A topographic ERG map of the retinal cone system can be produced using a multifocal ERG (mfERG). The stimulus consists of multiple hexagons, smaller in the center than the periphery to reflect cone photoreceptor density, each of which flashes with a pseudorandom sequence. Cross-correlation techniques are used to calculate the small ERGs corresponding to each hexagon. Overall stimulus size usually is approximately 50 degrees. For patients with stable and accurate fixation (a crucial point!), mfERG can determine objectively whether macular dysfunction is present, for example, in the early detection of hydroxychloroquine toxicity (Fig 3-3). Such tests may also help evaluate or compare treatment responses in various macular conditions.

Pattern ERG

The pattern ERG (PERG) is the retinal response to an isoluminant alternating checkerboard stimulus presented to the macula. The stimulus is thus primarily a contrast stimulus. The responses are small, and signal averaging is used to record the PERG. When important technical factors are taken into account, reliability is similar to full-field ERG. There are 2 main components, P50 and N95, with most subjects showing an earlier negative component, N35. N95 arises in the retinal ganglion cells (RGCs) and thus acts as a direct measure of central retinal ganglion cell function. The P50 component is consequent upon macular photoreceptor function, even though approximately 70% of it arises in the RGCs; the amplitude of P50 is clinically useful as an objective index of macular function. The image must be in focus on the macula, and PERGs are typically recorded with a conductive fiber or foil electrode that touches the cornea; contact lens electrodes are not recommended because of adverse effects on the optics of the eye. As it is evoked by a stimulus similar to that used for visual evoked potential (VEP) recording (discussed later in the chapter), knowledge of the PERG facilitates accurate interpretation of an abnormal VEP. PERG is also useful in primary ganglion cell disease such as dominantly inherited optic atrophy or Leber hereditary optic neuropathy.

Holder GE. Pattern electroretinography (PERG) and an integrated approach to visual pathway diagnosis. *Prog Retin Eye Res.* 2001;20(4):531–561.

Clinical Considerations

The ERG provides objective retinal functional data and is therefore important in the diagnosis, management, and follow-up of retinal disease (eg, see Chapter 12, Table 12-1 for applications in inherited disease). Symptomatic indications include night blindness, in which the potentially blinding rod–cone dystrophies must be distinguished from the relatively benign congenital stationary night blindness. The potentially blinding dystrophies are associated with markedly abnormal a-waves in the dark-adapted bright-flash ERGs, and the relatively benign form is associated with a "negative" ERG (see Fig 3-2). Other symptomatic indications include photophobia, which can result from generalized cone dysfunction as in a cone dystrophy, and photopsia or shimmering, which can signal the

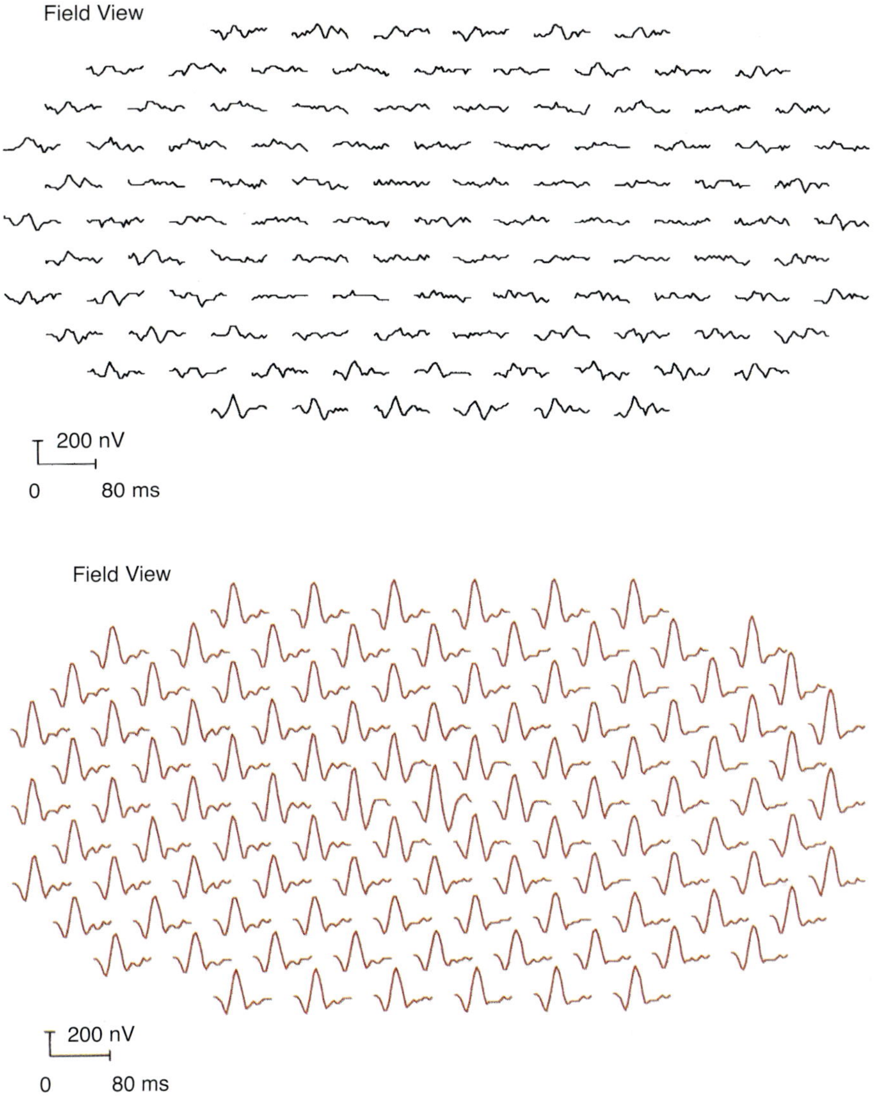

A B

Figure 3-3 Multifocal ERG tracings of the right eye of a patient with hydroxychloroquine toxicity. The central macular region has marked decreased waveform amplitudes **(A)** compared with the reference traces **(B)**. *(Courtesy of Carl Regillo, MD.)*

development of autoimmune retinopathy, possibly paraneoplastic. There is increasing use of the ERG in the assessment and monitoring of inflammatory disorders such as birdshot uveitis, for which the objective functional data allow management decisions to be taken with more confidence. The ERG provides an objective measure of disease severity, aiding decisions for when and how to treat, and it can then provide a valuable measure of treatment efficacy that is more sensitive than conventional clinical parameters.

ERGs must always be taken in the clinical context and to enable accurate ERG diagnosis, a careful clinical history should include previous drug and/or surgical treatment as well as a family history. Results are diagnostic only for 3 relatively rare inherited disorders in which there are pathognomonic findings: bradyopsia (mutation in *RGS9* or *R9AP*), enhanced S-cone syndrome (*NR2E3),* and cone dystrophy with supernormal rod ERG *(KCNV2).*

The ERG can be useful in vascular disease. The negative ERG that characteristically follows central retinal artery occlusion (CRAO) reflects the dual blood supply to the retina; the photoreceptors are supplied via choroidal circulation, but the central retinal artery supplies the inner nuclear layer. Thus, the b-wave is reduced but the a-wave is relatively preserved. In eyes with CRVO, a negative ERG or delay in the 30-Hz flicker ERG response is suggestive of significant ischemia.

The ERG can be helpful in determining the carrier state of individuals with X-linked disease. For example, carriers of X-linked RP will often have significant ERG abnormalities, caused by lyonization, despite having a normal-appearing fundus. However, in choroideremia, carriers usually exhibit a normal ERG despite having an abnormal fundus appearance (also because of lyonization).

ERGs can be obtained in children of all ages. To do so, sedation, general anesthesia, or eyelid electrodes may be used. Interpretation of pediatric ERGs involves special considerations. First, the ERG may reveal retinal abnormalities before the development of clear-cut ophthalmoscopic signs. Second, adult ERG values are not reached until 6–9 months of age. Third, if general anesthesia is used, its effect on ERG patterns must be considered.

Johnson MA, Marcus S, Elman MJ, McPhee TJ. Neovascularization in central retinal vein occlusion: electroretinographic findings. *Arch Ophthalmol.* 1988;106(3):348–352.

Vincent A, Robson AG, Holder GE. Pathognomonic (diagnostic) ERGs. A review and update. *Retina.* 2013;33(1):5–12.

Electro-oculography

The electro-oculogram (EOG) assesses the health of the RPE, as well as the interaction between the RPE and the photoreceptors, by measuring the changes in the corneoretinal standing potential that occur during scotopic or photopic adaptation. The standing potential, which reflects the voltage differential across the RPE, is positive at the cornea (Fig 3-4). Estimates of trans-RPE potential range from 1 to 10 mV.

During the test, the patient makes fixed 30° lateral eye movements during 15 minutes of dark adaptation, and again during a 12-minute period of light adaptation (Fig 3-5). The eye movements are made for approximately 10 seconds each minute. The amplitude of the signal recorded between electrodes positioned at medial and lateral canthi reaches a minimum after approximately 12 minutes of dark adaptation—the dark trough—and a maximum at approximately 8 minutes of light adaptation—the light peak. The EOG is quantified by expressing the size of the light peak in relation to the dark trough as a percentage known as the *Arden index* (or *ratio*). A normal EOG Arden index will be greater than 170%.

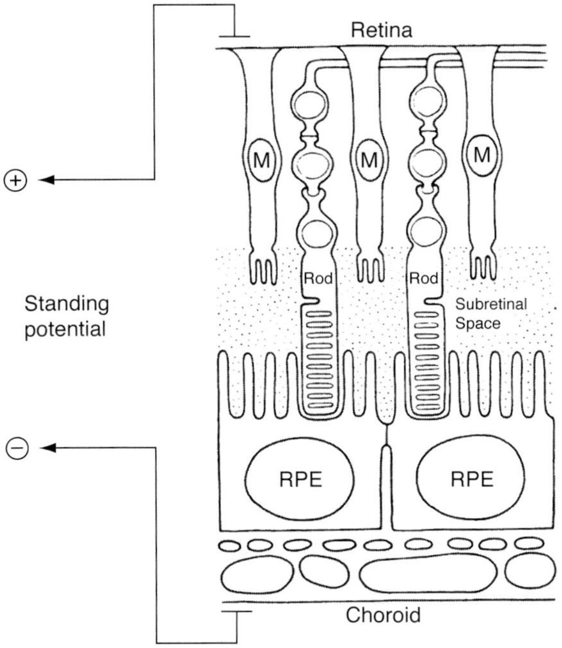

Figure 3-4 Electrical circuit of the standing potential. The retinal pigment epithelium (RPE) cells generate a voltage from apex to base because of the different ionic permeability characteristics on each surface and the presence of impermeable tight junctions between the cells. Changes in the voltage across the apical or basal RPE membrane are reflected in the standing potential and are measurable clinically as the c-wave on ERG or with electro-oculography. M = Müller cells. *(Modified with permission from Steinberg RH. Monitoring communications between photoreceptors and pigment epithelial cells: effects of "mild" systemic hypoxia. Friedenwald Lecture.* Invest Ophthalmol Vis Sci. *1987;28(12):1888–1904.)*

The development of a normal light peak requires normally functioning photoreceptors in contact with a normally functioning RPE. The light peak is generated by progressive depolarization of the RPE basal membrane via mechanisms that are not fully understood; the protein bestrophin is implicated in the final opening of chloride channels.

Any disorder that affects rod photoreceptor function will affect the EOG. The light rise is typically severely reduced in any widespread photoreceptor degeneration, including RP. However, the principal use of the EOG in clinical practice is in the diagnosis of Best vitelliform macular dystrophy (see Chapter 12). In this condition, a severely reduced or absent EOG light rise is accompanied by a normal ERG. The EOG in adult vitelliform macular dystrophy may be mildly subnormal but is not reduced to the same extent as it is in Best disease. Severe loss of the EOG light rise is also seen in autosomal recessive bestrophinopathy (ARB). ARB is a recessively inherited progressive retinal dystrophy and, like Best disease, is consequent upon mutation in *BEST1*. However, unlike in Best disease, affected patients have abnormal ERGs—but not sufficiently abnormal to explain the profound degree of EOG light rise reduction. In addition, unlike in Best disease, ARB carriers do not show an EOG abnormality.

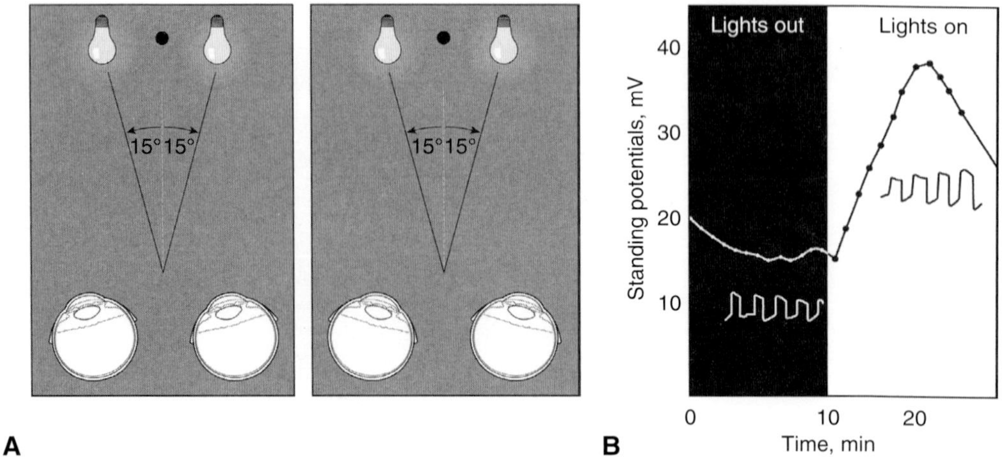

Figure 3-5 The clinical electro-oculogram (EOG). **A,** After electrodes are fixed to an area near the medial and lateral canthi, the subject is asked to look back and forth between 2 fixation targets (dimly lit lights), which are separated by a distance that results in a 30° horizontal eye movement. As each eye moves, the voltage between skin electrodes varies in proportion to the size of the standing potential of the eye (the voltage differential across the RPE). **B,** Plot of the amplitude of the oscillations. As the eyes turn toward the positive electrodes, an increased potential is measured, thus the slow back and forth motions result in the relatively square-looking voltage curve. During testing, the standing potential diminishes to a minimum in the dark (the *dark trough*) and then rises to a maximum after the light is turned on (the *light peak*). In clinical practice, the EOG result is usually reported as the ratio between the light peak and the dark trough expressed as a percentage, the Arden index or ratio. *(Illustrations by Mark Miller.)*

Arden GB, Constable PA. The electro-oculogram. *Prog Retin Eye Res.* 2006;25(2):207–248.

Burgess R, Millar ID, Leroy BP, et al. Biallelic mutation of *BEST1* causes a distinct retinopathy in humans. *Am J Hum Genet.* 2008;82(1):19–31.

Heckenlively, JR, Arden GB, eds. *Principles and Practice of Clinical Electrophysiology of Vision.* 2nd ed. Cambridge, MA: MIT Press; 2006.

Visual Evoked Cortical Potentials

The *visual evoked potential (VEP;* also *VECP* or *VER,* for *visual evoked cortical potential* or *response)* is recorded using scalp electrodes placed over the occipital scalp in response to stimulation of the retina by either light flashes or patterned stimuli (usually a reversing black-and-white checkerboard on a TV monitor). Computerized signal averaging extracts the VEP from the larger background electroencephalogram by averaging the responses to multiple reversals or flashes. Pattern-reversal VEPs, in which the black-and-white squares interchange without a change in luminance and the stimulus is displayed constantly, have a similar waveform across a population and a remarkably consistent timing; amplitudes show greater variability. Flash VEPs are far more variable across a population than pattern-reversal VEPs but can be useful in comparing eyes or hemispheric responses in the same patient; a hemispheric comparison requires multiple recording channels. A normal pattern-reversal VEP (Fig 3-6) contains a major positive component at approximately 100 ms, P100. Measurement is usually taken of P100 amplitude and peak time (sometimes called *latency*).

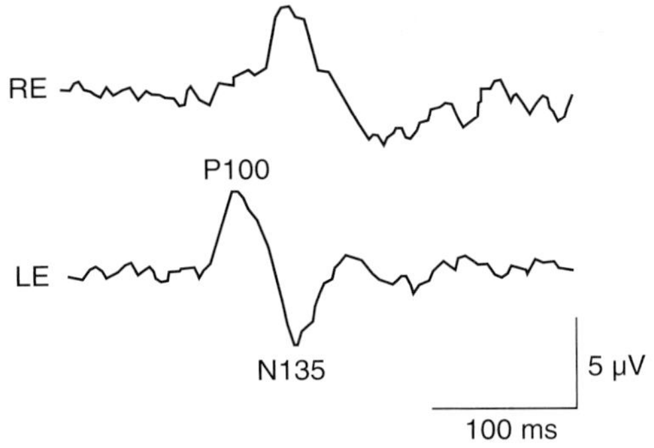

Figure 3-6 Pattern-reversal visual evoked potential from a patient with a 4-month history of right eye (RE) optic neuritis and recovery of right visual acuity to 20/20. Left eye (LE) response is normal; RE P100 component shows profound delay with preservation of amplitude and waveform.

VEPs are often used to demonstrate optic nerve conduction delay, particularly in suspected multiple sclerosis, in which the VEP can be delayed even in patients without history or signs of previous optic neuritis; patients with demyelinating optic neuritis almost invariably show VEP delay even when visual acuity recovers (see Fig 3-6). Most optic nerve diseases will exhibit VEP delay, but the abnormality can be confined to amplitude (interocular asymmetry) in nonarteritic anterior ischemic optic neuropathy. VEPs are indispensable in patients with nonorganic vision loss, demonstrating normal function even though symptoms suggest abnormalities. It must always be remembered that a delayed VEP is not diagnostic of optic nerve disease. Macular dysfunction can cause similar abnormalities, and assessment of macular function with mfERG or PERG greatly improves VEP interpretation.

VEPs can also be recorded in response to pattern-appearance stimuli, in which the stimulus appears from a uniformly gray background and then disappears, maintaining isoluminance throughout. Pattern-appearance VEPs are particularly useful in the detection of intracranial misrouting associated with ocular or oculo-cutaneous albinism (requiring multiple recording channels), as they are much less affected by nystagmus than are reversal VEPs. Flash stimulation is used to assess albinism misrouting in babies and infants who cannot maintain adequate fixation on a pattern stimulus. Appearance VEPs can also be used to assess visual system resolution objectively, providing a surrogate measure of visual acuity.

Psychophysical Testing

Although electrophysiologic testing objectively measures cell layers and cell types in the visual pathway, it does not always allow testing of localized responses and may not be sensitive to small degrees of visual dysfunction. Psychophysical tests can be exceedingly sensitive, but they are subjective and are usually not level-specific; perception represents an integration of information provided by different parts of the visual pathway. Psychophysical tests relevant to retinal disease include testing of

- visual acuity
- visual field
- contrast sensitivity
- color vision
- dark adaptation

Contrast sensitivity, dark adaptation, and color vision testing are discussed in this chapter. See BCSC Section 3, *Clinical Optics,* for discussion of visual acuity and additional technical information on contrast sensitivity, and BCSC Section 10, *Glaucoma,* for a discussion of visual field testing.

Dingcai C. Color vision and night vision. In: Ryan SJ, Schachat AP, Wilkinson CP, Hinton DR, Sadda SR, Wiedemann P, eds. *Retina.* 5th ed. Philadelphia: Elsevier/Saunders; 2013:285–299.

Contrast Sensitivity

Contrast sensitivity (CS) is a very important concept to understand. The loss of CS often results in visual difficulties and dysfunction out of proportion to the measured visual acuity. For example, patients with nonexudative macular degeneration or diabetic macular edema may have a fairly good measured visual acuity of 20/30 or better but experience major difficulties in performing routine visual tasks such as reading the newspaper and navigating stairways. Because a conventional Snellen visual acuity is based on high-contrast, achromatic, square-wave stimuli, it does not measure the ability to perceive subtleties of light. However, the visual system codes much of what is seen on the basis of *contrast* rather than spatial resolution, with subtleties of light and dark providing much of the richness of visual perception. For instance, dusk, fog, or smoke can reduce contrast, making it very difficult for anyone to resolve ordinary objects. Similarly, when the ability to perceive contrast under ordinary conditions is lost, as occurs in many retinal diseases or with media opacities, visual function is adversely impacted.

Testing of contrast sensitivity

Several clinical tests of CS are available. Most relate CS to *spatial frequency,* which refers to the size of the light–dark cycles. Individuals are normally most sensitive to contrast for objects that have a spatial frequency between 2 and 5 cycles per degree (Fig 3-7), but this sensitivity can change in disease. Some tests use letters or optotypes of varying dimness and size to provide a more clinical context.

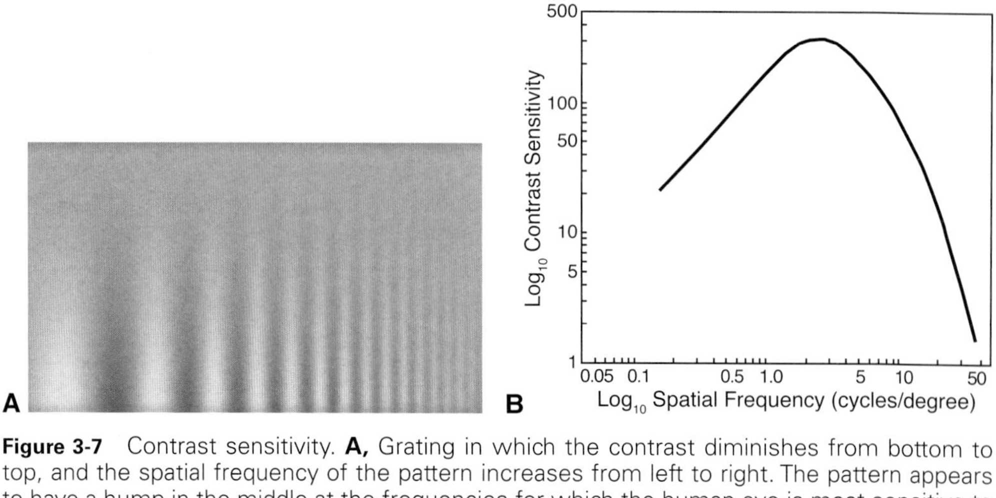

Figure 3-7 Contrast sensitivity. **A,** Grating in which the contrast diminishes from bottom to top, and the spatial frequency of the pattern increases from left to right. The pattern appears to have a hump in the middle at the frequencies for which the human eye is most sensitive to contrast. **B,** Plot of the contrast sensitivity function. *(Part A courtesy of Brian Wandell, PhD.)*

The *Pelli-Robson test* measures contrast sensitivity using a single, large letter size (20/60 optotype), with contrast varying across groups of letters (Fig 3-8). Patients read the letters, starting with the highest contrast, and continue until they are unable to read 2 or 3 letters in a single group. The subject is assigned a score based on the contrast of the last group in which 2 or 3 letters were correctly read. The Pelli-Robson score is a logarithmic measure of the subject's contrast sensitivity. Thus, a score of 2.0 means that the subject was able to read at least 2 of the 3 letters with a contrast of 1% (contrast sensitivity = 100%, or $\log_{10} 2$); in other words, a score of 2.0 indicates normal contrast sensitivity of 100%. A Pelli-Robson contrast sensitivity score of less than 1.5 is consistent with visual impairment, and a score of less than 1.0 represents visual disability.

Contrast sensitivity testing is discussed further in BCSC Section 3, *Clinical Optics,* and Section 5, *Neuro-Ophthalmology.*

Owsley C. Contrast sensitivity. *Ophthalmol Clin North Am.* 2003;16(2):171–177.

Rubin GS. Visual acuity and contrast sensitivity. In: Ryan SJ, Schachat AP, Wilkinson CP, Hinton DR, Sadda SR, Wiedemann P, eds. *Retina.* 5th ed. Philadelphia: Elsevier/Saunders; 2013:300–306.

Color Vision

The normal human retina has 3 cone types, each containing a different outer segment visual pigment: short-wavelength sensitive (S cone; formerly, *blue*), medium-wavelength

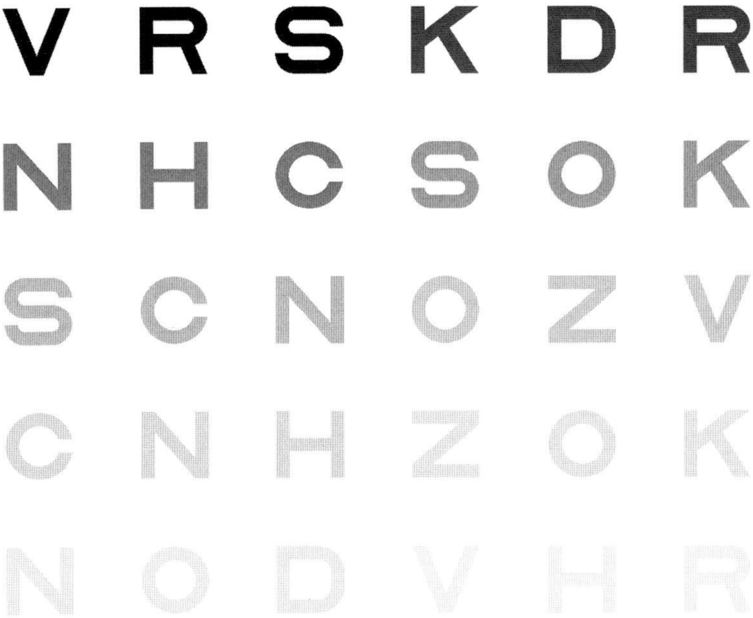

Figure 3-8 Pelli-Robson contrast sensitivity chart. The top 5 of 8 lines of a standard Pelli-Robson contrast sensitivity chart are shown. The top left 3-letter block has a log contrast value of 0.05, and there is a log contrast change of 0.15 with each 3-letter block. In the full 8-line chart, the lowest contrast letters have a log value of 2.3; 2.0 represents normal contrast sensitivity. *(Used with permission from Pelli DG, Robson JG, Wilkins AJ. The design of a new letter chart for measuring contrast sensitivity.* Clin Vision Sci. *1988;2(3):187–199.)*

(M cone; formerly, *green*), and long-wavelength sensitive (L cone; formerly, *red*) cones, commonly referred to as the initiators of color vision. However, the integrative cells in the retina and higher visual centers are organized primarily to recognize *contrasts* between light or colors, and the receptive fields of color-sensitive cells typically have regions that compare the intensity of red versus green or blue versus yellow.

The classification and the testing of dysfunctional color vision are based upon this contrast-recognition physiology. Red-green color deficiency, which occurs commonly through X-linked inheritance in males (6%–8% incidence), has traditionally been separated into protan and deutan categories, which refer to absent or defective long-wavelength–sensitive pigment or medium-wavelength–sensitive pigment, respectively. These distinctions have some clinical value in terms of what patients perceive, even though individuals with normal color vision often have a duplication of pigment genes, and color-deficient individuals do not necessarily have single or simple gene defects. Blue-yellow color deficiency is rarely inherited and can be an important early marker for acquired diseases. Inherited color vision defects are described in Chapter 11.

Testing of color vision

The most accurate instrument for classifying congenital red-green color defects is the *anomaloscope*, but it is not widely used. The patient views a split screen and is asked to match the yellow appearance of one half by mixing varying proportions of red and green light in the other half. Individuals with red-green color deficiency use abnormal proportions of red and green to make the match.

The most common tests of color vision use colored tablets or diagrams. These color tests are accurate only if done under proper lighting, usually blue-white illumination that mimics sunlight. Pseudoisochromatic plates, such as the *Ishihara* plates (which assess color discrimination along protan [red] and deutan [green] axes only) and *Hardy-Rand-Rittler* plates (which assess color discrimination along protan, deutan, and tritan [blue] axes), depict colored numbers or figures that stand out from a background of colored dots (Fig 3-9). The colors of the test figure and background are purposely pale and carefully

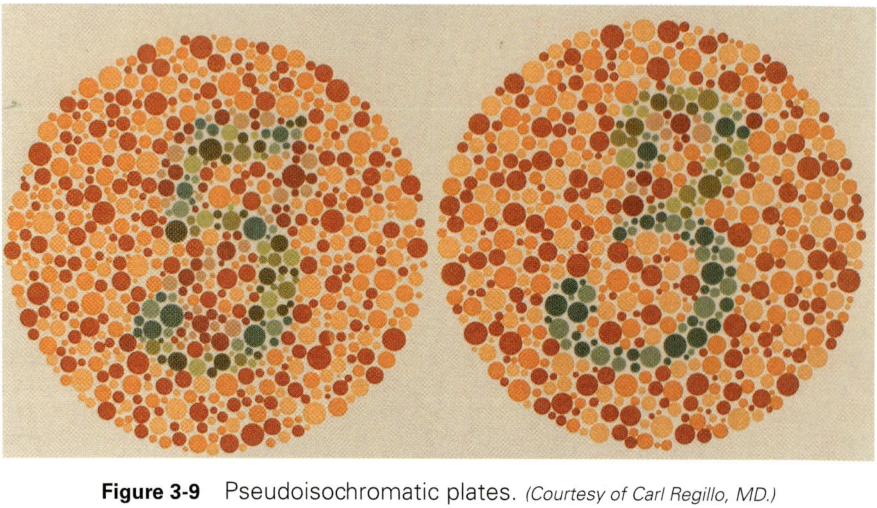

Figure 3-9 Pseudoisochromatic plates. *(Courtesy of Carl Regillo, MD.)*

chosen from hues that are difficult for a color-deficient person to distinguish. Individuals with defective color vision see either no pattern at all or an alternative pattern based on brightness rather than hue. The tests are quick to perform and sensitive for screening color vision, but they are not effective in classifying the deficiency.

The panel tests, including the Farnsworth-Munsell 100 and Farnsworth Panel D-15 hue tests, are more accurate in classifying color deficiency. The *Farnsworth-Munsell 100-hue test* is very sensitive because the difference in hues between adjacent tablets approximates the minimum that a normal observer is able to distinguish (1–4 nm). The spectrum is divided into 4 parts of 25 colored tablets each, and the patient is asked to discriminate between subtle shades of similar colors. However, the test is fatiguing and time-consuming.

The *Farnsworth Panel D-15 test* (Fig 3-10) is considerably quicker and more convenient for routine clinical use because it consists of only a single box of 15 colored tablets. The hues are more saturated, and they cover the spectrum so that patients will confuse colors for which they have deficient perception (such as red and green). The patient is asked to arrange the tablets in sequence, and errors can be plotted very quickly on a simple circular diagram to define the nature of the color deficiency. The D-15 test may miss mildly affected individuals, but its speed and accuracy make it useful. The relative insensitivity may also be an asset in judging the practical significance of mild degrees of color deficiency. For example, individuals who fail testing with the Ishihara plates but pass the D-15 test will probably not have color discrimination problems under most circumstances and in most jobs. Desaturated versions of the D-15 test, which recognize more subtle degrees of color deficiency, are also available. Enlarged versions (PV-16 tests) are also available for use in patients with reduced visual acuity.

The D-15 test is useful in the assessment of retinal diseases because it enables discrimination between congenital and acquired defects. Individuals with major congenital color deficiencies typically make errors that show a very precise protan or deutan pattern on the D-15 scoring graph, whereas those with acquired optic nerve or retinal disease show an irregular pattern of errors. The D-15 test shows tritan errors (blue-yellow confusion) very clearly; these results usually signify acquired disease. The S cones are fewer in number than the L and M cones and seem to be preferentially affected in many diseases. Although it is sometimes stated that optic nerve diseases usually cause red-green defects and retinal diseases blue-yellow defects, this distinction is not reliable.

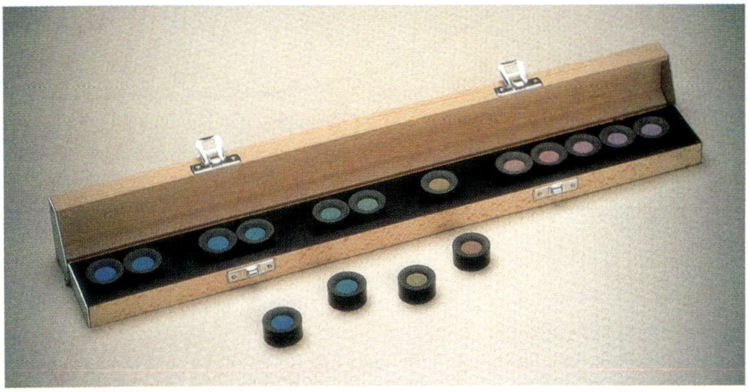

Figure 3-10 Panel D-15 test. *(Courtesy of Luneau Ophtalmologie.)*

The *Sloan achromatopsia test* is designed to test for complete achromatopsia. The test consists of 7 plates, each with a series of gray rectangles whose reflection increases gradually across the card. In the center of each rectangle appears a colored circle of fixed hue and reflectance. Patients with complete achromatopsia can find an exact match of the colored circle with one of the rectangles on each card. Observers who do not have complete achromatopsia can make only a brightness match of the colored circle to a rectangle.

Neitz M, Green DG, Neitz J. Visual acuity, color vision, and adaptation. In: Albert DM, Miller JW, Azar DT, Blodi BA, eds. *Albert & Jakobiec's Principles and Practice of Ophthalmology.* 3rd ed. Philadelphia: Saunders; 2008:chap 123.

Dark Adaptation

The sensitivity of the human eye extends over a range of 10–11 $\log_{10}$ units. Cones and rods adapt to different levels of background light through neural mechanisms and through the bleaching and regeneration of visual pigments. Clinical dark adaptometry measures primarily the absolute thresholds of cone and rod sensitivity.

Dark adaptation is most commonly tested with the *Goldmann-Weekers adaptometer.* The patient is first light-adapted to a bright background light. This light is then extinguished, and the patient, now in the dark, is presented with a series of dim-light targets approximately 11° below fixation. The intensity of the test lights is controlled by neutral-density filters, and the threshold at which the test light is first perceived is plotted against time. Under these conditions, the dark-adaptation curve, illustrated in Figure 3-11, shows

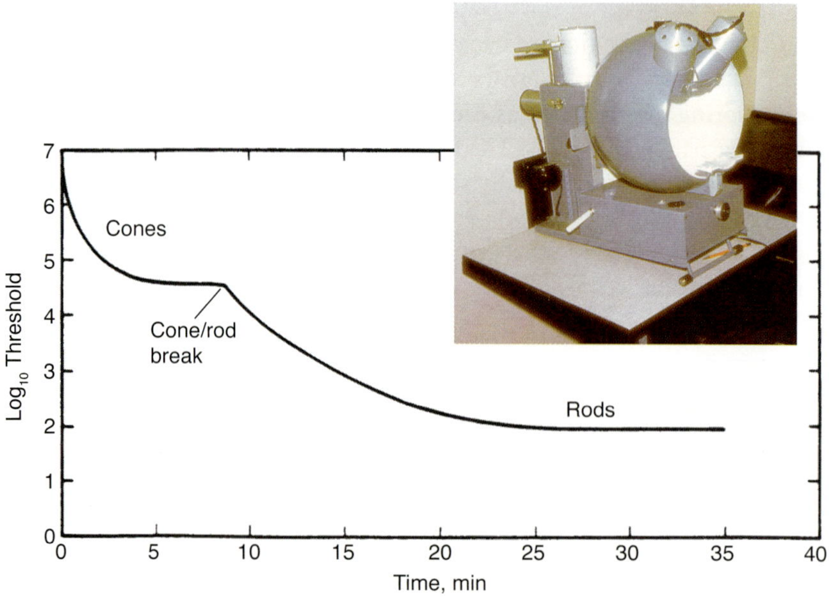

Figure 3-11 Dark-adaptation testing with the Goldmann-Weekers adaptometer *(inset)* yields a biphasic curve after preadaptation to bright light. *(Adapted with permission from Marmor MF. Clinical physiology of the retina. In: Peyman GA, Sanders DR, Goldberg MF, eds.* Principles and Practice of Ophthalmology. *Philadelphia: Saunders. 1980:823–856.)*

2 plateaus: the first represents the cone threshold, which is usually reached in 5–10 minutes, and the second represents the rod threshold, which is reached after approximately 30 minutes. If the clinical interest is limited to rod sensitivity in the dark, the test can be shortened by eliminating the first step of adaptation to bright light and recording only an endpoint rod threshold.

Dark adaptometry is useful in evaluating night blindness. Although the test is subjective, poor cooperation or malingering is easily recognized. A record of dark adaptation is complementary to the ERG because adaptometry is a *focal test* (a point to remember in interpreting results from patients with patchy, as opposed to diffuse, retinal disease), and thus it may in some instances be a more sensitive indicator of pathologic conditions than the ERG. Dark adaptometry can also demonstrate the degree of cone adaptation in the evaluation of cone dysfunction syndromes.

Photostress Recovery Time

The simple test of photostress recovery time aims to assist in the differentiation between optic nerve dysfunction and macular dysfunction, such as occurs from age-related macular degeneration or secondary to macular edema. The macula is exposed to bright light for 10 seconds via an ophthalmoscope, and the time taken for Snellen visual acuity to return to within 1 line of prebleach levels is noted. A normal subject will take 1 minute or less. Patients with macular dysfunction may take 2–3 minutes, whereas patients with optic nerve disease will have times similar to normal control values. Recovery time increases with age, and age-related normative data are used.

PART II

Disorders of the Retina and Vitreous

CHAPTER 4

Age-Related Macular Degeneration and Other Causes of Choroidal Neovascularization

This chapter reviews age-related macular degeneration and other conditions commonly associated with choroidal neovascularization.

Age-Related Macular Degeneration

Age-related macular degeneration (AMD) is the leading cause of blindness in the developed world in people over 50 years of age. It is estimated that among North Americans, 15 million (85%–90% of all AMD patients) currently have "dry" (nonneovascular, or nonexudative) AMD and 1.7 million people (10%–15% of all AMD patients) have "wet" (neovascular) AMD. An estimated 200,000 new cases of neovascular AMD develop each year in North America.

Normal aging results in a spectrum of changes in the macula, many clinically undetected, that affect the outer retina, retinal pigment epithelium (RPE), Bruch membrane, and choriocapillaris:

- Photoreceptors are reduced in density and distribution.
- Ultrastructural changes in the pigment epithelium include loss of melanin granules, formation of lipofuscin granules, and accumulation of residual bodies.
- Basal laminar/linear deposits accumulate; these deposits consist of granular, lipid-rich material and widely spaced collagen fibers collecting between the plasma membrane of the RPE cell and the inner collagenous layer of the Bruch membrane on either side of the basement membrane of the RPE (Fig 4-1; discussed later in the chapter).
- Progressive involutional changes occur in the choriocapillaris.

All of these changes represent aging and may not be part of AMD. Abnormalities associated with AMD that are not necessarily part of normal aging may be classified as nonneovascular or neovascular.

Population-based studies have demonstrated that of the risk factors for AMD, age is the first and foremost; in resource-rich countries, 10% of people over the age of 65 years

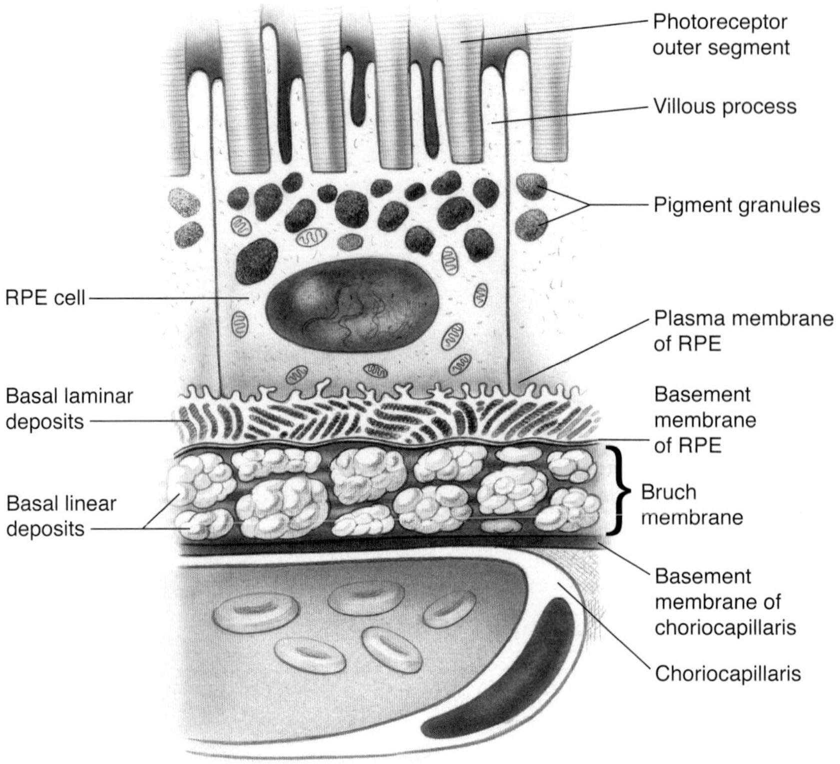

Figure 4-1 Schematic illustration of basal laminar deposits and basal linear deposits that result in a thickened inner collagenous layer of the Bruch membrane. RPE = retinal pigment epithelium. *(Illustration by Christine Gralapp.)*

and 25% over the age of 75 years have AMD. Additional risk factors include female sex, hypertension, hypercholesterolemia, cardiovascular disease, positive family history, cigarette smoking, hyperopia, and light iris color. Racial origin is another important risk factor. The 10-year longitudinal Multi-Ethnic Study of Atherosclerosis (MESA) found a prevalence of AMD highest in whites (5.4%) and lowest in African Americans (2.4%); prevalence was intermediate in Hispanics (4.2%) and Asians (4.6%).

Genetics and AMD

The etiology of AMD remains poorly understood. Development of the disorder involves interplay between genetic predisposition and other risk factors. A meta-analysis of multiple genome-wide association studies (GWAS) identified 19 genes with mutations that are associated with AMD. These genes harbor mutations that affect various biochemical pathways, including the complement cascade, lipid transport and metabolism (eg, *APOE*), modulation of the extracellular collagen matrix (eg, *COL8A1, COL10A1, TIMP3*), clearance of all-*trans*-retinaldehyde from photoreceptors *(ABCA4),* and angiogenesis (eg,

VEGFA). The alternate complement pathway includes the highest number of known AMD risk alleles, including *CFH, CFI, C2/CFB, C3,* and *C7.*

The 2 major susceptibility genes for AMD are *CFH* (1q31), which codes for complement factor H, and *ARMS2* (10q26), for which the gene product and function are poorly understood. The *CFH* Y402H mutation confers a 4.6-fold increased risk for AMD when heterozygous and a 7.4-fold increased risk when homozygous. The *ARMS2* A69S mutation confers a 2.7-fold increased risk for AMD when heterozygous and an 8.2-fold increased risk when homozygous. When both of these genes are homozygous for the aforementioned mutations in an individual, the risk for AMD is increased to 50-fold.

Genetic testing is available for AMD and usually includes testing for many of the known risk alleles. However, the interpretation and usefulness of the results remain controversial. The risk models used either are poorly validated or add little to the risk that can already be estimated from clinical findings and assessment of the patient's risk factors (eg, smoking history, family history). Pharmacogenomic testing is also possible; it aims to predict the optimal pharmacologic or nutritional-supplement interventions for a given patient. At this time, evidence to support this approach is only beginning to emerge, and validation studies are lacking. However, this is a fast-moving area of research, and progression to useful testing is likely.

Ratnapriya R, Chew EY. Age-related macular degeneration—clinical review and genetics update. *Clin Genet.* 2013:84(2):160–166.

Nonneovascular AMD

The prototypical lesion of the nonneovascular form of AMD is the druse. Other indicators are abnormalities of the RPE, including hyperpigmentation and atrophy.

Drusen

Clinically, drusen are small, round, yellow lesions located at the level of the RPE, mostly in the postequatorial retina (Fig 4-2). Histologically, this material corresponds to the abnormal thickening of the inner aspect of the Bruch membrane shown in Figure 4-1. Ultrastructurally, basal *laminar* deposits (granular, lipid-rich material and widely spaced collagen fibers between the plasma membrane and basement membrane of the RPE cell) and basal *linear* deposits (phospholipid vesicles and electron-dense granules within the inner collagenous zone of the Bruch membrane) are present (see Fig 4-1).

The thickened inner aspect of the Bruch membrane, along with the RPE, may separate from the rest of the Bruch membrane, resulting in a pigment epithelial detachment (PED). When small, such a detachment may be identified as a large or soft druse, and when larger, it may be recognized as a drusenoid PED.

Because drusen variably affect the overlying photoreceptors, there can be associated mild to moderate vision loss, decreased contrast sensitivity and color vision, and impairment of dark adaptation. Increasing size, number, and confluence of the drusen confer increasing risk of progression to choroidal neovascularization (CNV) or geographic atrophy (GA), referred to as stage 4 or the advanced stage of AMD by the Age-Related Eye Disease

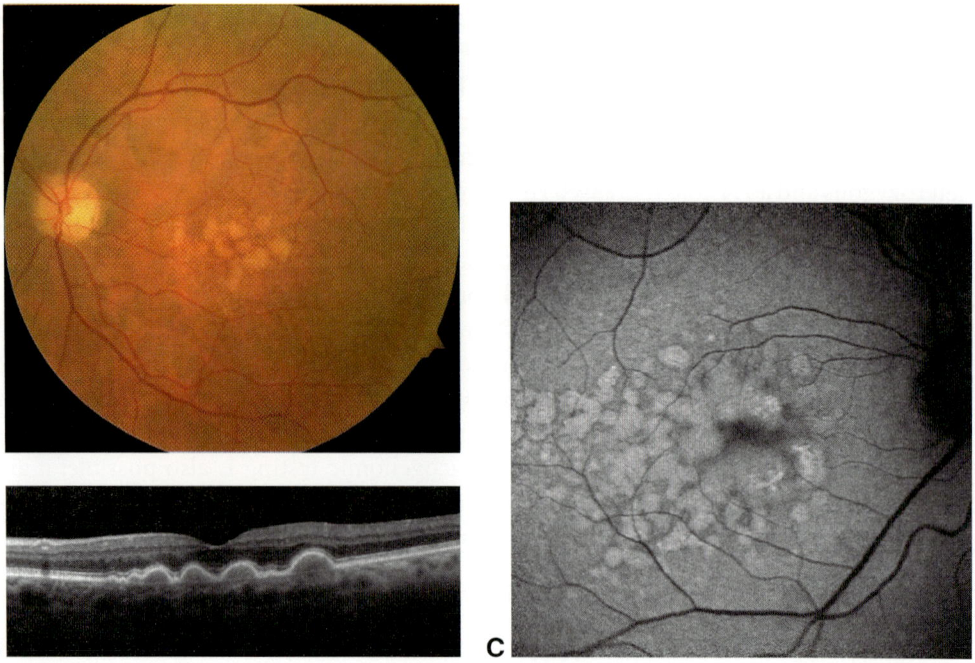

Figure 4-2 **A,** Color fundus photograph showing soft, confluent, large drusen in a patient with nonneovascular (dry) age-related macular degeneration (AMD). **B,** Corresponding spectral-domain optical coherence tomography (SD-OCT) image of the soft drusen. **C,** Autofluorescence image of an eye with areas of confluent drusen. *(Courtesy of David Sarraf, MD.)*

Study (AREDS). Drusen have been categorized as small (usually <64 μm diameter), intermediate (usually 63–124 μm), or large (usually ≥125 μm). *Drusenoid PEDs* are confluent large drusen that coalesce into a PED (>350 μm diameter). In AREDS, the risk of progression to stage 4 AMD over a 5-year period for patients with early AMD (many small drusen or few intermediate drusen, stage 2) was 1.3%. By contrast, the risk in patients with many intermediate drusen or even a single large druse (stage 3) was 18%.

In addition, the boundaries of drusen have been described as hard (discrete and well demarcated), soft (amorphous and poorly demarcated; see Fig 4-2A, B), or confluent (contiguous drusen without clear boundaries; see Fig 4-2C). Hard drusen are well-defined focal areas of lipidization or hyalinization of the RPE–Bruch membrane complex. Soft drusen are associated with the presence of diffuse thickening of the inner aspects of the Bruch membrane, that is, basal linear deposits. An eye with soft, and perhaps confluent, drusen is more likely to progress to atrophy or CNV than an eye with only hard drusen.

An additional type of drusen deposition is referred to as *reticular pseudodrusen,* also known as *subretinal drusenoid deposits,* because of the reticular-like network appreciated on fundus autofluorescence (Fig 4-3). These lesions are smaller than soft drusen and distribute typically in the superior macular region; they have been associated with progressive atrophy of the photoreceptor layer, GA, and a greater risk of CNV.

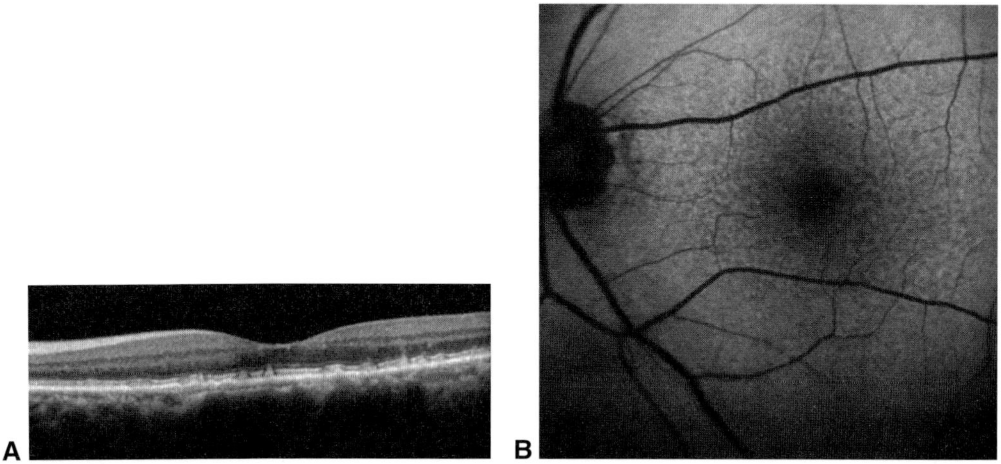

Figure 4-3 **A,** SD-OCT image demonstrating the location of reticular drusen above the RPE. **B,** Corresponding autofluorescence image showing the reticular network of these drusen. *(Courtesy of David Sarraf, MD.)*

Drusen occurring in patients younger than 50 years of age are referred to as *familial* or *early-onset* drusen and include 3 entities: large colloid drusen, malattia leventinese, and cuticular drusen. For more detail, see the section Early-Onset Drusen in Chapter 12.

Fluorescein angiography of drusen Typically, small hard drusen hyperfluoresce early in fluorescein angiography (FA) studies because of a window defect, whereas larger soft and confluent drusen and drusenoid PEDs slowly and homogenously stain late because of pooling of the fluorescein dye in the sub-PED compartment. However, there is some variability in how drusen appear on FA.

Optical coherence tomography of drusen Spectral-domain optical coherence tomography (SD-OCT) imaging of small and large drusen typically reveals sub-RPE nodular elevations or even small RPE detachments with a notable absence of intraretinal and subretinal fluid (see Fig 4-2). Reticular pseudodrusen are identified above the RPE and beneath the inner segment ellipsoid layer and are graded according to their degree of elevation (see Fig 4-3).

Enhanced depth imaging (EDI) of the choroid using OCT has permitted more detailed analysis of the choroid in AMD. Choroidal thickness values are typically normal or reduced in nonneovascular AMD.

Abnormalities of the RPE

Several patterns of RPE abnormalities characterize nonneovascular AMD, including focal hyperpigmentation, nongeographic atrophy, and geographic atrophy. Increased pigmentation at the level of the outer retina corresponds to focal hyperpigmentation of the RPE. On FA, these areas typically show blockage, and on SD-OCT, show hyperreflective outer retinal foci. The incidence of focal hyperpigmentations increases with age, and their presence indicates greater risk of progression to the more advanced forms of AMD.

Nongeographic atrophy refers to atrophy that does not cover a contiguous area and may appear as an area of mottling or depigmentation. When the area of absent or attenuated RPE is contiguous, the condition is termed *geographic atrophy* of the RPE. In areas of GA, the unmasked choroidal vessels are more readily visible, the overlying outer retina may appear thin, and the choriocapillaris is attenuated or atrophied. On FA, GA shows well-circumscribed round to oval window defects, whereas on SD-OCT, loss of the RPE and the overlying inner segment ellipsoid and photoreceptor layer can be seen. Dense hypoautofluorescence occurs in areas of GA. Fundus autofluorescence is a practical and noninvasive tool to monitor progression of GA (Fig 4-4).

Geographic atrophy often spares the fovea until late in the course of the disease. It may first present as one or more noncontiguous patches of atrophy around the fovea. These patches enlarge and coalesce and may be associated with a dense paracentral scotoma,

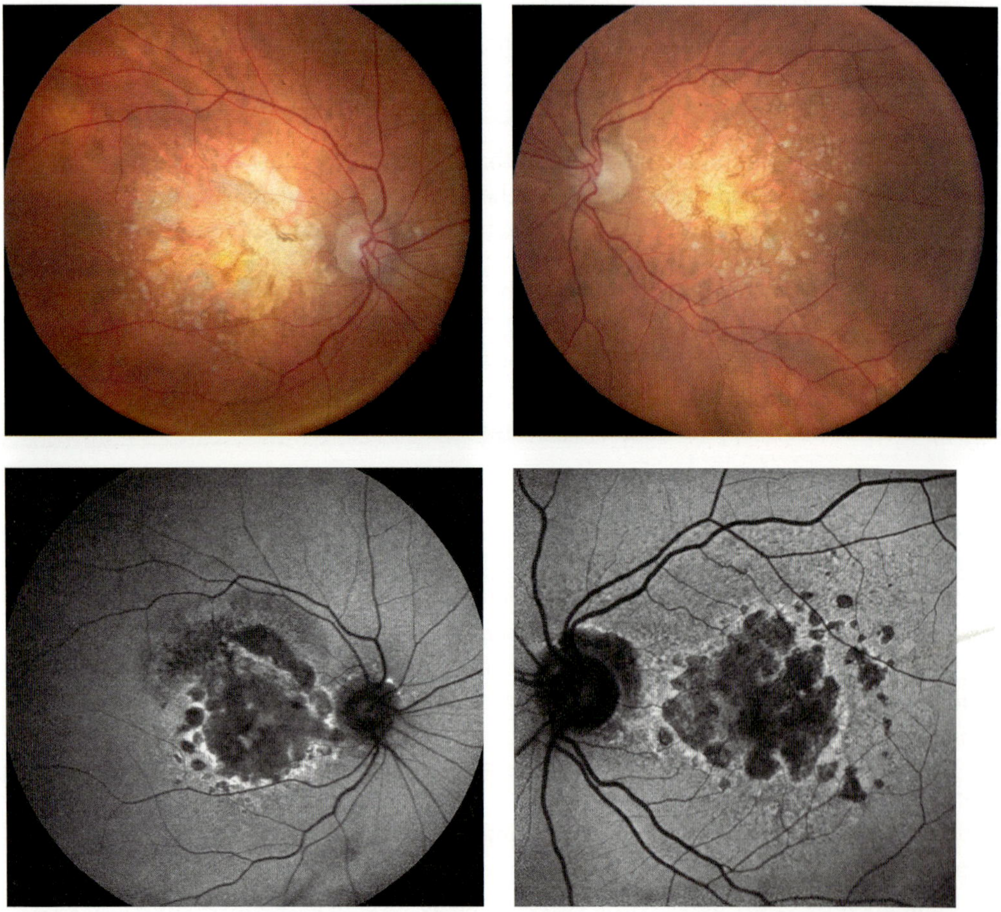

Figure 4-4 *Top,* Color fundus photographs of right *(left panel)* and left *(right panel)* eyes, demonstrating advanced geographic atrophy (GA). *Bottom,* corresponding autofluorescent images of GA in the same patient with atrophic AMD. *(Courtesy of David Sarraf, MD.)*

thereby limiting tasks such as reading. Patients with GA may demonstrate good visual acuity (VA) until late in the course of the disease, when the fovea becomes progressively atrophic, leading to severe visual acuity decline from central blindness and forcing the patient to use noncentral retina and eccentric fixation to read and perform other visual tasks.

Although not all eyes with drusen or PED will develop atrophy, the incidence of atrophy appears to increase with age. Twelve to 20% of patients with GA have severe vision loss, and 10% of patients with AMD and a visual acuity of 20/200 or less have GA.

Other abnormalities Chronic nonneovascular AMD can lead to regressed, drusen-associated, progressive RPE atrophy and GA. Dystrophic lipidization and calcification (refractile drusen) may occur, resulting in the development of refractile or crystalline lesions in the macula. Furthermore, pigment or pigment-laden cells (either RPE cells or macrophages that have ingested the pigment) may migrate to the photoreceptor level, resulting in focal clumps or a reticulated pattern of hyperpigmentation.

Differential diagnosis of nonneovascular AMD

A variety of disorders that include RPE abnormalities can be confused with nonneovascular AMD. Central serous chorioretinopathy (CSC; discussed in Chapter 9) may cause RPE changes similar to those in AMD. In patients with CSC, EDI-OCT shows a thickened choroid in the affected and fellow eyes, in contrast to the findings in AMD. Pattern dystrophy of the RPE may include one or more areas of reticular or butterfly-shaped hyperpigmentation, and it may present symmetrically in the macula of each eye. Alternatively, yellow subretinal material (ie, adult-onset vitelliform maculopathy) may be noted underneath the outer retina and best appreciated on SD-OCT as a hyperreflective, dome-shaped central lesion (Fig 4-5). FA shows early blocked fluorescence with a surrounding zone of hyperfluorescence. Late staining of the vitelliform material may occur and may help distinguish these cases from AMD. These features may occur in younger individuals

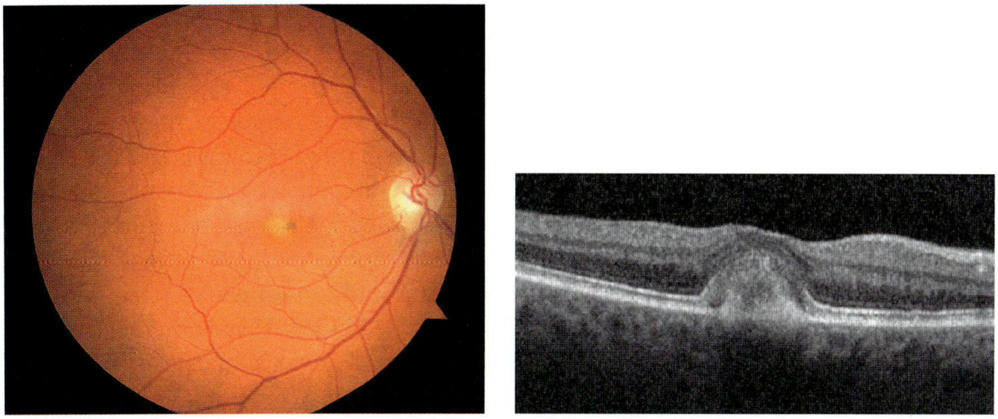

Figure 4-5 Color fundus photograph *(left)* and corresponding SD-OCT image *(right)* of adult-onset vitelliform macular dystrophy. *(Courtesy of David Sarraf, MD.)*

(less than 50 years of age). On the other hand, these changes may be present in older individuals who have the more typical drusen and abnormalities of the RPE associated with AMD.

The retinal signs of *drug toxicity,* such as bull's-eye macular atrophy caused by hydroxychloroquine toxicity, may resemble nongeographic or geographic atrophy of AMD, and central RPE mottling associated with deferoxamine toxicity may resemble nonneovascular AMD. A history of specific drug ingestion and lack of large drusen may help differentiate these abnormalities from AMD (see Chapter 14).

Management of nonneovascular AMD

Education and follow-up Eyes with soft drusen and RPE hyperpigmentation are at increased risk of developing GA and CNV. As such, patients with nonneovascular AMD should be educated about the symptoms of advanced AMD and instructed to contact an ophthalmologist promptly should these symptoms occur; ophthalmology office staff should respond to these reports without delay. If reduced visual acuity or reduced vision function (difficulty reading despite good measured visual acuity) is noted, a low vision evaluation should be considered. Periodic examinations are advised to monitor for concurrent, treatable eye disease (eg, cataract, glaucoma) and to reevaluate low vision needs. To assist patients whose visual function could be aided or enhanced by vision rehabilitation, refer to resources listed at the American Academy of Ophthalmology SmartSight website (http://one.aao.org/smart-sight-low-vision).

Amsler grid The Amsler grid is a test card for patient home-monitoring use; it contains white grid lines on a black background and a central dot for fixation. Each eye is tested *individually* with reading glasses and at reading distance to check for any new metamorphopsia, scotoma, or other significant changes in central vision. Any changes noted by the patient should be evaluated urgently.

Micronutrients Ophthalmologists should counsel patients about various epidemiologic studies that have demonstrated positive associations between the intake of certain micronutrients and a decreased risk of AMD, although only some micronutrients have been studied.

AREDS first established the benefit of vitamin and zinc supplementation in reducing the risk of vision loss in nonexudative AMD. In the study, supplementation with the antioxidant vitamins C (500 mg) and E (400 IU), beta carotene (15 mg), and the micronutrient zinc (80 mg zinc oxide and 2 mg cupric oxide to prevent zinc-induced anemia) in patients with intermediate or advanced AMD showed a 25% risk reduction for progression to more-advanced stages of AMD and a 19% risk reduction in rates of moderate vision loss (≥3 lines of visual acuity) at 5 years. In the study, intermediate (stage 3) AMD was defined as the presence of at least 1 large druse (≥125 μm), 10 or more intermediate drusen (63–124 μm diameter), or nonsubfoveal GA; and advanced (stage 4) AMD was defined as vision loss due to neovascular AMD or GA in only 1 eye. At 10 years, 44% of placebo recipients compared with 34% of the supplement recipients had advanced AMD (a 27% risk reduction). Among participants with no AMD or only early AMD (a few small drusen), there was no measurable benefit. There was no increased mortality among patients taking the AREDS formula.

A simplified 4-point grading scale was developed by AREDS for classifying the severity of AMD and predicting the disease course based on the following findings:

- presence of 1 or more large (>125-μm diameter) drusen (1 point)
- presence of any pigment abnormalities (1 point)
- for patients with no large drusen, presence of bilateral intermediate (63–124 μm) drusen (1 point)
- presence of neovascular AMD (2 points)

Risk factors were summed across both eyes to reach a number between 0 and 4 that could be used to estimate the 5- and 10-year risk of developing advanced AMD in 1 eye (Table 4-1).

Large population-based studies suggest that supplementation with the xanthophylls lutein and zeaxanthin as well as omega-3 long-chain polyunsaturated fatty acids (LCPUFAs: docosahexaenoic acid [DHA] and eicosapentaenoic acid [EPA]) may also help reduce AMD progression. The AREDS2 study was designed to test whether these observations could be confirmed in a prospective trial. Among the 4000 participants, the study confirmed the overall risk reduction found in the original AREDS study, concluded that lutein and zeaxanthin had similar effects to beta carotene, and found 80 mg of zinc to be the appropriate dose for AMD prophylaxis. Furthermore, LCPUFAs were not found to decrease the rate of progression to advanced AMD. A nonocular effect detected was an increased rate of lung cancer among current and former smokers using beta carotene, a finding other nonophthalmic studies had previously reported. As a result, the study's final recommendations for AREDS supplementation were to replace beta carotene with lutein and zeaxanthin and not to add LCPUFAs (Table 4-2). Currently, all patients with stage 3 or 4 AMD are advised to take the AREDS2 supplement.

Table 4-1 Five- and 10-Year Risks* of Advanced AMD in One Eye

Number of Risk Factor Points	5-Year Risk, %	10-Year Risk, %
0	0.5	1
1	3	7
2	12	22
3	25	50
4	50	67

AMD = age-related macular degeneration.
*Risks are based on the number of Age-Related Eye Disease Study (AREDS) risk factors (see text).

Table 4-2 AREDS2 Recommendations for Nutritional Supplementation*

Nutrient	Daily Dose
Vitamin C	500 mg
Vitamin E	400 IU
Lutein	10 mg
Zeaxanthin	2 mg
Zinc	80 mg

AREDS2 = Age-Related Eye Disease Study 2.
*Recommendations for nutritional supplementation are based on the AREDS 2 study (see text).

Age-Related Eye Disease Study 2 Research Group. Lutein + zeaxanthin and omega-3 fatty acids for age-related macular degeneration: the Age-Related Eye Disease Study 2 (AREDS2) randomized clinical trial. *JAMA.* 2013;309(19):2005–2015.
Ferris FL, Davis MD, Clemons TE, et al; Age-Related Eye Disease Study (AREDS) Research Group. A simplified severity scale for age-related macular degeneration: AREDS report no. 18. *Arch Ophthalmol.* 2005;123(11):1570–1574.

Lifestyle changes With increasing evidence that environment and health habits influence the development and progression of AMD, patients should be counseled to alter behaviors that put them at risk. Of particular importance are smoking cessation, obesity reduction, and blood pressure control. Cataract surgery has not been linked consistently to the progression of AMD, nor is there strong evidence linking UV (UV-A or UV-B) light exposure to the progression of AMD. It should be noted, however, that there are no negative effects of wearing UV-protective glasses.

Experimental treatments for nonneovascular AMD

Recent interest has been generated over phase II studies of lampalizumab (also known as *anti-factor D*), which selectively inhibits activation of the alternative complement pathway and may hold promise as a therapy to reduce the rate of progression of GA. Studies are also evaluating various regenerative medicine strategies, including whether adult RPE cells or embryonic-derived RPE stem cells can be transplanted to treat GA.

Disproven treatment approaches for nonneovascular AMD

Macular laser photocoagulation has been shown to cause drusen resolution or reduction, but there is no associated change in the natural course of vision loss or CNV development. Rheopheresis has not been demonstrated to have a role in treatment of nonneovascular AMD.

Neovascular AMD

The hallmark of the neovascular form of AMD is the presence of CNV. Degenerative changes in the Bruch membrane—such as the accumulation of drusen and the progressive thickening of the membrane's inner aspect that characterize the nonneovascular form of AMD—can be associated with a proangiogenic environment, including neovascularization that originates from the choriocapillaris and perforates the outer aspect of the Bruch membrane. These new vessels are accompanied by fibroblasts, resulting in a fibrovascular complex that can leak and bleed and may disrupt and destroy the normal architecture of the RPE–photoreceptor complex, ultimately leading to the formation of a hypertrophic fibrotic disciform scar.

Signs and symptoms of neovascular AMD

Patients with neovascular AMD describe the sudden onset of decreased vision, metamorphopsia, and/or paracentral scotomata. Amsler grid self-testing by patients is highly effective for early detection of neovascular AMD. Clinical signs of CNV may include subretinal or intraretinal fluid, exudate and/or blood, a pigment ring or gray-green membrane, irregular elevation of the RPE or a PED, an RPE tear, and/or a sea fan pattern of subretinal vessels.

Intraretinal blood and cystoid macular edema (CME) may indicate the presence of type 3 neovascularization, which originates from the deep capillary plexus of the retinal circulation.

Anatomical classification of CNV

Three types of CNV are now recognized. In type 1 neovascularization, new vessels originating from the choriocapillaris grow through a defect in the Bruch membrane into the sub–pigment epithelial space (Fig 4-6). Leakage and bleeding can lead to the development of a vascularized serous or fibrovascular PED. The fibrovascular PEDs are often seen to have an irregular surface contour. In type 2 neovascularization, the CNV occupies the subneurosensory compartment between the RPE and the outer segments of the retina. On examination, the membrane will appear as a lacy or gray-green lesion; in AMD, this finding is less common than is type 1 neovascularization. Type 3 neovascularization results from new blood vessels sprouting from the deep capillary plexus of the retina and growing downward toward the RPE. Because of their intraretinal growth, these lesions were originally termed *retinal angiomatous proliferations* (RAP). On examination, they appear as a small area of red discoloration, often associated with retinal exudate.

Ultimately, if untreated, these neovascular processes may evolve into a hypertrophic, fibrotic, disciform scar. The retina overlying the scar loses its normal outer retinal architecture, which can lead to severe, permanent central vision loss.

Fluorescein angiographic patterns of CNV FA patterns of CNV may include classic or occult CNV or combinations of both. Classic CNV is an area of bright, lacy, and well-defined hyperfluorescence that is identified in the early phase and progressively leaks by the late phases (Fig 4-7). Occult CNV consists of 2 forms: (1) PED, either fibrovascular PED or

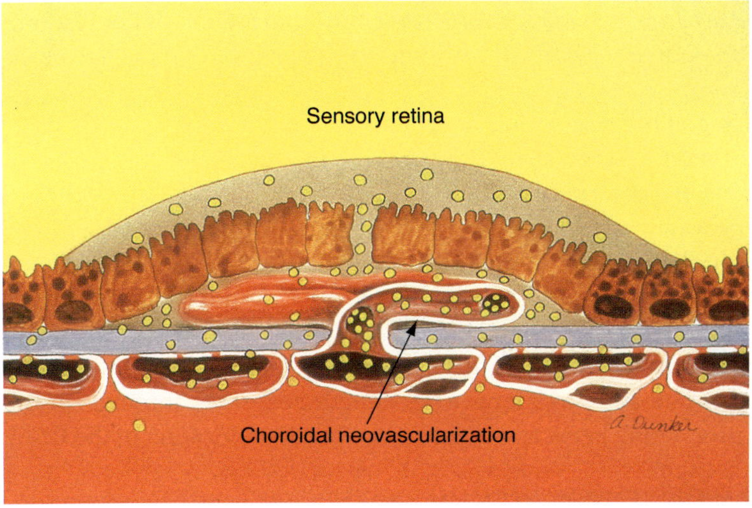

Figure 4-6 Schematic drawing of type 1 choroidal neovascularization (CNV) originating from the choriocapillaris, breaking through the Bruch membrane, and proliferating in the sub–pigment epithelial space. *(Used with permission from Bressler NM, Bressler SB, Fine SL. Age-related macular degeneration.* Surv Ophthalmol. *1988;32(6):375–413.)*

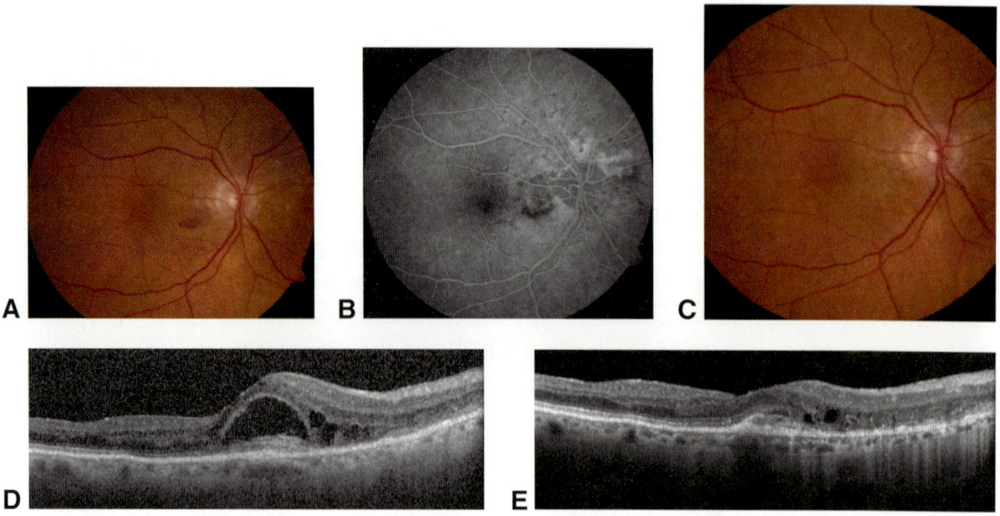

Figure 4-7 Color fundus photograph **(A)** and fluorescein angiography (FA) image **(B)** of classic extrafoveal CNV. **C,** Color fundus photograph showing regression of CNV and resolution of hemorrhage after intravitreal bevacizumab therapy. SD-OCT images before **(D)** and after **(E)** bevacizumab therapy for type 2 neovascularization. Note resolution of subretinal fluid and contraction of type 2 neovascular membrane. *(Courtesy of David Sarraf, MD.)*

vascularized serous PED, and (2) late leakage from an undetermined source. See Chapter 2, Fig 2-5.

Fibrovascular PED refers to an irregular elevation of the RPE with progressive, stippled leakage on FA. Alternatively, the PED may pool dye rapidly in a homogenous ground-glass pattern that is consistent with a serous PED but has a notch, or hot spot, indicating vascular tissue in the PED—a vascularized serous PED (Fig 4-8).

Late leakage from an undetermined source refers to regions of fluorescence at the level of the flat RPE that are ill defined early and best appreciated in the late phases of the angiographic study.

The angiographic description of occult CNV may be anatomically related to type 1 neovascularization, whereas that of classic CNV may be related to type 2 neovascularization; this relation is not a hard-and-fast rule, however.

Type 3 neovascularization, or RAP, may be signaled by the presence of a spot of retinal hemorrhage in the macula. FA and indocyanine green (ICG) angiography may demonstrate a focal hot spot and late CME; associated pooling into a PED may also be present.

The presence of thick blood, pigment, scar tissue, or a PED may block fluorescence and obscure any underlying CNV. ICG angiography, which employs a dye that is almost fully protein bound and has a longer wavelength nearer the infrared spectrum, may be valuable in penetrating heme and pigment to allow identification of the CNV, which may appear as a hot spot.

SD-OCT patterns of CNV Type 1 neovascular membranes demonstrate elevation of the RPE and a PED on SD-OCT. A serous PED appears as a sharply elevated, dome-shaped lesion

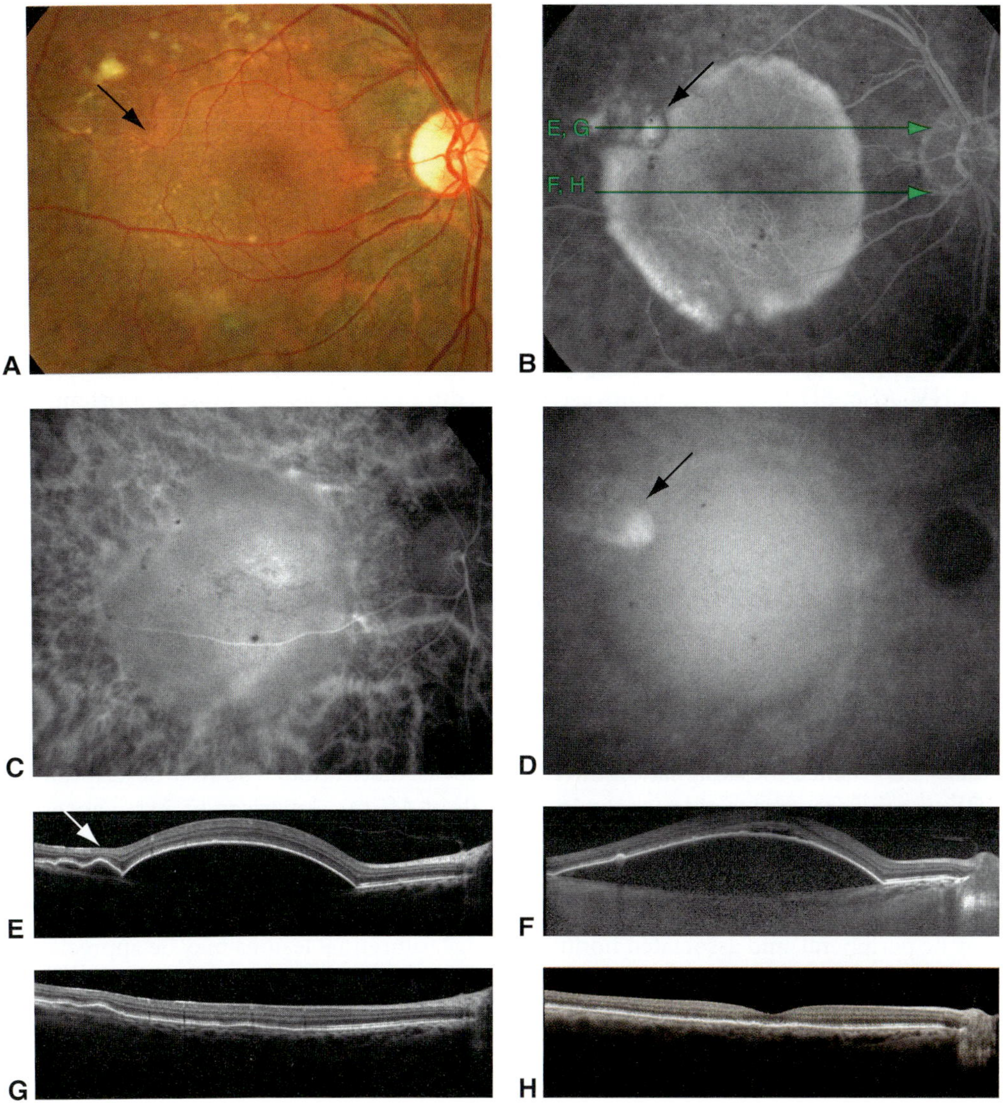

Figure 4-8 **A,** Color fundus photograph of a vascularized serous pigment epithelial detachment (PED) with a notch *(arrow)* that corresponds to a hot spot on FA (*black arrow* in **B**). *Green letters and arrows* in **B** indicate the SD-OCT scan locations for parts **E** through **H.** Indocyanine green (ICG) angiography images early **(C)** and late **(D)** showing pooling of the serous PED and hyperfluorescence of the hot spot (*arrow* in **D**). **E, F,** SD-OCT images of the large serous PED. Note the irregular portion of the PED (*arrow* in **E**), which corresponds to the hot spot and harbors the type 1 neovascular membrane. **G, H,** SD-OCT images showing that the PED has resolved after therapy with anti–vascular endothelial growth factor. *(Used with permission from Mrejen S, Sarraf D, Mukkamala SK, Freund KB. Multimodal imaging of pigment epithelial detachment: a guide to evaluation.* Retina. *2013;33(9):1735–1762.)*

with hollow internal reflectivity and typically no associated subretinal or intraretinal fluid. A fibrovascular PED may or may not be sharply elevated and typically demonstrates a lacy or polyplike hyperreflective lesion on the undersurface of the RPE, with or without signs of contraction. A chronic fibrovascular PED has a multilayered appearance, and a complex fibrovascular scar may be appreciated in the sub-PED compartment, with or without associated subretinal and/or intraretinal fluid.

Type 2 neovascular membranes appear as a hyperreflective band or plaque in the subneurosensory space, with associated subretinal and/or intraretinal fluid. Type 3 neovascular membranes are best appreciated with SD-OCT as a hyperreflective focus emanating from the deep capillary plexus of the retina, with or without associated CME and PED. Recognition of these SD-OCT patterns is crucial for the diagnosis and classification of CNV. Also, SD-OCT is a noninvasive procedure as well as the most important and practical modality for monitoring the response of therapy by assessing regression of the neovascular membrane and resolution of subretinal and intraretinal fluid.

Mrejen S, Sarraf D, Mukkamala SK, Freund KB. Multimodal imaging of pigment epithelial detachment: a guide to evaluation. *Retina.* 2013;33(9):1735–1762.

Polypoidal choroidal vasculopathy Polypoidal choroidal vasculopathy (PCV), initially described as *posterior uveal bleeding syndrome,* is a variant of choroidal neovascularization (type 1) and is characterized by multiple, recurrent serosanguineous RPE detachments. A network of polyps with associated feeder vessels, similar in appearance to a string of pearls, can be identified with SD-OCT adherent to the RPE monolayer of the fibrovascular PED—hence the designation of type 1 neovascularization. The first description of PCV was the occurrence of lesions in individuals of African American or Asian ancestry, typically hypertensive middle-aged women. It is now believed to occur in women and men of all races and to be a variant of neovascular AMD, with the same genetic profile. The areas of serosanguineous detachment are often peripapillary and multifocal but may be peripheral, and associated nodular, orange, subretinal lesions may be appreciated. Vitreous hemorrhage may occur more frequently than in classic AMD, and the typical soft drusen of AMD may or may not be present. The natural history and visual acuity outcomes of PCV may be better than those of CNV associated with AMD (Fig 4-9). ICG angiography and SD-OCT are important techniques for identifying the polyps.

Differential diagnosis of neovascular AMD

A variety of conditions can mimic the neovascular changes of AMD and typically include any disorder that is associated with disruption of the Bruch complex and secondary CNV.

The subretinal fluid of central serous chorioretinopathy can be confused with subretinal fluid or edema associated with CNV and AMD. However, patients with CSC are usually younger and usually do not have associated subretinal hemorrhage unless a secondary CNV has developed. CSC can be further differentiated by characteristic signs including patches of RPE mottling that may assume a geographic or gutterlike gravitational configuration on wide-field angiographic or autofluorescent imaging and a thick choroid best visualized with EDI-OCT.

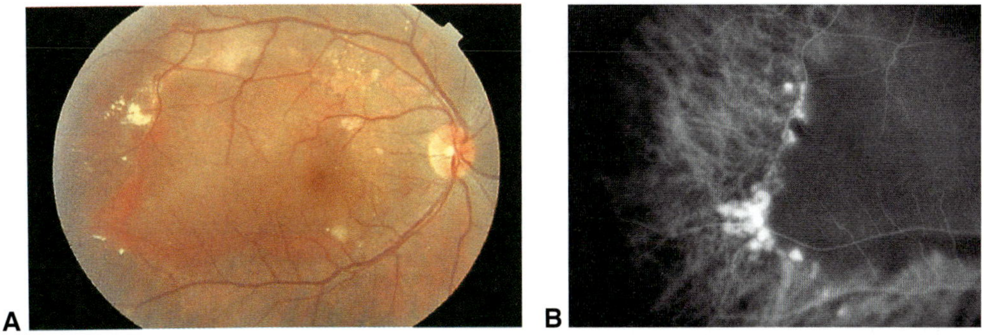

Figure 4-9 Polypoidal choroidal vasculopathy. **A,** Fundus photograph showing a large RPE detachment with multiple yellow-orange nodular lesions temporally. **B,** The ICG angiogram demonstrates the characteristic polypoidal lesions temporally. *(Courtesy of Lawrence A. Yannuzzi, MD.)*

Management of neovascular AMD

If neovascular AMD is suspected on clinical grounds, FA and OCT studies can be obtained. SD-OCT is the most efficient and reliable tool in diagnosing and distinguishing types 1, 2, and 3 neovascularization and in monitoring response to therapy.

Laser photocoagulation (thermal laser) From the 1980s through 2000, laser therapy was the primary treatment for classic extrafoveal CNV with well-defined boundaries. However, outcomes were poor because of high recurrence rates, as demonstrated in the Macular Photocoagulation Studies. The use of thermal laser treatment is now rare except to treat extrafoveal lesions that are sufficiently far from the foveal center to have minimal risk of iatrogenic foveal laser damage and a lower rate of recurrence.

Photodynamic therapy PDT was introduced in 2000 as a less-destructive modality for treating CNV than thermal laser and entails the systemic administration of a photosensitizing drug followed by an application of light of a particular wavelength to the affected tissue to incite a localized photochemical reaction. This reaction generates reactive oxygen species, leading to capillary endothelial cell damage and vessel thrombosis. Studies showed that PDT slowed progression but did not prevent significant vision loss in eyes with CNV that had certain lesion characteristics. Use of PDT in the management of exudative AMD is now rare except in recalcitrant cases or eyes with PCV.

Antiangiogenic therapies Angiogenesis—the formation of new blood vessels that occurs via sprouting or splitting from existing vessels—is characterized by a complex cascade of events. The first step in the cascade involves vasodilation of existing vessels and increased vascular permeability. This process is followed by degradation of the surrounding extracellular matrix, which facilitates migration and proliferation of endothelial cells. The endothelial cells join together to form a lumen, which becomes a new capillary. The vessels subsequently mature and undergo remodeling to form a stable vascular network. The successful execution of this cascade requires a balanced interplay of growth-promoting and growth-inhibiting angiogenic factors. Identified activators of angiogenesis include vascular endothelial growth factor (VEGF), fibroblast growth factor (FGF), transforming growth factor α (TGF-α) and TGF-β, angiopoietin-1, and angiopoietin-2. Inhibitors of angiogenesis include thrombospondin, angiostatin, endostatin, and pigment epithelium–derived factor (PEDF).

The majority of recent antiangiogenesis research has focused on the inhibition of VEGF. VEGF expression is increased in pigment epithelial cells during the early stages of AMD, suggesting that VEGF plays a causal role in the initiation of neovascularization. In addition, high concentrations of VEGF have been observed in excised CNV and vitreous samples from AMD patients. VEGF is a homodimeric glycoprotein that is a heparin-binding growth factor specific for vascular endothelial cells. It can induce angiogenesis, vascular permeability, and lymphangiogenesis and may act as a survival factor for endothelial cells by preventing apoptosis. There are at least 4 major VEGF isoforms, of which $VEGF_{165}$ is thought to be the most dominant in AMD.

Pegaptanib Pegaptanib, an RNA oligonucleotide ligand (or aptamer) that binds human $VEGF_{165}$ with high affinity and specificity, was the first intravitreal anti-VEGF therapy approved by the US Food and Drug Administration (FDA), in 2004. Studies showed that it slowed vision loss, but it has since been supplanted by far more effective agents.

Ranibizumab Ranibizumab is a recombinantly produced, humanized antibody fragment (Fab) that binds VEGF. Unlike pegaptanib, ranibizumab binds to and inhibits all active isoforms of VEGF-A and their active degradation products. Two studies, MARINA (Minimally Classic/Occult Trial of the Anti-VEGF Antibody Ranibizumab in the Treatment of Neovascular AMD) and ANCHOR (Anti-VEGF Antibody for the Treatment of Predominantly Classic Choroidal Neovascularization in AMD), demonstrated that, at 12 months, 95% of ranibizumab-treated patients experienced vision stabilization or improvement compared with 62% of sham-treated patients and 64% of patients treated with PDT, respectively. More important, approximately 30%–40% of ranibizumab-treated patients experienced vision improvement of 15 letters or more compared with control participants in each study, with an average letter gain of approximately 10 letters (Fig 4-10, Clinical Trials 4-1, 4-2). Almost 80% of patients maintained or improved vision after 24 months.

Similar to the MARINA and ANCHOR study results, the mean change in visual acuity from baseline in the PIER (Phase 3b, Multicenter, Randomized, Double-Masked, Sham Injection-Controlled Study of the Efficacy and Safety of Ranibizumab in Subjects With Subfoveal Choroidal Neovascularization With or Without Classic Choroidal Neovascularization Secondary to AMD) and EXCITE (Efficacy and Safety of Ranibizumab in Patients With Subfoveal Choroidal Neovascularization Secondary to AMD) studies improved over the first 3 months; however, the treatment effect declined in the ranibizumab recipients during quarterly dosing (ie, every 3 months) but not with monthly dosing intervals. These data clarified that quarterly treatment appears to be suboptimal. In general, there are 2 accepted treatment schemes that deviate from the FDA-approved labeling of monthly injections: "treat-and-observe," or "as-needed," and "treat-and-extend" approaches to anti-VEGF therapy. In the treat-and-observe method, regular treatment is administered until the macula is dry by clinical and OCT-determined criteria, followed by treatment only for signs of recurrent exudation during the maintenance phase. This approach is in contrast to the treat-and-extend regimen, in which regular monthly treatment is continued until

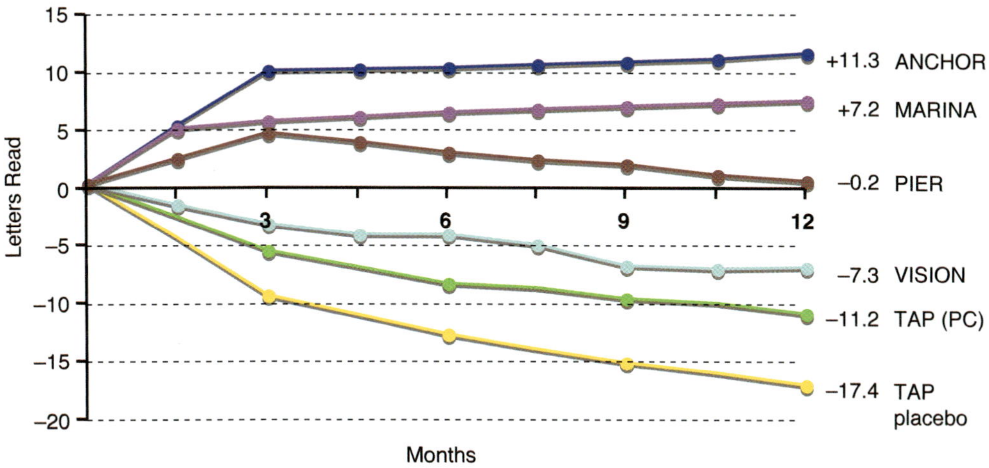

Figure 4-10 Graph illustrating the mean change in vision (number of letters read) from several phase 3 clinical trials. Comparison of data between different trials should be interpreted with caution because the potentially different study inclusion criteria and baseline characteristics of eyes for different studies may affect the stated visual acuity gains. ANCHOR = Anti-VEGF Antibody for the Treatment of Predominantly Classic Choroidal Neovascularization in AMD; MARINA = Minimally Classic/Occult Trial of the Anti-VEGF Antibody Ranibizumab in the Treatment of Neovascular AMD; PC = predominantly classic; PIER = Phase 3b, Multicenter, Randomized, Double-Masked, Sham Injection-Controlled Study of the Efficacy and Safety of Ranibizumab in Subjects With Subfoveal Choroidal Neovascularization With or Without Classic Choroidal Neovascularization Secondary to AMD; TAP = Treatment of AMD with Photodynamic Therapy; VISION = VEGF Inhibition Study in Ocular Neovascularization. *(Courtesy of Peter K. Kaiser, MD.)*

CLINICAL TRIAL 4-1

Minimally Classic/Occult Trial of the Anti-VEGF Antibody Ranibizumab in the Treatment of Neovascular AMD (MARINA)

Objective: To determine if monthly intravitreal ranibizumab injection can reduce the risk of vision loss in patients with subfoveal, minimally classic or occult with no classic CNV compared with placebo-controlled sham treatment.

Participants: Eyes with new or recurrent subfoveal CNV, minimally classic or occult with no classic CNV with evidence of recent disease progression defined as new subretinal hemorrhage, recent growth of CNV on FA, or recent visual acuity loss, CNV >50% of lesion, size ≤12 disc areas, no prior PDT, blood <50% of the lesion, and visual acuity of 20/40 to 20/320.

Outcome measures: Visual acuity loss of <15 letters at 1 year. Secondary outcomes included visual acuity loss of <30 letters, quality of life, and morphologic outcomes.

Results: 95% of study eyes experienced visual acuity improvement or stabilization vs 62% of control eyes. Close to 40% of study eyes had visual acuity improvement of >15 letters compared with control eyes.

Present status: See Clinical Trial 4-2.

CLINICAL TRIAL 4-2

Anti-VEGF Antibody for the Treatment of Predominantly Classic Choroidal Neovascularization in AMD (ANCHOR) Study

Objective: To determine if monthly intravitreal ranibizumab injection can reduce the risk of vision loss in patients with predominantly classic subfoveal CNV compared with photodynamic therapy with verteporfin treatment.

Participants: Eyes with new or recurrent subfoveal CNV, predominantly classic CNV, CNV >50% of lesion, size ≤9 disc areas, no prior PDT, blood <50% of the lesion, and visual acuity of 20/40 to 20/320.

Outcome measures: Visual acuity loss of <15 letters at 1 year. Secondary outcomes included visual acuity loss of <30 letters, contrast threshold function, quality of life, and morphologic outcomes.

Results: 95% of ranibizumab-treated eyes vs 64% of PDT-treated eyes maintained or improved vision (<15-letter loss in visual acuity) at 12 months. 90% of ranibizumab-treated patients lost <15 letters of visual acuity compared with 65.7% of PDT-treated eyes at 24 months. 40.3% of ranibizumab-treated eyes improved >3 lines after 24 months. Almost 80% of patients maintained or improved vision after 24 months.

Present status: Sixty-five AMD patients from the MARINA, ANCHOR, and HORIZON studies were evaluated approximately 7 years after baseline recruitment. Of these patients, 23% achieved a best-corrected visual acuity (BCVA) of 20/40 or better, while 37% had BCVA of 20/200 or worse, and almost one-half (43%) of eyes had an unchanged or improved letter score versus baseline. Active fluid was detected by SD-OCT in 68% of study eyes, and macular atrophy, the area of which correlated with vision loss, was detected by fundus autofluorescence in 98% of eyes.

Rofagha S, Bhisitkul RB, Boyer DS, Sadda SR, Zhang K; SEVEN-UP Study Group. Seven-year outcomes in ranibizumab-treated patients in ANCHOR, MARINA, and HORIZON: a multicenter cohort study (SEVEN-UP). *Ophthalmology.* 2013;120(11):2292–2299.

the macula is dry, after which treatment continues at gradually increasing intervals. In this second approach, injections are administered even with inactive CNV. The goal of this therapy is to cautiously extend the time between injections as far apart as tolerated as long as there are no signs of recurrence.

Several clinical trials have evaluated as-needed approaches to anti-VEGF therapy: PrONTO (Prospective Optical Coherence Tomography Imaging of Patients With Neovascular AMD Treated With Intraocular Ranibizumab), SAILOR (Study to Evaluate Ranibizumab in Subjects With Choroidal Neovascularization Secondary to AMD), SUSTAIN (Study of Ranibizumab in Patients with Subfoveal Choroidal Neovascularization Secondary to AMD), and HORIZON (Open-Label Extension Trial of Ranibizumab for Choroidal

Neovascularization Secondary to AMD). All of these studies utilized 3 monthly injections followed by various as-needed treatment regimens, determined on the basis of clinical and OCT-guided criteria, and all showed vision and OCT outcomes that were comparable to or reduced from those obtained with MARINA and ANCHOR. The HORIZON study was a continuation trial of patients enrolled in prior ranibizumab AMD trials. Eyes that had gained 10.2 letters on the ETDRS (Early Treatment Diabetic Retinopathy Study) eye chart during ANCHOR or MARINA after 2 years of monthly injections declined in visual acuity and ended with only a mean 2.0-letter gain compared with baseline (ie, they lost nearly 8 letters once the regimen was switched from monthly injections to an as-needed protocol). Experts believed that the major reason the HORIZON study showed such a decline in visual acuity was because of its protocol: unlike the other treatment-as-needed studies, HORIZON included no re-treatment guidelines for investigators, and patients received only a mean of 3.6 ranibizumab injections in the 12 months of the extension trial. HARBOR (A Study of Ranibizumab Administered Monthly or on an As-Needed Basis in Patients With Subfoveal Neovascular AMD) compared higher-dose (2.0 mg) with standard-dose (0.5 mg) ranibizumab therapy and failed to find any difference in visual acuity or anatomical outcomes between the 2 dosages.

Safety data have been favorable for intravitreal ranibizumab therapy. Intravitreal injections are occasionally associated with minor local complications such as subconjunctival hemorrhage and local irritation. However, the incidence of severe, visually compromising complications such as vitreous hemorrhage, retinal detachment, or endophthalmitis is exceedingly low across numerous trials including those just described. Systemic arteriothrombotic events can arise during the course of ranibizumab therapy, but no study has conclusively determined an increased incidence of these events related to injection of the drug.

Eyes with fibrovascular PEDs may be at increased risk for the development of an RPE tear after anti-VEGF therapy, and this risk may be especially significant with PEDs greater than 600 µm in height. The mechanism of the tear may relate to contraction of the type 1 neovascular membrane beneath the PED that occurs as a result of the anti-VEGF injection.

Aflibercept Aflibercept (also known as *VEGF Trap*) is a soluble protein that acts as a VEGF receptor decoy; it combines the ligand-binding elements of the extracellular domains of *VEGFR1* and *VEGFR2* fused to the constant region (Fc) of immunoglobulin G (IgG). Aflibercept binds both VEGF and placental-like growth factor and fully penetrates all retinal layers.

In the studies VIEW 1 and 2 (VEGF Trap-Eye: Investigation of Efficacy and Safety in Wet AMD 1 and 2), patients received aflibercept in monthly or every-second-month regimens, and a comparison group received monthly ranibizumab treatment. The primary endpoint of the studies, noninferiority compared with ranibizumab monthly treatment, was met by all aflibercept treatment regimens. Patients receiving monthly aflibercept, 2 mg, gained 10.9 letters on average, whereas those receiving monthly ranibizumab, 0.5 mg, had a mean 8.1-letter gain ($P < .01$). All other dose groups of aflibercept in the VIEW 1 study and all dose groups in the VIEW 2 study had results at this secondary endpoint of 52 weeks that were not statistically different from results for patients receiving ranibizumab, indicating that after 3 monthly doses, aflibercept could be administered every 2 months with similar efficacy to ranibizumab administered monthly.

At 96 weeks, mean letter increase was 7.6 letters in the 2-mg aflibercept group treated every 8 weeks and 7.9 letters in the monthly ranibizumab group; patients with 3-line increases comprised from 30% to 33% for each arm of the study. Anatomical response, as measured by a decrease in OCT-determined central retinal thickness, was maintained through 2 years and was not significantly different among the 4 groups. A favorable safety profile was observed for both aflibercept and ranibizumab therapy.

Bevacizumab Bevacizumab is a full-length monoclonal antibody against VEGF that was approved by the FDA in 2004 for the treatment of metastatic colorectal cancer. It has been described for "off-label" use via intravitreal and intravenous administration for the treatment of AMD. Both bevacizumab and ranibizumab are manufactured by the same pharmaceutical company, and there are important differences between the drugs: bevacizumab is larger and has 2 antigen-binding domains compared with the single domain for ranibizumab, and cost differences between them are substantial, potentially affecting access to treatment for some patients. Because fragment antibodies in general have shorter systemic half-lives than those of full-length antibodies (2.2 hours for ranibizumab vs ~21 days for bevacizumab), intravitreal injections of ranibizumab have a shorter systemic half-life than intravitreal injections of bevacizumab.

Because of the 50-fold lower cost and the purported similar efficacy of bevacizumab compared with ranibizumab, several comparative efficacy studies have been conducted. These studies include CATT (Comparison of Age-Related Macular Degeneration Treatments Trials) in the United States, IVAN (Randomised Controlled Trial of Alternative Treatments to Inhibit VEGF in Age-Related Choroidal Neovascularisation) in the United Kingdom, MANTA (Randomized Observer and Subject Masked Trial Comparing the Visual Outcome After Treatment With Ranibizumab or Bevacizumab in Patients With Neovascular Age-Related Macular Degeneration Multicenter Anti-VEGF Trial in Austria), and GEFAL (Groupe d'Evaluation Français Avastin vs Lucentis) in France.

CATT was the first and largest multicenter, randomized clinical trial to compare the relative safety and efficacy of ranibizumab with bevacizumab for the treatment of neovascular AMD. The trial was funded by the US National Eye Institute and studied 1208 patients. Results showed that bevacizumab was noninferior to ranibizumab therapy in monthly or as-needed delivery schedules over 2 years. Mean letters gained from baseline did not differ statistically among the 4 arms of the study: 8.8 letters in the ranibizumab-monthly group, 7.8 letters in the bevacizumab-monthly group, 6.7 letters in the ranibizumab as-needed group, and 5.0 letters in the bevacizumab as-needed group (see Clinical Trial 4-3 for 1-year results). Systemic adverse events were significantly greater in the bevacizumab (39.9%) than in the ranibizumab (31.7%) group, but death and arteriothrombotic events were not statistically different between the 2 drugs.

The IVAN trial included more than 500 patients in the United Kingdom, had a very similar design to that of CATT, and also found that visual and anatomical outcomes were

CLINICAL TRIAL 4-3

Comparison of Age-Related Macular Degeneration Treatment Trials (CATT) Study

Objective: To assess the relative efficacy and safety of ranibizumab and bevacizumab and to determine whether an as-needed regimen would compromise long-term visual acuity, as compared with a monthly regimen.

Participants: 1208 patients at 44 clinical centers in the United States. Eligibility criteria included age ≥50 years, presence in the study eye (1 eye per patient) of previously untreated active CNV due to AMD, and visual acuity between 20/25 and 20/320.

Outcome measures: Primary outcome: mean change in visual acuity at 1 year. Secondary outcomes included proportion of patients with ≥15 letters gained and SD-OCT anatomical outcomes such as the change in central macular thickness at 1 year.

Results: Bevacizumab administered monthly was equivalent to ranibizumab administered monthly, with 8.0 and 8.5 letters gained, respectively. Bevacizumab administered as needed was equivalent to ranibizumab as needed, with 5.9 and 6.8 letters gained, respectively. The proportion of patients who gained ≥15 letters did not differ significantly among the groups, ranging from 24.9% in the group that received ranibizumab as needed to 34.2% in the group that received ranibizumab monthly ($P = .09$). The mean decrease in central retinal thickness was greater in the ranibizumab-monthly group (196 μm) than in the other groups (152–168 μm, $P = .03$).

Conclusions: At 1 year, bevacizumab and ranibizumab had equivalent effects on visual acuity when administered according to the same schedule. Different schedules, monthly versus as needed, for the same agent did not result in a significant different visual acuity outcome.

Two-year results: Among patients following the same regimen for 2 years, mean gain in visual acuity was similar for both drugs (bevacizumab–ranibizumab difference, −1.4 letters; $P = .21$). Mean gain was greater for monthly treatment than for the as-needed regimen (difference, −2.4 letters; $P = .046$).

CATT Research Group, Martin DF, Maguire MG, et al. Ranibizumab and bevacizumab for neovascular age-related macular degeneration. *N Engl J Med.* 2011;364(20):1897–1908.

CATT Research Group, Martin DF, Maguire MG, et al. Ranibizumab and bevacizumab for treatment of neovascular age-related macular degeneration: two-year results. *Ophthalmology.* 2012;119(7):1388–1398.

not statistically different between bevacizumab and ranibizumab therapy for neovascular AMD. The GEFAL study comparatively assessed as-needed treatment following 3 monthly injections of bevacizumab and ranibizumab among 501 patients and found no significant difference in efficacy (ie, established noninferiority). The MANTA study compared as-needed bevacizumab with ranibizumab and found similar visual acuity and anatomical outcomes for the 2 regimens among 321 patients studied.

A few high-profile clusters of severe vision loss after bevacizumab injection in the United States related to substandard and erroneous compounding practices raised concerns about the off-label use of this drug. In response, legislative changes have led to improved regulation and increased monitoring of compounding pharmacies.

Combination treatment CNV is a multifactorial condition that involves all components of a wound-healing response, including inflammation, angiogenesis, and fibrosis. Certain trials (eg, RADICAL [Reduced Fluence Visudyne-Anti-VEGF-Dexamethasone in Combination for AMD Lesions] and DENALI [Safety and Efficacy of Verteporfin PDT Administered in Conjunction With Ranibizumab Versus Ranibizumab Monotherapy in Patients With Subfoveal CNV Secondary to AMD]) found that combining ranibizumab therapy with PDT reduced re-treatment rates compared with ranibizumab monotherapy. However, visual outcomes were inferior to monotherapy. Some cases of PCV recalcitrant to anti-VEGF therapy can benefit from this combination strategy. Similarly combining radiation with ranibizumab therapy may reduce the injection burden but lead to inferior visual outcomes compared with monotherapy.

Surgical treatments Submacular surgery, in which the CNV is removed from under the fovea, and macular translocation surgery, in which the fovea is moved to healthier RPE using complex surgical techniques, have been abandoned because of poor visual outcomes and complexities, respectively, particularly in comparison with the pharmacologic interventions described.

Low vision therapies Despite the success of intravitreal anti-VEGF pharmacotherapy, a significant number of patients with AMD will ultimately develop bilateral central blindness for which few therapeutic options exist. Recently, an implantable miniature telescope was approved by the FDA that can provide magnification up to a factor of 2.7; in pivotal FDA trials, its use resulted in 2 lines of vision gained in 90% of patients. Eyes need to be monitored carefully for corneal decompensation caused by endothelial cell loss; the corneal transplant rate is projected to be close to 5% at 5 years after the implantation surgery.

Low vision rehabilitation Vision loss of any degree has a profound effect on a patient's activities of daily living including driving and reading. Although the patient and doctor may be focused on therapies, sufficient attention should be given to low vision strategies that improve function and quality of life.

Severe vision loss and central blindness resulting from AMD can be devastating, but low vision rehabilitation and the use of optical and nonoptical devices can improve the patient's functional status and quality of life (see BCSC Section 3, *Clinical Optics*). Even patients who have undergone successful anti-VEGF therapy may sustain reduced visual acuity in the 20/50–20/70 range and can benefit from low vision interventions such as use of magnification (eg, high-plus lenses, closed-circuit television), improved lighting, and enhanced contrast. Training and visual rehabilitation to use eccentric foci shifted outside of the central scotoma caused by the disciform scar may also be very helpful. To accomplish some of these rehabilitation strategies and best meet patients' needs, clinicians are encouraged to consider referring patients for low vision consultation and to local low vision centers or state services for the blind, available in many US states.

In addition, the American Academy of Ophthalmology SmartSight website (available at http://one.aao.org/smart-sight-low-vision) provides guidelines for recognizing the need for vision rehabilitation and for implementing various strategies of low vision therapy. It also provides a patient handout and information for referring patients for additional vision rehabilitation beyond those interventions provided by the ophthalmologist.

Brown DM, Kaiser PK, Michels M, et al; ANCHOR Study Group. Ranibizumab versus verteporfin for neovascular age-related macular degeneration. *N Engl J Med.* 2006; 355(14):1432–1444.

Heier JS, Brown DM, Chong V, et al. Intravitreal aflibercept (VEGF trap-eye) in wet age-related macular degeneration. *Ophthalmology.* 2012;119(12):2537–2548.

Other Causes of Choroidal Neovascularization

The following discussion includes various conditions that are important causes of central vision loss, either from macular degenerative changes (not AMD) or from the development of CNV and its sequelae. CNV in most of these conditions was formerly treated with laser photocoagulation, usually guided by results of the macular photocoagulation studies (MPS), and with PDT. Currently, however, intravitreal anti-VEGF agents are usually used following the same principals used in treating neovascular AMD; this approach may be associated with significant gains in visual acuity.

Ocular Histoplasmosis Syndrome

Infection with the yeast form of the fungus *Histoplasma capsulatum* is endemic to the Mississippi and Ohio River valleys. Humans inhale the fungus, which is then disseminated into the bloodstream. The systemic infection eventually subsides, leaving chorioretinal scarring. Most of the visual symptoms occur years after initial infection.

Ocular histoplasmosis syndrome (OHS) has also been referred to as *presumed ocular histoplasmosis syndrome* (POHS) because the causal relationship between the fungus and the eye disease had been previously considered tenuous; however, the relationship is supported by epidemiologic and histologic data. For example, more than 90% of patients with the typical fundus appearance react positively to histoplasmin skin testing, and the highest prevalence of OHS is found where the population has the greatest percentage of positive skin reactors. In one community with endemic histoplasmosis (where 60% of the total population tested positive to histoplasmin skin testing), the characteristic peripheral lesions of OHS occurred in 2.6% of the total population surveyed and in 4.4% of the positive skin test responders. Only 1 individual with peripheral lesions showed disciform macular disease. The organism has been identified histologically in the choroid of 5 patients with

OHS. Nevertheless, other etiologies besides *H capsulatum* may produce a similar phenotype (see also the section "Multifocal choroiditis" in Chapter 10).

The clinical appearance of OHS includes small, atrophic, "punched-out" chorioretinal scars in the midperiphery and posterior pole ("histo spots"), linear peripheral atrophic tracks, and juxtapapillary chorioretinal scarring with or without CNV in the macula (Fig 4-11). The changes are bilateral in more than 60% of patients, and no vitreous inflammation is present. Most patients with OHS are asymptomatic until CNV develops. Vision loss, metamorphopsia, and paracentral scotomata are the sequelae of CNV. FA and OCT findings will guide the diagnosis and response to therapy. Other diseases with features similar to those of OHS include multifocal choroiditis and panuveitis, as discussed in BCSC Section 9, *Intraocular Inflammation and Uveitis.*

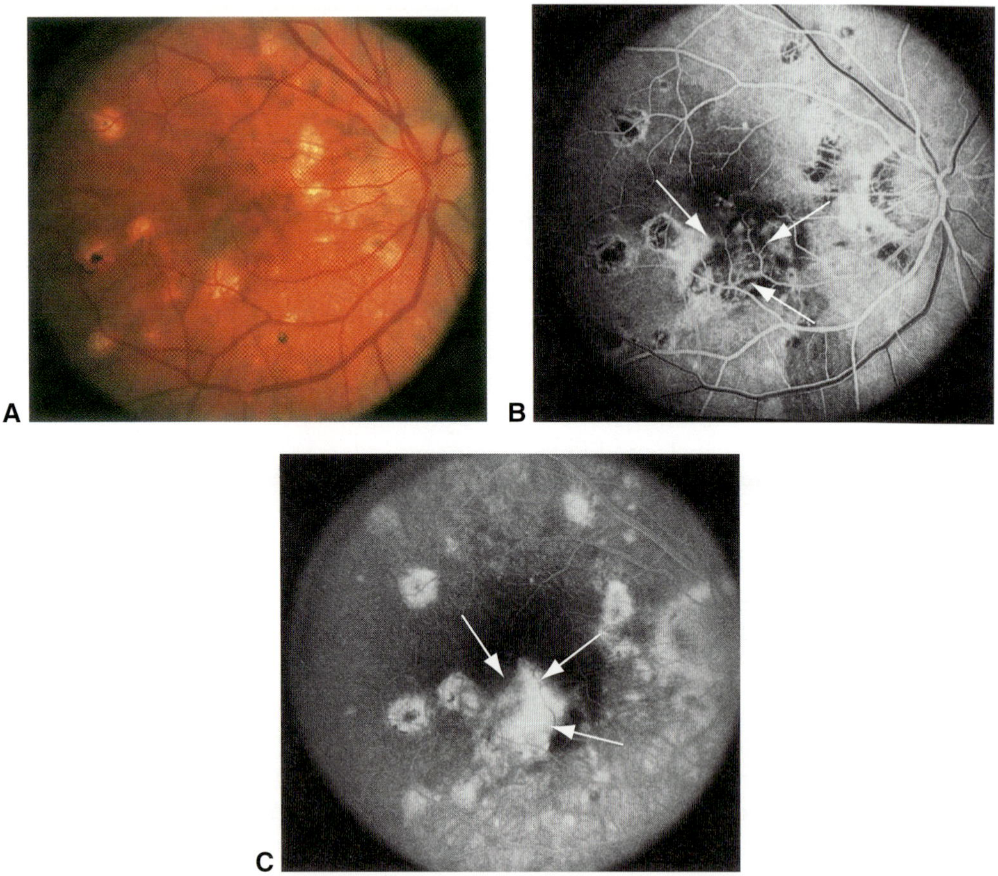

Figure 4-11 Ocular histoplasmosis syndrome with CNV. **A,** Fundus photograph shows peripapillary atrophy and numerous atrophic scars. **B,** Transit frame of the angiographic study reveals blocked fluorescence from blood and pigment as well as hyperfluorescence resulting from the CNV *(arrows)* and choroidal transmission in areas of atrophy. **C,** Leakage from the choroidal neovascular membrane *(arrows)* late in the study, as well as staining of the sclera beneath atrophic scars.

Management of OHS

There is no specific management necessary for OHS. When complicated by CNV, anti-angiogenic therapy has supplanted the use of laser treatment or PDT, as noted previously.

Nielsen JS, Fick TA, Saggau DD, Barnes CH. Intravitreal anti–vascular endothelial growth factor therapy for choroidal neovascularization secondary to ocular histoplasmosis syndrome. *Retina.* 2012;32(3):468–472.

Angioid Streaks

Dark red or brown subretinal bands of irregular contour that radiate from the optic nerve head are known as *angioid streaks* because they mimic blood vessels. On FA, characteristic window defects with late staining are noted that result from discontinuities or breaks in a thickened and calcified Bruch membrane (Fig 4-12).

The systemic disease most commonly associated with angioid streaks is *pseudoxanthoma elasticum* (PXE), or Grönblad-Strandberg syndrome, a predominantly autosomal recessive disorder inherited through mutation in the *ABCC6* gene located on band 16p13.1. Additional fundus findings associated with PXE include optic disc drusen, peripheral round atrophic scars with a "comet" sign, and a mottled RPE appearance referred to as *peau d'orange* ("skin of an orange"). *Paget disease* of bone, *beta thalassemia, sickle cell anemia* (SS), and *Ehlers-Danlos syndrome* may also be associated with angioid streaks.

Angioid streaks usually are asymptomatic unless they are subfoveal. Visual disturbances may develop due to submacular hemorrhage resulting from trauma, but these disturbances may resolve spontaneously if there is no CNV. The most significant visual complication is the development of CNV.

The use of safety glasses may be advised for patients with angioid streaks because of high susceptibility to choroidal rupture after even minor blunt injury. Consultation is

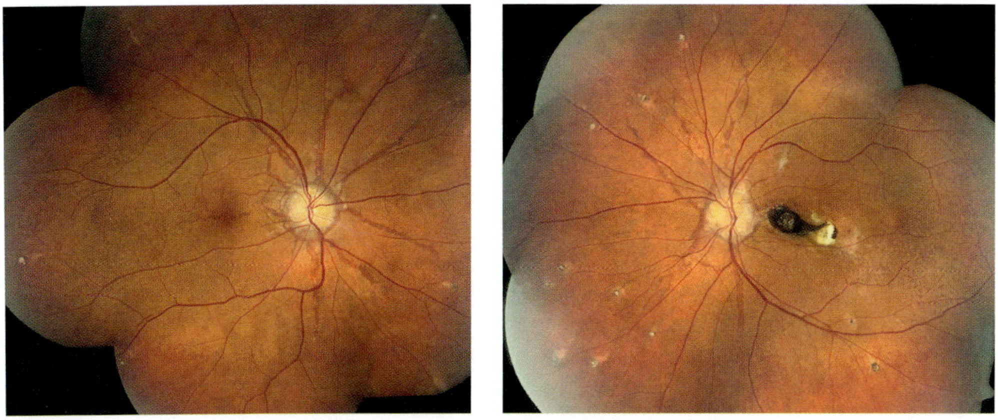

Figure 4-12 Color montages of fundus photographs from a patient with pseudoxanthoma elasticum showing, in both eyes, angioid streaks radiating from the optic nerve head, a "peau d'orange" appearance of the fundus temporal to the macula, optic nerve head drusen, mid-peripheral comet lesions, and in the left eye an old, inactive CNV. *(Courtesy of Stephen J. Kim, MD.)*

indicated to evaluate for systemic manifestations of PXE including "plucked chicken" skin appearance, calcific arteriosclerosis of coronary arteries, and gastrointestinal and cerebrovascular bleeding.

When CNV develops, treatment with antiangiogenic agents has supplanted the use of laser treatment or PDT, as noted previously.

Chang LK, Spaide RF, Brue C, Freund KB, Klancnik JM Jr, Slakter JS. Bevacizumab treatment for subfoveal choroidal neovascularization from causes other than age-related macular degeneration. *Arch Ophthalmol.* 2008;126(7):941–945.

Heier JS, Brown D, Ciulla T, et al. Ranibizumab for choroidal neovascularization secondary to causes other than age-related macular degeneration: a phase I clinical trial. *Ophthalmology.* 2011;118(1):111–118.

Pathologic Myopia

Myopia is the most common ocular abnormality, affecting 25% of the US population. In contrast, *high myopia,* defined as a spherical equivalent of greater than –6.00 D or an axial length greater than 26.5 mm, is uncommon, occurring in roughly 2% of the population. Whereas incidence rates are low in African Americans, they have reached epidemic proportions in the Asian population. Eyes with pathologic myopia have progressive elongation of the eye and associated thinning and degeneration of the retina, RPE, and choroid, and the prevalence and severity of these abnormalities correlate directly with the magnitude of myopia.

Fundus manifestations in pathologic myopia may include tilting of the optic disc with peripapillary atrophy. Nonexudative macular findings include lacquer cracks—spontaneous ruptures of the elastic lamina of the Bruch membrane that appear as yellow-white, irregular, subretinal lines in the posterior pole (Fig 4-13). FA can help identify subtle lacquer cracks as window defects. More significant atrophic features can develop,

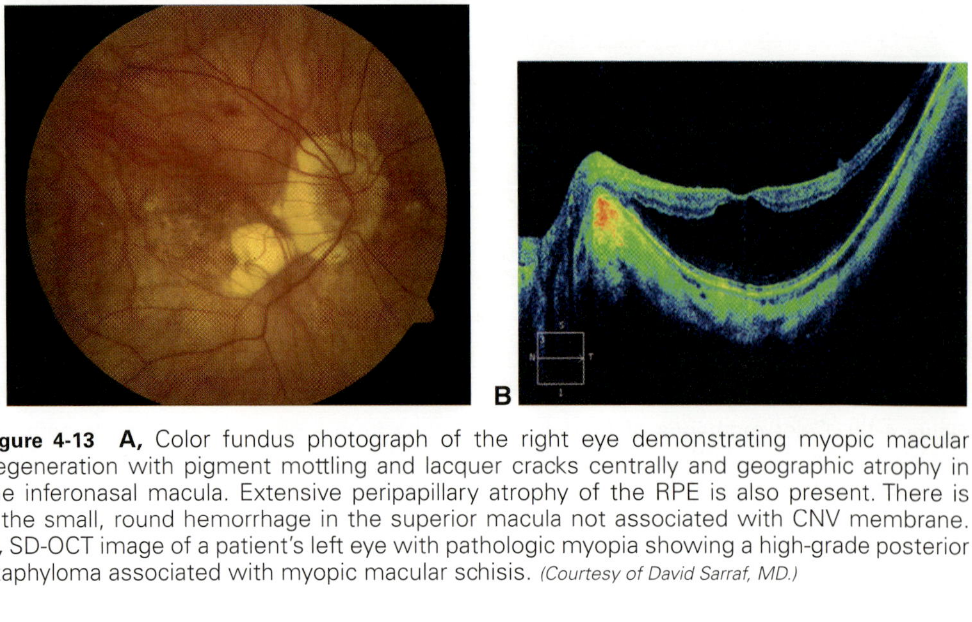

A B

Figure 4-13 **A,** Color fundus photograph of the right eye demonstrating myopic macular degeneration with pigment mottling and lacquer cracks centrally and geographic atrophy in the inferonasal macula. Extensive peripapillary atrophy of the RPE is also present. There is a the small, round hemorrhage in the superior macula not associated with CNV membrane. **B,** SD-OCT image of a patient's left eye with pathologic myopia showing a high-grade posterior staphyloma associated with myopic macular schisis. *(Courtesy of David Sarraf, MD.)*

including geographic atrophy. SD-OCT imaging of eyes with high myopia may confirm the presence of posterior staphyloma, the severity of which correlates with various macular complications such as vitreomacular traction, epiretinal membrane, and macular schisis. Isolated round or coin-shaped subretinal hemorrhages can develop but may resolve spontaneously if they result from the presence or extension of a lacquer crack. FA and OCT imaging may be helpful in excluding CNV. Other possible findings include Forster-Fuchs spots, which are dark lesions due to subretinal or intraretinal RPE hyperplasia that presumably develop in response to a small CNV that has spontaneously regressed.

CNV in myopia

CNV may develop in 5%–10% of eyes with an axial length of more than 26.5 mm, often in conjunction with widespread chorioretinal degeneration and lacquer cracks in the posterior pole. Laser therapy may be complicated by vision loss due to atrophic creep or long-term extension of the laser scar through the foveal center. Results of the Verteporfin in Photodynamic Therapy (VIP) trial showed that PDT of subfoveal lesions in eyes with pathologic myopia was beneficial in preventing vision loss up to 3 years after initiating treatment. However, studies of anti-VEGF therapies including ranibizumab and bevacizumab have been described with excellent visual and anatomical outcomes, and intravitreal anti-VEGF injection has become the gold standard of care for subfoveal and even extrafoveal CNV associated with myopia. Several studies have noted sustained regression of myopic CNV, with stabilization or improvement of visual acuity after only 1 or 2 injections.

A meta-analysis summarizing the results of several randomized and nonrandomized controlled trials found that intravitreal anti-VEGF therapy was superior to PDT for the treatment of myopic CNV and was associated with an average of 2 lines gained of visual acuity. The study recommended that anti-VEGF therapy should be the first line of therapy for myopic CNV.

Recently, 2 important European prospective trials have confirmed the benefit of ranibizumab therapy for myopic CNV. The REPAIR study (Efficacy and Safety of Ranibizumab [0.5mg] in Patients With Choroidal Neovascularisation Secondary to Pathological Myopia) demonstrated an average visual gain of 13.8 letters and a median number of 3 injections at 12 months in eyes with myopic CNV treated with ranibizumab therapy. The RADIANCE study (Randomized Controlled Study of Ranibizumab in Patients with Choroidal Neovascularization Secondary to Pathologic Myopia) showed significant superiority at 3 months of ranibizumab therapy (average, 10.5 letters gained) to PDT (average, 2.2 letters gained) for patients with CNV secondary to myopia.

SD-OCT imaging in patients with high myopia and vision loss is essential for identifying myopic macular schisis, which can be complicated by macular hole and even rhegmatogenous retinal detachment, warranting surgical intervention with vitrectomy.

Wang E, Chen Y. Intravitreal anti–vascular endothelial growth factor for choroidal neovascularization secondary to pathologic myopia: systematic review and meta-analysis. *Retina.* 2013;33(7):1375–1392.

Idiopathic CNV and Miscellaneous Causes of CNV

CNV may complicate a large spectrum of disorders that damage the Bruch membrane, including inflammatory chorioretinopathies, choroidal neoplasms, traumatic choroidal rupture, optic disc abnormalities, and others (Table 4-3). It also may develop without apparent risk factor or predisposing lesion (ie, idiopathic CNV). Although the results of the MPS trials may be extrapolated to apply to use of thermal laser ablation to treat extrafoveal CNV—because of its low cost and high convenience—this approach must be balanced against the possible development of a dense paracentral scotoma and the high recurrence rate. Therefore, in most instances of CNV associated with these conditions, anti-VEGF agents are now used for treatment.

Heier JS, Brown D, Ciulla T, et al. Ranibizumab for choroidal neovascularization secondary to causes other than age-related macular degeneration: a phase I clinical trial. *Ophthalmology.* 2011;118(1):111–118.

Kang HM, Koh HJ. Intravitreal anti–vascular endothelial growth factor therapy versus photodynamic therapy for idiopathic choroidal neovascularization. *Am J Ophthalmol.* 2013;155(4): 713–719.

Table 4-3 Conditions Associated With Choroidal Neovascularization

Degenerative
- Age-related macular degeneration
- Myopic degeneration
- Angioid streaks

Heredodegenerative
- Vitelliform macular dystrophy
- Fundus flavimaculatus
- Optic nerve head drusen

Inflammatory
- Ocular histoplasmosis syndrome
- Multifocal choroiditis
- Serpiginous-like choroiditis (also called *multifocal serpiginoid choroiditis*)
- Toxoplasmosis
- Toxocariasis
- Rubella
- Vogt-Koyanagi-Harada syndrome
- Behçet disease
- Sympathetic ophthalmia

Tumor
- Choroidal nevus
- Choroidal hemangioma
- Metastatic choroidal tumors
- Hamartoma of the RPE

Traumatic
- Choroidal rupture
- Intense photocoagulation

Idiopathic

CHAPTER 5

Retinal Vascular Disease: Diabetic Retinopathy

Diabetic retinopathy is a leading cause of blindness worldwide among patients aged 20–64 years. This chapter provides a foundation for the evaluation and treatment of diabetic retinopathy; additional information is available in the following selected references.

American Academy of Ophthalmology Retina/Vitreous Panel. Preferred Practice Pattern Guidelines. *Diabetic Retinopathy.* San Francisco: American Academy of Ophthalmology; 2014. Available at http://one.aao.org/guidelines.

Diabetic Retinopathy Clinical Research Network (DRCR.net) public website. http://drcrnet.jaeb.org. Accessed July 15, 2014.

Scott IU, Flynn HW Jr, Smiddy WE, eds. *Diabetes and Ocular Disease: Past, Present, and Future Therapies.* 2nd ed. Ophthalmology Monographs 14. New York: Oxford University Press; 2010.

Terminology and Classification

Diabetes Terminology

The terminology used for types of diabetes mellitus has evolved over the years. The American Diabetes Association (ADA) classifies diabetes mellitus as *type 1 diabetes mellitus,* formerly known as *insulin-dependent diabetes mellitus* (IDDM), and *type 2 diabetes mellitus,* formerly known as *non–insulin-dependent diabetes mellitus* (NIDDM). In type 1 diabetes mellitus, there is β-cell destruction, usually leading to absolute insulin deficiency. This process is either idiopathic or immune mediated. Type 2 diabetes mellitus ranges from a condition characterized as predominantly insulin resistance with relative insulin deficiency to one that is predominantly an insulin secretory defect with insulin resistance. Other forms of diabetes mellitus are recognized, including a genetically mediated form secondary to endocrinopathies and drug- or chemical-induced diabetes mellitus.

Diabetic Retinopathy Terminology

The classification of diabetic retinopathy is based upon clinical features. *Nonproliferative diabetic retinopathy* (NPDR) refers to the presence of intraretinal vascular changes prior to the development of extraretinal fibrovascular tissue; it is staged as mild, moderate, or severe. NPDR is also referred to as *background diabetic retinopathy,* a term that is still commonly used but not recommended. *Clinically significant diabetic macular edema* (CSME) is defined as macular edema that meets certain minimal severity criteria for size and location. The term *center-involving macular edema* is used when the fovea appears thickened on optical coherence tomography (OCT). *Proliferative diabetic retinopathy* (PDR) is defined by the presence of neovascularization, the result of diabetes-induced ischemia and its associated complications. PDR is staged as early, high-risk, or advanced. In the BCSC, study results are reported using the terminology of the particular study being described, even though such usage may not conform to current terminology.

Epidemiology of Diabetic Retinopathy

The prevalence of all types of diabetic retinopathy in the diabetic population increases with the duration of the disease and patient age. Diabetic retinopathy is rare in children younger than 10 years of age; however, the risk of developing diabetic retinopathy increases after puberty.

The Wisconsin Epidemiologic Study of Diabetic Retinopathy

The Wisconsin Epidemiologic Study of Diabetic Retinopathy (WESDR) is an ongoing epidemiologic study of the progression of diabetic retinopathy; progression is monitored by stereoscopic fundus photographs taken in 7 standard fields along with measurements of glycosylated hemoglobin levels and visual acuity. An important epidemiologic finding of the WESDR was the direct association of an increased prevalence of diabetic retinopathy, in both type 1 and type 2 forms, with the duration of diabetes mellitus. After 20 years of diabetes mellitus, nearly 99% of patients with type 1 and 60% with type 2 disease demonstrated some degree of diabetic retinopathy. Proliferative diabetic retinopathy was found in 50% of type 1 patients who had 20 years' duration of disease and in 25% of type 2 patients who had 25 years' duration of disease. Furthermore, 3.6% of younger-onset patients (aged <30 years at diagnosis, an operational definition of type 1 diabetes mellitus) and 1.6% of older-onset patients (aged ≥30 years at diagnosis, an operational definition of type 2 diabetes mellitus) were found to have a visual acuity of 20/200 or worse. Such vision loss was attributable to diabetic retinopathy in 86% of the younger-onset patients and in 33% of the older-onset group.

WESDR epidemiologic data were based largely on white populations of northern European descent and therefore are not entirely applicable to other racial groups. According to the National Health and Nutrition Examination Survey (NHANES) III, in 2011, the age-adjusted percentage of adults with diagnosed diabetes mellitus who reported visual impairment was 20.7% for blacks, 17.1% for whites, and 15.6% for Hispanics.

Centers for Disease Control and Prevention. Diabetes Public Health Resource. Age-adjusted percentage of adults aged 18 years or older with diagnosed diabetes reporting visual impairment, by race/ethnicity, United States, 1997–2011. http://www.cdc.gov/diabetes/statistics/visual/fig5.htm. Accessed July 15, 2014.

Klein R, Lee KE, Gangnon RE, Klein BE. The 25-year incidence of visual impairment in type 1 diabetes mellitus: the Wisconsin Epidemiologic Study of Diabetic Retinopathy. *Ophthalmology.* 2010;117(1):63–70.

Klein R, Lee KE, Knudtson MD, Gangnon RE, Klein BE. Changes in visual impairment prevalence by period of diagnosis of diabetes: the Wisconsin Epidemiologic Study of Diabetic Retinopathy. *Ophthalmology.* 2009;116(10):1937–1942.

University of Wisconsin Madison School of Medicine and Public Health. Wisconsin Epidemiologic Study of Diabetic Retinopathy (WESDR). http://www.epi.ophth.wisc.edu/content/wesdr. Accessed July 15, 2014.

Pathogenesis of Diabetic Retinopathy

Although the exact cause of diabetic microvascular disease remains poorly understood, exposure to hyperglycemia over an extended period results in biochemical and physiologic changes that ultimately cause endothelial damage. Specific retinal capillary changes such as basement membrane thickening and selective loss of pericytes favor capillary occlusion and retinal nonperfusion (Fig 5-1). In addition, endothelial barrier decompensation leads

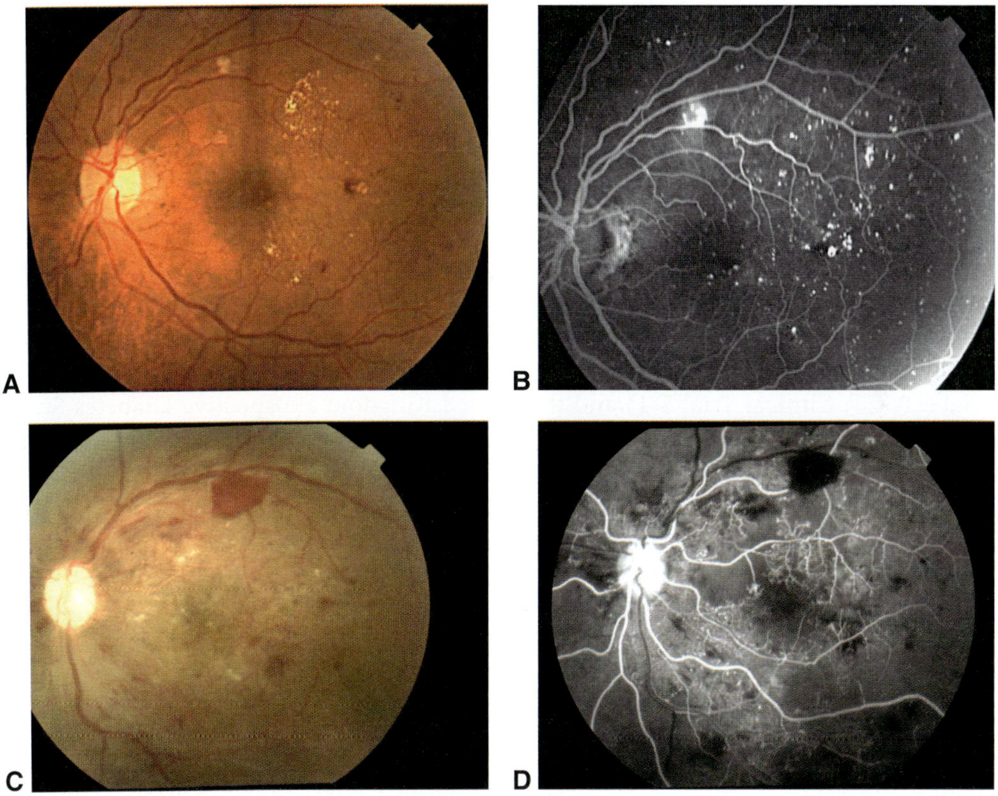

Figure 5-1 Capillary nonperfusion in diabetic retinopathy. **A,** Fundus photograph from a patient with severe nonproliferative diabetic retinopathy (NPDR). **B,** Corresponding mid–venous-phase fluorescein angiogram shows multiple microaneurysms and focal areas of capillary nonperfusion. Clinically difficult to appreciate, evidence of early neovascularization is revealed on the angiogram by dye leakage in the superior nasal aspect of the macula. **C,** Fundus photograph of a patient with early proliferative diabetic retinopathy. **D,** Corresponding early-phase fluorescein angiogram shows severe capillary nonperfusion. Clinically difficult to appreciate, evidence of early neovascularization is revealed on the angiogram by dye leakage at the disc. *(Parts A and B courtesy of Richard B. Rosen, MD; parts C and D courtesy of Colin A. McCannel, MD.)*

to serum leakage and retinal edema. The stages of disease result from continuous progression of the retinovascular damage, which leads to clinical manifestation that ranges from mild to advanced proliferative lesions. The pace of the progression varies among patients and depends mainly on systemic factors such as blood glucose levels, blood pressure, blood lipid profiles, and others.

Numerous hematologic and biochemical abnormalities correlate with the prevalence and severity of retinopathy:

- increased platelet adhesiveness
- increased erythrocyte aggregation
- abnormal levels of serum lipids
- defective fibrinolysis
- abnormal levels of growth hormone
- upregulation of vascular endothelial growth factor (VEGF)
- abnormalities in serum and whole-blood viscosity
- local and systemic inflammation

The precise role of each of these abnormalities in the pathogenesis of retinopathy—individually or in combination—is not well defined.

Antonetti DA, Klein R, Gardner TW. Diabetic retinopathy. *N Engl J Med.* 2012;366(13): 1227–1239.

Systemic Medical Management of Diabetic Retinopathy

Good glycemic control was found to be the most important factor in the medical management of diabetic retinopathy in both the Diabetes Control and Complications Trial (DCCT; Clinical Trial 5-1) and the United Kingdom Prospective Diabetes Study (UKPDS; Clinical Trial 5-2). Intensive glycemic control was associated with a reduced risk of newly diagnosed retinopathy and reduced progression of existing retinopathy in people with diabetes mellitus (type 1 in the DCCT and type 2 in the UKPDS). In addition, the DCCT showed that intensive glycemic control (compared with conventional treatment) was associated with reductions in progression to severe NPDR and PDR, incidence of macular edema, and need for panretinal and focal photocoagulation. The UKPDS showed that control of hypertension was also beneficial in reducing progression of retinopathy and loss of vision. Figure 5-2, adapted from published results of the DCCT, illustrates the interplay of sustained glycemic control, as represented by hemoglobin A_{1c} (HbA_{1c}) levels, time, and progression of diabetic retinopathy. Even small changes in sustained HbA_{1c} levels were found to have a large impact on diabetic retinopathy progression.

Hypertension, when poorly controlled over many years, is usually associated with a higher risk of progression of diabetic retinopathy and diabetic macular edema (DME). *Severe carotid artery occlusive disease* may result in advanced PDR as part of the ocular

CLINICAL TRIAL 5-1

Diabetes Control and Complications Trial (DCCT)

Study questions:

1. Primary prevention study: Will intensive control of blood glucose level slow development and subsequent progression of diabetic retinopathy (neuropathy and nephropathy)?
2. Secondary intervention study: Will intensive control of blood glucose level slow progression of diabetic retinopathy (neuropathy and nephropathy)?

Enrollment:

1. 726 patients with type 1 diabetes mellitus (1–5 years' duration) and no diabetic retinopathy.
2. 715 patients with type 1 diabetes mellitus (1–15 years' duration) and mild to moderate diabetic retinopathy.

Study groups: Intensive control of blood glucose level (multiple daily insulin injections or insulin pump) vs conventional management.

Outcome variables: Development of diabetic retinopathy or progression of retinopathy by 3 steps using a modified Airlie House classification scale; neuropathy, nephropathy (albuminuria, microalbuminuria), and cardiovascular outcomes were also assessed.

Results: In the primary prevention cohort, intensive control reduced the risk of developing retinopathy by 76%, and in the secondary intervention cohort, it slowed progression of retinopathy by 54%. In the 2 cohorts combined, intensive control reduced the risk of clinical neuropathy by 60% and albuminuria (nephropathy) by 54%.

CLINICAL TRIAL 5-2

United Kingdom Prospective Diabetes Study (UKPDS)

Study questions:

1. Will intensive control of blood glucose level, in patients with type 2 diabetes mellitus, reduce the risk of microvascular complications of diabetes, including the risk of retinopathy progression?
2. Will intensive control of blood pressure, in patients with type 2 diabetes mellitus and elevated blood pressure, reduce the risk of microvascular complications of diabetes, including the risk of retinopathy progression?

(Continued on next page)

(continued)

Enrollment:

1. 4209 patients with newly diagnosed type 2 diabetes mellitus.
2. 1148 patients with hypertension and newly diagnosed type 2 diabetes mellitus.

Randomization:

1. Patients were randomly assigned to conventional policy starting with diet (1138 patients) or to intensive policy starting with a sulfonylurea—chlorpropamide (788 patients), glibenclamide (615 patients), or glipizide (170 patients)—or with insulin (1156 patients). If overweight and in the intensive group, patients were assigned to start treatment with metformin (342 patients).
2. Patients were randomly assigned to tight control of blood pressure (400 with angiotensin-converting enzyme [ACE] inhibitor and 398 with beta blockers) or to less tight control (390 patients).

Outcome variables: Development of any of 3 aggregate adverse outcomes and specific retinopathy-related outcomes (worsening of retinopathy on a modified Airlie House scale, retinal photocoagulation, vitreous hemorrhage, and worsening of visual acuity).

Results:

1. Intensive control of blood glucose level slowed progression of retinopathy and reduced the risk of other microvascular complications of diabetes mellitus. Sulfonylureas did not increase the risk of cardiovascular disease.
2. Intensive control of blood pressure slowed progression of retinopathy and reduced the risk of other microvascular and macrovascular complications of diabetes mellitus. No clinically or statistically significant difference was found in the comparison of blood pressure lowering with ACE inhibitors versus beta blockers.

ischemic syndrome. Controversy exists as to whether or not mild or moderate carotid artery occlusive disease may have a protective effect on the development and severity of diabetic retinopathy. *Advanced diabetic nephropathy* and *anemia* also may be markers of advanced diabetic retinopathy.

Pregnancy is associated with a worsening of retinopathy; therefore, women with diabetes mellitus who become pregnant require more frequent retinal evaluations. Vision loss may occur from NPDR with DME or from the complications of PDR. Although some regression of retinopathy may occur after delivery, photocoagulation treatment is generally recommended if high-risk PDR develops during pregnancy.

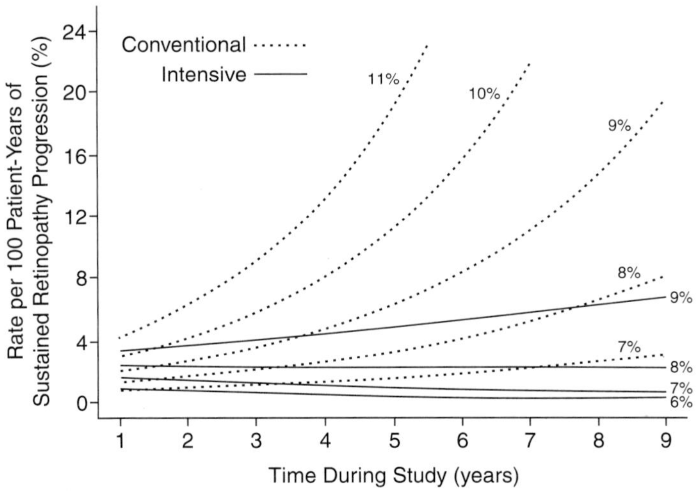

Figure 5-2 Comparison of results from the intensive *(solid lines)* and conventional *(dotted lines)* treatment groups of the Diabetes Control and Complications Trial (DCCT). The graph of the results from the DCCT show the risk of sustained retinopathy progression as a function of the mean hemoglobin A_{1c} level (percentage) during the study (years), based upon risk regression models of sustained progression as a function of time and glycemic exposure during the DCCT. *(Used with permission from Lachin JM, Genuth S, Nathan DM, Zinman B, Rutledge BN; DCCT/EDIC Research Group. Effect of glycemic exposure on the risk of microvascular complications in the Diabetes Control and Complications Trial—revisited.* Diabetes. *2008;57(4):995–1001.)*

Brown GC. Arterial occlusive disease. In: Regillo CD, Brown GC, Flynn HW Jr, eds. *Vitreoretinal Disease: The Essentials.* New York: Thieme; 1999:97–117.

Chew EY, Mills JL, Metzger BE, et al. Metabolic control and progression of retinopathy: the Diabetes in Early Pregnancy Study. National Institute of Child Health and Human Development Diabetes in Early Pregnancy Study. *Diabetes Care.* 1995;18(5):631–637.

Davis MD, Fisher MR, Gangnon RE, et al. Risk factors for high-risk proliferative diabetic retinopathy and severe visual loss: Early Treatment Diabetic Retinopathy Study report 18. *Invest Ophthalmol Vis Sci.* 1998;39(2):233–252.

Diabetes Control and Complications Trial Research Group. Progression of retinopathy with intensive versus conventional treatment in the Diabetes Control and Complications Trial. *Ophthalmology.* 1995;102(4):647–661.

Diabetes Control and Complications Trial Research Group. The effect of intensive treatment of diabetes on the development and progression of long-term complications in insulin-dependent diabetes mellitus. *N Engl J Med.* 1993;329(14):977–986.

Klein R, Klein BE, Moss SE, Cruickshanks KJ. Association of ocular disease and mortality in a diabetic population. *Arch Ophthalmol.* 1999;117(11):1487–1495.

UK Prospective Diabetes Study Group. Tight blood pressure control and risk of macrovascular and microvascular complications in type 2 diabetes: UKPDS 38. *Br Med J.* 1998;317(7160): 703–713.

United Kingdom Prospective Diabetes Study Group. Intensive blood-glucose control with sulphonylureas or insulin compared with conventional treatment and risk of complications in patients with type 2 diabetes (UKPDS 33). *Lancet.* 1998;352(9131):837–853.

Abnormalities Associated With Vision Loss From Diabetic Retinopathy

Vision loss in patients with diabetic retinopathy can be associated with the following abnormalities:

- capillary leakage (macular edema)
- capillary occlusion (macular ischemia, diabetic papillopathy)
- sequelae from ischemia-induced neovascularization (vitreous hemorrhage, tractional retinal detachment, neovascular glaucoma)

Nonproliferative Diabetic Retinopathy

Retinal microvascular changes that occur in NPDR are limited to the retina and do not extend beyond the internal limiting membrane (ILM). Characteristic findings in NPDR include microaneurysms, cotton-wool spots (boundary sentinels of infarction), areas of capillary nonperfusion, intraretinal microvascular abnormalities (IRMAs), "dot-and-blot" intraretinal hemorrhages, retinal edema, hard exudates, arteriolar abnormalities, and dilation and beading of retinal veins. NPDR can affect visual function through 2 mechanisms: (1) increased intraretinal vascular permeability, resulting in macular edema, and (2) variable degrees of intraretinal capillary closure, resulting in macular ischemia.

McLeod D. Why cotton wool spots should *not* be regarded as retinal nerve fibre layer infarcts. *Br J Ophthalmol.* 2005;89(2):229–237.

Wiley HE, Ferris FL III. Nonproliferative diabetic retinopathy and diabetic macular edema. In: Ryan SJ, Schachat AP, Wilkinson CP, Hinton DR, Sadda SR, Wiedemann P, eds. *Retina.* 5th ed. Philadelphia: Elsevier/Saunders; 2013:940–968.

Diabetic Macular Edema

Retinal edema threatening or involving the fovea often results in vision loss. It is an important consequence of abnormal retinal vascular permeability in diabetic retinopathy (Fig 5-3). The diagnosis of DME is made when retinal thickening is observed with slit-lamp biomicroscopy or on OCT. Important observations include the

- location of retinal thickening relative to the foveal center
- presence and location of exudates
- presence of cystoid macular edema

Fluorescein angiography is useful in demonstrating the breakdown of the blood–retina barrier by showing retinal capillary leakage. However, examination with OCT or slit-lamp biomicroscopy using a contact lens is the appropriate means to evaluate eyes for the presence or absence of macular thickening. Leakage shown on the angiogram may occur in the absence of macular retinal thickening and is thus not considered macular edema.

DME may manifest as focal or diffuse retinal thickening, with or without exudates. Although some overlap occurs, the 2 general categories of macular edema—focal and diffuse—are clinically useful descriptions. *Focal macular edema* is characterized by areas

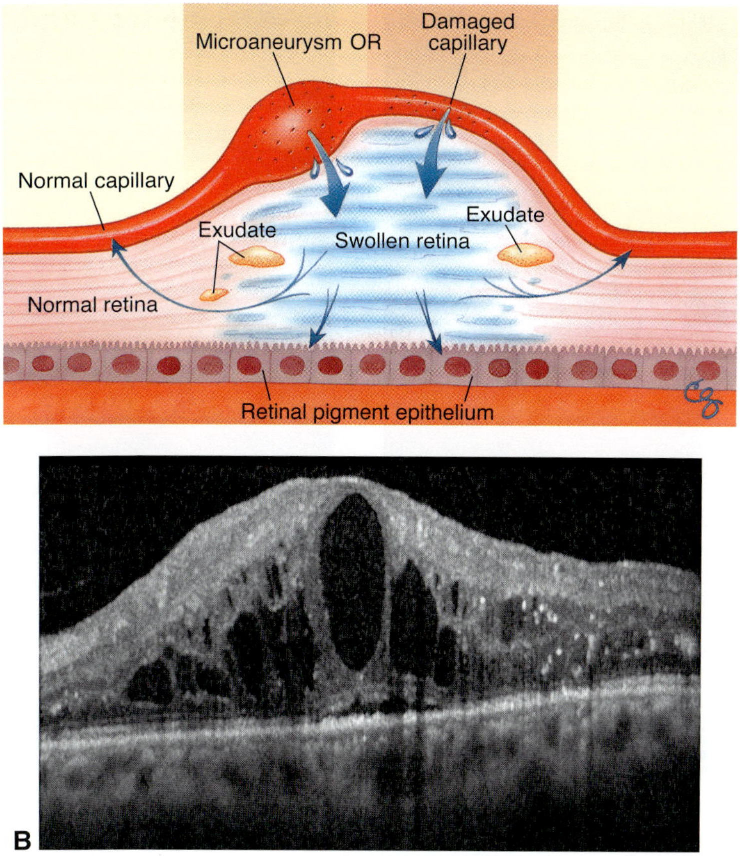

A

B

Figure 5-3 **A,** Artist's rendering of the mechanism of diabetic macular edema, demonstrating development of thickening from a breakdown of the blood–retina barrier. **B,** Spectral-domain optical coherence tomography scan of diabetic macular edema. Whereas there are extensive cystic changes in the outer plexiform and outer nuclear layers, the external limiting membrane line appears intact across the extent of the scan. Note the foveal detachment. *(Part A from Ginsburg LH, Aiello LM. Diabetic retinopathy: classification, progression, and management.* Focal Points: Clinical Modules for Ophthalmologists. *San Francisco: American Academy of Ophthalmology; 1993, module 7. Illustration by Christine Gralapp. Part B courtesy of Colin A. McCannel, MD.)*

of focal fluorescein leakage from capillary lesions, such as microaneurysms (Fig 5-4A, B). Focal macular edema may be associated with hard exudates, which are precipitates of plasma lipoproteins. Because resorption of extravascular aqueous occurs at a faster rate than that of plasma lipids, lipid residues often remain behind after the fluid has resorbed. These yellow-to-white lipid deposits accumulate within the outer and inner plexiform layers or occasionally beneath the sensory retina itself.

Diffuse macular edema is characterized by extensive retinal capillary leakage and widespread breakdown of the blood–retina barrier, often accumulating in a cystoid configuration in the perifoveal macula (cystoid macular edema) (Fig 5-4C, D). Whether the pattern of macular edema is focal or diffuse, treatment decisions are based upon lesions meeting defined size and location criteria that determine clinical significance.

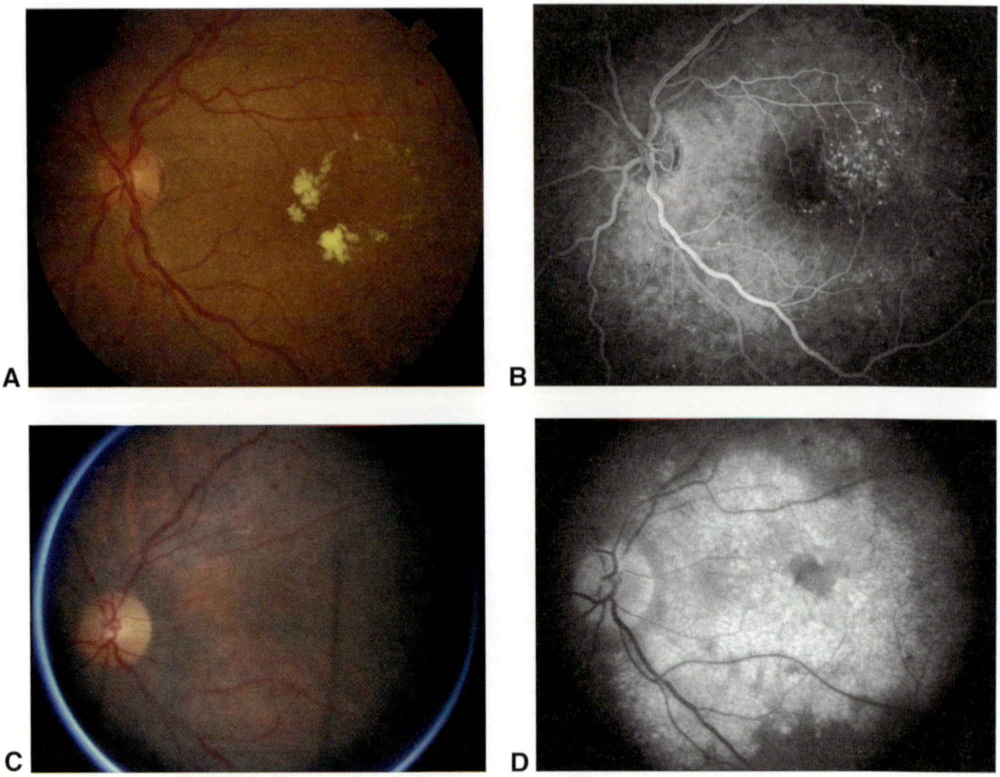

Figure 5-4 Focal and diffuse macular edema. **A,** Color fundus photograph showing circinate hard exudates surrounding a group of microaneurysms in an example of focal macular edema. **B,** Fluorescein angiogram confirming the microaneurysms, which appear as a group of punctate foci of hyperfluorescence. **C,** Color fundus photograph shows diffuse macular edema demonstrating diffuse thickening of the retina with glistening surface. **D,** Fluorescein angiogram confirming the diffuse intraretinal leakage. *(Courtesy of Hermann D. Schubert, MD.)*

Clinically significant diabetic macular edema

The Early Treatment Diabetic Retinopathy Study (ETDRS) was the first prospective, randomized clinical trial of photocoagulation in diabetic patients with less than high-risk PDR to establish standard treatment paradigms for managing DME (Clinical Trial 5-3). It defined *clinically significant diabetic macular edema* as the indication for focal laser photocoagulation treatment in the following settings:

- retinal thickening located at or within 500 µm of the center of the macula
- hard exudates at or within 500 µm of the center if associated with thickening of adjacent retina
- a zone of thickening larger than 1 disc area if located within 1 disc diameter of the center of the macula (Fig 5-5)

Studies now use the term *center-involving macular edema* or similar terminology, based on whether or not the fovea appears thickened on OCT scans. Most algorithms for pharmacologic intervention use this simplified, OCT-based definition.

CLINICAL TRIAL 5-3

Early Treatment Diabetic Retinopathy Study (ETDRS)

Study questions:

1. Is photocoagulation effective for treating DME?
2. Is photocoagulation effective for treating diabetic retinopathy?
3. Is aspirin effective for preventing progression of diabetic retinopathy?

Eligibility: Mild nonproliferative diabetic retinopathy through early proliferative diabetic retinopathy, with visual acuity 20/200 or better in each eye.

Randomization: 3711 participants: 1 eye randomly assigned to photocoagulation (scatter and/or focal) and 1 eye assigned to no photocoagulation; patients randomly assigned to 650 mg/day aspirin or placebo.

Outcome variables: Visual acuity less than 5/200 for at least 4 months; visual acuity worsening by doubling of initial visual angle (eg, 20/40 to 20/80); retinopathy progression.

Macular edema results:

1. Focal photocoagulation for DME decreased risk of moderate vision loss (doubling of initial visual angle).
2. Focal photocoagulation for DME increased chance of moderate vision gain (halving of initial visual angle).
3. Focal photocoagulation for DME reduced retinal thickening.

Early scatter photocoagulation results:

1. Early scatter photocoagulation resulted in a small reduction in the risk of severe vision loss (<5/200 for at least 4 months).
2. Early scatter photocoagulation is not indicated for eyes with mild to moderate diabetic retinopathy.
3. Early scatter photocoagulation may be most effective in patients with type 2 diabetes mellitus.

Aspirin use results:

1. Aspirin use did not alter progression of diabetic retinopathy.
2. Aspirin use did not increase risk of vitreous hemorrhage.
3. Aspirin use did not affect visual acuity.
4. Aspirin use reduced risk of cardiovascular morbidity and mortality.

Treatment of diabetic macular edema

In parallel to medical management and optimizing of health habits, ocular therapies should be considered to maximize visual function and prevent progressive vision loss. These therapies include ocular pharmacologic management and laser photocoagulation

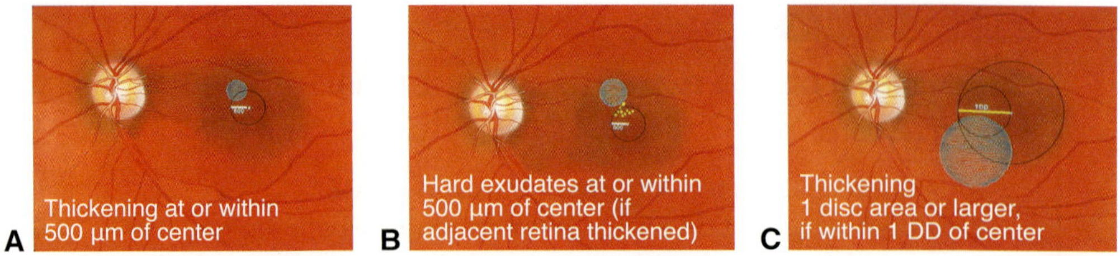

Figure 5-5 Clinically significant macular edema treatment criteria as established by the Early Treatment Diabetic Retinopathy Study (ETDRS). **A,** Retinal edema located at or within 500 µm of the center of the macula. **B,** Hard exudates at or within 500 µm of the center of the macula, if associated with thickening of the adjacent retina. **C,** A zone of thickening larger than 1 disc area, if located within 1 disc diameter (DD) of the center of the macula. *(Courtesy of the ETDRS.)*

treatment. Treatment is typically indicated when the macular edema is clinically significant or center involving. In most instances, visual acuity will be affected. For patients who are asymptomatic or have normal visual acuity, the decision-making process for treatment is more complex. Factors that should be considered include proximity of exudates to the fovea, the status and course of the fellow eye, anticipated cataract surgery, presence of high-risk PDR, and treatment risks. It is preferable to initiate DME treatment before performing scatter photocoagulation and prior to cataract surgery in an attempt to reduce the risk of DME resulting from these interventions.

Ocular pharmacologic management of diabetic macular edema Anti-VEGF drugs and corticosteroids have come to the forefront of DME management as clinical evidence accrues demonstrating their benefit and superiority in visual outcomes.

ANTI-VEGF DRUGS Currently available anti-VEGF drugs include ranibizumab, bevacizumab, pegaptanib, and aflibercept (also called *VEGF Trap*). Ranibizumab has undergone the most extensive studies to date with the completion of 2 parallel phase 3 trials, RISE and RIDE (identical study designs, both titled Ranibizumab Injection in Subjects With CSME With Center Involvement Secondary to Diabetes Mellitus). Results indicated ranibizumab rapidly and sustainably improved vision, reduced the risk of further vision loss, and improved macular edema in patients with DME, with low rates of complications. At 36 months, the pooled data of these studies showed that the proportion of patients who gained 15 or more letters from baseline in the initially sham/later 0.5 mg, 0.3 mg, and 0.5 mg ranibizumab groups were 20.6%, 44.0%, and 40.9%, respectively. Similarly, aflibercept treatment resulted in substantial visual acuity gains compared with laser photocoagulation in the 2-year results of VISTA (Phase 3 Study of Efficacy and Safety of Intravitreal Administration of VEGF Trap-Eye in Patients With DME).

DIABETIC RETINOPATHY CLINICAL RESEARCH NETWORK STUDIES Sponsored by the US National Eye Institute, the Diabetic Retinopathy Clinical Research Network (DRCR.net) was developed to conduct prospective, randomized trials that involve community practices as well as academic centers to assess the expanding number of management options and their combinations in a "real-world" setting. The DRCR.net Protocol I demonstrated that intravitreal ranibizumab combined with prompt or deferred (≥24 weeks) focal/grid laser treatment was more effective at 1 year in increasing visual acuity than was focal/grid laser treatment alone or in combination with triamcinolone acetonide injections for the treatment of center-involving DME. During the extension study, these results held up at 2 years. The latest publication from Protocol I included follow-up through the third year for only patients originally assigned to 1 of the 2 ranibizumab groups. In the second and third years of the study, despite a decreased number of injections given, the ranibizumab plus deferred laser treatment group showed no decline in visual acuity, and the ranibizumab plus prompt laser treatment group showed only a slight decline from results at the 1-year to 3-year visit (Fig 5-6). These results suggest that focal/grid laser treatment at the initiation of intravitreal ranibizumab is no better, and is possibly worse, for vision outcomes than deferring laser treatment for 24 weeks or more in eyes with vision impairment and DME involving the fovea. Focal macular laser treatment alone or in combination with triamcinolone, as used in this study, resulted in worse outcomes and is therefore no longer recommended for

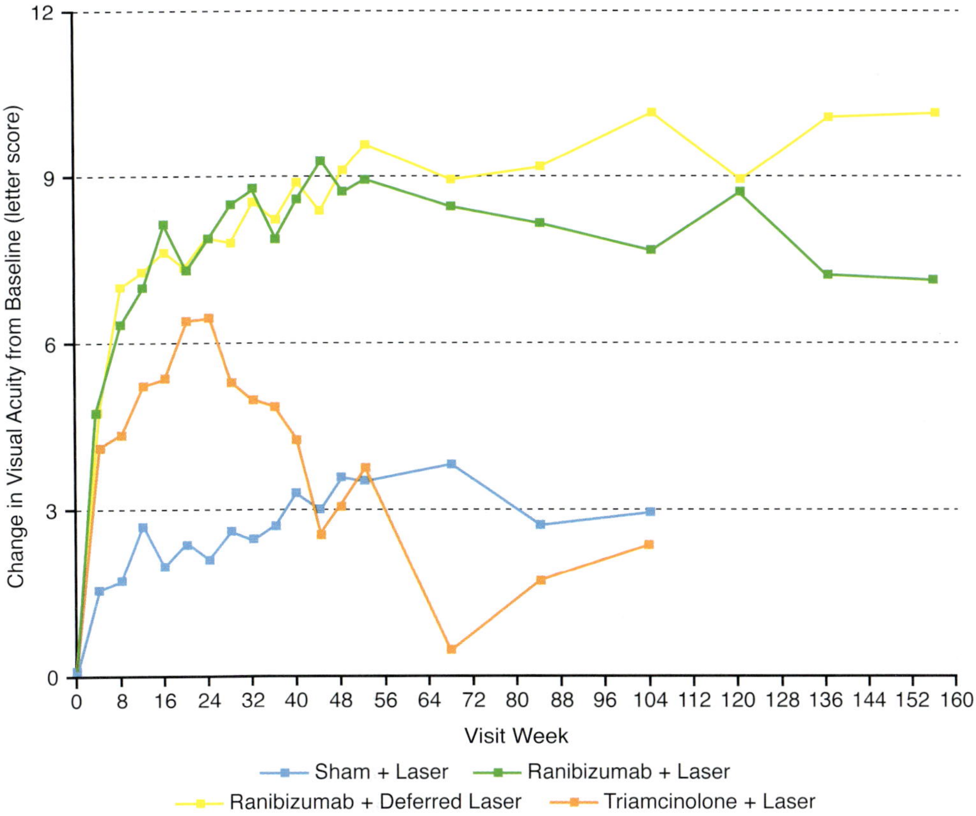

Figure 5-6 Results of the Diabetic Retinopathy Clinical Research Network (DRCR.net) Protocol I through 3 years demonstrating the superior visual acuity outcomes of treatment with ranibizumab, with either prompt or deferred laser treatment, compared with laser alone or in combination with triamcinolone through 2 years. In the third year, only patients originally assigned to a ranibizumab group were followed up. Treatment with ranibizumab plus prompt laser therapy proved to be no better and possibly worse than ranibizumab with deferred laser treatment. *(From Diabetic Retinopathy Clinical Research Network, Elman MJ, Qin H, Aiello LP, et al. Intravitreal ranibizumab for diabetic macular edema with prompt versus deferred laser treatment: three-year randomized trial results.* Ophthalmology. *2012;119(11):2312–2318.)*

center-involving DME when ranibizumab is an available treatment alternative. DRCR.net Protocol T is a study comparing effectiveness of aflibercept, bevacizumab, and ranibizumab for the treatment of DME. The agents had overall similar clinical efficacy; however, aflibercept treatment resulted in a statistically significant 2-letter ETDRS visual acuity gain beyond that with ranibizumab treatment.

CORTICOSTEROIDS Use of intravitreal triamcinolone acetonide in patients with refractory DME has been reported to have beneficial effects in a number of small series. However, at 2 years into the DRCR.net Protocol B trial, treatment with focal/grid photocoagulation was found to be more effective and had fewer adverse effects than 1-mg or 4-mg doses of preservative-free intravitreal triamcinolone. DRCR.net Protocol I also showed that at 2 years, treatment with intravitreal triamcinolone acetonide in combination with laser was substantially inferior to treatment with ranibizumab with or without laser, as well as to laser alone.

Diabetic Retinopathy Clinical Research Network (DRCR.net), Beck RW, Edwards AR, Aiello LP, et al. Three-year follow-up of a randomized trial comparing focal/grid photocoagulation and intravitreal triamcinolone for diabetic macular edema. *Arch Ophthalmol.* 2009;127(3):245–251.

Diabetic Retinopathy Clinical Research Network, Elman MJ, Aiello LP, Beck RW, et al. Randomized trial evaluating ranibizumab plus prompt or deferred laser or triamcinolone plus prompt laser for diabetic macular edema. *Ophthalmology.* 2010;117(6): 1064–1077.

Diabetic Retinopathy Clinical Research Network, Elman MJ, Qin H, Aiello LP, et al. Intravitreal ranibizumab for diabetic macular edema with prompt versus deferred laser treatment: three-year randomized trial results. *Ophthalmology.* 2012;119(11):2312–2318.

Gillies MC, Sutter FK, Simpson JM, Larsson J, Ali H, Zhu M. Intravitreal triamcinolone for refractory diabetic macular edema: two-year results of a double-masked, placebo-controlled, randomized clinical trial. *Ophthalmology.* 2006;113(9):1533–1538.

Ho AC, Scott IU, Kim SJ, et al. Anti–vascular endothelial growth factor pharmacotherapy for diabetic macular edema: a report by the American Academy of Ophthalmology. *Ophthalmology.* 2012;119(10):2179–2188.

Surgical management of diabetic macular edema In the management of DME, laser surgery is a well-proven treatment with very good efficacy, whereas the exact role of vitrectomy continues to evolve.

LASER TREATMENT OF DME The ETDRS demonstrated a treatment benefit in eyes with CSME that underwent treatment with focal- or grid-pattern macular argon laser photocoagulation (macular laser) compared with a similar control group of untreated eyes. The primary outcome measurement in the ETDRS was moderate visual loss (MVL) between baseline and follow-up examinations. MVL was defined as a doubling of the visual angle (eg, decline to 20/40 from 20/20 or 20/100 from 20/50), a decrease of 15 or more letters on an ETDRS visual acuity chart, or a decrease of 3 or more lines of Snellen visual acuity equivalent. Laser photocoagulation treatment of CSME reduced the risk of MVL, increased the chance of visual improvement, and was associated with only minor visual field loss. Eyes with less than CSME showed no treatment benefit over controls at 2 years.

In clinical practice, laser treatment of such eyes can be delayed until progression of edema threatens the center of the macula.

The ETDRS also demonstrated that subretinal fibrosis occurred less often in laser-treated eyes than in untreated control eyes. Subretinal fibrosis, a sheetlike retinal pigment epithelial metaplasia, was associated with the presence and severity of hard exudates in the macula. Table 5-1 lists the adverse effects of photocoagulation for macular edema.

Clinical features associated with poorer visual acuity outcomes after photocoagulation treatment for DME include the following:

- diffuse macular edema with center (foveal) involvement
- macular ischemia (extensive perifoveal capillary nonperfusion)
- hard exudates in the fovea

The patient's fluorescein angiogram along with OCT thickness map is used to guide laser treatment for CSME. Laser parameters typically used include spot sizes of 50–100 µm and burn durations of 0.1 second or less. For focal leakage, direct laser treatment using green or yellow wavelengths is applied to all leaking microaneurysms between 500 and 3000 µm from the center of the macula, with the goal of whitening or darkening them.

For diffuse leakage or zones of capillary nonperfusion adjacent to the macula, a light-intensity grid pattern can be applied. Burns are typically separated by 1 burn width, and green- or yellow-wavelength laser is used. Treatment should include areas of diffuse leakage more than 500 µm from the center of the macula and 500 µm from the temporal margin of the optic disc. Sub–threshold-intensity burns may be effective and may reduce retinal pigment epithelial and choroidal atrophy. Treatment sessions repeated over many months are frequently necessary for resolution of DME.

Early Treatment Diabetic Retinopathy Study Research Group. Treatment techniques and clinical guidelines for photocoagulation of diabetic macular edema. ETDRS report number 2. *Ophthalmology.* 1987;94(7):761–774.

PARS PLANA VITRECTOMY FOR DME Pars plana vitrectomy with detachment of the posterior hyaloid may also be useful for treating DME, particularly when there is evidence of posterior hyaloidal traction and diffuse DME. The DRCR.net Protocol D was a prospective observational case series that confirmed that after vitrectomy, retinal thickening was reduced in most eyes; however, median visual acuity remained unchanged over the 6-month follow-up period. Hence, the exact role of vitrectomy in the treatment of DME remains to be determined.

Table 5-1 Focal Laser Photocoagulation: Adverse Effects and Complications

Paracentral scotomata
Transient increase of edema/decrease in vision
Photocoagulation scar expansion
Subretinal fibrosis at site of laser scar
Choroidal neovascularization
Inadvertent foveolar burns

Used with permission from Kim JW, Ai E. Diabetic retinopathy. In: Regillo CD, Brown GC, Flynn HW Jr, eds. *Vitreoretinal Disease: The Essentials.* New York: Thieme; 1999:147. ©Thieme.

Diabetic Retinopathy Clinical Research Network Writing Committee; Haller JA, Qin H, Apte RS, et al. Vitrectomy outcomes in eyes with diabetic macular edema and vitreomacular traction. *Ophthalmology.* 2010;117(6):1087–1093.

Kaiser PK, Riemann CD, Sears JE, Lewis H. Macular traction detachment and diabetic macular edema associated with posterior hyaloidal traction. *Am J Ophthalmol.* 2001;131(1):44–49.

Diabetic Macular Ischemia

Retinal capillary nonperfusion is a feature commonly associated with moderate to severe NPDR. Fluorescein angiography can reveal the extent of capillary nonperfusion. The foveal avascular zone may gradually appear irregular and enlarged as the innermost capillaries become nonperfused. Microaneurysms may cluster along the borders of zones of capillary nonperfusion. Closure of retinal arterioles may result in larger areas of nonperfusion and progressive ischemia. Foveal avascular zones greater than 1000 µm in diameter generally correlate with central vision loss.

Severe Nonproliferative Diabetic Retinopathy

To help clinicians identify patients at greatest risk of progression to PDR and high-risk PDR, the ETDRS investigators developed the 4:2:1 rule, which is largely based on results from the ETRDS Report 9 (see Clinical Trial 5-3). Severe NPDR was defined as having any 1 of the following features:

- severe intraretinal hemorrhages and microaneurysms in *4* quadrants (Fig 5-7)
- venous beading in *2* or more quadrants (Fig 5-8)
- IRMAs in *1* or more quadrants (Fig 5-9)

Severe NPDR was found to have a 15% chance of progression to high-risk PDR within 1 year. Very severe NPDR, defined as having 2 or more of these features, increased the chance of progression to high-risk PDR within 1 year to 45%. Patients with severe NPDR or worse should be considered for early treatment with panretinal photocoagulation.

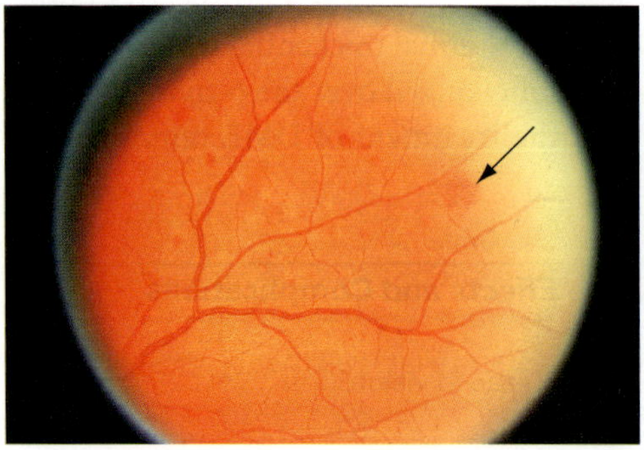

Figure 5-7 Fundus photograph showing diffuse intraretinal hemorrhages *(arrow)* and microaneurysms in nonproliferative diabetic retinopathy (NPDR). *(Standard photograph 2A, courtesy of the ETDRS.)*

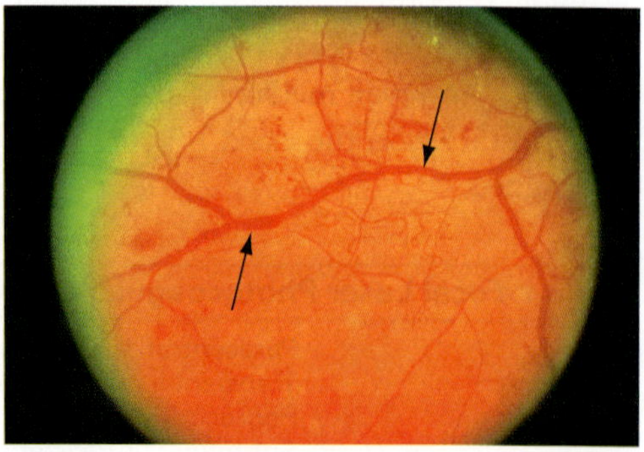

Figure 5-8 Fundus photograph of venous beading in NPDR *(arrows)*. *(Standard photograph 6B, courtesy of the ETDRS.)*

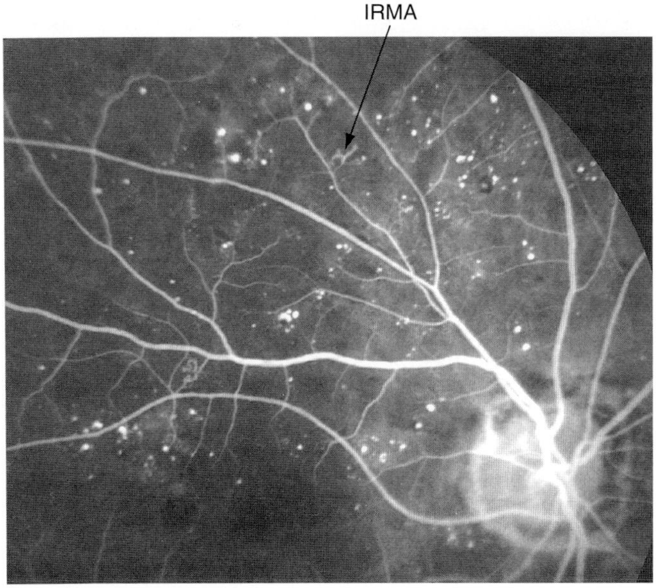

Figure 5-9 Intraretinal microvascular abnormalities (IRMAs) in NPDR. Fluorescein angiography image showing microaneurysms, areas of nonperfusion, and intraretinal capillary remodeling *(arrow)*. *(Courtesy of Hermann D. Schubert, MD.)*

As the retinopathy progresses, capillary damage and nonperfusion increases, worsening retinal ischemia and release of vasoproliferative factors. VEGF is one of the major vasoproliferative factors isolated from vitrectomy specimens of patients with PDR. This factor can stimulate neovascularization of the retina, optic nerve head, or anterior segment.

Aiello LP, Avery RL, Arrigg PG, et al. Vascular endothelial growth factor in ocular fluid of patients with diabetic retinopathy and other retinal disorders. *N Engl J Med.* 1994;331(22): 1480–1487.

Chew EY, Ferris FL III, Csaky KG, et al. The long-term effects of laser photocoagulation treatment in patients with diabetic retinopathy: the early treatment diabetic retinopathy follow-up study. *Ophthalmology.* 2003; 110(9):1683–1689.

Early Treatment Diabetic Retinopathy Study Research Group. Early photocoagulation for diabetic retinopathy. ETDRS report number 9. *Ophthalmology.* 1991;98(5 suppl): 766–785.

Proliferative Diabetic Retinopathy

Extraretinal fibrovascular proliferation defines PDR and progresses through 3 stages:

1. Fine new vessels with minimal fibrous tissue cross and extend beyond the ILM.
2. The new vessels increase in size and extent, containing an increased fibrous component.
3. The new vessels regress, leaving residual fibrovascular tissue that uses the posterior hyaloid as a scaffold.

PDR is graded as early, high-risk, or advanced, according to the extent of proliferation. Neovascular proliferation is categorized by location as either on the disc (NVD, neovascularization of the disc) or elsewhere (NVE, neovascularization elsewhere). High-risk PDR was defined in the Diabetic Retinopathy Study (DRS) as having any 1 of the following findings:

- mild NVD with vitreous hemorrhage
- moderate to severe NVD with or without vitreous hemorrhage (≥DRS standard 10A, showing one-fourth to one-third disc area of NVD) (Fig 5-10)
- moderate (one-half disc area) NVE with vitreous hemorrhage (Fig 5-11)

OR any 3 of the 4 following findings:

1. vitreous or preretinal hemorrhage
2. new vessels
3. new vessels located on or near the optic disc
4. moderate to severe extent of new vessels

Advanced diabetic retinopathy is also associated with a risk of cardiovascular disease and its effects, such as myocardial infarction, cerebrovascular accident, diabetic nephropathy, amputation, and death.

Management of Proliferative Diabetic Retinopathy and Its Complications

The management of proliferative diabetic retinopathy is aimed at controlling ischemia and reducing VEGF levels in the eye so that neovascularization can involute or regress. This control can be accomplished with anti-VEGF drugs, or preferably, with ablation of ischemic retina by photocoagulation. Because of the contracture of fibrovascular tissue, treatment may be followed by increased vitreoretinal traction, vitreous hemorrhage,

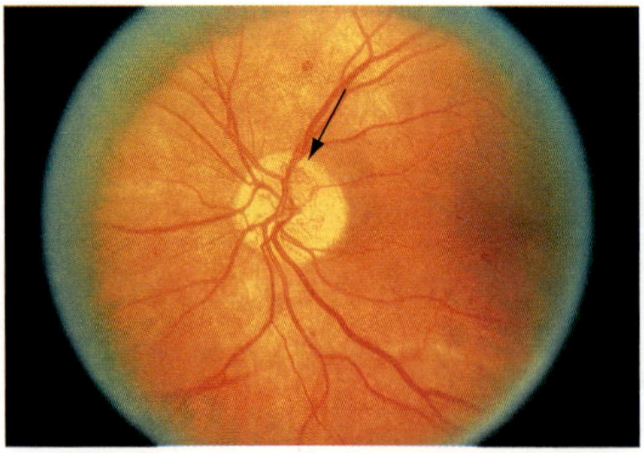

Figure 5-10 Fundus photograph of a left eye demonstrating neovascularization of the disc (NVD, *arrow*) with a small amount of vitreous hemorrhage. Even without vitreous hemorrhage, this degree of NVD is the lower limit of moderate NVD and is considered high-risk PDR. *(Standard photograph 10A, courtesy of the Diabetic Retinopathy Study [DRS].)*

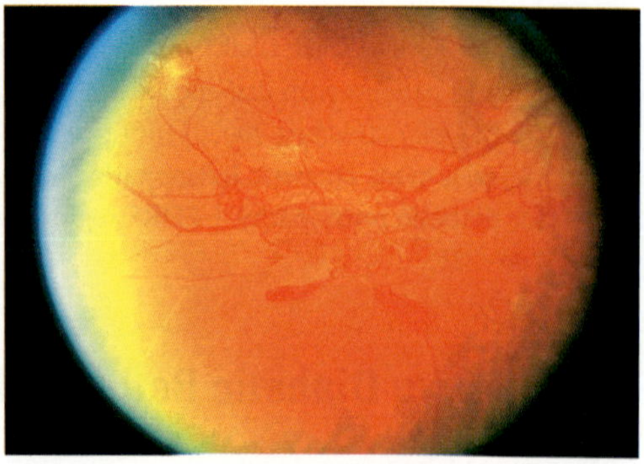

Figure 5-11 Fundus photograph of a right eye showing cotton-wool spots and moderate neovascularization elsewhere (NVE) with preretinal hemorrhage. *(Standard photograph 7, courtesy of the DRS.)*

tractional retinal detachment, and combined tractional and rhegmatogenous retinal detachment. In addition, the contracting fibrovascular tissue and resultant chronic traction can cause recurrent or intermittent vitreous hemorrhages.

The complications of proliferations or their treatment—vitreous hemorrhage and tractional retinal detachment—can be addressed with vitreoretinal surgical interventions, when appropriate.

Nonsurgical management of proliferative diabetic retinopathy

Anti-VEGF drugs Numerous, mostly uncontrolled, studies involving bevacizumab collectively suggest that anti-VEGF drugs may have a role in the management of PDR. Intravitreal anti-VEGF drugs can temporarily decrease leakage and cause regression of diabetic neovascular complexes in newly diagnosed and refractory disease. Anti-VEGF drugs may expedite resolution of vitreous hemorrhage and have been reported to cause regression of anterior segment neovascularization. When administered preoperatively, these drugs may be helpful as an adjunct to vitrectomy for diabetic tractional retinal detachment by reducing intraoperative bleeding and allowing for easier dissection. Potential complications from anti-VEGF drugs in the management of PDR include precipitating tractional retinal detachments, causing retinal tears and combined tractional and rhegmatogenous retinal detachments related to the induced rapid contracture of the fibrovascular tissue. Currently, DRCR.net Protocol S has 305 patients enrolled in a 2-year study comparing treatment with prompt panretinal photocoagulation (PRP) with that of intravitreal ranibizumab and deferred PRP.

Surgical management of proliferative diabetic retinopathy

Laser surgery The mainstay of treatment for PDR is thermal laser photocoagulation in a panretinal pattern to induce regression of neovascularization. The treatment indications are still largely based on findings in the DRS (Clinical Trial 5-4), a pivotal clinical trial. For patients with high-risk PDR, treatment with PRP is almost always recommended. The goal of PRP is regression or involution of neovascularization. PRP destroys ischemic retina and increases oxygen tension in the eye. Ischemic retina is known to produce growth factors, such as VEGF, that promote disease progression. Increased oxygen tension is achieved by 2 mechanisms: decreased consumption resulting from the purposeful retinal destruction, and increased diffusion of oxygen from the choroid in the areas of the photocoagulation scars. Collectively, these changes result in the regression of existing neovascular tissue and prevent progressive neovascularization.

Treatment may be accomplished in a single or over multiple sessions. The DRCR .net found no long-term vision benefit of multiple- over single-session laser administration. However, transient declines in vision occasionally occurred after single-session treatment. The use of automated pattern scan laser systems has been increasing in recent years; these systems possibly have a reduced risk of visual disturbance when complete treatment is provided in a single session. After the initial PRP, additional therapy can be applied incrementally in an attempt to achieve complete regression of persistent or recurrent neovascularization.

Full PRP, as used in the DRS (see Clinical Trial 5-4) and ETDRS (see Clinical Trial 5-3), included 1200 or more 500-μm burns using argon green or blue-green laser,

CLINICAL TRIAL 5-4

Diabetic Retinopathy Study (DRS)

Study question: Is photocoagulation (argon or xenon arc) effective for treating diabetic retinopathy?

Eligibility: PDR or bilateral severe NPDR, with visual acuity 20/100 or better in each eye.

Randomization: 1742 participants: 1 eye randomly assigned to photocoagulation (argon or xenon arc) and 1 eye assigned to no photocoagulation.

Outcome variable: Severe vision loss (SVL), ie, visual acuity less than 5/200 for at least 4 months, at 5 years.

Results: At 5 years of follow-up, eyes treated with PRP had a reduction of 50% or more in rates of SVL compared with untreated control eyes. Thus, photocoagulation (argon or xenon) reduces risk of SVL compared with no treatment. Treated eyes with high-risk PDR achieved the greatest benefit (Fig 5-12). Complications of argon laser PRP in the DRS were generally mild but included a decrease in visual acuity by 1 or more lines in 11% and visual field loss in 5%.

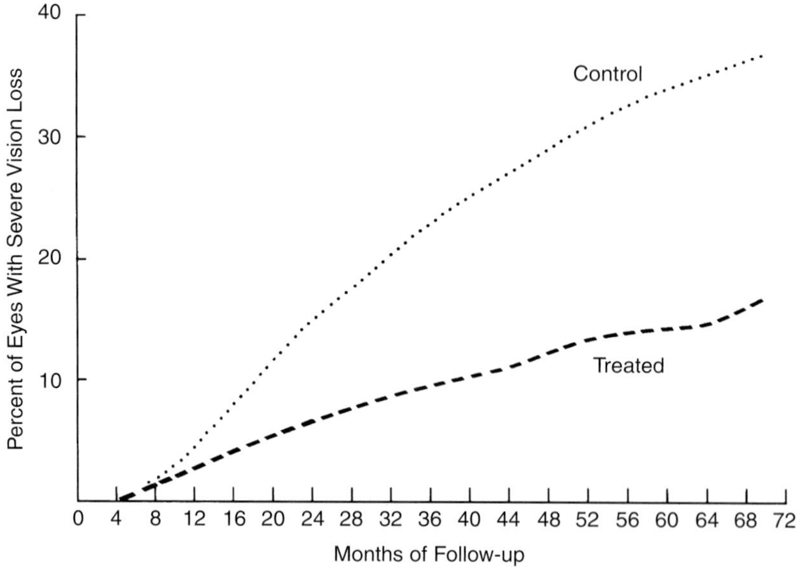

Figure 5-12 Comparison of treated versus control groups showing cumulative percentage of eyes experiencing severe vision loss during the period of follow-up in the Diabetic Retinopathy Study for argon laser and xenon arc treatment groups combined. *(From Diabetic Retinopathy Study Research Group (DRS). Photocoagulation treatment of proliferative diabetic retinopathy. Clinical application of Diabetic Retinopathy Study findings. DRS report number 8.* Ophthalmology. *1981;88(7):583–600.)*

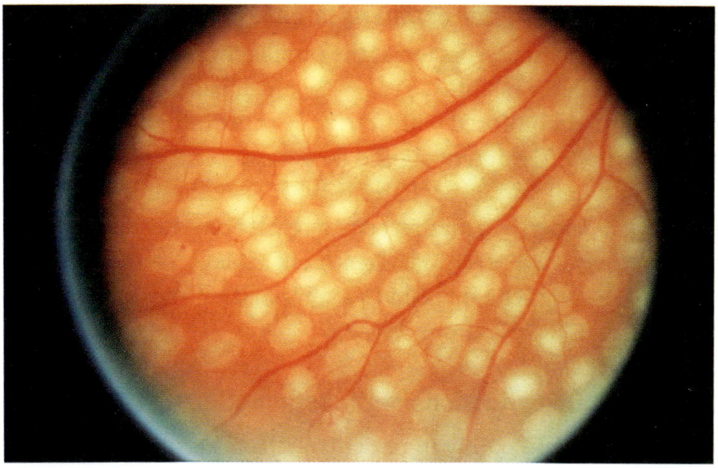

Figure 5-13 Fundus photograph showing full-scatter panretinal photocoagulation (PRP) treatment used in the DRS and the ETDRS. Included are 1200 or more 500-µm burns, separated by one-half burn width. The burns in this photograph are brighter than they would appear during treatment because the image was taken immediately following the laser session. Several spots have a surrounding ring of edema, making many of the burns appear confluent. *(Courtesy of Harry W. Flynn, Jr, MD.)*

separated from each other by one-half burn width (Fig 5-13). Uncontrolled studies have demonstrated that pattern scan laser treatments may not be equivalent in their treatment effect on a burn-for-burn comparison; the burn-count target for equivalent treatment effect with pattern scan laser treatment may need to be higher.

Adverse effects of scatter PRP include decreases in night vision, color vision, contrast sensitivity, peripheral vision, and rarely pupillary dilation. Some patients may experience a transient loss of 1 or 2 lines of visual acuity or increased glare following treatment. Other transient adverse effects include loss of accommodation, loss of corneal sensitivity, and photopsias. Macular edema may also be precipitated or worsened by PRP. Sparing the horizontal meridians, that is, the path of the long ciliary vessels and nerves, protects accommodation pupillary function and corneal innervation. Heavy treatment, when necessary, should be performed in areas of the retina where vision loss is less noticed by patients or that are associated with less morbidity. In particular, the lightest treatment should be in the nasal and superior retina, as those areas correspond to important temporal and inferior peripheral vision. Great care must be taken to avoid foveal photocoagulation, especially when using image-inverting lenses.

Diabetic Retinopathy Clinical Research Network; Brucker AJ, Qin H, Antoszyk AN, et al. Observational study of the development of diabetic macular edema following panretinal (scatter) photocoagulation given in 1 or 4 sittings. *Arch Ophthalmol.* 2009;127(2):132–140.

Diabetic Retinopathy Study Research Group. Photocoagulation treatment of proliferative diabetic retinopathy. Clinical application of Diabetic Retinopathy Study (DRS) findings, DRS report number 8. *Ophthalmology.* 1981;88(7):583–600.

Early Treatment Diabetic Retinopathy Study Research Group. Early photocoagulation for diabetic retinopathy. ETDRS report number 9. *Ophthalmology.* 1991;98(5 suppl):766–785.

Management of neovascularization of the iris or anterior chamber angle

Small, isolated tufts of neovascularization at the pupillary border are relatively common in eyes of patients with diabetes mellitus. Eyes with small, isolated tufts can have treatment withheld and be carefully monitored with relatively short intervals between slit-lamp and gonioscopic examinations. Treatment should be considered in eyes with contiguous neovascularization of the pupil and iris collarette, with or without inclusion of the anterior chamber angle, and if wide-field fluorescein angiography reveals widespread nonperfusion or peripheral neovascularization. Treatment usually consists of PRP. Intravitreal injection of anti-VEGF drugs can be used as a temporizing measure to reduce neovascularization until definitive PRP is administered.

Vitrectomy Surgery for Complications of Diabetic Retinopathy

Indications for pars plana vitrectomy in patients with diabetes mellitus are

- nonclearing (>1–6 months) vitreous hemorrhage
- tractional retinal detachment involving or threatening the macula
- combined tractional and rhegmatogenous retinal detachment
- diffuse DME associated with posterior hyaloidal traction
- significant recurrent vitreous hemorrhage despite use of maximal PRP
- red blood cell–induced (erythroclastic) glaucoma and “ghost cell” glaucoma
- anterior segment neovascularization with media opacities preventing PRP
- dense premacular subhyaloid hemorrhage

Vitreous hemorrhage

The Diabetic Retinopathy Vitrectomy Study (DRVS) was a prospective, randomized clinical trial investigating the role of vitrectomy in managing eyes with severe PDR. Outcome measurements were the percentages of eyes with 10/20 and 10/50 visual acuity at 2- and 4-year follow-ups. Benefits of early (1–6 months after onset of vitreous hemorrhage) versus late (1 year after onset) vitrectomy were evaluated. Eyes of patients with type 1 diabetes mellitus and severe vitreous hemorrhage clearly demonstrated a benefit from earlier vitrectomy, whereas eyes in patients with type 2 or mixed diabetes did not. Early vitrectomy was superior to conventional management for eyes with very severe PDR.

If PRP has not been performed previously, earlier intervention is usually recommended. Patients with previous, well-placed, complete PRP who have vitreous hemorrhage secondary to PDR may be observed for a longer period of time prior to initiating intervention. Frequent echography (ultrasound) studies are necessary to monitor for retinal detachment in patients with dense, nonclearing vitreous hemorrhage. If a retinal detachment is discovered, the timing of vitrectomy depends upon detachment characteristics. Patients with bilateral severe vitreous hemorrhage should undergo vitrectomy in 1 eye as soon as possible for visual rehabilitation.

Advances in vitreoretinal surgery have led to the modification of surgical indications beyond the DRVS results. These advances include the routine use of intraocular endolaser, perioperative anti-VEGF injections, and smaller-gauge instrumentation. Collectively, they have led to reduced surgical morbidity, facilitating earlier intervention.

Diabetic Retinopathy Vitrectomy Study Research Group. Early vitrectomy for severe proliferative diabetic retinopathy in eyes with useful vision. Results of a randomized trial—Diabetic Retinopathy Vitrectomy Study report 3. *Ophthalmology.* 1988;95(10):1307–1320.

Diabetic Retinopathy Vitrectomy Study Research Group. Early vitrectomy for severe vitreous hemorrhage in diabetic retinopathy. Two-year results of a randomized trial. Diabetic Retinopathy Vitrectomy Study report 2. *Arch Ophthalmol.* 1985;103(11):1644–1652.

Recchia FM, Scott IU, Brown GC, Brown MM, Ho AC, Ip MS. Small-gauge pars plana vitrectomy: a report by the American Academy of Ophthalmology. *Ophthalmology.* 2010;117(9): 1851–1857.

Tractional retinal detachment

Complications from PDR are exacerbated by vitreous attachment to and traction on fibrovascular proliferative tissue, often elevating the retina. Partial posterior vitreous detachment frequently develops in eyes with fibrovascular proliferation, resulting in traction on the new vessels and vitreous or preretinal hemorrhage. Tractional complications such as vitreous hemorrhage, retinal schisis, retinal detachment, or macular heterotopia may ensue, as may progressive fibrovascular proliferation. Contraction of the fibrovascular proliferation and vitreous may result in retinal breaks and subsequent rhegmatogenous retinal detachment. The presence of chronic retinal detachment in eyes with PDR contributes to retinal ischemia and may account for the increased risk of anterior segment neovascularization in such eyes.

Tractional retinal detachment not involving the macula may remain stable for many years. When the macula becomes involved, prompt vitrectomy is generally recommended. Combined tractional and rhegmatogenous retinal detachment may progress rapidly, and urgent surgery should be considered for these patients.

A more extensive discussion of the surgical management of tractional retinal detachments secondary to PDR appears in Chapter 19.

Silva PAS, Cavallerano JD, Sun JK, et al. Proliferative diabetic retinopathy. In: Ryan SJ, Schachat AP, Wilkinson CP, Hinton DR, Sadda SR, Wiedemann P, eds. *Retina.* 5th ed. Philadelphia: Elsevier/Saunders; 2013:969–1000.

Cataract Surgery in Patients With Diabetes Mellitus

Patients with diabetes mellitus enrolled in the ETDRS who underwent cataract surgery usually had improved visual acuity postoperatively. However, various studies suggest that diabetic retinopathy may progress after cataract surgery. In DRCR.net Protocol P, patients with NPDR but no history of DME were found to have a substantial risk of postoperative DME. Protocol Q enrolled patients with preexisting DME, and as many as half of the eyes had either no meaningful improvement or worsening of visual acuity. Only a small percentage of eyes had substantial visual acuity loss or definitive worsening in central retinal thickening. Therefore, in clinical practice, it is common and appropriate for patients with CSME about to undergo cataract surgery to receive an anti-VEGF drug injection preoperatively or steroid injection perioperatively.

Patients with severe NPDR or PDR should be considered for scatter photocoagulation before undergoing cataract removal if the ocular media are sufficiently clear to allow for treatment. If the density of the cataract precludes adequate evaluation of the retina or treatment, prompt postoperative retinal evaluation and treatment are recommended. In general, all patients with preexisting diabetic retinopathy should be reevaluated after cataract surgery.

Cataract surgeons should be mindful of the need for regular retinal evaluations and the possibility of future surgical interventions in eyes of patients with diabetes mellitus; thus, they need to plan capsulorrhexis accordingly to avoid capsular phimosis and a resultant, very small, anterior capsular opening that may limit the view of the posterior segment. Anticipating the possible need for future vitrectomy, the cataract surgeon should avoid the use of silicone lenses in these eyes because fluid condensation interferes with visualization during air-exchange procedures, and silicone oil tamponade results in implant opacification.

BCSC Section 11, *Lens and Cataract,* briefly discusses considerations the cataract surgeon must take into account in patients with diabetes mellitus.

Diabetic Retinopathy Clinical Research Network Authors/Writing Committee; Baker CW, Almukhtar T, Bressler NM, et al. Macular edema after cataract surgery in eyes without preoperative central-involved diabetic macular edema. *JAMA Ophthalmol.* 2013;131(7): 870–879.

Diabetic Retinopathy Clinical Research Network Authors/Writing Committee; Bressler SB, Baker CW, Almukhtar T, et al. Pilot study of individuals with diabetic macular edema undergoing cataract surgery. *JAMA Ophthalmol.* 2014;132(2):224–226.

Recommended Diabetes-Related Ophthalmic Examinations

In the first 5 years following diagnosis of type 1 diabetes mellitus, retinopathy is rare. By contrast, at the time of initial diagnosis of type 2 diabetes mellitus, a large percentage of patients have established retinopathy and require concomitant ophthalmic examination. Because pregnancy poses a risk of diabetic retinopathy progression, an eye examination is recommended in the first trimester and thereafter at the discretion of the ophthalmologist (Table 5-2). The frequency of follow-up visits depends on the

Table 5-2 Recommended Eye Examination Schedule for Patients With Diabetes Mellitus

Diabetes Type	Recommended Time of First Eye Examination	Routine Minimum Follow-up Interval
Type 1	5 years after diagnosis	Annually
Type 2	Upon diagnosis	Annually
Type 1 or 2 and Pregnancy	Soon after conception or early in first trimester	No retinopathy to mild or moderate NPDR: every 3–12 months Severe NPDR or worse: every 1–3 months

NPDR = nonproliferative diabetic retinopathy.

Modified from American Academy of Ophthalmology Retina/Vitreous Panel. Preferred Practice Pattern Guidelines. *Diabetic Retinopathy.* San Francisco: American Academy of Ophthalmology; 2014. Available at http://one.aao.org/guidelines.

severity of the retinopathy, history of blood glucose levels, and blood pressure control, as well as the threat to visual function from potentially missed opportunities to treat (Table 5-3).

American Academy of Ophthalmology Retina/Vitreous Panel. Preferred Practice Pattern Guidelines. *Diabetic Retinopathy.* San Francisco: American Academy of Ophthalmology; 2014. Available at http://one.aao.org/guidelines.

Table 5-3 Recommended Eye Examination Schedule Based on Diabetic Retinopathy Severity

Diabetic Retinopathy Severity	Presence of Macular Edema	Suggested Follow-up Interval (months)
Normal or minimal NPDR	No	12
Mild NPDR	No	12
	ME	4–6
	CSME*	1
Moderate NPDR	No	6–12
	ME	3–6
	CSME*	1
Severe NPDR†	No	4
	ME	4
	CSME*	1
Non–high-risk PDR†	No	4
	ME	2–4
	CSME*	1
High-risk PDR†	No	4
	ME	4
	CSME*	1
Inactive/involuted PDR	No	6–12
	Yes*	4

CSME = clinically significant diabetic macular edema; ME = macular edema; NPDR = nonproliferative diabetic retinopathy; PDR = proliferative diabetic retinopathy.

*Consider macular intravitreal anti–vascular endothelial growth factor drug injection.

†Consider panretinal scatter laser surgery.

Modified from American Academy of Ophthalmology Retina/Vitreous Panel. Preferred Practice Pattern Guidelines. *Diabetic Retinopathy.* San Francisco: American Academy of Ophthalmology; 2014. Available at http://one.aao.org/guidelines.

CHAPTER 6

Retinal Vascular Diseases Associated With Cardiovascular Disease

This chapter discusses retinal vascular diseases that are associated, some strongly, some more loosely, with cardiovascular disease. Most of these conditions, however, have additional causes or associations that are important to consider while evaluating patients.

Systemic Arterial Hypertension

Systemic arterial hypertension affects more than 65 million people in the United States. It is currently defined by a series of stages: prehypertension encompasses blood pressure readings of 120–139 mm Hg systolic or 80–89 mm Hg diastolic; stage 1 hypertension includes readings of 140–159 mm Hg systolic or 90–99 mm Hg diastolic pressure; and stage 2 hypertension is 160 mm Hg or higher systolic and 100 mm Hg or higher diastolic pressure.

Together with heart, kidneys, and brain, the eye is a target organ of systemic hypertension. Ocular effects of hypertension can be observed in the retina, choroid, and optic nerve. Retinal changes can be described and classified using ophthalmoscopy and angiography. Recognition of the posterior segment vascular changes by the ophthalmologist may prompt the initial diagnosis of hypertension and alert the patient to potential complications from this condition. BCSC Section 1, *Update on General Medicine,* discusses hypertension in more detail.

Kim SK, Mieler WF, Jakobiec F. Hypertension and its ocular manifestations. In: Albert DM, Miller JW, Azar DT, Blodi BA, eds. *Albert & Jakobiec's Principles and Practice of Ophthalmology.* 3rd ed. Philadelphia: Saunders; 2008:4367–4384.

Hypertensive Retinopathy

Hypertension affects precapillary arterioles and capillaries, the anatomical loci of autoregulation and nonperfusion. An acute hypertensive episode may produce focal intraretinal periarteriolar transudates (FIPTs) at the precapillary level. The presence of cotton-wool spots (sometimes referred to as *soft exudates*) indicates ischemia of the retinal nerve fiber layer (Fig 6-1). Uncontrolled systemic hypertension leads to nonperfusion at various

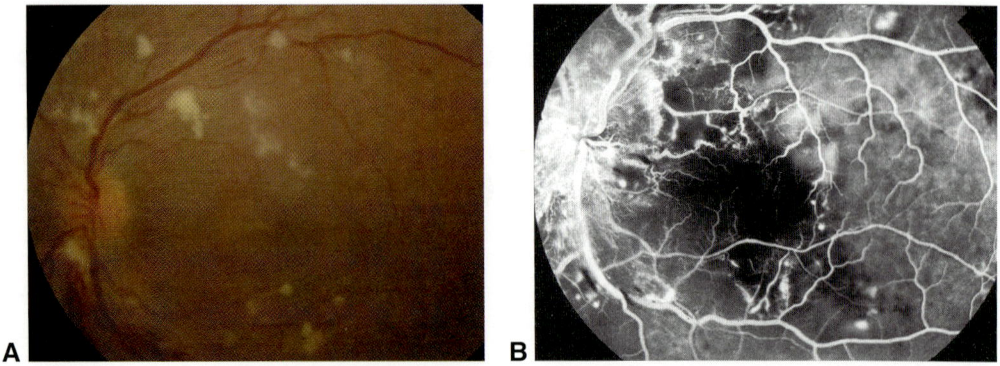

Figure 6-1 Severe hypertensive retinopathy. **A,** Fundus photograph from a 25-year-old man with renal hypertension showing large superficial and white cotton-wool spots contrasting with small, tan, and deep focal intraretinal periarteriolar transudates (FIPTs). **B,** The angiography image shows areas of nonperfusion corresponding to the cotton-wool spots and punctuate hyperfluorescence corresponding to the FIPTs. *(Courtesy of Hermann D. Schubert, MD.)*

retinal levels and to neuronal loss and related scotomata. Other, more chronic, hypertensive retinal lesions include microaneurysms, intraretinal microvascular abnormalities (IRMAs), blot hemorrhages, lipid exudates (sometimes referred to as *hard exudates*) venous beading, and new retinal vessels. The relationship between hypertensive vascular changes and the changes of arteriosclerotic vascular disease is complex, with wide variation related to duration of hypertension, severity of dyslipidemia, age, and history of smoking. Hence, classification of retinal vascular changes caused strictly by hypertension is difficult, and the often-cited focal arteriolar narrowing and arterial venous nicking have been shown to have little predictive value for actual hypertension. Nonetheless, one historical classification of mostly arteriolosclerotic retinopathy is the Modified Scheie Classification of Hypertensive Retinopathy:

Grade 0	No changes
Grade 1	Barely detectable arterial narrowing
Grade 2	Obvious arterial narrowing with focal irregularities
Grade 3	Grade 2 plus retinal hemorrhages and/or exudates
Grade 4	Grade 3 plus disc swelling

Hypertension may be complicated by branch retinal artery occlusion (BRAO), branch retinal vein occlusion (BRVO), central retinal vein occlusion (CRVO), and retinal arterial macroaneurysms (all discussed later in the chapter). The coexistence of hypertension and diabetes mellitus results in more severe retinopathy because precapillary and capillary insults act in combination.

Cheung CYL, Wong TY. Hypertension. In: Ryan SJ, Schachat AP, Wilkinson CP, Hinton DR, Sadda SR, Wiedemann P, eds. *Retina.* 5th ed. Philadelphia: Elsevier/Saunders; 2013: 1001–1005.

Wong TY, Mitchell P. The eye in hypertension. *Lancet.* 2007;369(9559):425–435.

Hypertensive Choroidopathy

Hypertensive choroidopathy typically occurs in young patients who experience an episode of acute, severe hypertension associated with preeclampsia, eclampsia, pheochromocytoma, or renal hypertension (see also Chapter 9). Lobular nonperfusion of the choriocapillaris may occur and initially results in tan, lobule-sized patches that, in time, become hyperpigmented and surrounded by margins of hypopigmentation—lesions known as *Elschnig spots* (Fig 6-2). Linear configurations of similar-appearing hyperpigmentations known as *Siegrist streaks* follow the meridional course of choroidal arteries. Fluorescein angiography shows focal choroidal hypoperfusion in the early phases and multiple subretinal areas of leakage in the late phases (Fig 6-3). Focal retinal pigment epithelium (RPE) detachments may occur, and extensive bilateral exudative retinal detachments may develop in severe cases.

Hypertensive Optic Neuropathy

Depending less on the degree than on the chronicity of the hypertension, hypertensive optic neuropathy has a variable presentation. Patients with severe hypertension may have linear peripapillary flame-shaped hemorrhages, blurring of the disc margins, florid disc edema with secondary retinal venous stasis, and macular exudates (Fig 6-4). The differential diagnosis for patients with this clinical appearance includes diabetic papillopathy, radiation papillopathy, CRVO, anterior ischemic optic neuropathy, and neuroretinitis. Treatment of systemic arterial hypertension is essential for reducing or reversing these ocular manifestations of the disease.

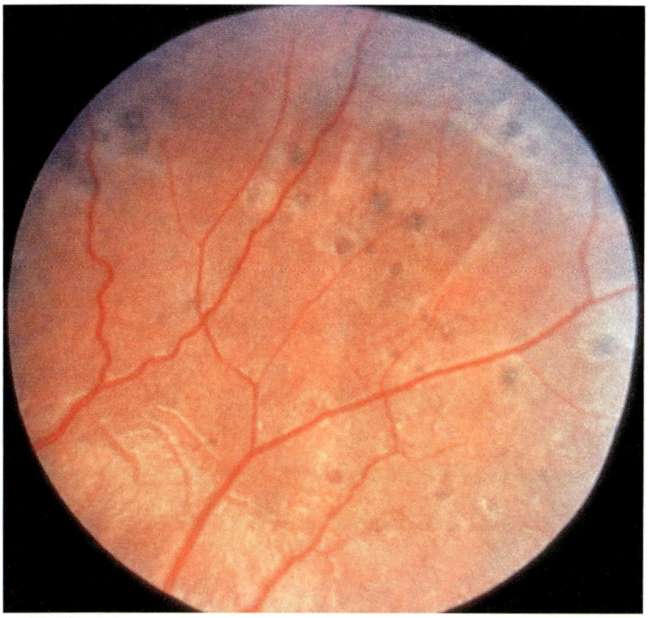

Figure 6-2 Fundus photograph showing Elschnig spots. *(Courtesy of Harry W. Flynn, Jr, MD.)*

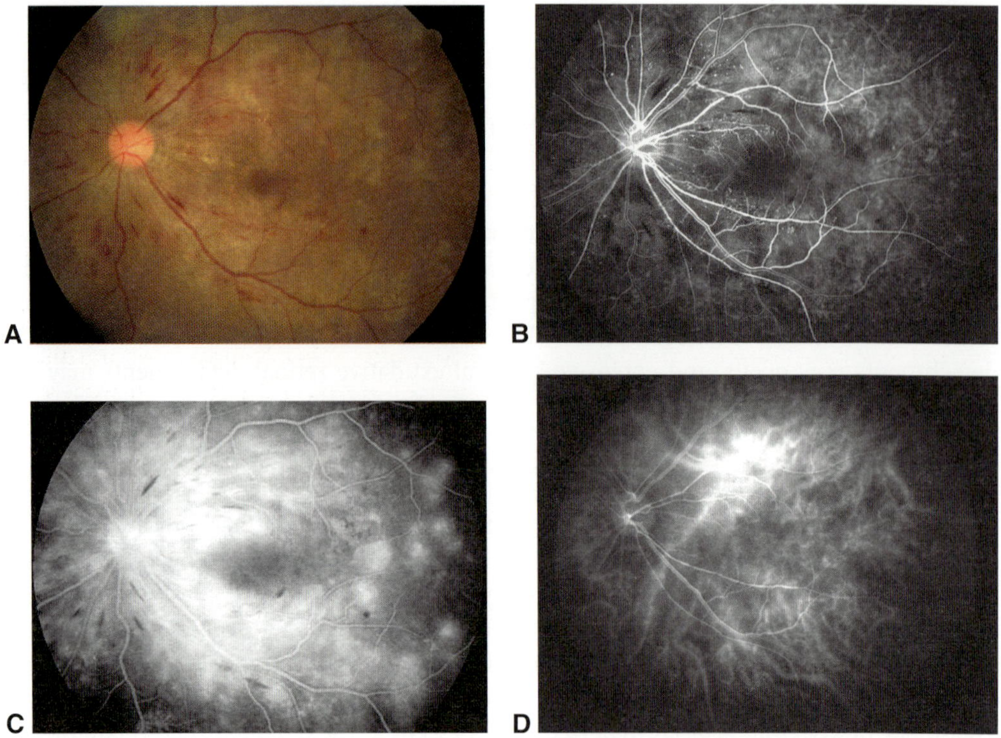

Figure 6-3 Malignant hypertension. **A,** Color fundus photograph of hypertensive retinopathy with shallow detachment of the macula, striae of the internal limiting membrane, splinter hemorrhages in the radial peripapillary net, hyperemia of the optic nerve, and a few lipid exudates in the macula. Multiple tan patches at the level of the retinal pigment epithelium (RPE) and inner choroid are due to hypertensive choroidopathy. **B,** Early fluorescein angiography image revealing retinal capillary nonperfusion, microaneurysms, and choroidal filling defects. **C,** Late angiography image showing intense vascular leakage as well as leakage from patches of hypertensive choroidopathy. **D,** Early indocyanine green (ICG) angiography image showing a "moth-eaten" appearance of the choriocapillaris. *(Courtesy of Richard Spaide, MD.)*

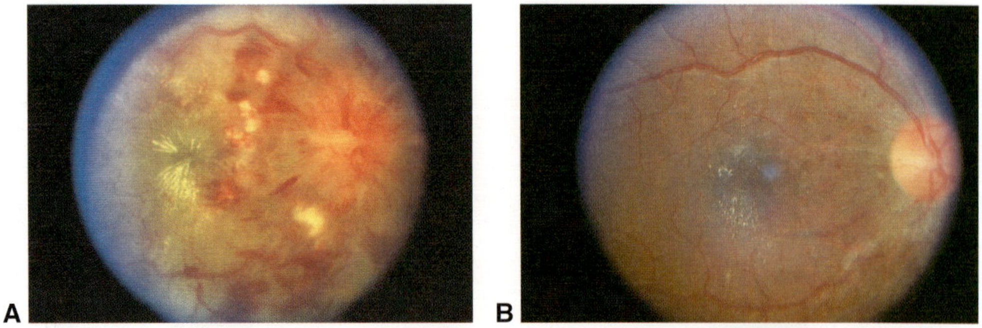

Figure 6-4 Severe hypertensive retinopathy with improvement. **A,** Fundus photograph from a 25-year-old patient with severe hypertension (210/140 mm Hg) and visual acuity loss to the 2/200 level. Note the disc edema, macular exudates, intraretinal hemorrhage with nerve fiber layer (NFL) infarct, and venous congestion. **B,** Fundus photograph from the same patient 10 weeks later, after treatment of hypertension and normalization of blood pressure. The optic disc is now normal, and minimal residual macular exudates are present. The visual acuity has returned to 20/50. *(Courtesy of Harry W. Flynn, Jr, MD.)*

Retinal Vein Occlusion

Retinal vein occlusion (RVO) is most commonly associated with advancing age and hypertension but also has uncommon or rare associations and causes. As such, evaluation of the patient for cardiovascular disease by an internist, or a search for other causative or predisposing systemic conditions, should be considered.

All RVO patients should undergo a complete ocular examination. BRVO and CRVO share ocular risk factors such as glaucoma, in both the open-angle and angle-closure forms (see also BCSC Section 10, *Glaucoma*). In suspected BRVO, vasculitis must be ruled out.

In both branch and central retinal vein occlusion, elevated retinal venous pressure and reduced blood flow occur. In the affected retina, intraretinal hemorrhages and dilated tortuous retinal vasculature are classic findings, and in severe cases, cotton-wool spots may be present (Fig 6-5). In acute disease, the level of visual acuity impairment depends on the severity of macular ischemia or edema and on the presence or absence of intraretinal hemorrhages affecting the fovea. Macular edema and ischemia are best assessed with optical coherence tomography and fluorescein angiography, respectively.

It is important to monitor cases of RVO for neovascularization. In BRVO, neovascularization most commonly occurs at the border of healthy and affected retina or at the optic nerve. In CRVO, posterior segment neovascularization is rare. Anterior segment neovascularization occurs in both branch and central retinal vein occlusions; however, it

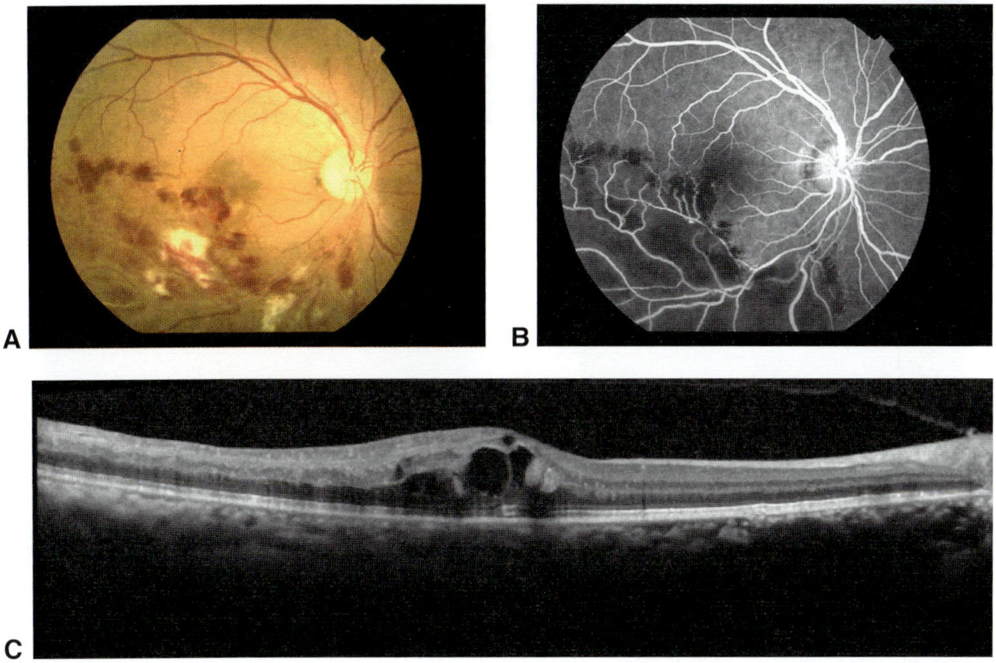

Figure 6-5 Branch retinal vein occlusion (BRVO) with ischemia. **A,** Inferotemporal BRVO. **B,** Fluorescein angiography image corresponding to **A** reveals pronounced retinal capillary nonperfusion in the distribution of the retina drained by the obstructed vein. **C,** Spectral-domain optical coherence tomography (SD-OCT) image of the same eye reveals cystoid macular edema. *(Courtesy of Neal H. Atebara, MD.)*

is a common complication of untreated ischemic CRVO (discussed later in the chapter). As such, undilated iris and gonioscopic angle examinations should be performed periodically in all RVO patients.

Improvement or spontaneous resolution can occur. Improvement is usually associated with the development of collateral blood flow. In BRVO, capillaries that cross the median raphe dilate and—to some degree—compensate for compromised venous drainage. In CRVO, small vessels that normally connect the retinal circulation to the choroidal circulation near the optic disc begin to enlarge, resulting in optociliary shunt vessels. In this way, venous drainage is redirected to the choroid, vortex veins, and superior and inferior ophthalmic veins in the orbit, thereby bypassing the occluded central retinal vein. Chronic, untreated venous occlusive disease commonly leads to development of retinal microvascular changes characterized by microaneurysms and telangiectasias (Fig 6-6).

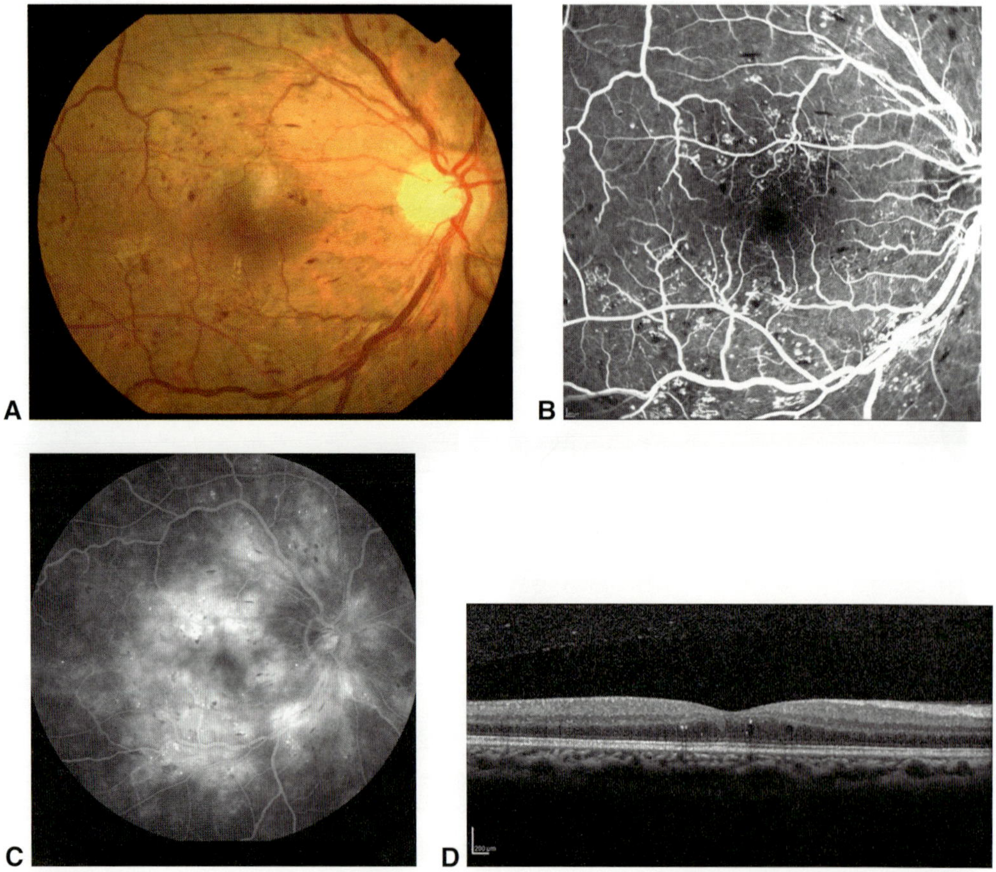

Figure 6-6 Chronic changes from nonischemic central retinal vein occlusion (CRVO) in a 30-year-old woman with a history of diabetes mellitus and blurry vision for 2 months. Visual acuity is 20/25. **A,** Color fundus photograph of a mild nonischemic, or perfused, CRVO. Dilated retinal veins and retinal hemorrhages are present, as are scant macular exudates; however, a foveolar reflex is still present. **B,** Fluorescein angiography image at 22 seconds after injection reveals capillary telangiectasias and microaneurysms throughout the posterior pole. **C,** Late angiogram at 9 minutes reveals diffuse retinal staining and microaneurysms. **D,** OCT scan reveals mild cystic changes and microaneurysms but minimal retinal thickening. *(Courtesy of Neal H. Atebara, MD.)*

Anti–vascular endothelial growth factor (VEGF) drugs have become the mainstay of RVO treatment because of their excellent efficacy and safety profiles. Best visual acuity outcomes are achieved by administering anti-VEGF treatment immediately upon diagnosis of RVO-related macular edema. It should be noted that anti-VEGF treatment suppresses neovascular complications of RVO. Intraocular steroid treatments and macular or scatter panretinal photocoagulation are also employed to manage vision loss from, and complications of, RVO.

Specific considerations for branch and central retinal vein occlusion are discussed in the following sections.

Goldman DR, Shah CP, Morley MG, Heier JS. Venous occlusive disease of the retina. In: Yanoff M, Duker JS, eds. *Ophthalmology.* 4th ed. Elsevier/Saunders; 2014: 526–534.

Branch Retinal Vein Occlusion

In BRVO, obstruction of the vein occurs most commonly at an arteriovenous crossing, where thickening of the arterial wall compresses the vein at a site of a common adventitial binding. When the occlusion does not occur at an arteriovenous crossing, the possibility of an underlying retinochoroiditis or retinal vasculitis should be considered. The quadrant most commonly affected is the superotemporal (63%); a clinical finding of nasal vascular occlusion is rare. The artery serving the area of occlusion may become narrowed and sheathed over time.

Risk factors for the development of BRVO

The mean age of patients at the time of occurrence is in the seventh decade. The Eye Disease Case-Control Study identified the following risk factors for the development of BRVO:

- increasing age
- history of systemic arterial hypertension
- history of smoking
- history of glaucoma

Diabetes mellitus was not a major independent risk factor.

Prognosis

In acute disease, the presence or absence of macular or foveal involvement determines the visual prognosis. Prior to the current routine use of pharmacologic intervention, the Branch Vein Occlusion Study (BVOS) determined that extensive retinal ischemia, defined as an area of at least 5 disc diameters in size, may result in neovascularization from the retina or optic nerve in 36% of eyes. Furthermore, vitreous hemorrhage will develop in 60%–90% of such eyes if laser photocoagulation is not performed.

Over the long term, permanent vision loss may be related to macular ischemia, cystoid macular edema, lipid exudates in the fovea (hard exudates), pigmentary macular disturbance, subretinal fibrosis, and epiretinal membrane formation. Less common is loss of vision as the result of vitreous hemorrhage, tractional retinal detachment, or rhegmatogenous retinal detachment. The latter typically develops after a break occurs in the retina adjacent to, or underlying, an area of retinal neovascularization secondary to vitreous traction.

Treatment of BRVO

Pharmacologic management of BRVO A growing arsenal of pharmacologic interventions is available for the management of BRVO.

INTRAVITREAL ANTI-VEGF THERAPY In BRAVO (Study of the Efficacy and Safety of Ranibizumab Injection in Patients With Macular Edema Secondary to Branch Retinal Vein Occlusion), *ranibizumab* was injected into eyes with BRVO with macular edema. At 6 months, after monthly injections of either 0.5- or 0.3-mg ranibizumab or monthly sham injections, overall results indicated 61.1%, 55.2%, and 28.8% of eyes gained 15 or more ETDRS (Early Treatment of Diabetic Retinopathy Study) letters, respectively. Similarly, roughly twice as many eyes receiving *aflibercept* injections gained 15 or more ETDRS letters compared with sham treatment (53% versus 23%) in VIBRANT (Study to Assess the Clinical Efficacy and Safety of VEGF Trap-Eye in Patients With Branch Retinal Vein Occlusion).

Uncontrolled studies of *bevacizumab* have also demonstrated substantial resolution of macular edema and improvement in visual acuity. In the CRAVE study (Comparison of Anti-VEGF Agents in the Treatment of Macular Edema from Retinal Vein Occlusion), 98 patients were randomized to receive either monthly bevacizumab or ranibizumab treatment for macular edema secondary to central and branch retinal vein occlusions. At the primary endpoint of 6 months, there were no significant differences in central foveal thickness reduction or visual acuity improvement between the treatment groups. In practice, anti–VEGF agent administration strategies for BRVO treatment include monthly dosing, as-needed treatment, and treat-and-extend approaches.

Brown DM, Campochiaro PA, Bhisitkul RB, et al. Sustained benefits from ranibizumab for macular edema following branch retinal vein occlusion: 12-month outcomes of a phase III study. *Ophthalmology.* 2011;118(8):1594–1602.

INTRAVITREAL CORTICOSTEROIDS Specific risks of intravitreal corticosteroids include cataract formation (common) and steroid-induced elevation in intraocular pressure (IOP) (fairly common). These risks must be weighed carefully against benefits and alternative treatments when making care decisions. In the BRVO arm of the SCORE study (Standard Care Versus Corticosteroid for Retinal Vein Occlusion), *intravitreal triamcinolone* injection was found to be comparable in efficacy to macular grid laser treatment with respect to 3 or more lines of visual acuity gain. Because eyes receiving triamcinolone were more likely to develop a cataract or experience elevated IOP, the study investigators pointed out that macular grid laser therapy remains the benchmark against which other treatments should be compared.

In the GENEVA study (Randomized, Sham-Controlled Trial of Dexamethasone Intravitreal Implant in Patients With Macular Edema due to Retinal Vein Occlusion), a *dexamethasone* (0.7-mg) intravitreal implant was used for the treatment of macular edema secondary to venous occlusive disease. Compared with sham-injection eyes, this treatment resulted in a significantly greater percentage of eyes gaining at least a 15-letter improvement. The effect was greater in CRVO eyes than in BRVO eyes. Trials are under way to evaluate efficacy of an injectable *fluocinolone* sustained-delivery implant over 36 months.

Haller JA, Bandello F, Belfort R Jr, et al; OZURDEX GENEVA Study Group. Randomized, sham-controlled trial of dexamethasone intravitreal implant in patients with macular edema due to retinal vein occlusion. *Ophthalmology.* 2010;117(6):1134–1146.

Scott IU, Ip MS, VanVeldhuisen PC, et al; SCORE Study Research Group. A randomized trial comparing the efficacy and safety of intravitreal triamcinolone with standard care to treat vision loss associated with macular edema secondary to branch retinal vein occlusion: the Standard Care vs Corticosteroid for Retinal Vein Occlusion (SCORE) study report 6. *Arch Ophthalmol.* 2009;127(9):1115–1128.

Surgical management of BRVO A number of laser and other surgical methods have been explored for the treatment of BRVO.

MACULAR LASER SURGERY In this treatment, laser photocoagulation is applied to areas of macular edema caused by the obstructed vein (Fig 6-7). The BVOS found that laser-treated eyes with intact foveal vasculature, macular edema, and visual acuity in the 20/40–20/200 range were more likely to gain 2 lines of visual acuity (65%) than were untreated eyes (37%). Furthermore, at 3-year follow-up, treated eyes were more likely than untreated eyes to have 20/40 or better visual acuity (60% vs 34%, respectively), with a mean visual acuity improvement of 1.3 ETDRS lines versus 0.2 line, respectively. In the BVOS, laser treatment of macular edema was delayed for at least 3 months to permit the maximum

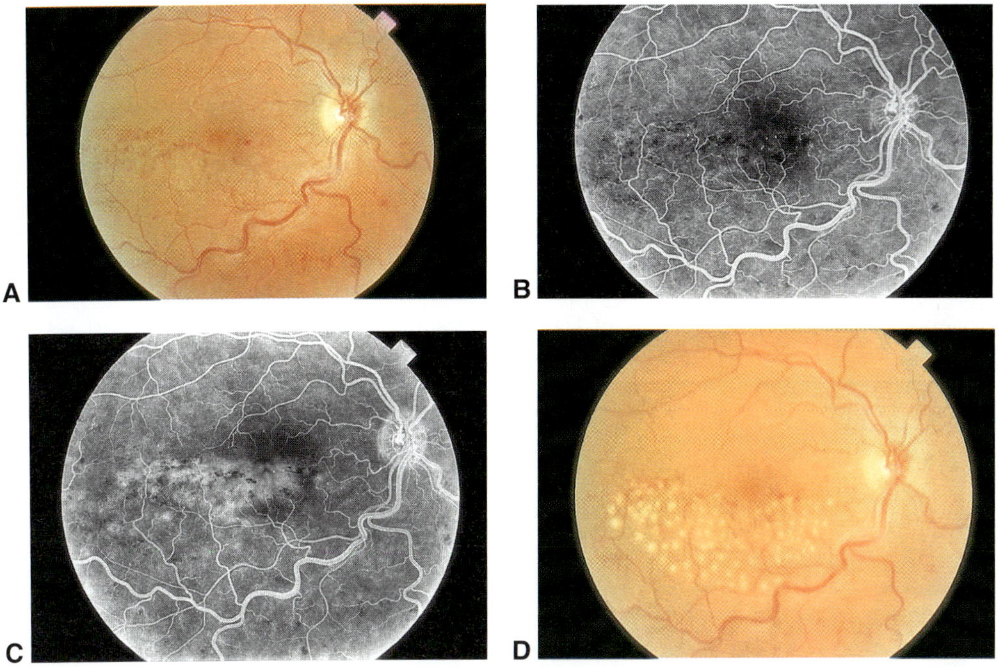

Figure 6-7 BRVO. **A,** Fundus photograph of inferotemporal BRVO. Corresponding fluorescein angiography images show, at 49 seconds after injection **(B)**, telangiectatic vessels in the distribution of the inferotemporal vein, and at 393 seconds after injection **(C)**, intraretinal leakage of dye from the capillaries in macular distribution of the vein occlusion *(white)*. **D,** Fundus photograph after treatment shows a grid of macular photocoagulation lesions in the affected area but sparing the foveal region. *(Courtesy of Gary C. Brown, MD.)*

spontaneous resolution of the edema and intraretinal blood. Although this practice may still be appropriate for macular laser therapy, treatment with pharmacologic agents may commence immediately upon diagnosis of BRVO.

SCATTER PHOTOCOAGULATION In the BVOS, scatter photocoagulation to the area of retinal capillary nonperfusion was shown to be effective in causing regression of the new vessels in eyes with retinal, disc, or iris neovascularization (Fig 6-8) and reduced the risk of vitreous hemorrhage from 60% to 30%. Although the BVOS showed that patients with large areas of nonperfusion (such as that shown in Figure 6-5) were found to be at significant risk of developing neovascularization, the study concluded that ischemia alone was not an indication for treatment, provided that follow-up could be maintained.

Clinically, it is important to distinguish neovascularization of the disc or retina from collateral vessels, which have a larger caliber and do not leak on fluorescein angiography. Neovascularization of the iris occurs in approximately 2% of eyes with BRVO. Scatter laser photocoagulation in the distribution of the occluded vein should be considered in such instances to prevent the development of neovascular glaucoma.

Fuller JJ, Mason JO III. Retinal vein occlusions: update on diagnostic and therapeutic advances. *Focal Points: Clinical Modules for Ophthalmologists.* San Francisco: American Academy of Ophthalmology; 2007, module 5.

PARS PLANA VITRECTOMY Vitrectomy may be indicated for eyes that develop nonclearing vitreous hemorrhage or retinal detachment (also see Chapters 15 and 19). Although vitrectomy with arteriovenous sheathotomy has been reported as a treatment for BRVO and macular edema, it lacks data to support its benefit. Consequently, this treatment is now performed rarely.

Central Retinal Vein Occlusion

In CRVO, vision loss is most commonly sudden, with severity ranging from mild (in nonischemic disease) to severe (in ischemic disease). Less commonly, patients may experience premonitory symptoms of transient obscuration of vision before overt retinal

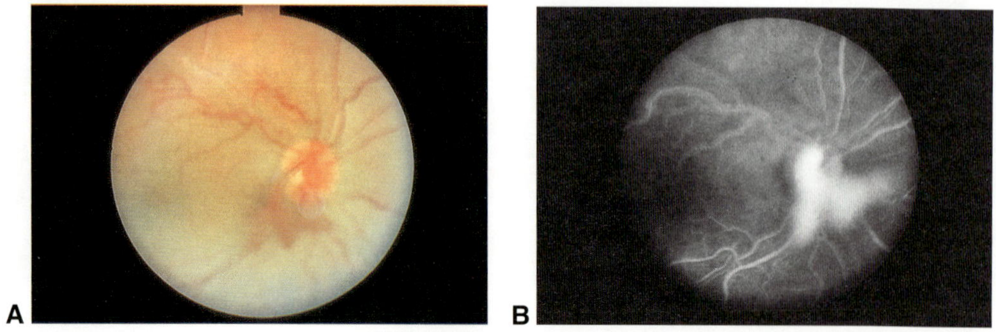

Figure 6-8 BRVO with neovascularization. **A,** Neovascularization of the disc occurring secondary to a superotemporal BRVO. **B,** Corresponding fluorescein angiography image at 18 seconds after injection reveals marked hyperfluorescence of the new vessels originating on the optic disc. *(Courtesy of Gary C. Brown, MD.)*

manifestations appear. CRVOs are said to be intermediate, or indeterminate, when they are neither clearly ischemic nor nonischemic; more than 80% of intermediate eyes progress to ischemic disease.

Nonischemic (mild) CRVO, sometimes referred to as *partial, perfused,* or *venous stasis retinopathy,* is characterized by good visual acuity, a mild or no afferent pupillary defect, and mild visual field changes. Ophthalmoscopy shows mild dilation and tortuosity of all branches of the central retinal vein as well as dot- and flame-shaped hemorrhages in all quadrants of the retina (Fig 6-9). Macular edema with decreased visual acuity and mild optic disc swelling may be present. Fluorescein angiography usually demonstrates prolongation of the retinal circulation time with breakdown of capillary permeability but minimal areas of nonperfusion. Anterior segment neovascularization is rare in mild CRVO. Chronic nonischemic changes from CRVO include telangiectasias, aneurysms, and macular pigment changes (see Fig 6-6).

Ischemic (severe) CRVO, also known as *complete, nonperfused,* or *hemorrhagic retinopathy,* is defined as having at least 10 disc areas of retinal capillary nonperfusion on fluorescein angiography on a posterior pole view. Ischemic cases are usually associated with poor vision, an afferent pupillary defect, and dense central scotoma. Marked venous dilation, more extensive 4-quadrant hemorrhage, retinal edema (Fig 6-10), and variable numbers of cotton-wool spots are frequently found as well. Fluorescein angiography typically has prolonged retinovascular circulation times and shows widespread capillary nonperfusion. A decreased electroretinographic bright-flash, dark-adapted b- to a-wave amplitude ratio is characteristic because of inner retinal dysfunction from the ischemia. The Central Vein Occlusion Study (CVOS) showed that visual prognosis is generally poor, with only approximately 10% of eyes achieving vision better than 20/400. With anti-VEGF treatment, the prognosis may be somewhat better in all but the most ischemic cases.

A hemiretinal vein occlusion, considered a variant of CRVO, is associated with a congenital variation in central vein anatomy; it may involve either the superior or inferior half of the retina (Fig 6-11).

Histologic studies suggest that most forms of CRVO share a common mechanism: thrombosis of the central retinal vein at and posterior to the level of the lamina cribrosa. It is postulated that, in some cases, a thickened central retinal artery may impinge on the central retinal vein, causing turbulence, endothelial damage, and thrombus formation.

Iris neovascularization in CRVO

Among eyes with very ischemic CRVO, the incidence of anterior segment neovascularization, iris and angle, is high (up to 60%); this development occurs a mean of 3–5 months after the onset of symptoms. If not detected promptly, neovascular glaucoma may develop. The CVOS found that the most important risk factor predictive of iris neovascularization in central venous occlusive disease is poor visual acuity. Other risk factors include large areas of retinal capillary nonperfusion and intraretinal blood.

Baseline and early natural history report. The Central Vein Occlusion Study. *Arch Ophthalmol.* 1993;111(8):1087–1095.

Klein R, Moss SE, Meuer SM, Klein BE. The 15-year cumulative incidence of retinal vein occlusion: the Beaver Dam Eye Study. *Arch Ophthalmol.* 2008;126(4):513–518.

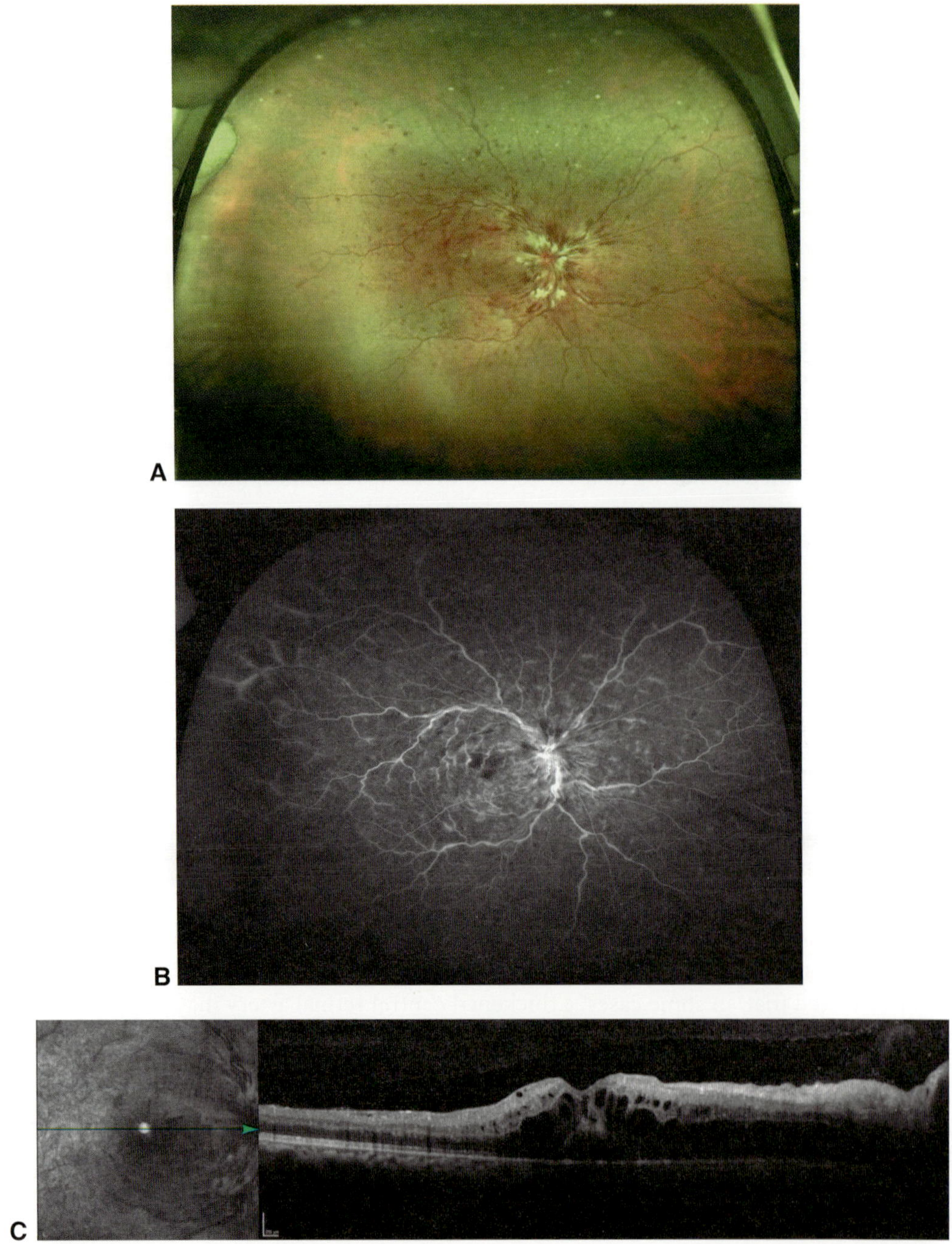

Figure 6-9 Moderate to severe nonischemic central retinal vein occlusion (CRVO). **A,** Ultra-wide-field fundus photograph of moderate to severe nonischemic, or perfused, CRVO in an eye with 20/80 vision. Dilated retinal veins and retinal hemorrhages are present in all 4 quadrants. Cotton-wool spots can be seen near the optic nerve head. **B,** A fluorescein angiography image at 1 minute, 8 seconds reveals relatively intact perfusion of the retinal capillary bed but dilated vessels and peripheral leakage from the large vessels. There are some areas of capillary nonperfusion in the superior macula. **C,** An SD-OCT scan shows severe cystoid retinal edema with a serous foveal detachment. After 2.5 years of anti-VEGF treatment with bevacizumab, the patient maintains a visual acuity of 20/40. *(Courtesy of Colin A. McCannel, MD.)*

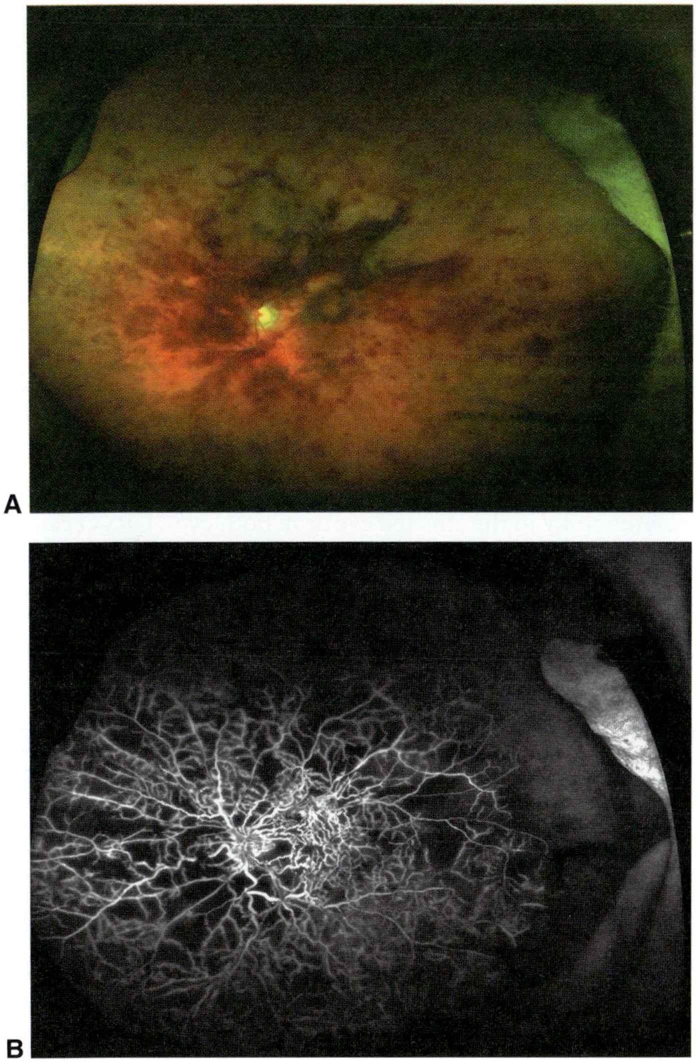

Figure 6-10 Ischemic CRVO. **A,** Ultra-wide-field fundus photograph of severe, or ischemic, CRVO in an eye with hand motions vision. The veins are dilated, and extensive retinal hemorrhages are present. **B,** Ultra-wide-field fluorescein angiography image corresponding to **A** at 40 seconds after injection reveals widespread retinal capillary nonperfusion, which causes the midsize and larger retinal vessels to stand out from the gray-black, nonperfused areas. *(Courtesy of Colin A. McCannel, MD.)*

Risk factors and causes of CRVO

The most important risk factor for the development of CRVO is age; 90% of patients are older than 50 years at the time of onset. Mild CRVOs generally occur at a younger age. The Eye Disease Case-Control Study found the following associations with CRVO:

- systemic arterial hypertension
- open-angle glaucoma
- diabetes mellitus
- hyperlipidemia

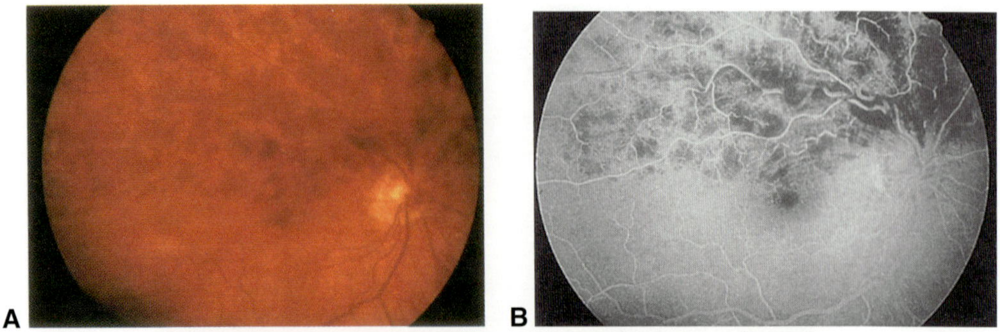

Figure 6-11 Hemiretinal vein occlusion. **A,** Fundus photograph showing superior involvement with intraretinal hemorrhage. **B,** Fluorescein angiography image showing blockage of underlying details in areas of hemorrhage. Note that the foveal avascular zone is largely intact.

It is common for patients presenting with CRVO to have elevated IOP or frank open-angle glaucoma, either only in the affected eye or in both eyes. CRVO can also be followed by a transient shallowing of the anterior chamber that, in some instances, leads to angle-closure glaucoma.

Oral contraceptives and diuretics have been implicated as risk factors for the development of CRVO. Although rare, predisposing hypercoagulable conditions may be present; these abnormalities include hyperhomocysteinemia, protein S deficiency, protein C deficiency, and disorders associated with vasculitis such as sarcoidosis and systemic lupus erythematosus. However, when CRVO occurs in patients more than 50 years of age, it is generally considered unnecessary to pursue an elaborate systemic workup for these rare causes.

Differential diagnosis of CRVO

It is particularly important to recognize that *hyperviscosity retinopathy* can mimic a typical CRVO. However, the retinal findings in hyperviscosity retinopathy are generally bilateral and usually related to dysproteinemia such as that associated with Waldenström macroglobulinemia, multiple myeloma, or blood dyscrasias (eg, polycythemia vera). In many cases, the hyperviscosity can be reversed by treating the underlying condition. To assess for these conditions, diagnostic testing may include complete blood count, serum protein electrophoresis, and a measure of whole-blood viscosity. *Ocular ischemic syndrome* can also mimic CRVO. Unusual diseases that affect the blood vessel wall or affect blood-clotting mechanisms and blood viscosity may be associated with a CRVO-like picture.

Central Vein Occlusion Study Group. Natural history and clinical management of central retinal vein occlusion. *Arch Ophthalmol.* 1997;115(4):486–491.

Fuller JJ, Mason JO III. Retinal vein occlusions: update on diagnostic and therapeutic advances. *Focal Points: Clinical Modules for Ophthalmologists.* San Francisco: American Academy of Ophthalmology; 2007, module 5.

Evaluation and management of CRVO

The examiner should attempt to determine whether the vein occlusion is nonischemic or ischemic. Assessments of visual acuity, visual fields, and relative afferent defect using techniques of ophthalmoscopy, fluorescein angiography, and electroretinography are helpful in making this determination. At follow-up, it is important to perform gonioscopy to check for angle neovascularization.

If the evaluation indicates that common risk factors for CRVO are absent, or if the patient is less than 50 years of age, a thorough investigation should be considered, possibly including a workup for thrombophilia.

Patients with CRVO should be warned of the possibility of worsening vision because eyes with initially perfused CRVO sometimes progress to an ischemic pattern. In the CVOS, 16% of initially nonischemic CRVOs converted to ischemia by 4 months of follow-up and by 36 months, the percentage was 34%.

Follow-up In the absence of treatment, patients with CRVO should be monitored on a monthly basis for progression and for at least 6 months for the development of anterior segment neovascularization or neovascular glaucoma. Patients treated with anti-VEGF agents should be observed for a similar duration after discontinuation of the drugs.

Complications The most common complications of CRVO are vitreous hemorrhage, anterior segment neovascularization, and neovascular glaucoma. Vitreous hemorrhage often occurs in the absence of neovascularization, and neovascular glaucoma can occur from angle neovascularization with or without iris neovascularization.

Stem MS, Talwar N, Comer GM, Stein JD. A longitudinal analysis of risk factors associated with central retinal vein occlusion. *Ophthalmology.* 2013;120(2):362–370.

Treatment of CRVO

Pharmacologic management of CRVO As for BRVO, a growing arsenal of pharmaceuticals is available for the management of CRVO. Most important, the visual acuity outcomes with these interventions can be dramatic compared with what could be achieved before their availability.

INTRAVITREAL ANTI-VEGF THERAPY In CRUISE (Study of the Efficacy and Safety of Ranibizumab Injection in Patients With Macular Edema Secondary to Central Retinal Vein Occlusion), ranibizumab was administered to eyes with CRVO with macular edema. At 6 months, following monthly injections of either 0.5 or 0.3 mg of *ranibizumab* or monthly sham injections, overall, 47.7%, 46.2%, and 16.9% of eyes gained 15 or more ETDRS letters, respectively. Similar results were achieved in the GALILEO (Vascular Endothelial Growth Factor Trap-Eye: Investigation of Efficacy and Safety in Central Retinal Vein Occlusion; conducted outside North America) and COPERNICUS (same protocol, but conducted within North America) studies investigating intravitreal *aflibercept* (also called *VEGF-Trap*) for the treatment of macular edema secondary to CRVO. The benefits were maintained during the second 6 months of these studies, during which an as-needed treatment strategy was employed. Uncontrolled studies of bevacizumab administration have also demonstrated substantial resolution of macular edema as well as improvement in visual acuity (Fig 6-12), and many practitioners use the 3 anti-VEGF drugs interchangeably. In practice, anti-VEGF agent administration strategies for CRVO treatment include monthly dosing, as-needed treatment, and treat-and-extend approaches. Intravitreal anti-VEGF

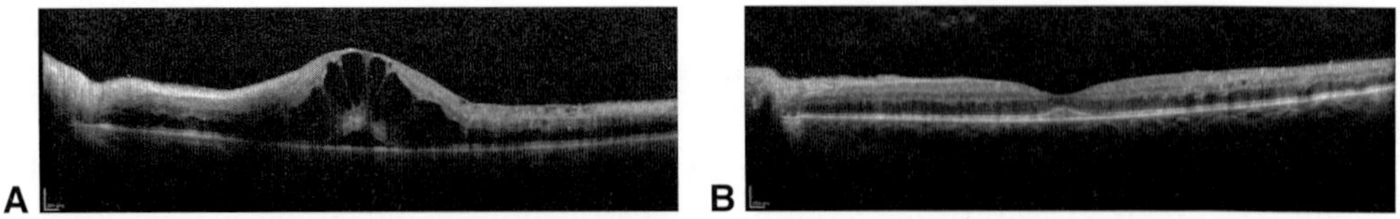

Figure 6-12 Cystoid macular edema (CME) secondary to CRVO before and after treatment. **A,** Spectral-domain optical coherence tomography scan showing severe CME with foveal detachment in a patient with a nonischemic CRVO. Visual acuity was 20/200. **B,** One month after intravitreal injection of bevacizumab, 1.25 mg, the cystic changes and foveal detachment had resolved, and the visual acuity measured 20/25. *(Courtesy of Colin A. McCannel, MD.)*

drugs may also be used to reduce iris neovascularization and treat neovascular glaucoma in the short term.

Campochiaro PA, Brown DM, Awh CC, et al. Sustained benefits from ranibizumab for macular edema following central retinal vein occlusion: twelve-month outcomes of a phase III study. *Ophthalmology.* 2011;118(10):2041–2049.

INTRAVITREAL CORTICOSTEROIDS Before using corticosteroids for treatment of venous occlusive disease, clinicians should consider the risk of complications such as glaucoma and cataract formation as well as possible alternative treatments and any benefits. However, steroid treatments have been shown to be effective in managing macular edema from CRVO. In the CRVO arm of the SCORE study, at 1 year, 27% of eyes treated with 1 mg of *triamcinolone* and 26% with 4 mg of triamcinolone had an improvement of 15 ETDRS letters or more compared with 7% of eyes in the observation group. The *dexamethasone* injectable intravitreal implant also improved visual acuity outcomes over a 6-month period. Clinical trials are currently assessing a fluocinolone acetonide intravitreal insert with longer-term steroid delivery for the treatment of retinal vein occlusion.

Scott IU, Ip MS, VanVeldhuisen PC, et al. A randomized trial comparing the efficacy and safety of intravitreal triamcinolone with standard care to treat vision loss associated with macular edema secondary to branch retinal vein occlusion: the Standard Care vs. Corticosteroid for Retinal Vein Occlusion (SCORE) study report 6. *Arch Ophthalmol.* 2009;127(9):1115–1128.

Systemic anticoagulation Systemic anticoagulation for the treatment or prevention of CRVO has been attempted and is now discouraged. There is no benefit, and to the contrary, reports have documented poorer visual acuity outcomes from such treatment due to more extensive intraretinal hemorrhages.

Surgical management of CRVO A number of laser and other surgical methods have been used for the treatment of CRVO.

MACULAR LASER SURGERY Grid-pattern photocoagulation for treatment of macular edema in CRVO was evaluated prospectively in the CVOS. Even though grid laser treatment of the macula reduced angiographic evidence of macular edema, visual acuity did not improve.

PANRETINAL PHOTOCOAGULATION In the CVOS, prophylactic panretinal photocoagulation (PRP) did not result in a statistically significant decrease in the incidence of iris neovascularization.

In fact, 20% of participants who had received the prophylactic PRP still developed iris neovascularization. Therefore, close monitoring of patients at high risk of iris neovascularization is necessary. The CVOS investigators recommended waiting until undilated gonioscopic examination revealed at least 2 clock-hours of iris neovascularization before performing PRP. In clinical practice, however, PRP is often performed at the first sign of iris neovascularization, particularly when close follow-up is not possible or seems unlikely. Wide-field angiography is enhancing visualization of peripheral nonperfusion in CRVO; however, no evidence to date supports altered treatment criteria based on this information.

Central Vein Occlusion Study Group. A randomized clinical trial of early panretinal photocoagulation for ischemic central vein occlusion. The Central Vein Occlusion Study Group N report. *Ophthalmology.* 1995;102(10):1434–1444.

PARS PLANA VITRECTOMY CRVOs complicated by vitreous hemorrhage may benefit from pars plana vitrectomy. Vitrectomy is used for purposes of vision rehabilitation or to accomplish retinal ablative treatment in the management of anterior segment neovascularization and neovascular glaucoma. For neovascular glaucoma, a glaucoma valve may be implanted concurrently.

OTHER SURGICAL APPROACHES Because of a lack of evidence for their efficacy, several surgical approaches have largely been abandoned. They include attempts to create an anastomotic connection between the retinal vein and the choroidal circulation using a high-power laser application, radial optic neurotomy involving sectioning of the posterior scleral ring to decompress the central retinal vein, and retinal vein cannulation with an infusion of tissue plasminogen activator (tPA).

Ocular Ischemic Syndrome and Retinopathy of Carotid Occlusive Disease

Ocular ischemic syndrome is the term used to describe ocular symptoms and signs attributable to chronic, severe ocular hypoperfusion caused by carotid artery obstruction. Chronic ophthalmic artery obstruction can cause a similar clinical picture.

Symptoms and Signs

Symptoms typically include gradual vision loss that develops over a period of weeks to months, aching pain localized to the orbital area of the affected eye, and prolonged vision recovery after exposure to a bright light. Anterior segment signs include iris neovascularization in two-thirds of eyes and an anterior chamber cellular response in about one-fifth of eyes. Although iris and angle neovascularization are common, only one-half of eyes with this condition show an increase in IOP; the low or normal IOP in the other half is most likely caused by impaired aqueous production.

Ocular ischemic syndrome can cause a retinopathy similar in appearance to a partial occlusion of the central retinal vein; therefore, it was originally called venous stasis retinopathy. Typical retinal findings include narrowed arteries, dilated but not very tortuous veins, hemorrhages, microaneurysms, and neovascularization of the optic disc, retina, or both (Fig 6-13). The retinal hemorrhages in carotid occlusive disease are usually deep, round, and more often located in the midperipheral retina. A helpful method for differentiating between the 2 entities is to measure the retinal artery pressure, either by using an ophthalmodynamometer, or by gently pushing on the eye during the examination and observing the central retinal artery. An eye with CRVO will have normal artery pressure, whereas one with carotid occlusive disease will have low artery pressure, and the artery would therefore collapse easily.

Fluorescein angiography reveals delayed choroidal filling in 60% of eyes, delayed arteriovenous transit time in 95% of eyes, and prominent vascular staining (particularly of the arteries) in 85% of eyes. Electroretinography will reveal global amplitude reduction in disorders that affect the blood supply to the photoreceptors, such as in carotid ischemic syndrome. In contrast, an electronegative ERG occurs if the blood supply to the inner retina is disturbed and that to the photoreceptors preserved, such as occurs in central retinal artery occlusion (CRAO) or can occur in CRVO.

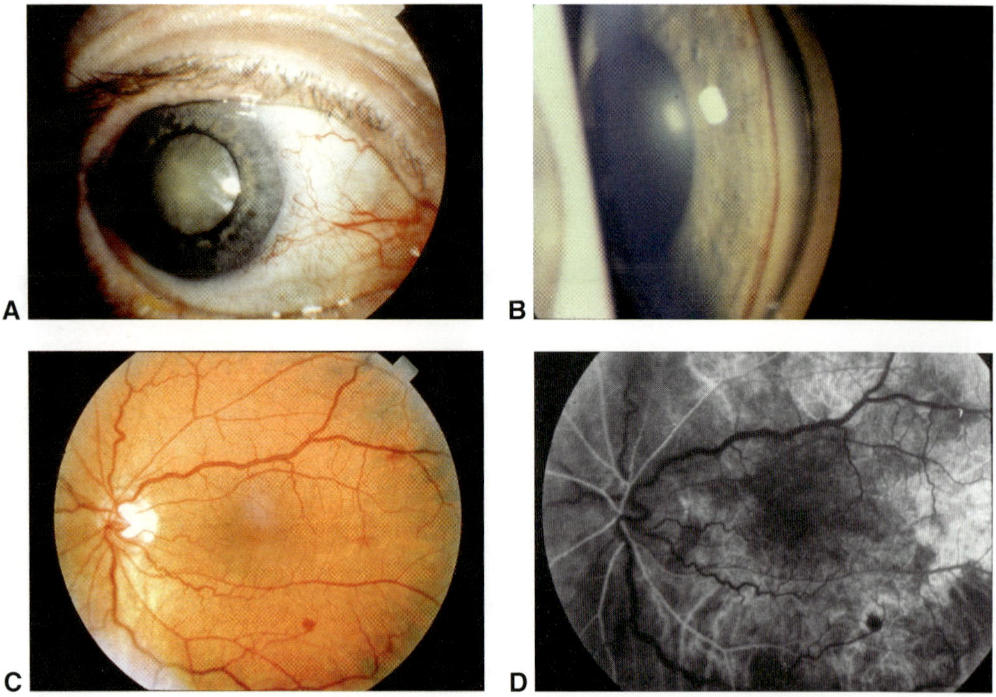

Figure 6-13 Ocular ischemic syndrome. **A,** Clinical photograph of an eye with ocular ischemic syndrome displaying features of conjunctival injection, cataract, and rubeosis irides. **B,** Gonioscopic appearance of neovascularization of the iridocorneal angle due to ocular ischemic syndrome. **C,** Fundus photograph of an eye with ocular ischemic syndrome showing features of venous dilation, midperipheral intraretinal hemorrhages, and attenuated arterioles. **D,** Fluorescein angiography image at 19 seconds (arterial phase) demonstrating a prolonged arm-to-retina circulation time and a patchy choroidal filling pattern. *(Courtesy of Neal H. Atebara, MD.)*

Etiology and Course

Atherosclerosis is the most common etiology, but other possible causes include Eisenmenger syndrome, giant cell arteritis, and other inflammatory conditions. Most patients are older than 55 years. Typically, a 90% or greater ipsilateral obstruction is necessary to cause the ocular ischemic syndrome. Both eyes are involved in approximately 20% of cases.

The visual prognosis of eyes with ocular ischemic syndrome is uncertain, but when rubeosis iridis is also present, visual acuity in more than 90% will decline to 20/200 or worse within 1 year after diagnosis. For this reason, timely diagnosis is essential.

Approximately one-half of patients with ocular ischemic syndrome also have ischemic cardiovascular disease; one-fourth have had a previous cerebrovascular accident; and one-fifth have peripheral atherosclerotic vascular disease so severe that a previous surgical procedure was necessary. The stroke rate is increased over that in the general population, and the 5-year mortality is approximately 40%, mostly from complications of cardiovascular disease.

Treatment of Ocular Ischemic Syndrome

The most definitive treatment for ocular ischemic syndrome appears to be carotid artery stenting and endarterectomy, although visual acuity outcomes are variable. Unfortunately, the procedures are ineffective when there is 100% obstruction, which is often the case. Extracranial to intracranial bypass surgery has been attempted in such cases but has been shown to be ineffective for preventing loss of vision or stroke. In eyes with iris neovascularization and low or normal IOP as a result of impaired ciliary body perfusion and decreased aqueous formation, carotid reperfusion can lead to increased aqueous formation and a severe rise in IOP. Full-scatter PRP results in regression of anterior segment neovascularization in approximately two-thirds of cases. Anti-VEGF treatments and local steroid therapy have not been investigated for the treatment of ocular ischemic syndrome.

Brown GC, Sharma S. Ocular ischemic syndrome. In: Ryan SJ, Schachat AP, Wilkinson CP, Hinton DR, Sadda SR, Wiedemann P, eds. *Retina*. 5th ed. Philadelphia: Elsevier/Saunders; 2013:1091–1103.

Arterial Occlusive Disease

The blood supply to the inner layers of the retina is derived entirely from the central retinal artery, unless a cilioretinal artery is present (20%–23% of eyes). Retinal ischemia results from disease processes affecting the afferent vessels anywhere from the common carotid artery to the intraretinal arterioles. The signs and symptoms of arterial obstruction depend on the vessel involved: occlusion of a peripheral extramacular arteriole may be asymptomatic, whereas an ophthalmic artery occlusion can cause total blindness.

Capillary Retinal Arteriole Obstruction (Cotton-Wool Spots)

Acute obstruction in the distribution of the radial peripapillary capillary net leads to the formation of a nerve fiber layer (NFL) infarct, or cotton-wool spot, thereby inhibiting axoplasmic transport in the NFL (Fig 6-14). These inner retinal ischemic spots are superficial, white, and typically one-fourth disc area or less in size. They usually fade in 5–7 weeks, although spots present in association with diabetic retinopathy often remain longer. A subtle retinal depression caused by inner retinal ischemic atrophy may develop in the area of prior ischemia. The effect on visual function, including loss of visual acuity and field defects, is related to the size and location of the occluded area.

The most common cause of cotton-wool spots is diabetic retinopathy (discussed in Chapter 5). Other causes include

- systemic arterial hypertension
- HIV-associated retinopathy
- anemia (severe)
- radiation retinopathy
- sickle cell retinopathy
- cardiac embolic disease
- carotid artery obstructive disease
- vasculitis
- collagen vascular disease
- leukemia

The observation of even 1 cotton-wool spot in the fundus in an otherwise apparently healthy eye should alert the clinician to initiate a workup for an underlying etiology.

Brown GC, Brown MM, Hiller T, Fischer D, Benson WE, Magargal LE. Cotton-wool spots. *Retina.* 1985;5(4):206–214.

Branch Retinal Artery Occlusion

Although an acute BRAO may not initially be apparent on ophthalmoscopic examination, within hours to days it leads to an edematous opacification caused by infarction of the inner retina in the distribution of the affected vessel (Fig 6-15). With time, the occluded vessel recanalizes, perfusion returns, and the edema resolves; however, a permanent visual field defect remains. A retinal arterial occlusion that occurs outside of the posterior pole may be clinically silent.

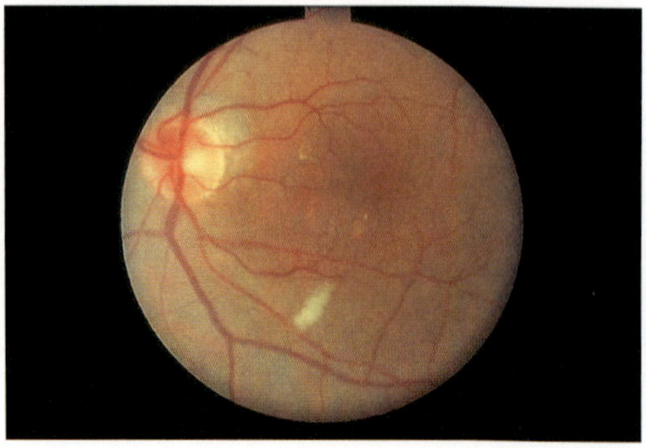

Figure 6-14 Fundus photograph showing a cotton-wool spot. *(Courtesy of Gary C. Brown, MD.)*

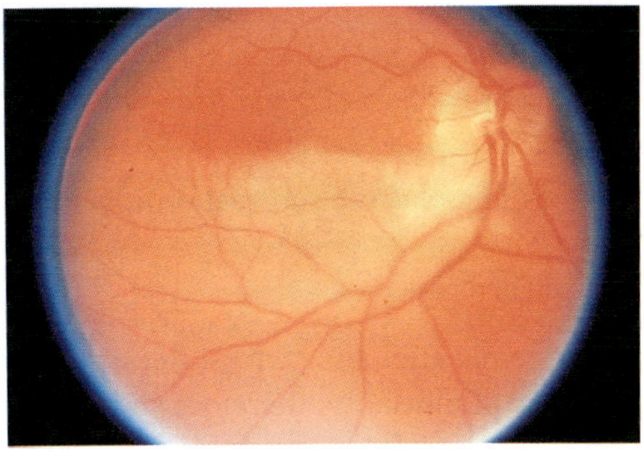

Figure 6-15 Inferotemporal branch retinal artery obstruction. The fundus photograph shows opacification of the retina in the distribution of the occluded vessel (inferior macula). In this case, the visual acuity was 20/30 at presentation but returned to 20/20 over several weeks. *(Courtesy of Gary C. Brown, MD.)*

Occlusion at any site is a result of embolization or thrombosis of the affected vessel. Three main varieties of emboli are recognized:

1. cholesterol emboli (Hollenhorst plaques) arising in the carotid arteries (Fig 6-16)
2. platelet-fibrin emboli associated with large-vessel arteriosclerosis
3. calcific emboli arising from diseased cardiac valves

Rare causes of emboli include cardiac myxoma, fat emboli from long-bone fractures, septic emboli from infective endocarditis, and talc emboli in intravenous drug users. Although rare, migraine can cause ocular arterial occlusions in patients younger than 30–40 years of age. Other associations include

- arrhythmias
- mitral valve prolapse

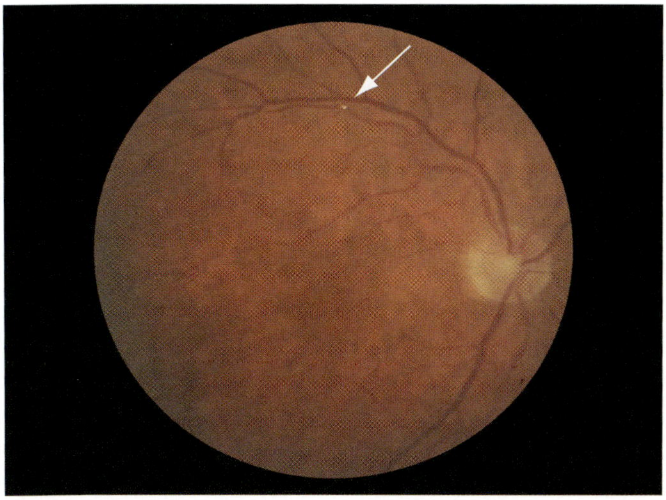

Figure 6-16 Hollenhorst plaque. Fundus photograph showing a Hollenhorst plaque lodged at a bifurcation of the superior arcade arteriole *(arrow)*. Hollenhorst plaques do not typically cause vascular obstruction and can remain at a bifurcation indefinitely. Occasionally, they can be observed to move with blood flow. *(Courtesy of Tara A. McCannel, MD, PhD.)*

- oral contraceptive use or pregnancy
- coagulation disorders
- trauma
- sickle cell disease
- inflammatory and infectious etiologies such as toxoplasmic retinochoroiditis and syphilis
- connective tissue disorders, including giant cell arteritis

Management is directed toward determining systemic etiologic factors. Retinal arterial emboli have been associated with an increased risk of mortality; therefore, a systemic and vascular evaluation should be considered. No specific ocular therapy has been found to be effective in improving the visual prognosis. Lowering the intraocular pressure and applying intermittent pressure on the globe ("ocular massage") may dislodge an embolus from a large central vessel toward a more peripheral location, but the efficacy of these maneuvers in improving vision outcomes is unknown.

Hayreh SS, Podhajsky PA, Zimmerman MB. Branch retinal artery occlusion: natural history of visual outcome. *Ophthalmology.* 2009;116(6):1188–1194.

Wang JJ, Cugati S, Knudtson MD, et al. Retinal arteriolar emboli and long-term mortality: pooled data analysis from two older populations. *Stroke.* 2006;37(7):1833–1836.

Cilioretinal Artery Occlusion

A distinct clinical entity is the occlusion of the cilioretinal artery. As their name suggests, cilioretinal arteries arise from the short posterior ciliary vessels rather than the central retinal artery. When present, they usually contribute to some portion of the macular circulation. Most commonly, their occlusion occurs in the setting of a central retinal vein occlusion; it is postulated that the increased hydrostatic pressure associated with CRVO can reduce blood flow in the cilioretinal artery to the point of stagnation.

When cilioretinal artery occlusion occurs in isolation, giant cell arteritis should be considered strongly.

Hayreh SS, Fraterrigo L, Jonas J. Central retinal vein occlusion associated with cilioretinal artery occlusion. *Retina.* 2008;28(4):581–594.

Central Retinal Artery Occlusion

Sudden, complete, and painless loss of vision in 1 eye is characteristic of CRAO. The retina becomes opaque and edematous, particularly in the posterior pole, where the nerve fiber and ganglion cell layers are thickest (Fig 6-17). The orange reflex from the intact choroidal vasculature beneath the foveola thus stands out in contrast to the surrounding opaque neural retina, producing the cherry-red spot. Some degree of macular vision may be preserved by a cilioretinal artery protecting an area of retina perfused by it (see Chapter 1, Fig 1-7).

With time, the central retinal artery reopens or recanalizes and the retinal edema clears; however, the effect on visual acuity is usually permanent because the inner retina has been infarcted. In one study, 66% of eyes had final visual acuity worse than 20/400, and 18% of eyes had 20/40 or better. Most cases of 20/40 or better visual acuity occur in

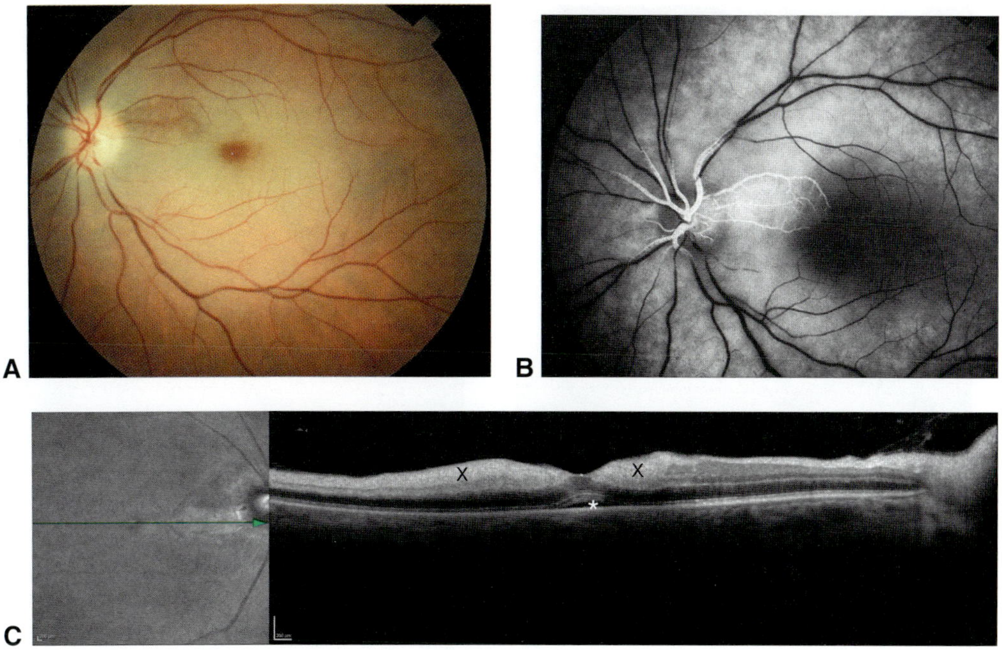

Figure 6-17 Central retinal artery occlusion (CRAO). **A,** Fundus photograph showing superficial macular opacification and a cherry-red spot in the foveola. **B,** Angiography image revealing preservation of a sector of superonasal macula related to cilioretinal vessels, perfused in this image. The patient had hand motions visual acuity. **C,** SD-OCT scan of a similar case of CRAO with cilioretinal artery sparing shows opacification of the inner two-thirds of the retina in the affected areas *(X)*. All retinal layers are identifiable in the area of retina perfused by the cilioretinal artery, adjacent to the optic nerve head. The retina in the fovea is spared from opacification, resulting in the appearance of a cherry-red spot on examination. Subfoveal fluid *(asterisk)* is variably present in these cases. *(Parts A and B courtesy of Hermann D. Schubert, MD; part C courtesy of Colin A. McCannel, MD.)*

the presence of a patent cilioretinal artery (see Fig 6-17; also see Chapter 1, Fig 1-7). Vaso-occlusive loss of vision to the level of no light perception is usually caused by choroidal vascular insufficiency from partial or complete ophthalmic artery occlusion or occlusions of the ciliary arteries in conjunction with occlusion of the central retinal artery (Fig 6-18). Studies in nonhuman primates have suggested that irreversible damage to the sensory retina occurs after 90 minutes of complete CRAO. Nevertheless, clinical return of vision can occur in some instances even if the obstruction has persisted for many hours.

CRAO is most often caused by embolization or atherosclerosis-related thrombosis occurring at the level of the lamina cribrosa. Less common causes are hemorrhage under an atherosclerotic plaque, thrombosis, spasm, and dissecting aneurysm within the central retinal artery.

Emboli within the carotid distribution may cause transient ischemic attacks, amaurosis fugax, or both. Bright cholesterol emboli, or Hollenhorst plaques, located typically at retinal arterial bifurcations, suggest a carotid atheromatous origin and, when accompanied by relevant symptoms and findings, may be an indication for carotid artery treatment. Systemic etiologic considerations, as outlined for BRAO, are important and require

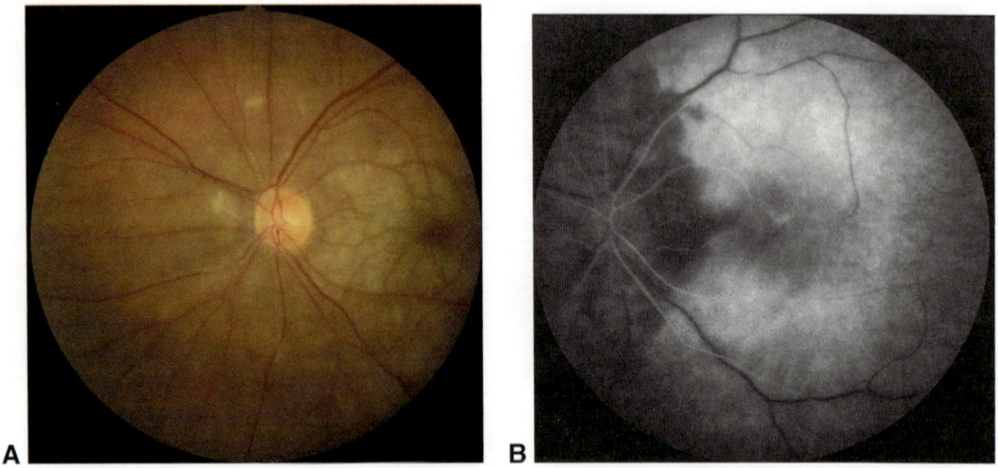

Figure 6-18 Central retinal and parent short ciliary artery occlusion. **A,** Fundus photograph of acute central retinal and short ciliary artery obstruction. Severe retinal opacification is present. The visual acuity was no light perception. **B,** Fluorescein angiography image at 3 minutes after injection reveals hypofluorescence of the retinal vessels, the nasal choroid, and the optic disc, corresponding to an occlusion of the central retinal artery and nasal parent ciliary artery. The latter results in ischemia in the distribution of the short posterior ciliary arteries with a vertical watershed of choroidal perfusion (also see Chapter 9, Fig 9-2). *(Courtesy of Hermann D. Schubert, MD.)*

evaluation. It should be noted that the leading cause of death in patients with retinal arterial obstruction is cardiovascular disease.

Giant cell arteritis (GCA) accounts for approximately 1%–2% of cases of CRAO. In cases of CRAO in which emboli are not readily visible, a thorough evaluation for GCA should be considered. The erythrocyte sedimentation rate (ESR) and C-reactive protein level—markers of inflammation—are usually elevated and should be checked. A complete blood count may detect an elevated platelet count, which is also suggestive of GCA, and aids in the interpretation of the ESR. If GCA is suspected as a cause, corticosteroid therapy should be instituted promptly because the second eye can become involved by ischemia within hours to days after the first; in addition, a temporal artery biopsy should be performed. See BCSC Section 5, *Neuro-Ophthalmology,* for further discussion of giant cell arteritis.

Falkenberry SM, Ip MS, Blodi BA, Gunther JB. Optical coherence tomography findings in central retinal artery occlusion. *Ophthalmic Surg Lasers Imaging.* 2006;37(6):502–505.

Management of CRAO

If therapy for CRAO is to be instituted, it should be undertaken without delay. Unfortunately, treatment efficacy is questionable. Simple therapeutic approaches, such as reducing IOP by administering IOP-lowering medications and performing ocular massage, are not unreasonable. However, both anterior chamber paracentesis and carbinogen (a mixture of 95% oxygen and 5% carbon dioxide) vasodilatory inhalation therapy have been shown to be ineffective and are no longer recommended. Hyperbaric oxygen therapy, catheterization of the ophthalmic artery with tPA infusion, and transvitreal Nd:YAG embolysis all lack good evidence of efficacy.

Iris neovascularization develops after acute CRAO in approximately 18% of eyes 1–12 weeks after the event, with a mean time interval of approximately 4–5 weeks. Full-scatter PRP results in regression of anterior segment neovascularization in approximately two-thirds of cases.

Ophthalmic Artery Occlusion

Ophthalmic artery occlusion is very rare. Clinically, the disorder typically produces vision loss to the level of light perception or no light perception because simultaneous nonperfusion of the choroid and retina results in ischemia of all retinal layers. A cherry-red spot is usually not present, as both the inner retina and outer retina become opacified from the infarction, and thus there is no contrast difference between foveal and perifoveal retina that would lead to such a spot.

Ophthalmic artery occlusion may be caused by dissection of the internal carotid artery, orbital mucormycosis, and embolization. In recent years, an increasing number of ophthalmic artery occlusions caused by various cosmetic facial-filler injections, particularly into the periocular and brow area, have been reported (Fig 6-19). In autopsy studies of patients who died during active giant cell arteritis, up to 76% had some degree of ophthalmic artery affected by vasculitis; clinically, however, ophthalmic artery occlusion is rare in GCA.

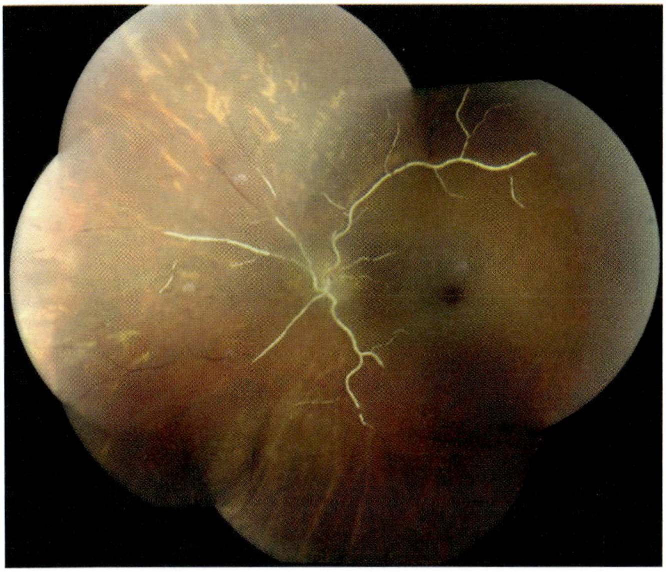

Figure 6-19 Fundus photographic montage of the left eye of a 44-year-old woman following an ipsilateral injection of synthetic calcium hydroxylapatite gel into her left lateral lower eyelid for cosmetic purposes. Sudden loss of vision ensued to the level of no light perception. An ophthalmic artery occlusion occurred from presumed retrograde flow of the injectable cosmetic filler into the ophthalmic artery by way of anastomotic arteries in the orbit bridging the internal and external carotid circulations. The white filler material is visible in the retinal circulation and choroidal blood vessels. *(Courtesy of Kathryn Sun, MD, PhD, Thomas F. Essman, MD, and Brenda Schoenauer, CDOS.)*

Arterial Macroaneurysms

Retinal arterial macroaneurysms are acquired ectasias of mostly second-order retinal arterioles. Large macroaneurysms can actually traverse the full thickness of the retina. Vision loss may occur from embolic or thrombotic occlusion of the end-arteriole (white infarct) or from sub–internal limiting membrane, intraretinal, subretinal, or vitreous hemorrhage. Other retinal findings may include capillary telangiectasia and remodeling, as well as retinal edema and exudate involving the macula. Frequently, there are multiple arterial macroaneurysms, although only 10% of cases are bilateral. Arterial macroaneurysms are associated with systemic arterial hypertension in about two-thirds of cases and may occur in the area of previous vascular occlusions. Sclerosis and spontaneous closure often accompany macroaneurysm-related hemorrhage; bleeding more than once is rare.

Laser photocoagulation treatment may be considered if increasing edema in the macula threatens central visual function. In most instances, moderate-intensity laser treatment of the retina—performed immediately adjacent to the macroaneurysm using 2–3 rows of large-spot-size (200–500 μm) applications—results in closure. Some specialists prefer direct treatment. Caution should be used when treating macroaneurysms that occur in macular arterioles because a primary complication of the disease and its therapy is thrombosis with retinal arterial obstruction distal to the macroaneurysm.

Lee EK, Woo SJ, Ahn J, Park KH. Morphologic characteristics of retinal arterial macroaneurysm and its regression pattern on spectral-domain optical coherence tomography. *Retina.* 2011;31(10):2095–2101.

Pitkänen L, Tommila P, Kaarniranta K, Jääskeläinen JE, Kinnunen K. Retinal arterial macroaneurysms. *Acta Ophthalmol.* 2014;92(2):101–104.

CHAPTER 7

Other Retinal Vascular Diseases

Sickle Cell Retinopathy

The sickle cell hemoglobinopathies of greatest ocular importance are those in which mutant hemoglobins S, C, or both are inherited instead of normal hemoglobin A (see BCSC Section 2, *Fundamentals and Principles of Ophthalmology*). Sickle cell hemoglobinopathies are most prevalent in the black population. In the US African American population, sickle cell trait (Hb AS) affects 8%; sickle cell disease (Hb SS), 0.4%; and hemoglobin SC disease, 0.2% (Table 7-1). Thalassemia, in which the α- or β-polypeptide chain is defective, is rare but frequently causes retinopathy. Although sickling and solubility tests (sickle cell preparations) are reliable indicators of the presence of hemoglobin S and are therefore excellent for screening, they do not distinguish between heterozygous and homozygous states. Hemoglobin electrophoresis testing should be performed for patients testing positive on sickle cell preparations.

Scott AW, Lutty GA, Goldberg MF. Hemoglobinopathies. In: Ryan SJ, Schachat AP, Wilkinson CP, Hinton DR, Sadda SR, Wiedemann P, eds. *Retina*. Vol 1. 5th ed. Philadelphia: Elsevier/Saunders; 2013:1071–1082.

Table 7-1 Incidence of Sickle Cell Hemoglobinopathies in North America

Hemoglobinopathy	Incidence in Population (%)	Incidence of Proliferative Retinopathy in Subgroups
Any sickle hemoglobin	10	—
Sickle cell trait (AS)	8	Uncommon
Hemoglobin C trait (AC)	2	Uncommon
Sickle cell homozygote (SS)	0.4	3%*
Sickle cell hemoglobin C (SC)	0.2	33%*
Sickle cell thalassemia (SThal)	0.03	14%*
Homozygous C (CC)	0.016	Unknown

* Approximate.

Used with permission from Fekrat S, Goldberg MF. Sickle retinopathy. In: Regillo CD, Brown GC, Flynn HW Jr, eds. *Vitreoretinal Disease: The Essentials.* New York: Thieme; 1999:333. ©Thieme.

Nonproliferative Sickle Cell Retinopathy

The retinal changes in nonproliferative sickle cell retinopathy (NPSR) are caused by arteriolar and capillary occlusion, similar to white or hemorrhagic infarcts of the central nervous system. Anastomosis and remodeling occur in the periphery, as does the resorption of blood in the area of the infarct. Salmon-patch hemorrhages represent areas of intraretinal hemorrhage occurring after a peripheral retinal arteriolar occlusion. Refractile spots are old, resorbed hemorrhages with hemosiderin deposition within the inner retina just beneath the internal limiting membrane (ILM) (Fig 7-1). Black "sunburst" lesions are localized areas of retinal pigment epithelial hypertrophy, hyperplasia, and pigment migration in the peripheral retina, probably caused by hemorrhage.

Occlusion of parafoveal capillaries and arterioles is one cause of decreased visual acuity in sickle cell retinopathy. Spontaneous occlusion of the central retinal artery may also develop in patients with sickle cell hemoglobinopathies.

Proliferative Sickle Cell Retinopathy

Serious ocular complications of proliferative sickle cell retinopathy (PSR) are more characteristic of sickle cell hemoglobin C (SC) and sickle cell thalassemia (SThal) than of SS disease, although SS disease results in more systemic complications. The ocular complications result from ischemia secondary to infarction of the retinal tissue by means of arteriolar, precapillary arteriolar, capillary, or venular occlusions, and they include retinal neovascularization, preretinal or vitreous hemorrhage, and tractional retinal detachment.

PSR has been classified into 5 stages based on the following pathogenetic sequence:

1. Peripheral arteriolar occlusions (stage 1) lead to peripheral nonperfusion and
2. peripheral arteriovenular anastomoses (stage 2), which are dilated, preexisting capillary channels.

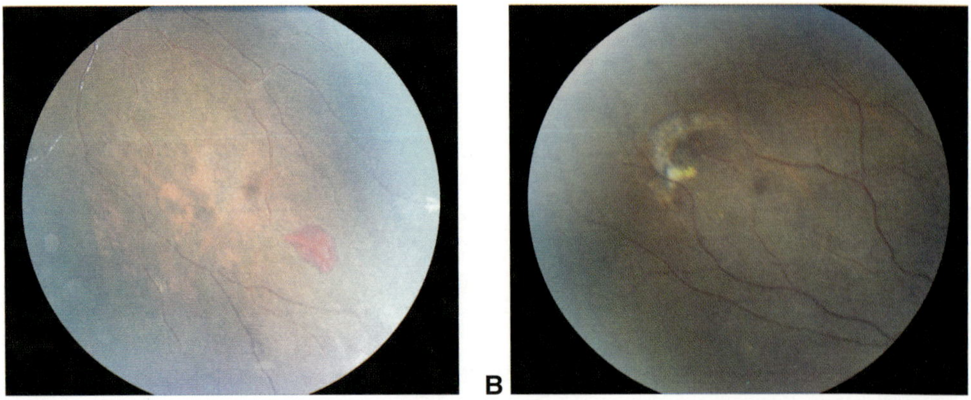

A B

Figure 7-1 Salmon patch in sickle cell retinopathy. **A,** Peripheral fundus photograph of a patient with sickle cell disease. The image shows a retinal hemorrhage unrelated to proliferation but the result of infarction of the retina from a vascular occlusion—a *salmon patch.* **B,** Peripheral fundus photograph of an iridescent, or retractile, patch that represents an area of previous, now resorbed, retinal hemorrhage (salmon patch). *(Courtesy of G. Baker Hubbard III, MD.)*

3. Preretinal sea fan neovascularization (stage 3) may occur at the posterior border of areas of nonperfusion and lead to
4. vitreous hemorrhage (stage 4) and
5. tractional retinal detachment (stage 5).

PSR is one of many retinal vascular diseases in which extraretinal fibrovascular proliferation occurs in response to retinal ischemia. Whereas the neovascularization in proliferative diabetic retinopathy (PDR) generally begins postequatorially, that in PSR is located more peripherally (Fig 7-2). Another way in which PSR differs from PDR is in

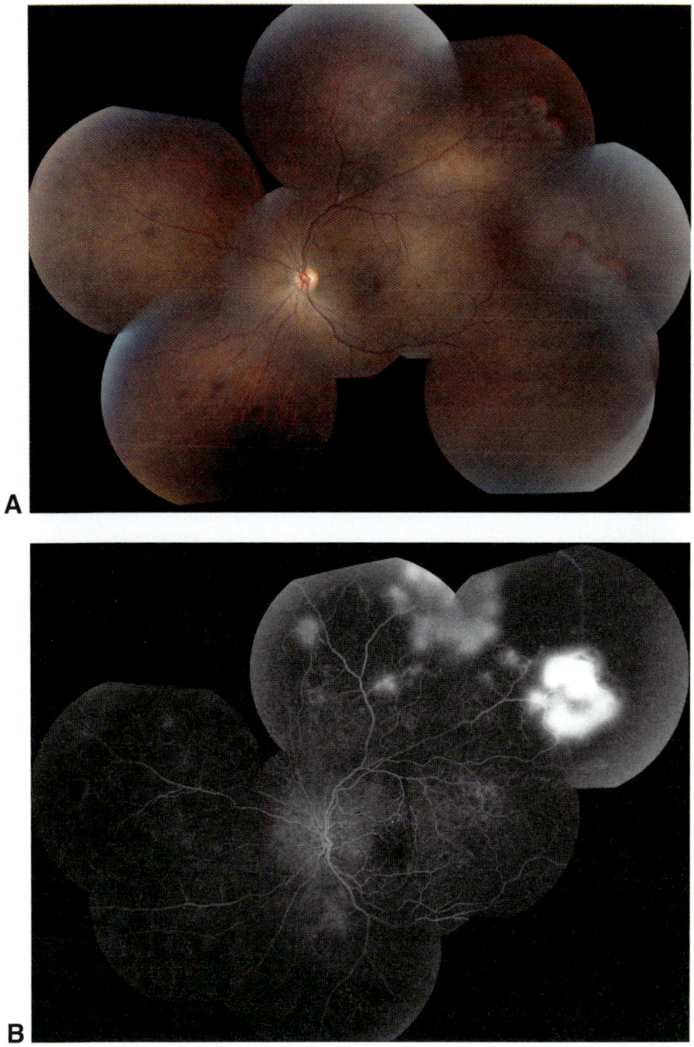

Figure 7-2 Wide-field fundus montage images of the left eye of a 26-year-old African American man with a history of SC sickle cell disease. **A,** Hemorrhaging has occurred at the anterior border of the proliferative lesions. **B,** The wide-field montage fluorescein angiogram shows leakage from the sea fan lesions in the periphery and peripheral nonperfusion anterior to the sea fans. *(Courtesy of Asheesh Tewari, MD.)*

the frequent occurrence in PSR of autoinfarction of the peripheral neovascularization, resulting in a white sea fan neovascularization (Fig 7-3). Table 7-2 presents a differential diagnosis of peripheral retinal neovascularization.

Elagouz M, Jyothi S, Gupta B, Sivaprasad S. Sickle cell disease and the eye: old and new concepts. *Surv Ophthalmol.* 2010;55(4):359–377.

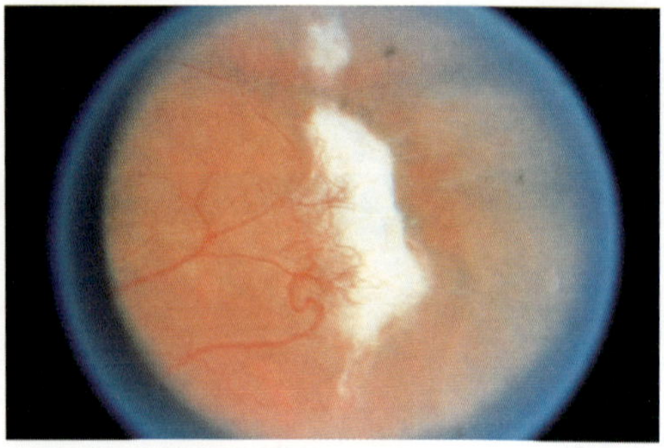

Figure 7-3 Fundus photograph of peripheral neovascularization (sea fan neovascularization) with autoinfarction, as illustrated by the white atrophic vessels. *(Courtesy of Harry W. Flynn, Jr, MD.)*

Table 7-2 Differential Diagnosis of Peripheral Retinal Neovascularization

Vascular diseases with ischemia
- Proliferative diabetic retinopathy (PDR)
- Branch retinal vein occlusion (BRVO)
- Branch retinal arteriolar occlusion (BRAO)
- Carotid cavernous fistula
- Sickling hemoglobinopathies (eg, SC, SS)
- Other hemoglobinopathies (eg, AC, AS)
- Idiopathic retinal vasculitis, aneurysms, and neuroretinitis (IRVAN)
- Retinal embolization (eg, talc emboli)
- Retinopathy of prematurity (ROP)
- Familial exudative vitreoretinopathy (FEVR)
- Hyperviscosity syndromes (eg, chronic myelogenous leukemia)
- Aortic arch syndromes/ocular ischemic syndromes
- Eales disease

Inflammatory diseases with possible ischemia
- Sarcoidosis
- Retinal vasculitis (eg, systemic lupus erythematosus)
- Uveitis, including pars planitis
- Birdshot uveitis
- Toxoplasmosis
- Multiple sclerosis

Miscellaneous conditions
- Incontinentia pigmenti
- Long-standing retinal detachment
- Choroidal melanoma
- Retinitis pigmentosa
- Retinoschisis
- Chronic retinal detachment

Modified from Jampol LM, Ebroon DA, Goldbaum MH. Peripheral proliferative retinopathies: an update on angiogenesis, etiologies, and management. *Surv Ophthalmol.* 1994;38(6):519–540.

Other Ocular Abnormalities in Sickle Cell Hemoglobinopathies

Many patients with SS or SC disease exhibit segmentation of blood in the conjunctival blood vessels. Numerous comma-shaped thrombi dilate and occlude capillaries, most often in the inferior bulbar conjunctiva and fornix (the comma sign). Similarly, small vessels on the surface of the optic disc can exhibit intravascular occlusions, manifested as dark red spots (the disc sign of sickling). Angioid streaks have been reported clinically in up to 6% of cases of SS disease and in persons with AS trait. The pathogenetic basis of this association is uncertain.

Management of Sickle Cell Retinopathy

All black patients presenting with a traumatic hyphema should be screened for a sickling hemoglobinopathy (including trait) because of the increased risk of complications in the presence of rigid sickled erythrocytes. Control of intraocular pressure (IOP) may be difficult, and ischemic optic neuropathy may result from short intervals of a modest increase in IOP. Some authors have recommended early anterior chamber washout in the presence of a hyphema with increased IOP. In addition, physicians must be cautious in the use of carbonic anhydrase inhibitors, which may worsen sickling through the production of systemic acidosis.

McLeod DS, Merges C, Fukushima A, Goldberg MF, Lutty GA. Histopathologic features of neovascularization in sickle cell retinopathy. *Am J Ophthalmol.* 1997;124(4):455–472.

Photocoagulation

Therapeutic approaches to PSR have included diathermy, cryopexy, and photocoagulation. Peripheral scatter photocoagulation, applying lower-intensity light burns to the ischemic peripheral retina, may cause regression of neovascular fronds and thus decrease the risk of vitreous hemorrhage. The decision to treat PSR with scatter photocoagulation should be made cautiously, however, as retinal tears and subsequent rhegmatogenous retinal detachment can occur and do so more commonly after such treatment in PSR than in proliferative diabetic retinopathy.

Elagouz M, Jyothi S, Gupta B, Sivaprasad S. Sickle cell disease and the eye: old and new concepts. *Surv Ophthalmol.* 2010;55(4):359–377.

Vitreoretinal surgery in PSR

Surgery may be indicated for nonclearing vitreous hemorrhage and for rhegmatogenous, tractional, schisis, or combined retinal detachment. Retinal detachment usually begins in the ischemic peripheral retina. The tears typically occur at the base of sea fans and are often precipitated by photocoagulation treatment. Anterior segment ischemia or necrosis has been reported in association with 360° scleral buckling procedures, particularly when combined with extensive diathermy or cryopexy. During surgery, care should be taken to ensure adequate patient hydration and supplemental nasal oxygenation. Precautions for vitrectomy also include the judicious use of expansile gases to minimize IOP elevations postoperatively, which increase the risk of vascular occlusions. The use of exchange transfusion before vitreoretinal surgery is no longer favored.

Vasculitis

Retinal vasculitis from any cause can lead to similar pathologic sequelae; it may be primarily ocular or be associated with inflammatory disease elsewhere in the body. The early clinical manifestations are generally nonspecific, consisting of perivascular infiltrates and sheathing of the retinal vessels (vascular wall thickening with vessel involution; Fig 7-4). Involvement of exclusively retinal arteries or veins is uncommon. Veins tend to be inflamed earlier and more frequently than arterioles, and combinations are the rule. Causes of retinal vasculitis include

- giant cell arteritis
- polyarteritis nodosa
- systemic lupus erythematosus
- Behçet disease
- inflammatory bowel disease
- multiple sclerosis
- pars planitis
- sarcoidosis
- syphilis
- toxoplasmosis
- viral retinitides
- Lyme disease
- cat-scratch disease
- certain medications, such as rifabutin

The masquerade syndromes should also be considered. See BCSC Section 9, *Intraocular Inflammation and Uveitis,* for further discussion of most of these conditions and Section 5, *Neuro-Ophthalmology,* for discussion of multiple sclerosis and giant cell arteritis.

A primary occlusive retinal vasculopathy for which no cause can be found is termed *Eales disease.* This condition is an occlusive vasculopathy that usually involves the peripheral retina of both eyes and often results in extraretinal neovascularization with vitreous hemorrhage. It typically occurs in males, and there may be associated tuberculin hypersensitivity.

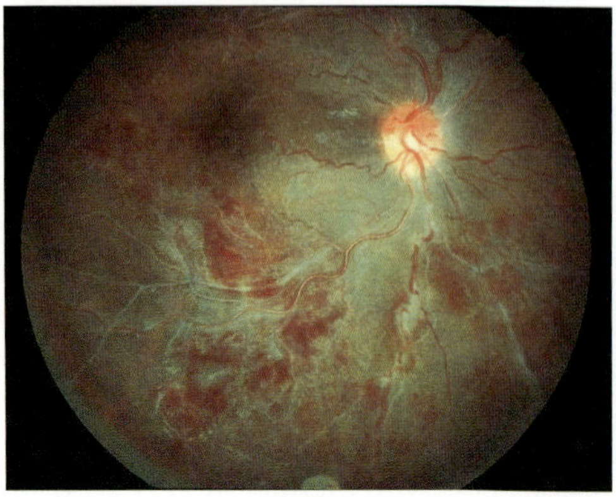

Figure 7-4 Fundus photograph of retinal vasculitis in an eye of a patient with Crohn disease. Retinal hemorrhages and edema are present, as is prominent sheathing of the retinal vessels. *(Courtesy of Gary C. Brown, MD.)*

Susac syndrome is characterized by multiple branch retinal arterial occlusions and can be associated with hearing loss and, rarely, with strokes. The syndrome is most commonly diagnosed in women in their third decade, and there is no known cause. Treatment is with corticosteroids or immunosuppression.

A clinical picture indistinguishable from past retinal vasculitis may result from chronic embolism or thrombosis without inflammation. Evaluation includes a search for possible causes: cardiac valvular disease, cardiac arrhythmias, ulcerated atheromatous disease of the carotid vessels, and hemoglobinopathies.

Idiopathic retinal vasculitis, aneurysms, and neuroretinitis (IRVAN) describes a syndrome characterized by the presence of retinal vasculitis, multiple macroaneurysms, neuroretinitis, and peripheral capillary nonperfusion. Systemic investigations are generally noncontributory, and oral prednisone has demonstrated little benefit. Capillary nonperfusion is often sufficiently severe to warrant panretinal photocoagulation (PRP).

Cystoid Macular Edema

Cystoid macular edema (CME) is characterized by intraretinal edema contained in honeycomb-like cystoid spaces. Fluorescein angiography shows the source of the edema to be abnormal perifoveal retinal capillary permeability, which is visible as multiple small focal fluorescein leaks and late pooling of the dye in extracellular cystoid spaces. Optical coherence tomography (OCT) findings in CME include diffuse retinal thickening with cystic areas of low reflectivity (reduced reflectivity), more prominently in the inner nuclear and outer plexiform layers. This finding correlates with histologic studies that indicate swelling in and between müllerian glia. On occasion, a nonreflective cavity is present beneath the neurosensory retina that is consistent with subretinal fluid accumulation (see Chapter 5, Fig 5-3B, and Chapter 6, Fig 6-12A). Because of the radial foveal arrangement of both glia and Henle inner fibers, this pooling classically forms a "flower-petal" (petaloid) pattern (Fig 7-5). Severe cases may be associated with vitritis (vitreous cells) and optic nerve head swelling.

Etiologies for CME

Abnormal permeability of the perifoveal retinal capillaries may occur in a wide variety of conditions, including diabetic retinopathy, central and branch retinal vein occlusion (CRVO, BRVO), any type of uveitis (particularly pars planitis), and retinitis pigmentosa. CME may occur after any ocular surgery, such as cataract extraction (in which case the CME is termed *Irvine-Gass Syndrome*), retinal detachment surgery, vitrectomy, glaucoma procedures, photocoagulation, and cryopexy. It can also be triggered by prostaglandin analogues used to treat glaucoma. Subretinal disease processes (choroidal neovascularization, choroidal hemangioma, subclinical retinal detachment) must also be considered when CME is detected; see Chapter 4. The nutritional supplement niacin has also been implicated as a cause of atypical CME.

Rare causes of cystic macular change of different pathogeneses (such as X-linked hereditary retinoschisis, Goldmann-Favre disease, some cases of retinitis pigmentosa, and

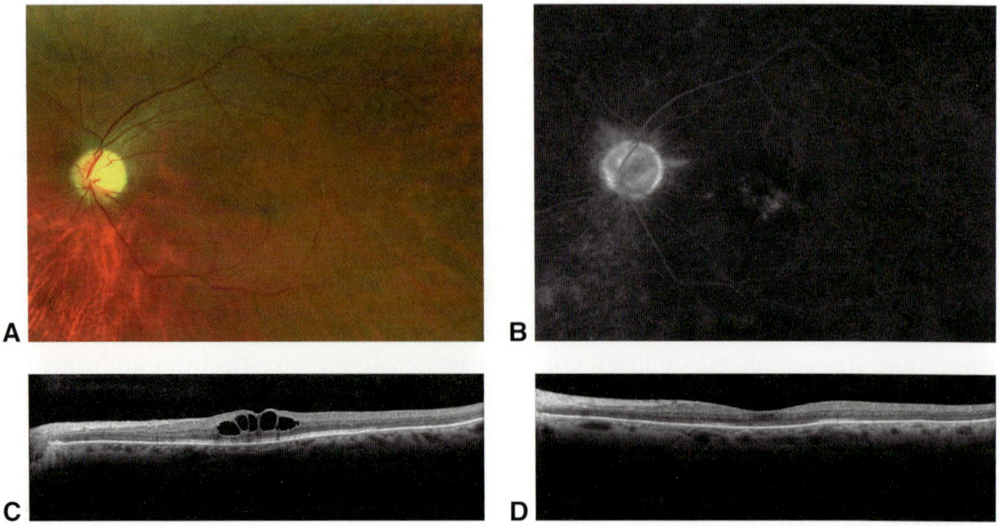

Figure 7-5 Cystoid macular edema (CME). Fundus photograph **(A)** and late fluorescein angiogram (at 5 minutes, 58 seconds) **(B)** demonstrate petaloid perifoveal hyperfluorescence in a patient with intermediate uveitis. Disc staining is commonly observed in intermediate uveitis. The small patchy areas of hyperfluorescence (leakage) throughout the fundus can also be present in inflammatory disorders. **C,** Corresponding optical coherence tomography (OCT) scan shows severe CME. **D,** Following treatment of patient's intermediate uveitis with an intravitreal dexamethasone sustained-delivery implant, OCT scan shows the CME is completely resolved. *(Courtesy of Colin A. McCannel, MD.)*

nicotinic acid maculopathy) are distinguishable by the clinical setting, family history, and lack of late-phase fluorescein leakage into the cystlike spaces, as well as by OCT.

Incidence of CME

For patients who have undergone intracapsular lens extraction, the incidence of CME is as high as 60%. Intraocular lens implantation at the time of extracapsular surgery does not appear to increase the incidence of CME. The peak incidence occurs 6–10 weeks postoperatively, with spontaneous resolution occurring clinically in approximately 95% of uncomplicated cases, usually within 6 months. Most such cases of CME are mild and asymptomatic, and distinguishing between symptomatic, or clinical, CME and edema that is apparent only on fluorescein angiography, termed *angiographic CME,* is relevant. More severe CME may result in permanent vision loss. The incidence of CME is affected by many factors. The presence of predisposing disease, as mentioned under etiologies, is an important factor. Factors affecting the incidence and severity of CME after intraocular, particularly cataract, surgery include the degree of postoperative inflammation and the presence or absence of surgical complications such as vitreous loss or iris prolapse. See also BCSC Section 11, *Lens and Cataract.*

Johnson MW. Etiology and treatment of macular edema. *Am J Ophthalmol.* 2009;147(1): 11–21.e1.

Treatment for CME

The effect of therapy on CME is difficult to evaluate because of the high rate of spontaneous resolution. Pharmacologic therapy using a combination of topical corticosteroids and nonsteroidal anti-inflammatory drugs (NSAIDs) has become commonplace for prophylaxis and is well supported by the medical literature for established edema. If CME is severe or refractory to topical therapy, periocular (eg, posterior sub-Tenon triamcinolone acetonide) or intraocular injection of steroid preparations are appropriate escalations of therapy. In chronic CME, systemic acetazolamide treatment can be successful, especially in cases associated with retinitis pigmentosa. For treating CME associated with diabetic retinopathy or ocular venous occlusive disease, also see Chapters 5 and 6.

If CME is associated with vitreous adhesions to the iris or a corneoscleral wound, interruption of the vitreous strands by vitrectomy or Nd:YAG laser treatment may be helpful.

Coats Disease

Coats disease is defined by the presence of vascular dilatations (retinal telangiectasia), including ectatic arterioles, microaneurysms, venous dilations (phlebectasias), and fusiform capillary dilatations, frequently associated with exudative retinal detachment. Usually only 1 eye is involved, and there is a marked male predominance (85%). To date, researchers have not identified an associated gene or chromosome or any hereditary pattern, and an association between Coats disease and systemic disease has not been found.

The abnormal vessels are incompetent, resulting in the leakage of serum and other blood components, which accumulate in and under the retina. Any portion of the peripheral and macular capillary system may be involved. Despite the presence of retinal capillary nonperfusion shown by angiography, posterior segment neovascularization is unusual. Variation in the clinical findings is wide, ranging from mild retinal vascular abnormalities and minimal exudation to extensive areas of retinal telangiectasia associated with massive leakage and exudative retinal detachment. The severity and rate of progression appear greater in children under the age of 4 years, in whom massive exudative retinal detachment with retina apposed to the lens may simulate retinoblastoma or other causes of leukocoria (Coats reaction; Fig 7-6; see BCSC 6, *Pediatric Ophthalmology and Strabismus,* for the differential diagnosis of leukocoria) or xanthocoria (yellow pupil).

Patients with peripheral areas of leaky vascular anomalies typically present with lipid deposition in an otherwise angiographically normal macula, as "hard" exudate tends to accumulate in the macula. Similar findings in adults probably represent late decompensation of preexisting vascular anomalies. Occasionally, a submacular lipogranuloma or subretinal fibrosis is the initial finding. The differential diagnosis may include

- dominant (familial) exudative vitreoretinopathy
- facioscapulohumeral muscular dystrophy
- retinopathy of prematurity (ROP)
- capillary hemangioma (von Hippel disease)

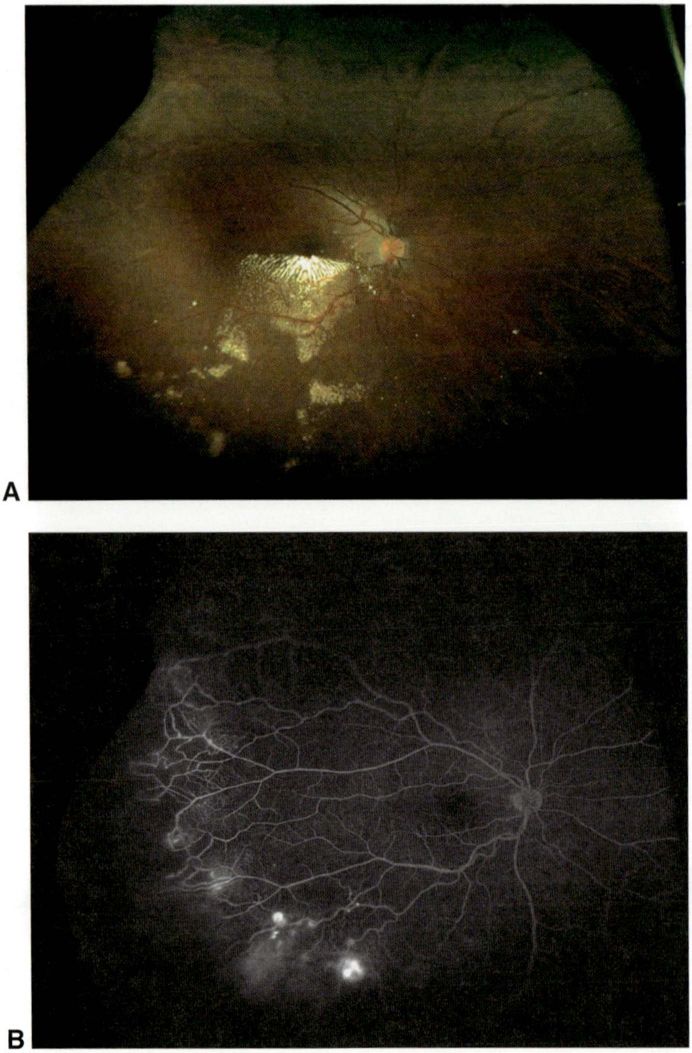

Figure 7-6 Coats disease. **A,** Ultra-wide-field fundus photograph of a patient with Coats disease showing dilated vessels with aneurismal changes in the inferior temporal periphery as well as moderate to severe accumulation of exudate in the macula. **B,** Corresponding fluorescein angiography image shows nonperfusion in the peripheral retina and around the abnormal blood vessels. The aneurisms, characteristic of Coats disease, hyperfluoresce brightly and leak. *(Courtesy of Colin A. McCannel, MD.)*

For milder cases of lipid exudation, additional considerations are diabetic retinopathy, BRVO, juxtafoveal retinal telangiectasia, and radiation retinopathy.

Treatment of Coats disease generally consists of photocoagulation, cryotherapy, and in severe cases, retinal reattachment surgery. Photocoagulation and cryotherapy are effective in obliterating the vascular anomalies and in halting progression. Several treatments may be necessary, and long-term follow-up is important to detect and treat recurrences.

Parafoveal (Juxtafoveal) Retinal Telangiectasia

Focal retinal gliosis and telangiectasia of the capillary bed, confined to the juxtafoveolar region of 1 or both eyes, may result in vision loss from capillary incompetence and exudation (Fig 7-7). Refractile changes ("retinal crystals") are visible in advanced cases. Histologic evidence suggests that this condition is not a true telangiectasia but rather consists of structural abnormalities similar to those of diabetic microangiopathy, with deposits of excess basement membrane within the retinal capillaries. The entity has been subdivided into 3 general types:

Type 1: unilateral parafoveal telangiectasia, congenital or acquired
Type 2: bilateral parafoveal telangiectasia (Fig 7-8)
Type 3: bilateral parafoveal telangiectasia with retinal capillary obliteration

Type 1, also referred to as *aneurysmal telangiectasia,* typically occurs in males and resembles a macular variant of Coats disease with a circinate type of exudate, also known as *Leber miliary aneurysm.* Type 2, or *perifoveal telangiectasia,* has no sex predilection and affects both eyes. Perifoveal retinal changes typically include thickening, loss of transparency with a grayish appearance, small telangiectatic vessels, and a cystic appearance of the fovea, all most pronounced in the temporal fovea. As the lesion ages, intralesional retinal pigment epithelium (RPE) migration is often present, and choroidal neovascularization may subsequently develop. Vision loss ranges from mild to severe. Approximately one-third of patients with this variant have an abnormal glucose tolerance test result. Cases in type 3 show progressive vision loss from obliteration of the perifoveal capillaries.

On fluorescein angiography, the telangiectatic vessels are readily apparent and usually leak. OCT imaging typically shows a thinned central macular retina, including the fovea, with inner lamellar oblong foveal cavitations in which the long axis is parallel to the retinal surface.

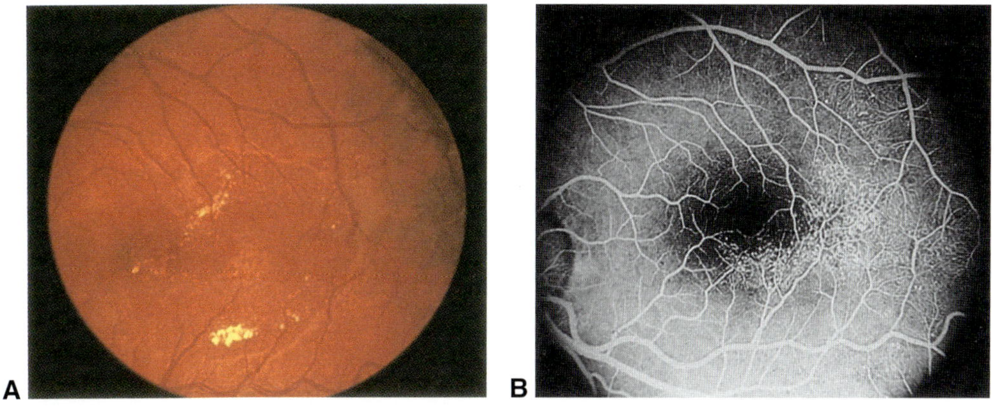

Figure 7-7 Parafoveal telangiectasia, type 1. **A,** Fundus photograph shows typical retinal capillary abnormalities in the temporal macula and retinal exudates. **B,** Fluorescein angiography image demonstrates more clearly the retinal capillary abnormalities.

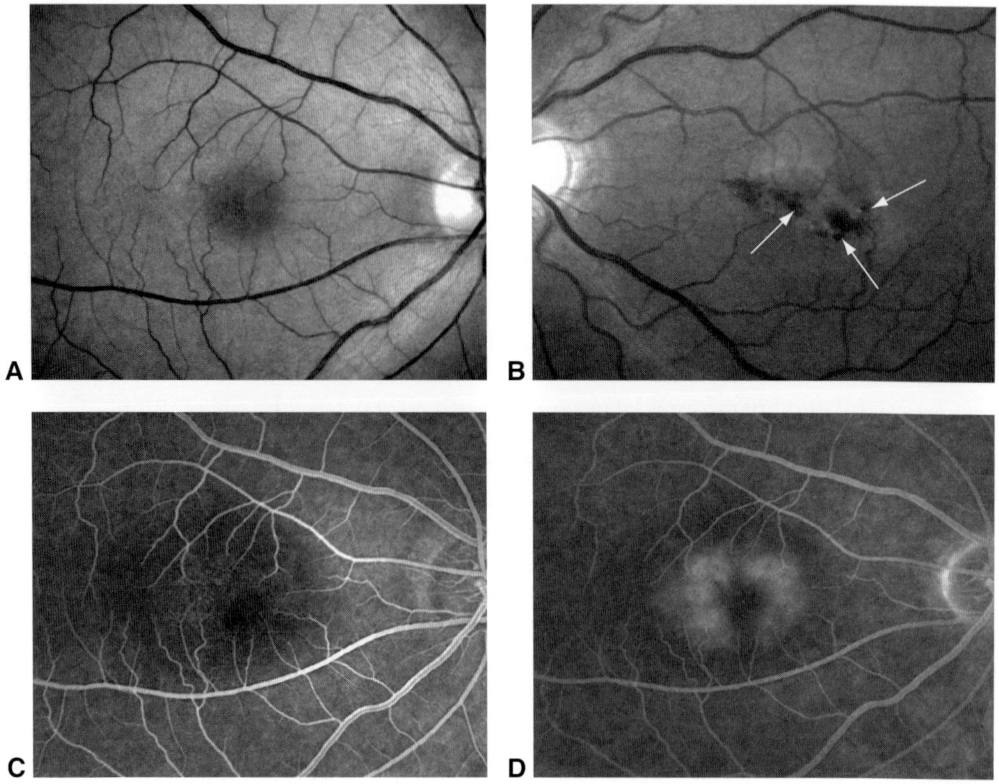

Figure 7-8 Parafoveal telangiectasia, type 2. Red-free photographs of right **(A)** and left **(B)** eyes, show bilateral parafoveal telangiectasia. Early right-angle branching and fine crystals are visible temporal to the fovea in each eye. *Arrows* point to the intraretinal pigment migration in the left eye **(B),** typically present as a late manifestation in this condition. Early **(C)** and late **(D)** fluorescein angiography images of the right eye. The early-phase image **(C)** demonstrates telangiectatic changes of the retinal capillaries temporal to the fovea. The late-phase image **(D)** demonstrates hyperfluorescence from inner retinal leakage of fluorescein in the perifoveal macula. *(Courtesy of Richard F. Spaide, MD.)*

Photocoagulation treatment may be indicated for type 1 cases and can be successful in resolving exudation. Type 2 and type 3 eyes typically do not respond to photocoagulation because leaky vessels are not the predominant feature. Small controlled and uncontrolled trials suggest limited success of management using intravitreal anti–vascular endothelial growth factor (VEGF) drugs. The differential diagnosis includes branch retinal vein or venule obstruction, diabetes mellitus, radiation retinopathy, cystoid macular edema (especially chronic), and carotid artery disease.

Clemons TE, Gillies MC, Chew EY, et al; MacTel Research Group. Baseline characteristics of participants in the natural history study of macular telangiectasia (MacTel) MacTel Project report no. 2. *Ophthalmic Epidemiol.* 2010;17(1):66–73.

Yannuzzi LA, Bardal AM, Freund KB, Chen KJ, Eandi CM, Blodi B. Idiopathic macular telangiectasia. *Arch Ophthalmol.* 2006;124(4):450–460.

Phakomatoses

Conventionally, a number of syndromes referred to as phakomatoses ("mother spot") are grouped loosely by the common features of ocular and extraocular or systemic involvement of a congenital nature. Most, but not all, are hereditary. With the exception of Sturge-Weber syndrome, the phakomatoses involve the neuroretina and its circulation. For further discussion of the phakomatoses, see BCSC Section 5, *Neuro-Ophthalmology,* and Section 6, *Pediatric Ophthalmology and Strabismus.*

Von Hippel–Lindau Disease

The phakomatosis *von Hippel–Lindau* (VHL) *disease* (also called *von Hippel–Lindau syndrome*) is caused by a tumor suppressor gene mutation on the short arm of chromosome 3 (3p26–p25), the inheritance of which is autosomal dominant with incomplete penetrance and variable expression. The disease is characterized by retinal and central nervous system hemangioblastomas and visceral manifestations (see BCSC Section 6, *Pediatric Ophthalmology and Strabismus*); the diagnosis can be confirmed with genetic testing. Central nervous system tumors include hemangioblastomas of the cerebellum, medulla, pons, and spinal cord in 20% of VHL disease patients. Visceral manifestations include renal cell carcinoma, meningiomas, pheochromocytomas, and cysts of the kidney, pancreas, liver, epididymis, and ovary. Diagnosis of a retinal hemangioblastoma warrants systemic workup and possibly genetic testing. The leading causes of death in patients with VHL disease are cerebellar hemangioblastoma and renal cell carcinoma. Patients may incur severe disability from central nervous system lesions and their treatments.

A fully developed retinal lesion is a spherical orange-red tumor fed by a dilated, tortuous retinal artery and drained by an engorged vein (Fig 7-9). Hemangioblastomas of the optic nerve head and peripapillary region are often flat and difficult to recognize. Multiple hemangioblastomas may be present in the same eye, and bilateral involvement occurs in 50% of patients. Leakage from a hemangioblastoma may cause decreased vision

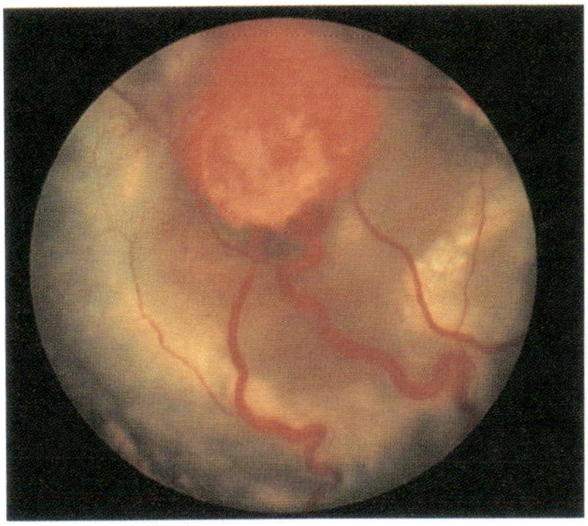

Figure 7-9 Fundus photograph from a patient with von Hippel disease, showing a peripheral retinal capillary hemangioblastoma with surrounding exudate and retinal detachment. The feeder arteriole and draining venule are dilated.

from macular exudates (Fig 7-10) with or without exudative retinal detachment. Vitreous hemorrhage or tractional detachment may also occur.

Ocular management includes treatment of all identified retinal angiomas with careful follow-up to detect recurrence or the development of new lesions. Successful treatment is facilitated by early diagnosis, as the lesions usually enlarge with time. Wide-angle fluorescein angiography can assist in detecting small, early lesions (Fig 7-11). Photocoagulation, photodynamic therapy with verteporfin, and cryotherapy are used to treat the angiomatous lesions directly. Successful treatment results in shrinkage of the angioma, attenuation of the afferent vessels, and resorption of the subretinal fluid. Cryotherapy may be used to treat larger lesions, but it can cause a temporary and marked increase in the amount of exudation and sometimes exudative retinal detachment.

Retinal hemangioblastomas may also occur sporadically without systemic involvement; these are termed *von Hippel lesions. Vasoproliferative tumors,* another form of retinal angiomas, are idiopathic or, rarely, may be present as a late complication of ROP, retinitis pigmentosa, or other conditions. These lesions do not have the dilated feeder and draining vessels seen with hemangioblastomas.

Atebara NH. Retinal capillary hemangioma treated with verteporfin photodynamic therapy. *Am J Ophthalmol.* 2002;134(5):788–790.

Gaudric A, Krivosic V, Duquid G, Massin P, Giraud S, Richard S. Vitreoretinal surgery for severe retinal capillary hemangiomas in von Hippel–Lindau disease. *Ophthalmology.* 2011; 118(1):142–149.

Wyburn-Mason Syndrome

In Wyburn-Mason syndrome, congenital retinal arteriovenous malformations occur in conjunction with similar ipsilateral vascular malformations in the brain, face, orbit, and

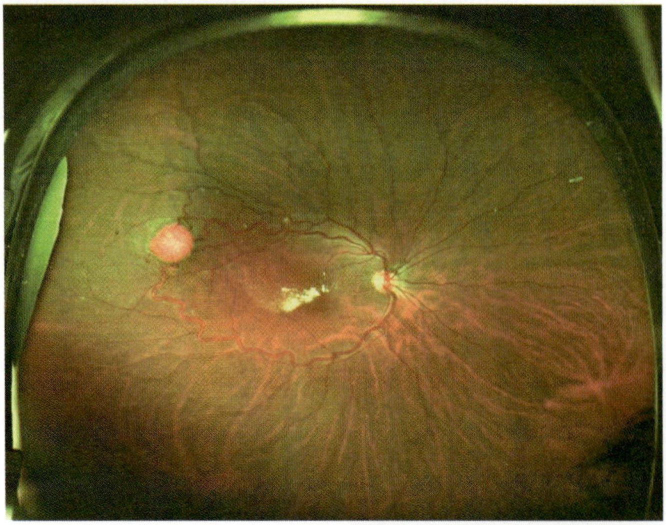

Figure 7-10 Von Hippel–Lindau disease. Ultra-wide-field fundus photograph of a patient with von Hippel–Lindau disease, showing retinal capillary hemangioblastoma in the near periphery and associated exudative maculopathy. *(Courtesy of Colin A. McCannel, MD.)*

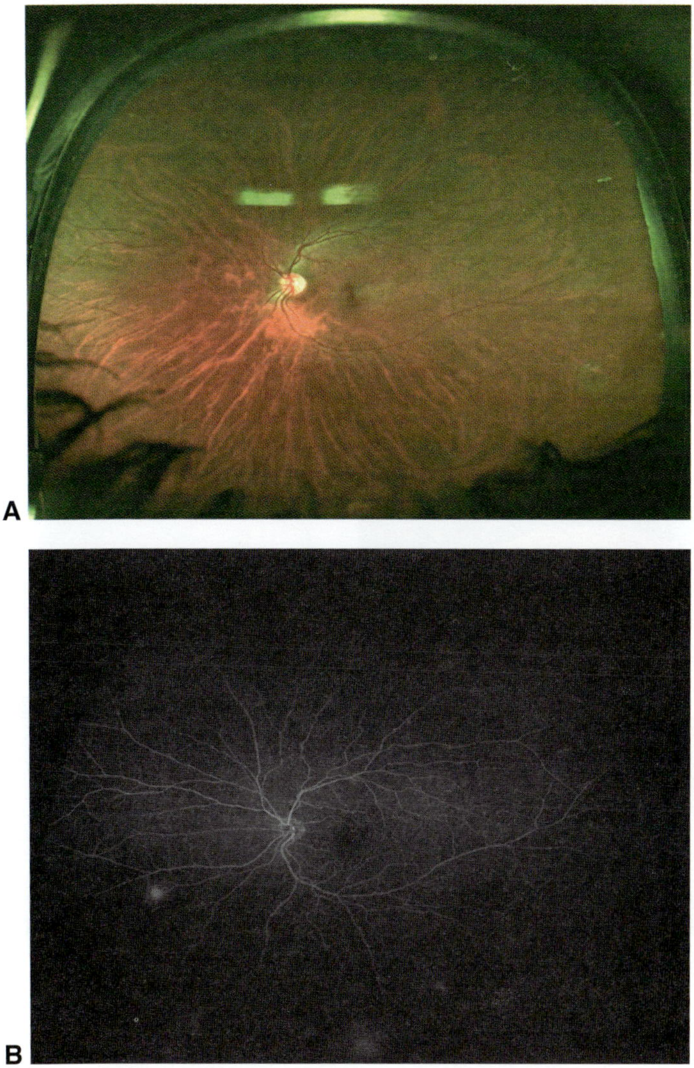

Figure 7-11 Von Hippel–Lindau disease. **A,** Ultra-wide-angle fundus image of the left eye of a 26-year-old woman with von Hippel–Lindau disease. No obvious lesions are visible. **B,** The corresponding ultra-wide-angle fluorescein angiography image demonstrates multiple foci of leakage that are early, small retinal hemangioblastomas, some of which are not visible on the photograph or clinically. *(Courtesy of Colin A. McCannel, MD.)*

mandible. The lesions are composed of blood vessels without an intervening capillary bed (racemose angioma). The abnormalities may range from a single arteriovenous communication to a complex anastomotic system. In the eye, the lesions are usually asymptomatic, unilateral, and located in the retina and optic nerve. Typically, they do not show leakage on fluorescein angiography. Intraosseous vascular malformations that may occur in the maxilla and mandible can lead to unexpected hemorrhaging during dental extractions. Most commonly, racemose angiomas in the retina are isolated and not part of the full syndrome.

Retinal Cavernous Hemangioma

Although most cases of cavernous hemangioma are sporadic and restricted to the retina or optic nerve head, they may occur in a familial (autosomal-dominant) pattern and may be associated with intracranial and skin hemangiomas. For this reason, cavernous hemangioma may be considered one of the phakomatoses.

Retinal cavernous hemangioma is characterized by the formation of grapelike clusters of thin-walled saccular angiomatous lesions in the inner retina or on the optic nerve head (Fig 7-12). The blood flow in these lesions is derived from the retinal circulation and is relatively stagnant, producing a characteristic fluorescein angiographic picture. These dilated saccular lesions fill slowly during angiography, and plasma-erythrocyte layering occurs as a result of the sluggish blood flow. Fluorescein leakage is characteristically absent, correlating with the absence of subretinal fluid and exudate in the retinal cavernous

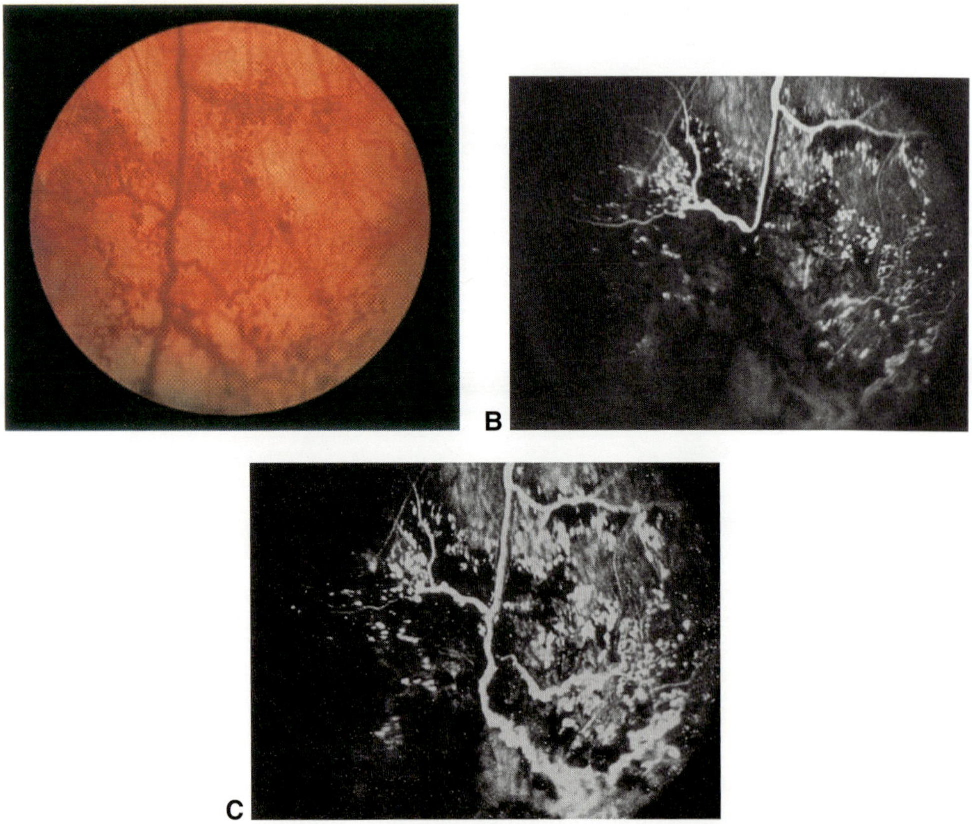

A B C

Figure 7-12 Retinal cavernous hemangioma. **A,** Fundus photograph of the right eye, showing a large retinal cavernous hemangioma in the inferior retina. Note the dilated and tortuous vein with grapelike saccular clusters of angiomatous lesions that could be mistaken for retinal neovascularization. These lesions are usually stable and require no treatment. **B,** Fluorescein angiography image (late transit at 43.3 seconds) shows poor blood flow and uneven filling of the vascular lesion. **C,** Even by 70.8 seconds, the vascular tree is not completely filled. Late phases typically show an accumulation of dye in the saccular lesions with no sign of leakage.

hemangioma and serving to differentiate the condition from retinal telangiectasia, retinal capillary hemangioblastomas, and racemose aneurysm of the retina.

Though rare occurrences, these hemangiomas may bleed into the vitreous but usually remain asymptomatic. Vitreous traction is thought to be the cause of hemorrhage in these cases. Treatment of retinal cavernous hemangiomas is usually not indicated unless vitreous hemorrhage is recurrent, in which case photocoagulation or cryotherapy may be effective. For further discussion, see BCSC Section 4, *Ophthalmic Pathology and Intraocular Tumors.*

Radiation Retinopathy

Exposure to ionizing radiation can damage the retinal vasculature. Radiation retinopathy typically has a delayed onset, is slowly progressive, and causes microangiopathic changes that clinically resemble diabetic retinopathy. Radiation retinopathy can occur after either external-beam or local plaque therapy, typically within months to years after radiation treatment. In general, radiation retinopathy is observed around 18 months after treatment with external-beam radiation and earlier with brachytherapy. Because radiation retinopathy is very similar to other vascular diseases, eliciting a history of radiation treatment is important in establishing the diagnosis. An exposure to doses of 30–35 grays (Gy) or more is usually required to induce clinical symptoms; occasionally, however, retinopathy may develop after as little as 15 Gy of external-beam radiation. Studies have shown retinal damage in 50% of patients receiving 60 Gy and in 85%–95% of patients receiving 70–80 Gy. The total dose, volume of retina irradiated, and fractionation scheme are important in determining the threshold dose for radiation retinopathy. See BCSC Section 4, *Ophthalmic Pathology and Intraocular Tumors,* for further discussion of these therapies, including sample dosages.

Clinically, affected patients may be asymptomatic or may describe decreased visual acuity. Ophthalmic examination may reveal signs of retinal vascular disease, including cotton-wool spots, retinal hemorrhages, microaneurysms, perivascular sheathing, capillary telangiectasis, macular edema, and disc edema. Capillary nonperfusion, documented by fluorescein angiography, is commonly present, and extensive retinal ischemia can lead to neovascularization of the retina, iris, or disc (Fig 7-13). Other complications may occur, such as optic atrophy, central retinal artery occlusion, central retinal vein occlusion, choroidal neovascularization, vitreous hemorrhage, neovascular glaucoma, and tractional retinal detachment. Vision outcome is primarily related to the extent of macular involvement with cystoid macular edema, exudative maculopathy, or capillary nonperfusion. Occasionally, vision loss may be caused by acute optic neuropathy. Although no clinical trials have been performed, the management of radiation retinopathy is similar to that for diabetic retinopathy and includes focal laser therapy to reduce macular edema or panretinal photocoagulation to treat zones of ischemia and neovascularization. Intravitreal administration of triamcinolone acetonide or anti-VEGF drugs can stabilize or improve visual acuity in some patients, but the effect might not be lasting.

Patel SJ, Schachat AP. Radiation retinopathy. In: Albert DM, Miller JW, Azar DT, Blodi BA, eds. *Albert & Jakobiec's Principles and Practice of Ophthalmology.* 3rd ed. Philadelphia: Saunders; 2008:chap 175.

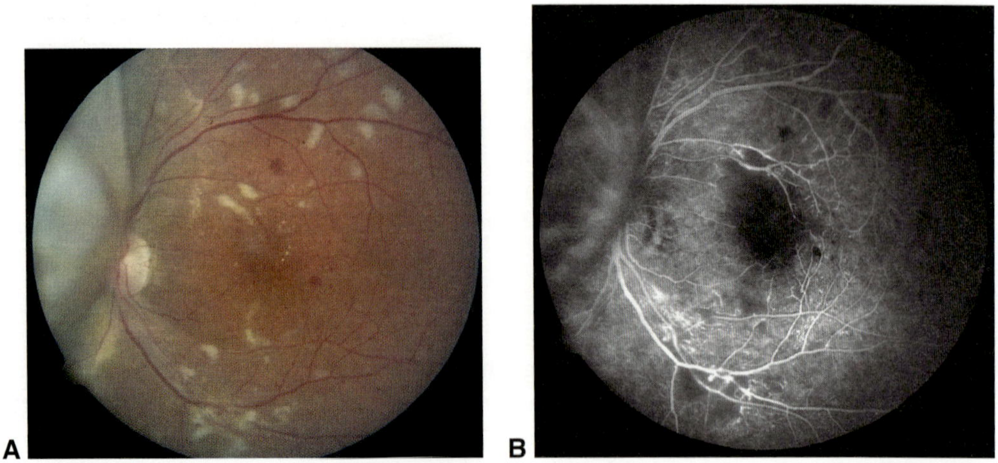

Figure 7-13 Radiation retinopathy. Images of an eye that has undergone plaque brachytherapy for treatment of choroidal melanoma. The melanoma can be seen nasally, obscuring part of the disc. Typical radiation retinopathy changes are apparent. **A,** In the fundus photograph, cotton-wool spots, exudates ("hard" exudates), and intraretinal blot hemorrhages are visible. **B,** The fluorescein angiography image shows microvascular abnormalities (representative of capillary nonperfusion) superior to the fovea and adjacent to an enlarged foveal avascular zone. Additional areas of nonperfusion are noted in the macula and near periphery. *(Courtesy of Tara A. McCannel, MD, PhD.)*

Valsalva Retinopathy

A sudden rise in intrathoracic or intra-abdominal pressure (such as accompanies coughing, vomiting, lifting, or straining for a bowel movement) may raise intraocular venous pressure sufficiently to rupture small superficial capillaries in the macula. The hemorrhage is typically located under the ILM, where it may create a hemorrhagic detachment of the ILM. Vitreous hemorrhage and subretinal hemorrhage may be present. Vision is usually only mildly reduced and the prognosis is excellent, with spontaneous resolution usually occurring within months after onset. The differential diagnosis of Valsalva retinopathy includes posterior vitreous separation, which may cause an identical hemorrhage or a macroaneurysm. Therefore, in all cases, a peripheral retinal tear or an aneurysm along an arteriole must be ruled out.

Purtscher Retinopathy and Purtscherlike Retinopathy

After acute compression injuries to the thorax or head, a patient may experience loss of vision associated with Purtscher retinopathy in 1 or both eyes. Large cotton-wool spots, hemorrhages, and retinal edema are found most commonly surrounding the optic disc, and fluorescein angiography shows evidence of arteriolar obstruction and leakage (Fig 7-14). Occasionally, patients present with disc edema and an afferent pupillary defect. Vision may be permanently lost from this infarction, and optic atrophy may develop.

Purtscher retinopathy is thought to be a result of injury-induced complement activation, which causes granulocyte aggregation and leukoembolization. This process in turn occludes small arterioles such as those in the peripapillary retina.

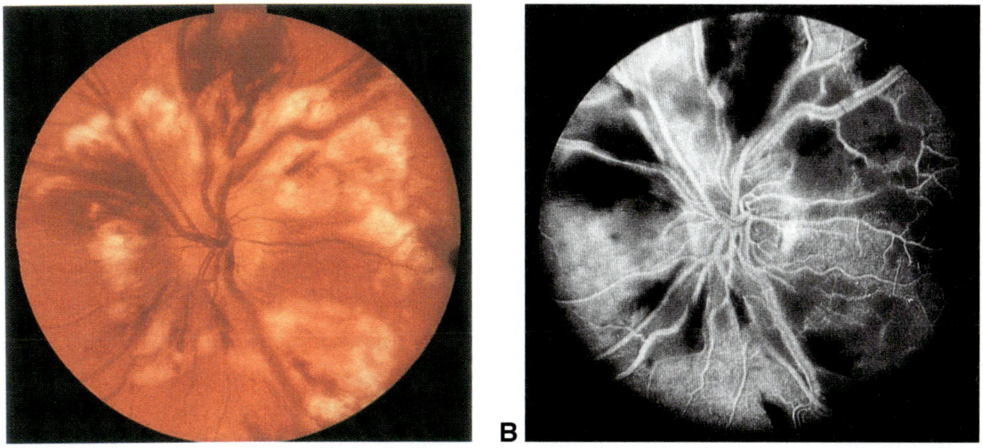

A B

Figure 7-14 Purtscher retinopathy following trauma to the head and face. **A,** Extensive cotton-wool spots and retinal hemorrhage appear in the fundus photograph. **B,** Fluorescein angiography image reveals capillary nonperfusion in areas of cotton-wool spots. *(From Burton TC. Unilateral Purtscher's retinopathy.* Ophthalmology. *1980;87(11):1096–1105.)*

Table 7-3 Conditions Associated With Purtscher or Purtscherlike Retinopathy

Trauma
Head injury
Chest compression
Long-bone fractures (fat embolism syndrome)
Acute pancreatitis
Chronic renal failure
Autoimmune diseases
Systemic lupus erythematosus
Thrombotic thrombocytopenic purpura
Scleroderma
Dermatomyositis
Sjögren syndrome
Amniotic fluid embolism
Retrobulbar anesthesia
Orbital steroid injection

Used with permission from Fekrat S, Goldberg MF. Sickle retinopathy. In: Regillo CD, Brown GC, Flynn HW Jr, eds. *Vitreoretinal Disease: The Essentials.* New York: Thieme; 1999:538. ©Thieme.

Even in the absence of trauma, various other conditions may activate complement and produce a similar fundus appearance. Because Purtscher's original description involved trauma, cases with similar fundus findings are termed *Purtscherlike retinopathy* (Table 7-3). For example, the retinopathy associated with acute pancreatitis, which appears identical to traumatic Purtscher retinopathy, is probably also caused by complement-mediated leukoembolization. Other conditions that may cause these changes include collagen-vascular diseases (such as systemic lupus erythematosus), childbirth, and amniotic fluid embolism.

Fat embolism following crushing injuries or long-bone fractures may cause similar retinal findings. Usually, intraretinal hemorrhages are scattered in the paramacular area, and the cotton-wool spots of fat embolism are generally smaller and situated more peripherally in the retina than they are in Purtscher retinopathy.

Terson Syndrome

Terson syndrome is recognized as vitreous and sub-ILM or subhyaloid hemorrhage caused by an abrupt intracranial hemorrhage. Although the exact mechanism is not known, it is suspected that the acute intracranial hemorrhage causes an acute rise in the intraocular venous pressure, resulting in a rupture of peripapillary and retinal vessels. Approximately one-third of patients with subarachnoid or subdural hemorrhage have associated intraocular hemorrhage, which may include intraretinal and subretinal bleeding. Terson syndrome occurs primarily in individuals between 30 and 50 years old, but it can occur at any age. In most cases, visual function is unaffected once the hemorrhage clears. Spontaneous improvement generally occurs, although vitrectomy is occasionally required to clear the ocular media.

Agarwal A. *Gass' Atlas of Macular Diseases.* 5th ed. Philadelphia: Saunders; 2012:724–726.

CHAPTER 8

Retinopathy of Prematurity

Introduction

Retinopathy of prematurity (ROP) is a complex disease process initiated in part by a lack of complete or normal retinal vascularization in premature infants. ROP has a typical progression pattern, but the earlier disease stages may regress spontaneously at any time. The absence of retinal vessels in portions of the immature retina can result in retinal ischemia, leading to the release of growth factors that promote vascular growth. Instead of the normal vascular-growth process, the growth pattern becomes disturbed and vessels proliferate into the vitreous cavity at the border of vascular and avascular retina. As the disease progresses, vitreous hemorrhage and tractional retinal detachment can occur. The end stage of untreated ROP is the development of a dense, white, fibrovascular plaque behind the lens and complete tractional retinal detachment. The former name of this condition, *retrolental fibroplasia,* is descriptive of the end stage of ROP. The main risk factors for developing this condition are prematurity and low birth weight. Also see BCSC Section 6, *Pediatric Ophthalmology and Strabismus,* for additional discussion of ROP.

Epidemiology

In the United States, ROP that is severe enough to require treatment occurs in approximately 1100–1500 infants annually. Among these infants, 400–600 will never achieve vision better than 20/200. In resource-limited regions of the world, there has been a recent rise in the incidence of ROP that corresponds to the establishment of neonatal intervention initiatives to treat premature infants who would not previously have survived. In many instances, there has been an unfortunate lag between successes in saving premature infants and successes in diagnosing and managing their subsequent ROP.

Terminology and Classification

For the purpose of consistently describing, staging, and studying ROP, an international classification of ROP was developed. Four classification concepts have prognostic and pathophysiologic importance: the location, or *zone,* of involvement; the disease severity, or *stage;* the *extent* of disease in clock-hours of involvement; and whether or not *plus disease* is present. This important terminology is detailed in Table 8-1.

Table 8-1 Descriptive Terminology for Acute Retinopathy of Prematurity

Location

Zone I: posterior retina within a 60° circle centered on the optic nerve

Zone II: from the posterior circle (zone I) to the nasal ora serrata anteriorly

Zone III: remaining temporal peripheral retina

Extent: number of clock-hours involved

Severity

Stage 0: immature retinal vasculature without pathologic changes

Stage 1: presence of a demarcation line between vascularized and nonvascularized retina (Fig 8-1)

Stage 2: presence of a demarcation line that has height, width, and volume (ridge); small, isolated tufts of neovascular tissue lying on the surface of the retina, commonly called "popcorn," may be present (Fig 8-2)

Stage 3: a ridge with extraretinal fibrovascular proliferation that may be mild, moderate, or severe, as judged by the amount of proliferative tissue present (Fig 8-3)

Stage 4: partial retinal detachment

A. extrafoveal

B. retinal detachment including fovea (Fig 8-4)

Stage 5: total retinal detachment with funnel configuration; combinations are listed in order of frequency: top row is the most common and bottom row the least common configuration (Fig 8-5)

Anterior	*Posterior*
Open	Open
Narrow	Narrow
Open	Narrow
Narrow	Open

Plus disease: vascular dilatation (venous) and tortuosity (arteriolar) of posterior retinal vessels in at least 2 quadrants of the eye; iris vascular dilatation and vitreous haze may be present (Fig 8-6)

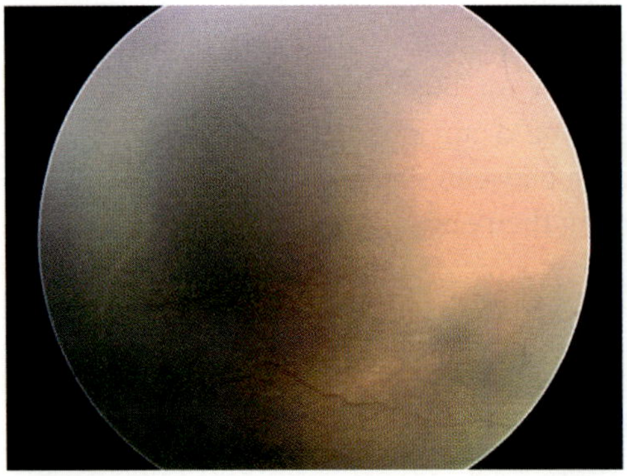

Figure 8-1 Stage 1 retinopathy of prematurity (ROP). Fundus photograph revealing a faint demarcation line present temporally. *(Courtesy of Colin A. McCannel, MD.)*

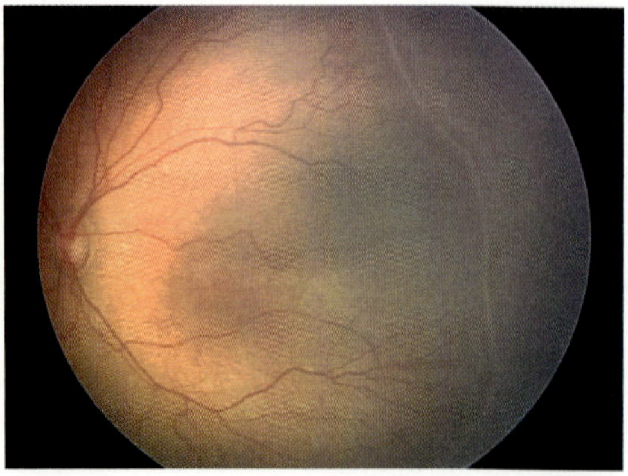

Figure 8-2 Stage 2 ROP. Fundus photograph showing an elevated ridge of mesenchymal tissue at the border of the vascularized (reddish) and avascular (grayish) retina. *(Courtesy of Colin A. McCannel, MD.)*

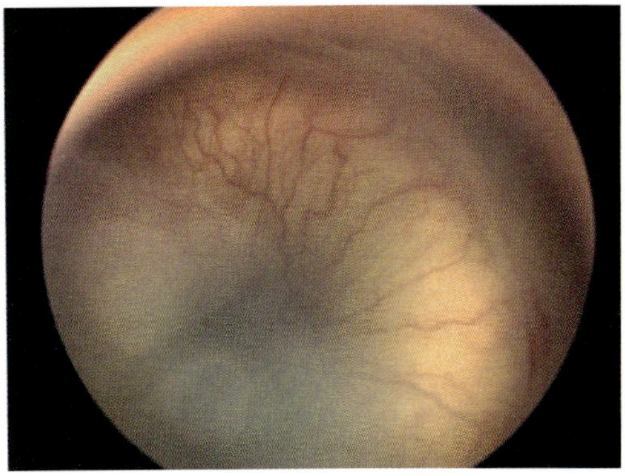

Figure 8-3 Stage 3 ROP. Fundus photograph of severe stage 3 ROP with marked preretinal proliferations. Some vitreous and preretinal hemorrhage is visible *(lower right)*. *(Courtesy of Colin A. McCannel, MD.)*

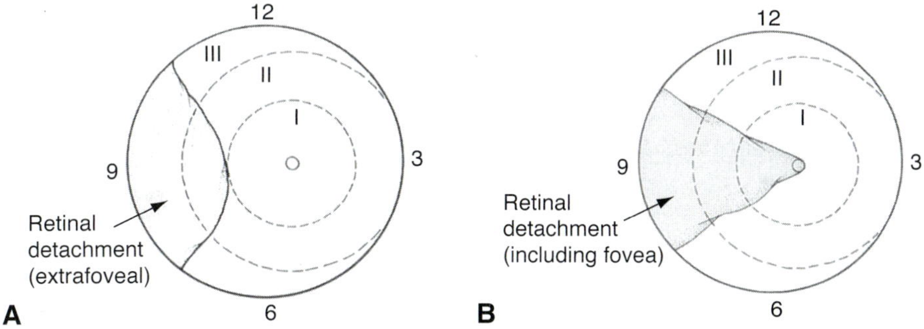

Figure 8-4 **A,** Schematic representation of stage 4A ROP. **B,** Stage 4B ROP representation. The roman numerals in each circle indicate the zones, as per the international classification, and the arabic numerals indicate clock-hours. *(Courtesy of J. Arch McNamara, MD.)*

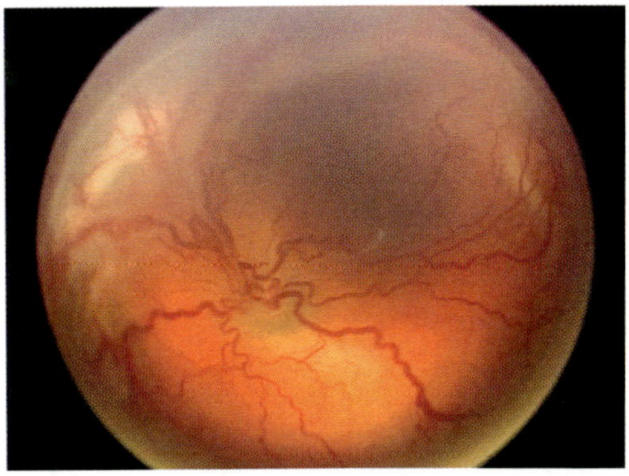

Figure 8-5 Stage 5 ROP. A total ROP retinal detachment can be appreciated in this fundus photograph. The marked contraction of the preretinal fibrosis can be seen to act like a purse string. Even at this stage—an open-funnel stage 5 retinal detachment—the arborizing pattern of the retinal blood vessels approaching the preretinal proliferation is visible. Additionally, tortuous dilated vessels, also called *plus disease,* are present. *(Courtesy of Colin A. McCannel, MD.)*

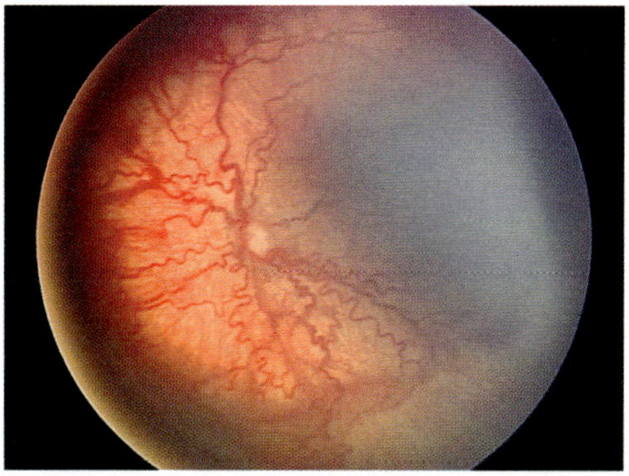

Figure 8-6 Pronounced plus disease in an eye with ROP. The retinal arteries and veins are dilated, and the arteries in particular are tortuous. The avascular retina and preretinal proliferations can be seen inferiorly and inferotemporally *(bottom right)*. *(Courtesy of Colin A. McCannel, MD.)*

Based on this terminology, ROP is classified into several disease stages and severities important for management and treatment decisions (Table 8-2). *Aggressive posterior ROP* (also referred to as *rush disease*) is said to be present when vascularization ends in zone I or very posterior zone II and is accompanied by plus disease. *Threshold disease* is characterized by more than 5 contiguous clock-hours of extraretinal neovascularization or 8 cumulative clock-hours of extraretinal neovascularization in association with plus disease and location of the retinal vessels within zone I or II (Fig 8-7). *Prethreshold disease* is a term coined by the Early Treatment for Retinopathy of Prematurity (ETROP) study;

Table 8-2 Classification of Acute Retinopathy of Prematurity (ROP)

Aggressive posterior ROP (rush disease)

Vascularization ends in zone I or very posterior zone II and is accompanied by plus disease; may progress rapidly

Threshold disease

5 contiguous clock-hours of extraretinal neovascularization

or

8 cumulative clock-hours of extraretinal neovascularization in association with plus disease and location of the retinal vessels within zone I or II

Prethreshold disease

All zone I and zone II changes, except zone II stage 1, and zone II stage 2 without plus disease, that do not meet threshold treatment criteria, and subdivided into type 1 and type 2 disease:

Type 1

zone I, any stage ROP with plus disease, or
zone I, stage 3 ROP without plus disease, or
zone II, stage 2 or 3 ROP with plus disease

Type 2

zone I, stage 1 or 2 ROP without plus disease, or
zone II, stage 3 ROP without plus disease

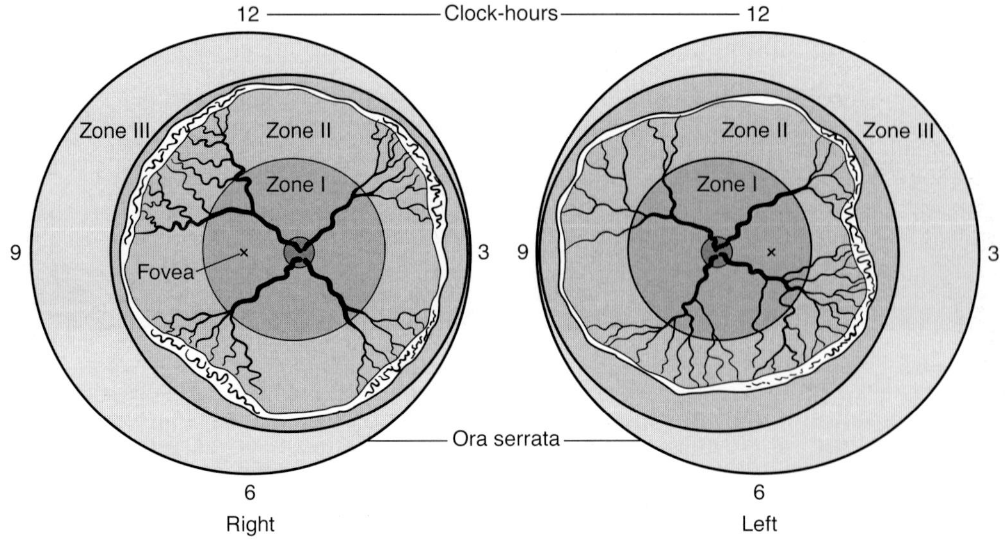

Figure 8-7 Examples of threshold disease, as characterized in the Multicenter Trial of Cryotherapy for Retinopathy of Prematurity. *Right,* 8 cumulative, noncontiguous clock-hours of stage 3 disease. *Left,* 5 contiguous clock-hours of proliferation. *(Illustration by Mark M. Miller.)*

it encompasses all zone I and zone II ROP changes, except zone II stage 1 and zone II stage 2 without plus disease, that do not meet threshold treatment criteria. It is further divided into high-risk prethreshold ROP, or *type 1 ROP,* and lower-risk prethreshold ROP, or *type 2 ROP* (see Table 8-2).

An eye is classified according to the most advanced disease noted; however, documentation should reflect all zones and stages observed, including their relative extent. Eyes with ROP in zone III typically have a good visual prognosis. The more posterior the zone at the time of recognition of the disease, the more nonperfused retina there is and thus the more worrisome the prognosis.

International Committee for the Classification of Retinopathy of Prematurity. The International Classification of Retinopathy of Prematurity revisited. *Arch Ophthalmol.* 2005;123(7):991–999.

Pathophysiology of ROP

Normally, retinal vascularization proceeds from the optic disc to the periphery, begins at approximately week 16 of gestation, and is completed nasally by approximately 36 weeks' gestation and temporally by 40 weeks' gestation. When the normal pattern of vascularization is interrupted and becomes abnormal, ROP may develop. Although the current understanding of the pathophysiology of ROP is incomplete, it is thought of as a 2-phase process. The first phase is characterized by the cessation of normal vascular development. Cessation occurs largely as the result of a decrease in the level of hormones and growth factors governing normal vascular development in the eye, such as vascular endothelial growth factor (VEGF) and insulin-like growth factor 1 (IGF-1). The cause for the drop in expression and levels of these growth factors is thought to be an increase in the infant's systemic oxygen tension that occurs following birth and commencement of breathing by the infant.

The second phase begins at approximately 31–34 weeks' postconceptional age. It is characterized by an abundance of growth factors secreted by the ischemic retina—particularly VEGF and IGF-1, among others—as well as by oxidative damage to endothelial cells, which leads to disorganized vascular growth. Initially, this process causes the formation of a visible tissue ridge (ROP stages 1, 2). As the disease progresses, vascular growth proliferates into the vitreous cavity (ROP stage 3). Eventually, growth factor and hormone shifts cause involution of the blood vessels with cicatricial contraction, which can lead to tractional retinal detachment (ROP stages 4, 5).

The more peripheral the neovascularization and the smaller its size and extent on the retina, the better is the outlook for spontaneous regression with minimal scarring. Active neovascularization with shunting of blood flow is associated with dilation and increased tortuosity of the retinal vessels posteriorly. A notable finding in active disease is increased and abnormal terminal arborization of retinal vessels as they approach the shunt or ridge. In addition, microvascular abnormalities (eg, microaneurysms, areas of capillary nonperfusion, and dilated vessels) may be visible posterior to the ridge.

In the vasoproliferative phase, new vessels varying widely in size and extent arise from retinal vessels just posterior to the shunt. These new vessels can induce contracture of the firmly attached vitreous gel, which results in progressive tractional retinal detachment. Vitreous hemorrhage can occur in stages 3–5, as can exudative retinal detachment.

Hartnett ME, Penn JS. Mechanisms and management of retinopathy of prematurity. *N Engl J Med.* 2012;367(26):2515–2526.

Natural Course

Although the systemic and/or local tissue factors that influence regression and progression of ROP are not known, the time course is predictable. ROP is a transient disease in the majority of infants, and spontaneous regression occurs in 85% of eyes. The initial clinical sign of regression is the development of a clear zone of retina beyond the shunt, followed by the development of straight vessels crossing the shunt and an arteriovenous feeder extending into the avascular retina.

Threshold ROP eventually develops in approximately 7% of infants with a birth weight of 1250 g or less. Eyes that demonstrate progression undergo a gradual transition from the active to the cicatricial stage of ROP, which is associated with variable degrees of fibrosis, contracture of the proliferative tissue, vitreous and retinal traction, macular distortion, and/or retinal detachment.

Associated Conditions and Late Sequelae

Conditions more likely to occur in eyes with regressed ROP include the following:

- myopia with astigmatism
- anisometropia
- strabismus
- amblyopia
- cataract
- glaucoma
- macular pigment epitheliopathy
- vitreoretinal scarring
- tractional retinal detachment
- anomalous foveal anatomy

Though rare, both angle-closure and pupillary-block glaucoma may occur in myopic eyes with cicatricial ROP. Angle-closure glaucoma typically occurs before 10 years of age, but it can occur well into adulthood in affected individuals. Rhegmatogenous retinal detachment, exudative retinopathy, and recurrent vitreous hemorrhages can also occur later in life. ROP and its sequelae can cause problems throughout a patient's life; therefore, long-term monitoring is crucial. The failure to diagnose and treat ROP and its complications in a timely fashion, combined with a statute of limitations of up to 20 years from the time of assessment or treatment in many US states, increases the legal exposure of physicians caring for children with ROP.

Day S, Menke AM, Abbott RL. Retinopathy of prematurity malpractice claims: the Ophthalmic Mutual Insurance Company experience. *Arch Ophthalmol.* 2009;127(6):794–798.

Screening Recommendations

The Cryotherapy for Retinopathy of Prematurity Cooperative Group determined that signs of ROP were present in 66% of infants with a birth weight of 1250 g or less and in 82% of infants with a birth weight of less than 1000 g. Recommendations for the screening of premature infants at risk of ROP have been issued in a joint statement of the American Academy of Pediatrics, Section on Ophthalmology; the American Association for Pediatric Ophthalmology and Strabismus; and the American Academy of Ophthalmology (available at http://one.aao.org/clinical-statement/screening-examination-of-premature-infants-retinop).

One caveat of paramount importance to recognize is that screening criteria and risk factors developed in one country do not necessarily apply in another country, especially if the level or quality of available medical or perinatal care is not comparable.

Screening Criteria

Screening consists of performing dilated funduscopic examinations using binocular indirect ophthalmoscopy on all infants with a birth weight of less than 1500 g or gestational age of 30 weeks or less. Additionally, screening applies to infants with a birth weight between 1500 g and 2000 g or a gestational age greater than 30 weeks, with an unstable clinical course, and who are believed to be at high risk by their attending pediatricians or neonatologists. The first examination should generally be performed between 4 and 6 weeks of postnatal age or, alternatively, between 31 and 33 weeks' postconceptional or postmenstrual age, whichever is later.

Systemic IGF-1 levels and weight gain are also associated with ROP risk. Taken together, the rate of weight gain and IGF-1 levels are more predictive of ROP development than is either value alone. A newer model—the weight, IGF-1, neonatal ROP (WINROP) algorithm—is being assessed for more targeted screening efforts, replacing the conventional screening criteria. In some studies, this model has been 100% sensitive in detecting at-risk infants while identifying as many as 90% of infants that do not need screening. The WINROP model has led to interest in developing other, preferably simpler, algorithms to identify infants at risk for ROP who thus require screening.

Screening Intervals

After each evaluation, the follow-up interval should be determined based on the disease features; more severe disease indicates a need for shorter follow-up intervals.

1-Week or Less Follow-up

- immature vascularization: zone I—no ROP
- immature retina extends into posterior zone II, near the boundary of zone I
- stage 1 or 2 ROP: zone I
- stage 3 ROP: zone II
- the presence or suspected presence of aggressive posterior ROP

1- to 2-Week Follow-up

- immature vascularization; posterior zone II
- stage 2 ROP: zone II
- unequivocally regressing ROP: zone I

2-Week Follow-up

- stage 1 ROP: zone II
- immature vascularization: zone II—no ROP
- unequivocally regressing ROP: zone II

2- to 3-Week Follow-up

- stage 1 or 2 ROP: zone III
- regressing ROP: zone III

Retinal screening examinations can usually be discontinued when any one of the following criteria is met:

- zone III retinal vascularization attained without previous zone I or II ROP (if there is examiner doubt about the zone or if the postmenstrual age is less than 35 weeks, confirmatory examinations may be warranted);
- full retinal vascularization in close proximity to the ora serrate for 360°—that is, the normal distance found in mature retina between the end of vascularization and the ora serrata. This criterion should be used for all cases treated for ROP solely with bevacizumab;
- postmenstrual age of 50 weeks and no prethreshold disease or worse ROP is present; or
- regression of ROP (care must be taken to be sure that there is no abnormal vascular tissue present that is capable of reactivation and progression in zone II or III).

Fierson WM; American Academy of Pediatrics Section on Ophthalmology; American Academy of Ophthalmology; American Association for Pediatric Ophthalmology and Strabismus; American Association of Certified Orthoptists. Screening examination of premature infants for retinopathy of prematurity. *Pediatrics.* 2013;131(1):189–195.

Fundus Photographic Screening of ROP

Ultra-wide-angle (120°) fundus photography of premature infant eyes is very useful, both to document the findings and to use in fundus photographic screening. Remote screening of photographic fundus images has established itself as an efficient and cost-effective method for screening premature infants for ROP. A study by the Photographic Screening for Retinopathy of Prematurity (Photo-ROP) Cooperative Group concluded that remote interpretation of weekly digital fundus images was a useful adjunct to conventional bedside ROP screening by indirect ophthalmoscopy. The study also concluded that because of limitations of image quality in some cases, there continued to be a need for the availability of an ophthalmologist skilled at examining premature infant eyes. In addition, the study established a definition of clinically significant ROP, the presence of which warrants evaluation by an ophthalmologist for assessment and possible treatment.

Prevention and Risk Factors

As ROP became a clinically distinct and recognized entity in the 1950s, supplemental oxygen administration was implicated as a major causative factor. The substantial reductions in oxygen utilization in neonatal intensive care units that followed indeed reduced the incidence of ROP dramatically. An unintended consequence of the oxygen restriction was that many of the infants incurred adverse neurologic outcomes, and infant death rates rose. Once oxygen was utilized more liberally again, neurologic outcomes and survival improved, at the price of a resurgence of ROP.

Preventing ROP begins with preventing prematurity through optimal pre-, peri-, and postnatal care. Avoiding extremely low birth weight and short gestational ages may be the most important factors. There is mounting evidence that the postnatal clinical course alters risk as well; that is, very sick premature infants are at greater risk of developing ROP. Specific factors shown to increase the risk of ROP are sepsis, blood transfusion, and slow rate of postnatal weight gain.

Recently, diet has been recognized as an additional risk factor. Several studies are currently under way to assess nutritional interventions for reducing the risk of ROP; one such intervention is addition of the sugar inositol to the neonate's diet (formula) or parenteral nutrition.

BOOST II United Kingdom Collaborative Group; BOOST II Australia Collaborative Group; BOOST II New Zealand Collaborative Group, Stenson BJ, Tarnow-Mordi WO, Darlow BA, et al. Oxygen saturation and outcomes in preterm infants. *N Engl J Med.* 2013;368(22): 2094–2104.

Treatment

In 1988, the Cryotherapy for ROP study demonstrated that ablation of avascular anterior retina in ROP eyes with threshold disease reduced by approximately half the incidence of an unfavorable outcome such as macular dragging, retinal detachment, or retrolental cicatrix formation. Treatment reduced these sequelae from 47% to 25% at 1 year follow-up, and visual results were shown to parallel anatomical results. At 10 years, eyes that received cryotherapy were still much less likely to be blind than untreated control eyes.

The ETROP trial randomly assigned 1 eye of infants with bilateral, high-risk, prethreshold ROP to receive early ablation of the avascular retina and the fellow eye to receive conventional management according to Cryotherapy for ROP study methods. High risk was determined using a computational model based on the natural history cohort of the Cryotherapy for ROP study; this model used demographic characteristics of the infants and clinical features of ROP to classify eyes with prethreshold ROP as high risk or low risk. In infants with high-risk prethreshold ROP, earlier treatment was associated with a reduction in unfavorable grating visual acuity outcomes (from 19.5% to 14.5%; $P = .01$) and a reduction in unfavorable structural outcomes (from 15.6% to 9.1%; $P < .001$) at 9 months. The study determined that the clinical categorization of prethreshold eyes into type 1 or type 2 ROP achieved very similar results to the computational model for risk assessment to prethreshold eyes.

Any eyes meeting the criteria for type 1 ROP should be considered for peripheral retinal ablative treatment, whereas type 2 ROP eyes can be monitored in short intervals and laser ablative treatment considered if they progress to type 1 ROP or threshold ROP. The authors of the ETROP study pointed out that the prethreshold treatment algorithm did not take into account all other known risk factors for progression, such as systemic disease, and that clinical judgment is still required for optimal management.

Early Treatment for Retinopathy of Prematurity Cooperative Group. Revised indications for the treatment of retinopathy of prematurity: results of the Early Treatment for Retinopathy of Prematurity Randomized Trial. *Arch Ophthalmol.* 2003;121(12):1684–1694.

Wallace DK. Retinopathy of prematurity. *Focal Points: Clinical Modules for Ophthalmologists.* San Francisco: American Academy of Ophthalmology; 2008, module 12.

Laser and Cryoablation Surgery

Ablation treatment of threshold or prethreshold type 1 ROP should be accomplished whenever possible with laser rather than cryoablation surgery, as laser surgery has less treatment-related morbidity. Treatment should be administered within 72 hours of determining its need and applied using the indirect ophthalmoscope in a confluent or subconfluent scatter fashion to the avascular retina anterior to the ridge (Fig 8-8). In the horizontal meridia, laser treatment should be applied in a lighter pattern to avoid damage to the long ciliary vessels and nerves. Damage to these structures can lead to severe anterior segment ischemia. Use of retinal cryoablation (Fig 8-9) is now rare (in the United States), but the technique may still have a role in the treatment of eyes with media opacities or persistent tunica vasculosa lentis, or when a laser is not available. Treatment should be performed in conjunction with pediatric consultation and with systemic monitoring because respiratory or cardiorespiratory arrest can occur in up to 5% of treated infants. Use of systemic analgesia is also advisable to minimize stress and risk to the infant. Some neonatologists prefer that infants undergo treatment with general anesthesia in an operating room.

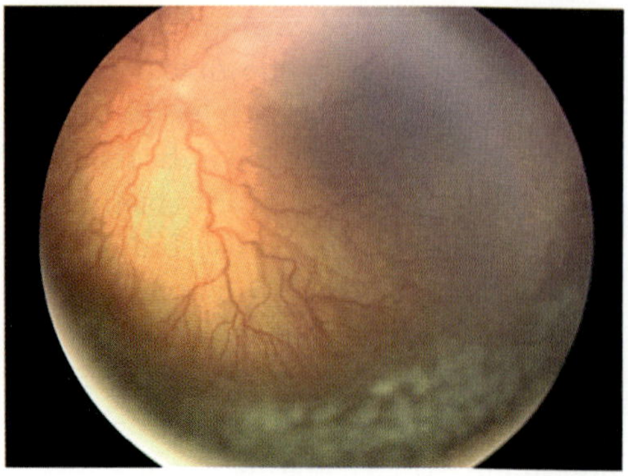

Figure 8-8 Wide-angle photographic view of fundus after laser photocoagulation for threshold ROP. Plus disease is visible posteriorly, and avascular retina is apparent in the inferior and inferior temporal fundus *(bottom right).* Arborization of the vasculature leading up to the ridge and associated fibrovascular proliferation is pronounced. *(Courtesy of Colin A. McCannel, MD.)*

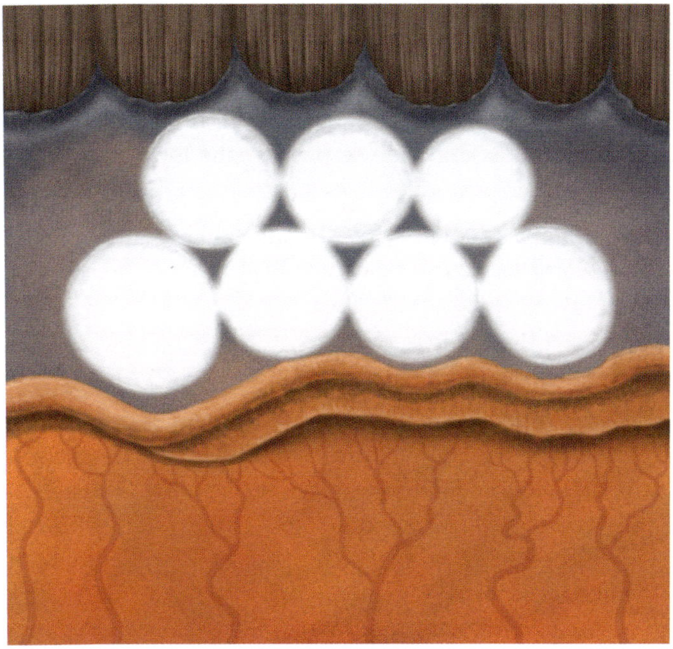

Figure 8-9 Schematic representation of cryotherapy to the avascular anterior retina in an eye with threshold ROP. Note the nonoverlapping, but near confluent, treatment pattern. Attempts are to treat all avascular retina. *(Illustration by Mark M. Miller.)*

Brown GC, Tasman WS, Naidoff M, Schaffer DB, Quinn G, Bhutani VK. Systemic complications associated with retinal cryoablation for retinopathy of prematurity. *Ophthalmology.* 1990;97(7):855–858.

Connolly BP, McNamara JA, Sharma S, Regillo CD, Tasman W. A comparison of laser photocoagulation with trans-scleral cryotherapy in the treatment of threshold retinopathy of prematurity. *Ophthalmology.* 1998;105(9):1628–1631.

Laser ROP Study Group. Laser therapy for retinopathy of prematurity. *Arch Ophthalmol.* 1994;112(2):154–156.

Anti-VEGF Drugs

The BEAT-ROP (Bevacizumab Eliminates the Angiogenic Threat of Retinopathy of Prematurity) Cooperative Group conducted a prospective, randomized, multicenter trial to assess intravitreal bevacizumab monotherapy for zone I or zone II posterior stage 3 ROP with plus disease. Compared with conventional laser therapy, a statistically significant treatment benefit for bevacizumab was demonstrated for zone I ROP, whereas zone II disease had similar outcomes with either treatment. Normal peripheral retinal vascularization continued after treatment with intravitreal bevacizumab, whereas laser therapy led to permanent destruction of the peripheral retina. Recurrences occurred significantly later with bevacizumab than with laser therapy. Therefore, prolonged, close follow-up is essential. The study was too small and the follow-up too short to allow proper evaluation of the safety of intravitreal bevacizumab for the treatment of ROP. The use of bevacizumab in eyes previously treated with laser is not recommended.

It is very likely that the results of this study, and other published evidence, will lead to a dramatic change in how zone I ROP, and probably all ROP, is treated. However, to date there are insufficient data to assess safety, especially the long-term safety, of using anti-VEGF drugs to treat ROP.

Mintz-Hittner HA, Kennedy KA, Chuang AZ; BEAT-ROP Cooperative Group. Efficacy of intravitreal bevacizumab for stage 3+ retinopathy of prematurity. *N Engl J Med.* 2011; 364(7):603–615.

Vitrectomy and Scleral Buckling Surgery

Eyes with stage 4 ROP (progressive, active-phase ROP) require surgical intervention using scleral buckling or a lens-sparing vitrectomy to alleviate the vitreoretinal traction causing retinal detachment. Eyes undergoing surgical intervention at stage 4A—rather than at later stages 4B or 5—have more favorable outcomes. Lens-sparing vitrectomy for stage 4A ROP may reduce the progression to stages 4B and 5 ROP and is therefore the preferred approach given the improved visual outcome.

For eyes with stage 5 disease, vitrectomy combined with dissection of the fibrovascular membranes and adherent vitreous has been successful in fully or partially reattaching the retina in approximately 30% of eyes. Nevertheless, only 25% of retinas in eyes with initial partial or total reattachment after surgery remained fully attached a median of 5 years later. Among the patients whose retinas were initially reattached, only 10% eventually have ambulatory vision. If a drainage retinotomy is performed or an iatrogenic retinal break occurs during a vitrectomy for ROP, the prognosis for that eye becomes uniformly poor.

Capone A Jr, Trese MT. Lens-sparing vitreous surgery for tractional stage 4A retinopathy of prematurity retinal detachments. *Ophthalmology.* 2001;108(11):2068–2070.

Quinn GE, Dobson V, Barr CC, et al. Visual acuity of eyes after vitrectomy for retinopathy of prematurity: follow-up at 5 1/5 years. The Cryotherapy for Retinopathy of Prematurity Cooperative Group. *Ophthalmology.* 1996;103(4):595–600.

CHAPTER 9

Choroidal Disease

This chapter describes noninflammatory choroidal diseases that also involve the retina. Inflammatory disorders of the retina and choroid are discussed in Chapter 10. See also BCSC Section 9, *Intraocular Inflammation and Uveitis.* Intraocular tumors, such as melanoma, are covered in BCSC Section 4, *Ophthalmic Pathology and Intraocular Tumors.*

Central Serous Chorioretinopathy

Central serous chorioretinopathy (CSC), also commonly known by the less-preferred names of *central serous retinopathy* or *central serous choroidopathy,* is an idiopathic condition characterized by the development of a typically well-circumscribed, serous detachment of the sensory retina. The detachment has been ascribed to altered barriers and defective pumping functions at the level of the retinal pigment epithelium (RPE), although the primary pathology is still under debate; malfunction of the choriocapillaris, choroidal hyperpermeability, and abnormal choroidal thickness are in contention for primacy. Some cases may include serous detachment of the RPE, usually underneath the superior half of the serous retinal detachment. Often, small whitish subretinal precipitates or gray-white subretinal sheets may be observed; they probably indicate the presence of shed outer segments or fibrin. Occasionally, a localized serous detachment of the RPE without overlying neurosensory elevation is present. CSC is often bilateral, with asymmetric findings.

Previous CSC episodes are often suggested by areas of macular and extramacular RPE atrophy, which are referred to as *runoff* or *guttering.* These areas are most easily identified using autofluorescence imaging. A recent report describes a group of patients who have similar RPE changes and choroidal thickening but no evidence of serous detachment; this condition, termed *pachychoroidal pigmentary retinopathy,* may be a forme fruste of CSC.

Very severe CSC can occur but is uncommon. Some patients may have multifocal disease extending to the periphery. Subtotal bullous serous retinal detachment, often bilateral, can also occur in CSC, although it is rare. These severe forms of CSC are challenging to manage, as any focal treatment may be difficult to administer through detached retina.

CSC occurs primarily in otherwise healthy men between 25 and 55 years of age. Most patients are asymptomatic unless the macula is affected. CSC is the fourth most common nonsurgical maculopathy after age-related macular degeneration, diabetic retinopathy, and branch retinal vein occlusion. Although various authors have reported different occurrence rates across racial populations, more recent reports do not confirm any predilection. Symptomatic patients describe the sudden onset of blurred and dim vision, micropsia (which causes objects to appear smaller than they are), metamorphopsia (which causes objects to appear distorted), paracentral scotomata, or decreased color vision. In general, visual acuity ranges from 20/20 to 20/200, but in most patients, it is better than 20/30. The decreased visual acuity can often be reversed with a hyperopic correction. In rare cases, these symptoms are accompanied by a migrainelike headache.

The etiology of CSC is unknown. Common associations include the use of exogenous steroids, a "type A" personality, stress, endogenous hypercortisolism (Cushing syndrome), organ transplantation, systemic lupus erythematosus, systemic hypertension, sleep apnea, gastroesophageal reflux disease, use of psychopharmacologic medications, and pregnancy.

Carvalho-Recchia CA, Yannuzzi LA, Negrão S, et al. Corticosteroids and central serous chorioretinopathy. *Ophthalmology.* 2002;109(10):1834–1837.

Desai UR, Alhalel AA, Campen TJ, Schiffman RM, Edwards PA, Jacobsen GR. Central serous chorioretinopathy in African Americans. *J Natl Med Assoc.* 2003;95(7):553–559.

Haimovici R, Koh S, Gagnon DR, Lehrfeld T, Wellik S; Central Serous Chorioretinopathy Case-Control Study Group. Risk factors for central serous chorioretinopathy: a case-control study. *Ophthalmology.* 2004;111(2):244–249.

Maruko I, Iida T, Sugano Y, Ojima A, Ogasawara M, Spaide RF. Subfoveal choroidal thickness after treatment of central serous chorioretinopathy. *Ophthalmology.* 2010;117(9): 1792–1799.

Tsai DC, Chen SJ, Huang CC, et al. Epidemiology of idiopathic central serous chorioretinopathy in Taiwan, 2001–2006: a population-based study. *PLoS One.* 2013;8(6): e66858.

Warrow DJ, Hoang QV, Freund KB. Pachychoroid pigment epitheliopathy. *Retina.* 2013;33(8): 1659–1672.

Optical Coherence Tomography

Optical coherence tomography (OCT) is an excellent, noninvasive method for use in the diagnosis and monitoring of CSC. Findings include serous retinal detachment, serous retinal pigment epithelial detachment (Fig 9-1), and a thickened choroid. To visualize the thickened choroid, spectral-domain OCT (SD-OCT), enhanced depth imaging OCT (EDI-OCT), or swept-source OCT (SS-OCT) may be necessary.

Fluorescein Angiography

CSC has characteristic fluorescein angiographic findings, including leakage from the RPE and irregular relative window defects. Leakage from the RPE typically occurs in 1 of the 3 following characteristic patterns: (1) expansile dot pattern, (2) smokestack pattern, or (3) diffuse pattern.

The *expansile dot pattern* of hyperfluorescence is the most common. It appears in the early phase of the fluorescein study and increases in size and intensity as the study progresses (see Fig 9-1). More than one dot may be present in some patients.

In the classic *smokestack pattern,* a focal spot of hyperfluorescence appears early in the study, spreading vertically and finally laterally as the study progresses to the late phases, resembling a plume of smoke. This unique pattern is thought to be secondary to convection currents and to a pressure gradient between the protein concentration of the

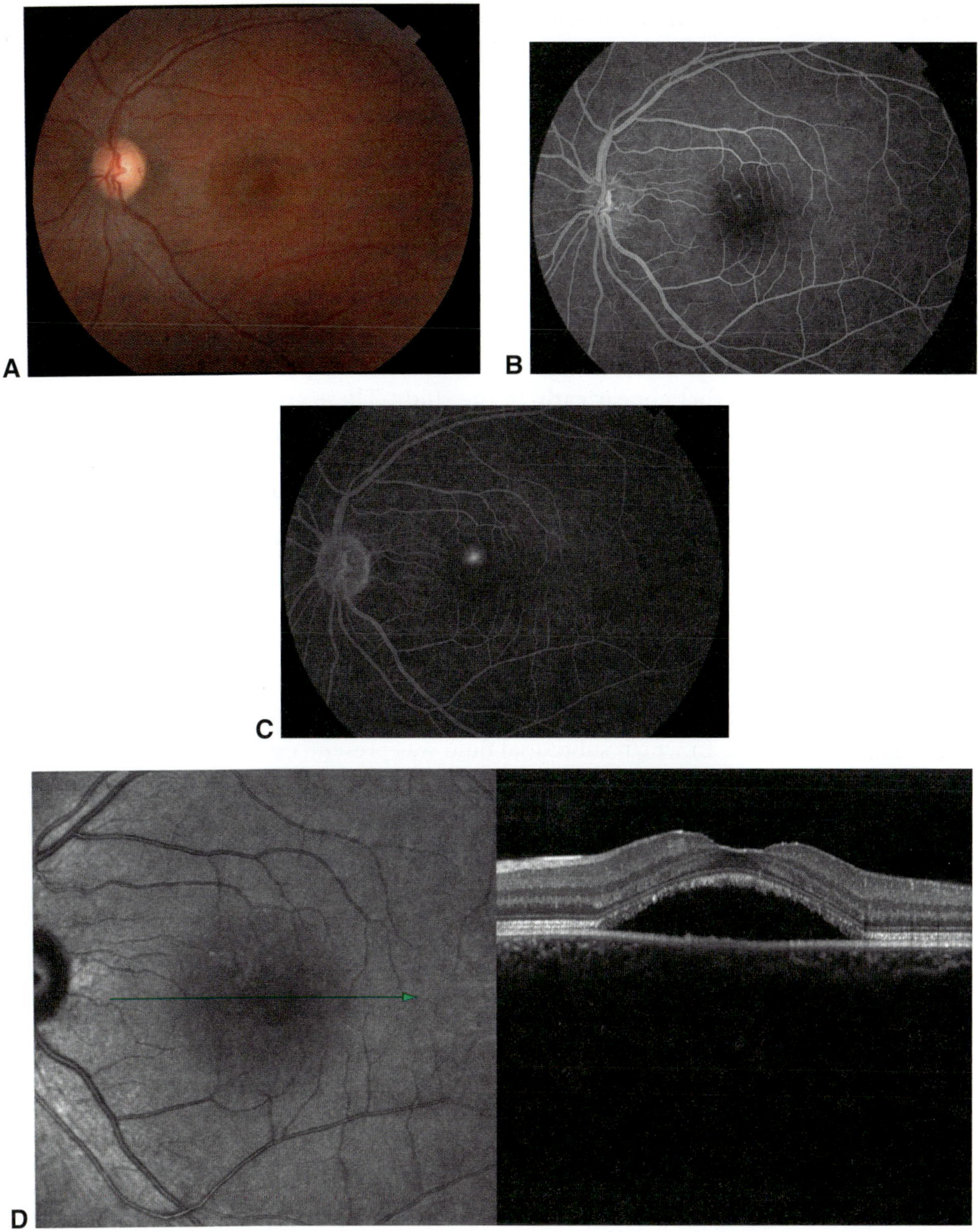

Figure 9-1 Central serous chorioretinopathy. **A,** Color fundus photograph from a patient with central serous chorioretinopathy. **B,** Early-phase fluorescein angiography image demonstrates pinpoint hyperfluorescence. **C,** Late-phase fluorescein angiography image shows the expansile dot pattern of the leakage. **D,** Corresponding optical coherence tomography (OCT) scan illustrates the subretinal fluid accumulation. Accumulation of deposits on the outer surface of the photoreceptors is visible. This material is thought to represent shed photoreceptor outer segments or fibrin. *(Courtesy of Richard B. Rosen, MD.)*

subretinal fluid and the fluorescein dye entering the detachment. Although characteristic, this angiographic presentation is present in only 10% of cases.

In rare cases, an extensive, often gravity-dependent serous detachment of the retina may develop from one or more leakage points outside the central area or may be associated with a *diffuse pattern* of fluorescein leakage. Often, there is no prominent leakage point.

Indocyanine Green Angiography

Indocyanine green (ICG) angiography can reveal choroidal vascular abnormalities, including filling delays in the choroidal arteries and choriocapillaris, venous dilation, hyperpermeability of the choroidal vessels, and characteristic multifocal choroidal hyperfluorescent patches that appear early in the study. These areas slowly enlarge during the angiographic study but are less prominent in late-phase views. In addition, a characteristic "washed-out" pattern is often evident that remains unchanged during clinically inactive phases. ICG angiography can be useful in helping distinguish atypical diffuse CSC in older patients from both occult choroidal neovascularization (CNV) in exudative age-related macular degeneration and idiopathic polypoidal choroidal vasculopathy.

Fundus Autofluorescence Imaging

Acutely, relative hypoautofluorescence can be observed corresponding to the site of the focal RPE leak depicted on fluorescein angiography (FA) and in the area of subretinal fluid. Chronically, areas in which subretinal fluid was present, especially for extended periods of time, can show mild to dramatic hypoautofluorescence. Fundus autofluorescence (FAF) imaging may show dramatic changes even when the clinical examination findings are normal or minimally abnormal, allowing visualization of the guttering mentioned earlier. Increased autofluorescence often observed in the area of serous detachment may be related to unmasking of RPE fluorescence by photoreceptor pigmentary atrophy.

Imamura Y, Fujiwara T, Margolis R, Spaide RF. Enhanced depth imaging optical coherence tomography of the choroid in central serous chorioretinopathy. *Retina.* 2009;29(10): 1469–1473.

Spaide RF, Klancnik JM Jr. Fundus autofluorescence and central serous chorioretinopathy. *Ophthalmology.* 2005;112(5):825–833.

Differential Diagnosis

Perhaps the most difficult differential diagnoses to distinguish from CSC are age-related macular degeneration and idiopathic polypoidal choroidal vasculopathy. The presence of blood or significant amounts of lipid strongly suggests the diagnosis of CNV or idiopathic polypoidal choroidal vasculopathy. In the absence of these signs, the angiographic patterns of fluorescence and disease course may help differentiate these conditions. Other considerations in the differential diagnosis include optic nerve pits, idiopathic uveal effusion syndrome (IUES), and Vogt-Koyanagi-Harada syndrome. Older patients presenting with CNV occasionally may show pigment epithelial changes that suggest previous episodes of CSC.

Natural Course and Management

The visual prognosis of CSC is generally good except in chronic, recurrent cases and in cases of bullous CSC. Most (80%–90%) eyes with CSC undergo spontaneous resorption of subretinal fluid within 3–4 months; recovery of visual acuity usually follows but can take up to 1 year. Mild metamorphopsia, faint scotomata, abnormalities in contrast sensitivity, and mild deficits in color vision frequently persist. Some eyes have permanently reduced visual acuity, and many (40%–50%) experience one or more recurrences.

Initially, observation is appropriate, unless the patient's livelihood is at risk because of the changes in vision. If fluid persists for more than 3–6 months, treatment using thermal laser photocoagulation, photodynamic therapy, or systemic medications should be considered.

Thermal laser photocoagulation at the site of fluorescein leakage can induce rapid remission; similar results have recently been reported for subthreshold laser photocoagulation to the leakage site. If laser photocoagulation is performed, a follow-up examination within 3–4 weeks may help detect the rare complication of postlaser CNV. Although rare, CNV has been reported to develop in as many as 2% of patients with typical CSC, even without laser treatment.

Verteporfin *photodynamic therapy* (PDT), using standard fluence (600 mW/cm^2) or reduced fluence (300 mW/cm^2), resolves the fluid leakage, which may also result in improved vision. In addition, several authors have described the use of sub–visible threshold or micropulse laser to help resolve the chronic serous fluid in CSC. These treatments, however, are not supported by level 1 evidence.

Several *systemic drugs* have been variably reported to be effective in resolving cases of chronic, recurrent, or resistant CSC; medications include mifepristone, finasteride, ketoconazole, spironolactone, valproic acid, and eplerenone. The rationale for their use rests largely on their impact on steroid metabolism.

Loo RH, Scott IU, Flynn HW Jr, et al. Factors associated with reduced visual acuity during long-term follow-up of patients with idiopathic central serous chorioretinopathy. *Retina.* 2002; 22(1):19–24.

Choroidal Perfusion Abnormalities

Although most of the blood flow to the eye goes to the choroid, perfusion abnormalities in the choroid are more difficult to diagnose. Retinal vascular occlusion is readily visible by ophthalmoscopy and corroborated by FA. Choroidal vascular occlusion, however, may produce changes that are quite subtle. In addition, it is not uncommon for choroidal vascular abnormalities to be obscured by overlying retinal vascular abnormalities such as cotton-wool spots and intraretinal hemorrhages. The entities that cause choroidal vascular abnormalities may affect the circulation from the ophthalmic artery to the choriocapillaris. Although individual variation is high, there often are a nasal and a temporal posterior ciliary artery, which have a vertical watershed that transects the fundus at or near the optic nerve head. From the posterior ciliary arteries arise the short and long posterior ciliary arteries, each of which supplies patches of choroid that are essentially triangular. Figure 9-2 illustrates a typical pattern of choroidal vascular distribution in the temporal fundus with its watershed areas. As a result of this anatomy, short posterior ciliary artery occlusions usually result in triangular areas of choroidal ischemia.

Hayreh SS. Posterior ciliary artery circulation in health and disease: the Weisenfeld lecture. *Invest Ophthalmol Vis Sci.* 2004;45(3):749–757; 748.

Increased Venous Pressure

Although rare, choroidal blood flow abnormalities may be related to venous outflow problems, including those caused by *dural arterial malformations* and *carotid cavernous fistulas.* Diagnosis of choroidal blood flow abnormalities often requires both fluorescein and ICG angiography, and occasionally a stethoscope, to detect a bruit.

Hypertension

The most commonly observed diseases that lead to choroidal vascular compromise are those that cause severe, acute elevations in blood pressure, such as in *malignant hypertension, eclampsia,* or severe cocaine abuse. In addition to retinal abnormalities, these disorders commonly lead to serous detachment of the retina associated with areas of yellow placoid discoloration of the RPE (Fig 9-3). The perfusion abnormalities may range from focal infarction of the choriocapillaris to fibrinoid necrosis of larger arterioles. Although

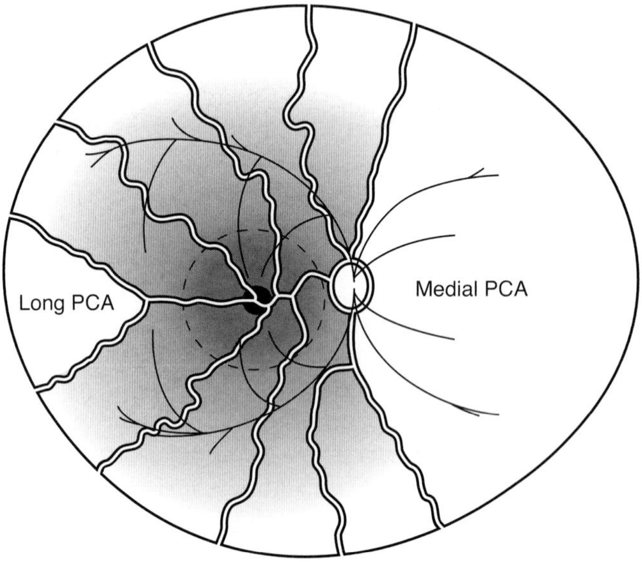

Figure 9-2 Diagrammatic representation of the choroidal distribution of the short posterior ciliary arteries (PCAs) and long PCA branches arising from the temporal (lateral) PCA, and their watershed zones. Details of the branches from the medial PCA are not indicated. *Dashed circle* indicates the macular region. *(Used with permission from Hayreh SS. Submacular choroidal vascular pattern: experimental fluorescein fundus angiographic studies.* Graefes Arch Clin Exp Ophthalmol. *1974;192(3):181–196.)*

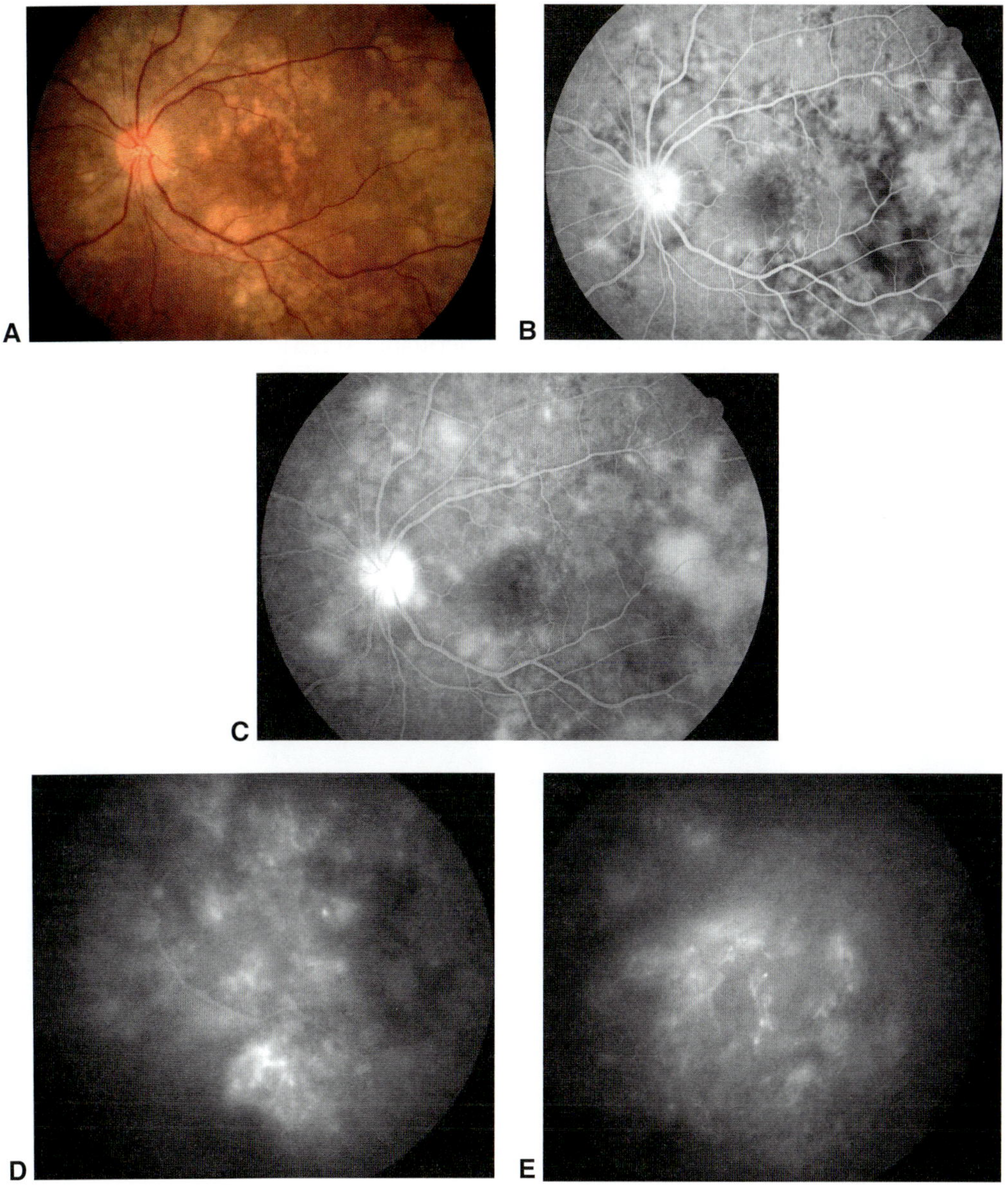

Figure 9-3 Preeclampsia with HELLP (*h*emolysis, *e*levated *l*iver enzymes, and *l*ow *p*latelet count) syndrome. **A,** Color fundus photograph of a patient reveals a serous detachment of the retina and multiple yellowish placoid areas at the level of the retinal pigment epithelium (RPE) and inner choroid. **B,** Early-phase fluorescein angiography image shows reticular patterns of decreased choroidal perfusion bordering areas of hyperfluorescence. Early leakage from the level of the RPE is evident and becomes more apparent in the later phases of the study **(C).** There is also staining of and leakage from the optic nerve. **D,** Indocyanine green (ICG) angiography image shows profound choroidal vascular filling defects alternating with areas of abnormal vessel leakage and staining, a rare finding. **E,** In the late phase, numerous arterioles show staining of their walls, indicating severe vascular damage. *(Used with permission from Spaide RF, Goldbaum M, Wong DW, Tang KC, Iida T. Serous detachment of the retina.* Retina. *2003;23(6):820–846.)*

the choroid has a rich circulation, the blood flows in a functionally terminal fashion at the level of the choriocapillaris, so there is very little collateral flow after a focal occlusion. Resolution of smaller infarcts, which initially appear tan in color, produces small patches of atrophy and pigmentary hyperplasia called *Elschnig spots*. Linear aggregations of these spots are called *Siegrist streaks*.

Inflammatory Conditions

Various types of arteritis may affect the choroidal circulation as well. *Giant cell arteritis* may cause occlusion of one or more short, posterior ciliary arteries, leading to broad triangular areas of choroidal nonperfusion in any meridian (Amalric sign) (Fig 9-4). Patients with this condition may have concurrent central retinal artery occlusion combined with nasal choroidal hypoperfusion, suggesting involvement of the first intraorbital segment of the ophthalmic artery. *Granulomatosis with polyangiitis* (formerly, Wegener granulomatosis) is a disorder characterized by necrotizing granulomatous lesions of the upper and lower respiratory tracts, glomerulonephritis, and generalized focal necrotizing vasculitis. Ocular manifestations occur in 30%–50% of patients and may include retinal vascular occlusion, choroidal vascular occlusion, or both (Fig 9-5). Other inflammatory conditions

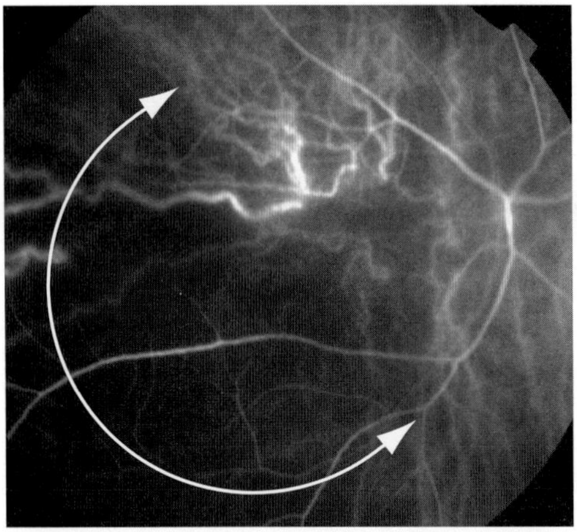

Figure 9-4 Giant cell arteritis. ICG angiography image 1 day after this patient had severe vision loss secondary to arteritic anterior ischemic optic neuropathy revealed a wedge-shaped area of choroidal nonperfusion *(curved arrow)*. The apex of the triangle (wedge) of nonperfusion points toward the area of the occluded short posterior ciliary artery. *(Courtesy of Richard F. Spaide, MD.)*

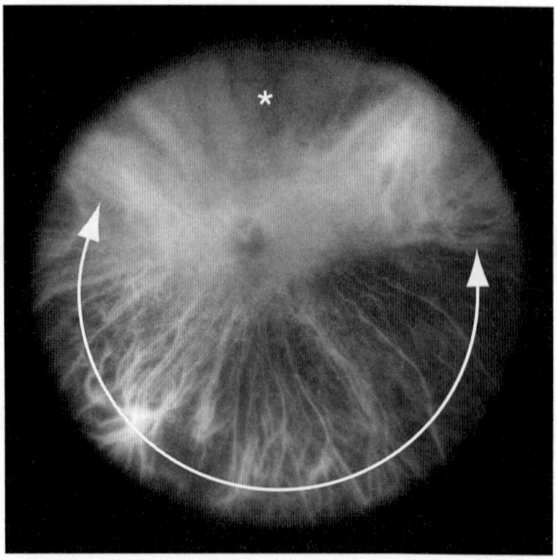

Figure 9-5 Granulomatosis with polyangiitis (formerly, Wegener granulomatosis). The early phase of wide-angle ICG angiography of the left eye reveals a widespread filling defect of the arterioles and choriocapillaris in the inferior fundus *(curved arrow)* and in a segmental area of the superior fundus *(asterisk)*. *(Used with permission from Iida T, Spaide RF, Kantor J. Retinal and choroidal arterial occlusion in Wegener's granulomatosis.* Am J Ophthalmol. *2002;133(1):151–152. Copyright © 2002, with permission from Elsevier.)*

reported to cause choroidal infarction include *systemic lupus erythematosus, polyarteritis nodosa,* and *antiphospholipid syndrome.*

Amalric P. Acute choroidal ischaemia. *Trans Ophthalmol Soc U K.* 1971;91:305–322.

Thromboembolic Disease

Vaso-occlusion by microemboli may occur in various diseases. In these entities, the choroidal circulation may also be affected and at somewhat greater risk than retinal circulation because it has a 10-fold higher volume of blood flow, which provides platelet emboli more opportunity to enter and become lodged within that circulation. *Thrombotic thrombocytopenic purpura* causes a classic pentad of findings: (1) microangiopathic hemolytic anemia, (2) thrombocytopenia, (3) fever, (4) neurologic dysfunction, and (5) renal dysfunction. Patients with this condition may also have multifocal yellow placoid areas and associated serous detachment of the retina. Similar fundus findings may occur in patients with *disseminated intravascular coagulation,* in which consumption of coagulation proteins, involvement of cellular elements, and release of fibrin degradation products lead to hemorrhage from multiple sites and ischemia from microthrombi.

Iatrogenic Abnormalities

Although rare, choroidal ischemia may result from iatrogenic causes. Thermal laser photocoagulation and photodynamic therapy have also, on rare occasions, caused choroidal vascular occlusion with resultant segmental ischemia. Ocular compression related to cataract surgery has caused choroidal ischemia in some patients. Other reported causes of emboli to the choroid include subcutaneous injection of micronized dermal matrix or fat in the forehead region (see Chapter 6, Fig 6-19), periocular corticosteroid injection, and intracisternal papaverine injection with resultant rapid and dramatic elevation of intracranial pressure.

Gaudric A, Coscas G, Bird AC. Choroidal ischemia. *Am J Ophthalmol.* 1982;94(4):489–498.

Iida T, Spaide RF, Kantor J. Retinal and choroidal arterial occlusion in Wegener's granulomatosis. *Am J Ophthalmol.* 2002;133(1):151–152.

Spaide RF, Goldbaum M, Wong DW, Tang KC, Iida T. Serous detachment of the retina. *Retina.* 2003;23(6):820–846.

Choroidal Hemangiomas

Isolated choroidal hemangiomas are reddish-orange, well-circumscribed tumors of varying thickness; they may be discovered during routine examinations or because of blurring of vision caused by hyperopia or related to serous detachment induced by the tumor. Circumscribed hemangiomas transilluminate readily and have distinctive echographic and angiographic characteristics (Fig 9-6). Large choroidal vessels are visible early during ICG angiography studies, and the tumors show a characteristic washed-out pattern in the later phases of the study.

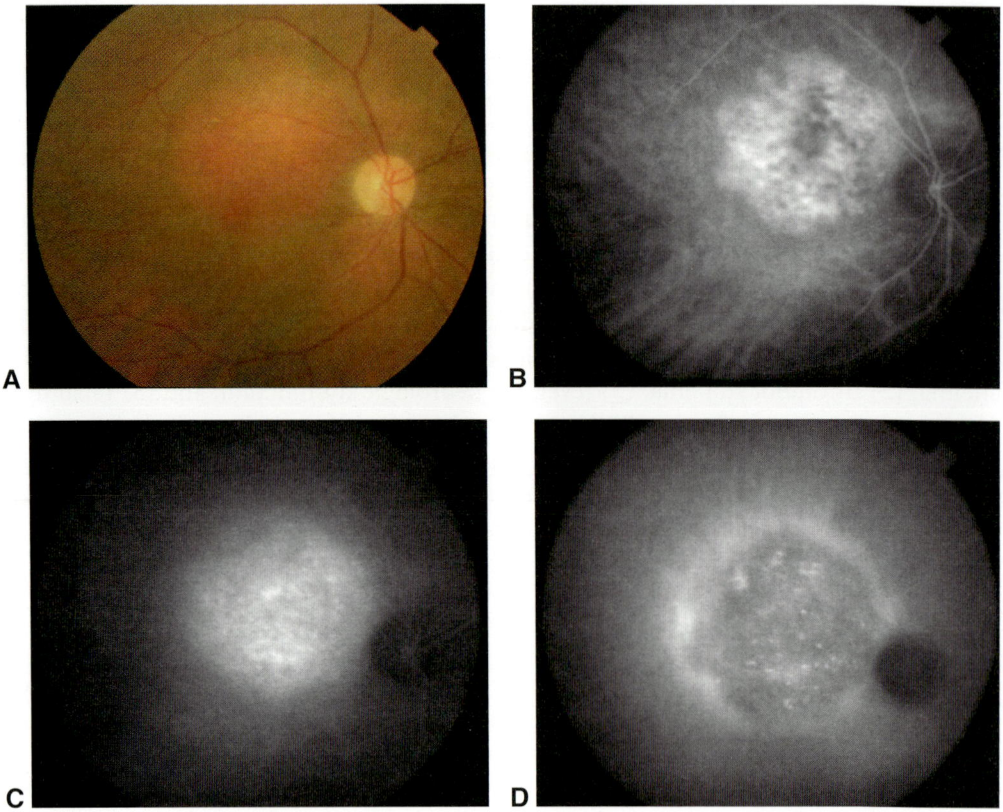

Figure 9-6 Choroidal hemangioma. **A,** Fundus photograph of the typical reddish-orange elevation of a circumscribed choroidal hemangioma. **B,** Soon after ICG injection, the vascular composition of the hemangioma is revealed. **C,** Hyperfluorescence of the tumor occurs in the middle phase of the angiogram study from a combination of dye within and leakage from the vessels of the hemangioma. **D,** In the late phase of the study, the dye "washes out" of the lesion, leaving hyperfluorescent staining in the adjacent tissues. *(Used with permission from Spaide RF, Goldbaum M, Wong DW, Tang KC, Iida T. Serous detachment of the retina.* Retina. *2003;23(6):820–846.)*

By contrast, the hemangioma associated with Sturge-Weber syndrome (encephalofacial cavernous hemangiomatosis) is diffuse and may present first as glaucoma or amblyopia in children. Biomicroscopically, the areas corresponding to the hemangioma have a typical tomato ketchup appearance, in which the underlying choroidal markings are not visible. The choroidal hemangiomas in Sturge-Weber syndrome may sometimes be overlooked because they are diffuse and may blend imperceptibly into adjacent normal choroid. An ipsilateral facial nevus flammeus (port-wine stain) is also typically present in patients with this syndrome.

The alterations to retina and pigment epithelium caused by choroidal hemangiomas range from cystic retinal edema to neurosensory detachment to formation of an epichoroidal membrane with calcification and ossification. The particular alterations ultimately determine the ophthalmoscopic appearance, which therefore is quite varied. Retinal vascular leakage in the form of hard exudate is not common.

Hemangiomas have been treated with various modalities, including laser photocoagulation, cryopexy, external-beam and plaque radiation, and photodynamic therapy. When applied before chronic retinal changes occur, each modality has had therapeutic success. Photodynamic therapy with verteporfin may have the lowest risk of treatment-related morbidity.

Beardsley RM, McCannel CA, McCannel TA. Recurrent leakage after Visudyne photodynamic therapy for the treatment of circumscribed choroidal hemangioma. *Ophthalmic Surg Lasers Imaging Retina.* 2013;44(3):248–51.

Blasi MA, Tiberti AC, Scupola A, et al. Photodynamic therapy with verteporfin for symptomatic circumscribed choroidal hemangioma: five-year outcomes. *Ophthalmology.* 2010;117(8):1630–1637.

Madreperla SA, Hungerford JL, Plowman PN, Laganowski HC, Gregory PT. Choroidal hemangiomas: visual and anatomic results of treatment by photocoagulation or radiation therapy. *Ophthalmology.* 1997;104(11):1773–1778.

Tsipursky MS, Golchet PR, Jampol LM. Photodynamic therapy of choroidal hemangioma in Sturge-Weber syndrome, with a review of treatments for diffuse and circumscribed choroidal hemangiomas. *Surv Ophthalmol.* 2011;56(1):68–85.

Uveal Effusion Syndrome

Net water movement across the vitreous cavity and posterior eye wall can be altered by reduced transscleral aqueous outflow. This alteration may be caused by abnormal scleral composition or thickness, as in nanophthalmos, scleritis, IUES, and other conditions. Hyperopia frequently accompanies such conditions, as does glaucoma. Choroidal and ciliary body thickening, RPE alterations, and exudative retinal detachment may occur transiently or permanently. FA usually shows a leopard spot pattern of hypofluorescence without focal leakage (Fig 9-7).

Posterior pole manifestations in uveal effusion syndrome may be accompanied by ciliochoroidal detachment and abnormal episcleral vessels. Visual function may fluctuate during the natural course of the disease. Although encouraging anatomical restitution can be obtained with surgical approaches such as scleral window surgery, the visual results may be less rewarding because of chronic, irreversible changes. A high index of suspicion for uveal effusion syndrome should be maintained for young patients with hyperopia whose disorder has been diagnosed as either CSC or retinal detachment without a retinal hole or tear.

Brockhurst RJ. Nanophthalmos with uveal effusion. A new clinical entity. *Arch Ophthalmol.* 1975;93(12):1989–1999.

Elagouz M, Stanescu-Segall D, Jackson TL. Uveal effusion syndrome. *Surv Ophthalmol.* 2010; 55(2):134–145.

Johnson MW, Gass JD. Surgical management of the idiopathic uveal effusion syndrome. *Ophthalmology.* 1990;97(6):778–785.

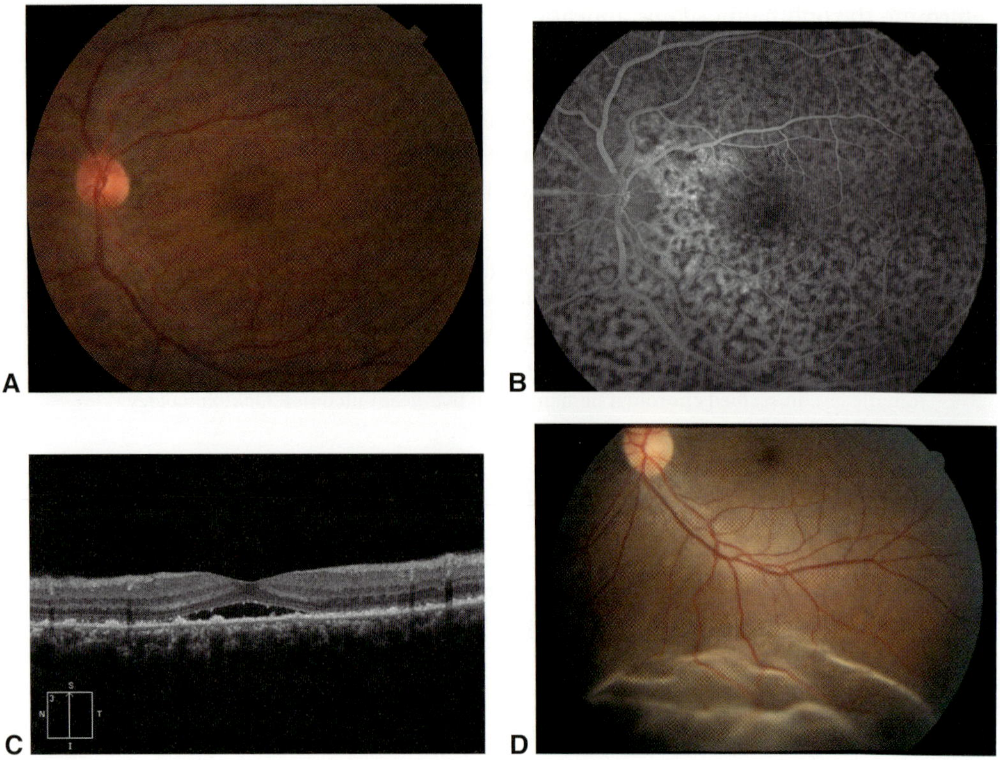

Figure 9-7 Idiopathic uveal effusion. **A–C,** In this patient's left eye, the visual acuity was reduced to 20/70, and systemic workup was negative. **A,** Fundus photograph demonstrates blunted foveal reflex and irregular, subtle subretinal deposits. **B,** Corresponding fluorescein angiography image reveals a diffuse leopard-spot pattern of blocking with intervening window defects involving the entire posterior pole. **C,** OCT scan reveals a small amount of subfoveal fluid and outer retinal deposits. Not shown is a peripheral serous retinal detachment. **D,** Fundus photograph from a separate case of recent-onset uveal effusion shows the typical appearance of serous retinal detachment syndrome as well as an underlying choroidal detachment, which is common for this condition. *(Parts A–C courtesy of Ronald C. Gentile, MD; part D courtesy of Colin A. McCannel, MD.)*

Bilateral Diffuse Uveal Melanocytic Proliferation

A rare paraneoplastic disorder affecting the choroid, bilateral diffuse uveal melanocytic proliferation (BDUMP) causes diffuse thickening of the choroid, reddish or brownish choroidal discoloration, serous retinal detachment, and cataracts. The bilateral proliferation of benign melanocytes is usually associated with or often heralds a systemic cancer. These proliferations can look like large nevi (Fig 9-8). Some BDUMP lesions appear as reddish areas of depigmentation of the RPE that have associated hyperfluorescence on FA. Common tumors associated with BDUMP are cancers of the ovary, uterus, and lung, but BDUMP may also occur with cancers of the colon, pancreas, gallbladder, and esophagus.

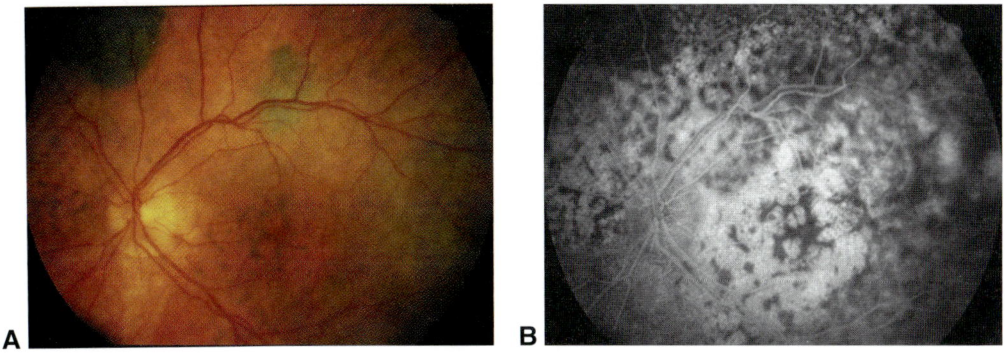

Figure 9-8 Bilateral diffuse uveal melanocytic proliferation. **A,** Note the large nevuslike regions of increased pigmentation and thickening of the choroid in this fundus photograph. **B,** Fluorescein angiography image demonstrates decreased fluorescence in the region of the melanocytic proliferation in the superonasal portion. There is a leopard spot pattern to the fluorescence in the posterior pole, secondary to chronic subretinal fluid. *(Courtesy of Mark Johnson, MD.)*

Gass JD, Gieser RG, Wilkinson CP, Beahm DE, Pautler SE. Bilateral diffuse uveal melanocytic proliferation in patients with occult carcinoma. *Arch Ophthalmol.* 1990;108(4):527–533.

Mets RB, Golchet P, Adamus G, et al. Bilateral diffuse uveal melanocytic proliferation with a positive ophthalmoscopic and visual response to plasmapheresis. *Arch Ophthalmol.* 2011; 129(9):1235–1238.

CHAPTER 10

Focal and Diffuse Choroidal and Retinal Inflammation

A variety of inflammatory disorders are associated with yellow-white lesions of the retina and choroid. This chapter highlights various focal and diffuse retinal and choroidal inflammatory disorders that can cause such lesions, including epidemiology and descriptions of clinical features. When the term *standard treatment* is used to describe therapy, options for autoimmune disease include corticosteroids in the acute phase and immunosuppressive agents for suppressive therapy. Other therapies or disease-specific treatment options are also outlined as appropriate. See BCSC Section 9, *Intraocular Inflammation and Uveitis,* for more in-depth information on these entities, further detail on treatment approaches, and additional illustrations.

Agarwal A. *Gass' Atlas of Macular Diseases.* 2 vols. 5th ed. Philadelphia: Saunders; 2012: 805–1064.

Foster CS, Vitale AT, Jakobiec FA. *Diagnosis and Treatment of Uveitis.* 2nd ed. New Delhi: Jaypee Brothers Medical Publishers; 2013.

Yannuzzi LA. *The Retina Atlas.* Philadelphia: Saunders; 2010:305–380.

Noninfectious Retinal and Choroidal Inflammation

White Dot Syndromes

The term *white dot syndromes* has been used to describe the following conditions:

- acute posterior multifocal placoid pigment epitheliopathy (APMPPE)
- serpiginous choroidopathy
- multiple evanescent white dot syndrome (MEWDS)
- birdshot uveitis
- multifocal choroiditis (MFC)
- multifocal choroiditis and panuveitis syndrome (MCP)
- punctate inner choroidopathy (PIC)

Many authorities now believe that MFC and PIC are part of a spectrum of the same condition; in this chapter, these entities are referred to as MFC (discussed in a later section). Acute zonal occult outer retinopathy (AZOOR), acute macular neuroretinopathy (AMN), and acute idiopathic maculopathy are often discussed along with the more classic white dot syndromes listed above because of their presumed inflammatory etiology and the frequently shared symptoms of decreased vision, scotomas, and photopsias.

Buggage RR. White dot syndrome. *Focal Points: Clinical Modules for Ophthalmologists.* San Francisco: American Academy of Ophthalmology; 2007, module 4.

Matsumoto Y, Haen SP, Spaide RF. The white dot syndromes. *Compr Ophthalmol Update.* 2007;8(4):179–200.

Acute posterior multifocal placoid pigment epitheliopathy

Acute posterior multifocal placoid pigment epitheliopathy (APMPPE; also known as *AMPPPE*) is an uncommon, bilateral inflammatory disorder characterized by the acute onset of blurred vision, scotomas, and, in some patients, photopsias. Approximately one-third of patients describe an antecedent flulike illness. Men and woman are affected equally, usually in youth to middle age. Mild anterior chamber and vitreous inflammation may be present. Lesions typically are multiple, yellow-white, placoid, and variable in size at the level of the outer retina (retinal pigment epithelium, RPE) and inner choroid (choriocapillaris) (Fig 10-1). Recurrences are uncommon. The etiology is unknown, although hypoperfusion of the choriocapillaris resulting in ischemic injury to the overlying RPE

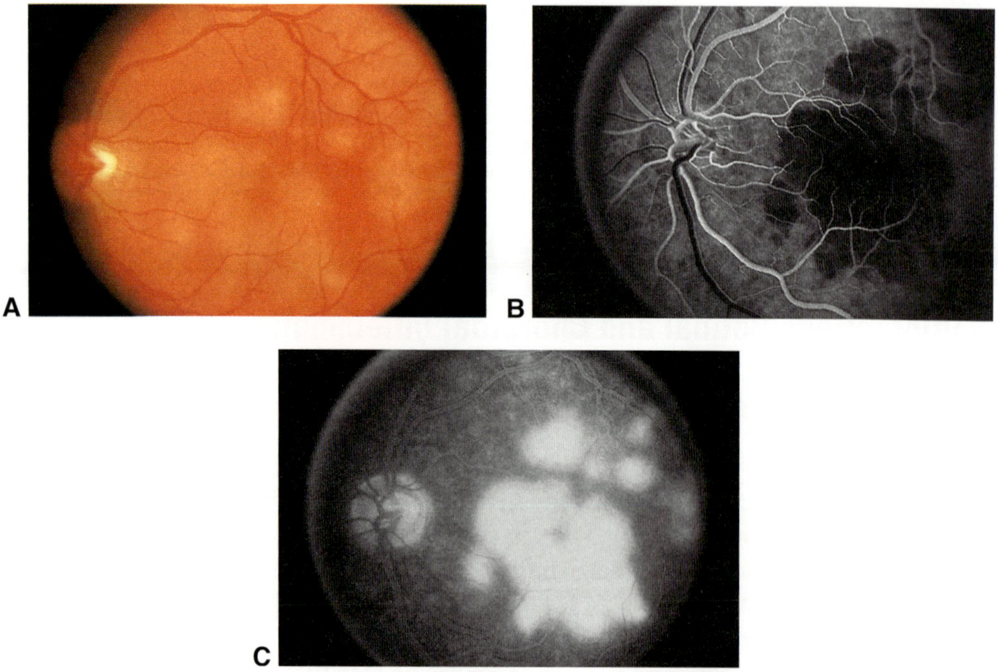

Figure 10-1 Acute posterior multifocal placoid pigment epitheliopathy (APMPPE). **A,** Color fundus photograph showing multiple, placoid yellowish lesions in the posterior pole. **B,** Early-phase angiography image demonstrates hypofluorescence resulting from both decreased perfusion of the choriocapillaris and thickening of the retinal pigment epithelium (RPE) lesions. **C,** Late-phase angiography image demonstrates hyperfluorescence in the areas involved. *(Courtesy of J. Donald M. Gass, MD.)*

characterizes the condition. Systemic involvement—especially cerebral vasculitis—can occur, although it is uncommon. APMPPE-like lesions can be present in patients with sarcoidosis, syphilis, and tuberculosis; therefore, testing should be done to exclude these conditions.

Acutely, fluorescein angiography (FA) of active lesions shows early blockage followed by progressive late leakage and staining. Indocyanine green (ICG) angiography shows early and late (persistent) hypofluorescence, corresponding to and often extending beyond lesions identified clinically and on FA. Ocular coherence tomography (OCT) images taken through active lesions reveal dome-shaped, outer-retinal lesions corresponding with disruption of the hyperreflective bands associated with the photoreceptors and RPE. Autofluorescence in and around active lesions varies over time and may be either increased or decreased at presentation; it tends to decrease as disease activity subsides. With time, hypoautofluorescence develops in areas of RPE disruption. The fundus appearance and visual symptoms typically improve within weeks. The long-term prognosis tends to be good, although faint scotomas may persist and central vision can be limited in eyes with central macular involvement.

Treatment for APMPPE is not typically indicated, although systemic corticosteroids may be considered in isolated cases involving central macular involvement or cerebral vasculitis. Severe APMPPE can sometimes be difficult to distinguish from serpiginous choroidopathy (discussed in the next section), leading to the introduction of the term *ampiginous* to characterize the APMPPE–serpiginous choroidopathy disease continuum. Other, related placoid disorders have also been described, including persistent placoid maculopathy, which is characterized by central macular involvement, a longer healing time, and a high risk of CNV formation, as well as relentless placoid chorioretinitis, which is characterized by the frequent occurrence of smaller, geographically distributed lesions that typically require immunosuppressive treatment.

Steiner S, Goldstein DA. Imaging in the diagnosis and management of APMPPE. *Int Ophthalmol Clin.* 2012;52(4):211–219.

Serpiginous choroidopathy

Serpiginous choroidopathy, also known as *geographic choroiditis* or *helicoid peripapillary choroidopathy,* is an uncommon, often vision-threatening, recurrent inflammatory disorder involving the outer retina (the RPE) and inner choroid (the choriocapillaris). Classically, lesions first appear at or near the disc and extend centrifugally in a serpentine pattern. With repeated recurrences, a serpiginous (pseudopodial) or geographic (maplike) pattern of chorioretinal scarring develops (Fig 10-2). Findings on clinical examination and through multimodal imaging of active serpiginous lesions resemble those of acute APMPPE. Lesions tend to occur near or adjacent to inactive scars from prior episodes of inflammation. Persistent scotomas and decreased central vision are common symptoms. Serpiginous choroidopathy tends to affect men slightly more often than women, typically in middle age. In endemic areas, such as India, tuberculosis is well recognized as producing serpiginous-like lesions, leading some clinicians to describe such lesions as *tubercular serpiginous-like choroiditis.* In addition to evaluation for tuberculosis, patients

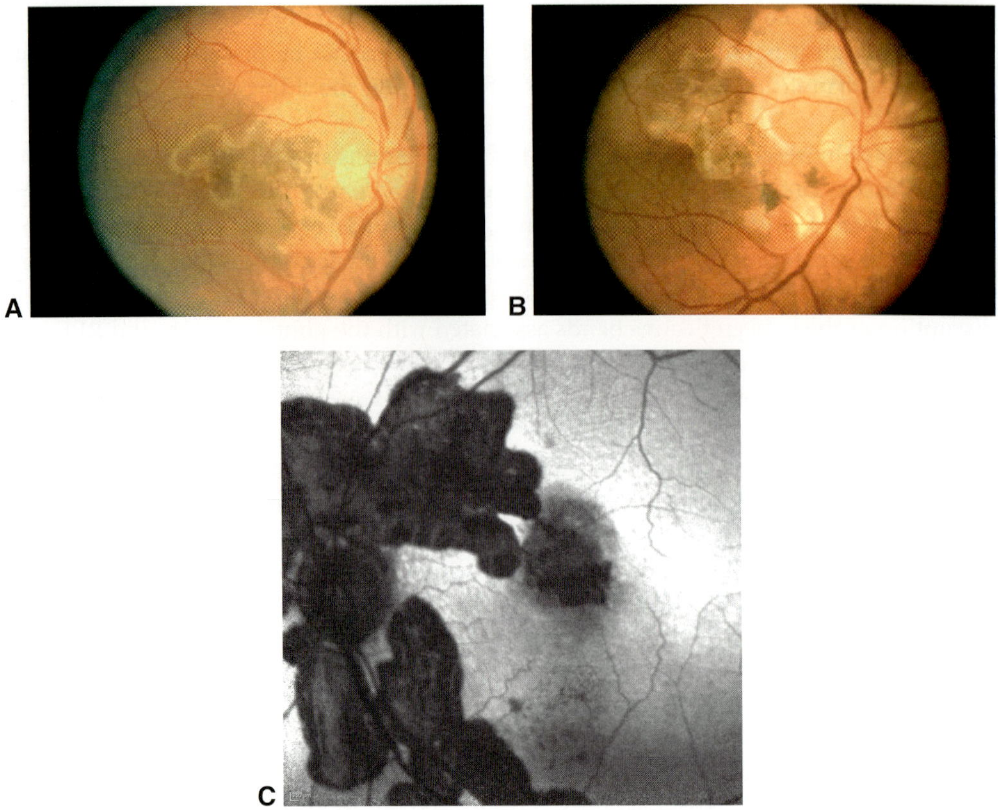

Figure 10-2 Serpiginous choroidopathy. **A,** Color fundus photograph of a chorioretinal scar with irregular borders and snakelike protrusion to the foveal region. **B,** Color fundus photograph of the same eye several years later, illustrating expansion of chorioretinal scarring that consumed most of the superior and nasal macula, characteristic of serpiginous choroidopathy. **C,** Autofluorescence image of an unrelated case illustrating the absence of autofluorescence in the area of chorioretinal scarring. *(Courtesy of Colin A. McCannel, MD.)*

with serpiginous-like lesions should be routinely evaluated for sarcoidosis and syphilis. Standard autoimmune disease treatment options are employed.

Bansal R, Gupta A, Gupta V. Imaging in the diagnosis and management of serpiginous choroiditis. *Int Ophthalmol Clin.* 2012;52(4):229–236.

Multiple evanescent white dot syndrome

Multiple evanescent white dot syndrome (MEWDS) is an acute-onset syndrome characterized by multiple small gray, white, or yellow-white dots at the level of the outer retina (RPE level) in and around the posterior pole (Fig 10-3). In some patients, an unusual transient foveal granularity consisting of tiny yellow-orange flecks at the level of the RPE also develops and is highly suggestive of the condition. Abnormalities on ICG angiography suggest simultaneous choroidal involvement. Mild anterior chamber cell reaction or vitritis may be present. Patients are typically young to middle aged and frequently have myopia; women are affected more often than men. Symptoms tend to be unilateral and

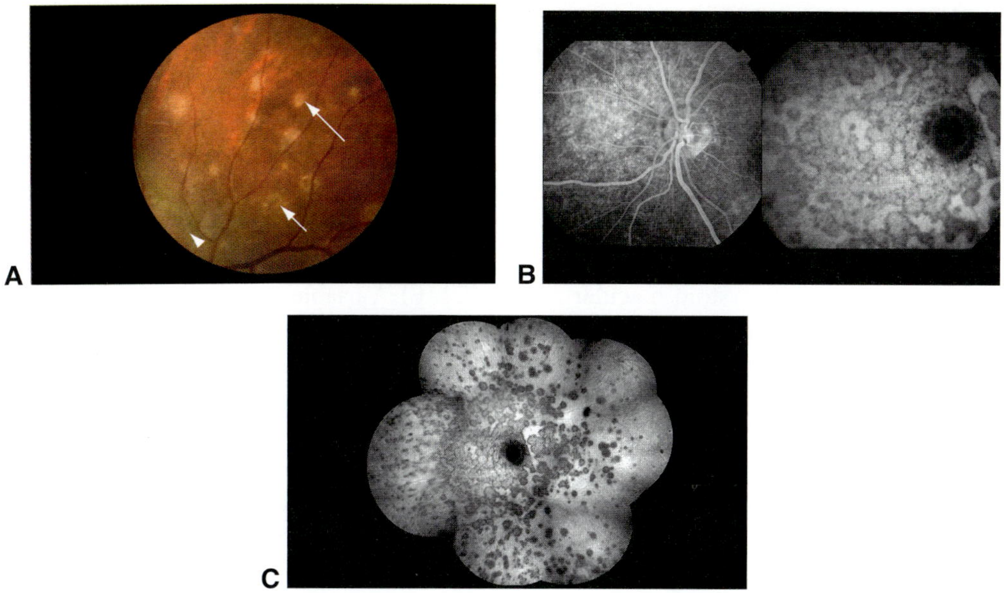

Figure 10-3 The gray-white dots in multiple evanescent white dot syndrome (MEWDS) resolve quickly. **A,** Acute lesions are gray-white *(long arrow);* they first resolve centrally *(short arrow),* leaving behind a subtle change in color *(arrowhead).* **B,** The fluorescein angiography image *(left)* shows wreaths of gray-white dots. The corresponding indocyanine green (ICG) angiography image *(right)* shows darker placoid lesions with bordering darker dots. **C,** Wide-angle ICG angiography image demonstrates that the extent of involvement is often much greater than that visible using ophthalmoscopy alone. *(Courtesy of Richard F. Spaide, MD.)*

include decreased vision, scotomas, and sometimes photopsias. Temporal visual field abnormalities and an enlarged blind spot are common, and an afferent pupillary defect is often present. The etiology is unknown, although one-third of patients describe a flulike prodrome.

Fluorescein angiography reveals multiple, punctate, hyperfluorescent dots associated with the spots observed clinically, typically in a wreathlike cluster. Mild, late leakage and staining of the disc is often observed. ICG angiography shows hypofluorescence around the disc as well as multiple hypofluorescent dots, which are typically more numerous than those observed either clinically or on FA. OCT images taken through active lesions reveal dome-shaped outer retinal lesions associated with disruption of the outer retinal hyperreflective bands. Fundus autofluorescence imaging often shows focal hyperautofluorescence in the area of the white dots. On electroretinogram (ERG) testing, some patients show delayed 30-Hz flicker responses and decreased bright-flash, dark-adapted a-wave amplitudes. The symptoms and fundus findings start to improve in most patients in 2–6 weeks without treatment. In rare cases, MEWDS can be recurrent or bilateral, cause persistent scotomas or visual field defects, or be associated with the late development of choroidal neovascularization (CNV).

dell'Omo R, Pavesio CE. Multiple evanescent white dot syndrome (MEWDS). *Int Ophthalmol Clin.* 2012;52(4):221–228.

Birdshot uveitis

Birdshot uveitis, or *vitiliginous chorioretinitis,* is bilateral and affects women slightly more often than men, typically in late middle age. Early symptoms include floaters and blurred or decreased vision. Later in the course of disease, nyctalopia, diminished contrast sensitivity, and decreased color vision may occur. Examination reveals vitreous inflammation, which is typically mild and associated with multiple yellow-white choroiditis spots that are often initially observed inferior to the disc (Fig 10-4). Fluorescein angiography often shows active retinal vasculitis with leakage from the retinal vessels and optic disc, frequently producing cystoid macular edema (CME). Variable amounts of outer retinal atrophy can also be present, resulting in window defects; when extensive, these defects can produce diffuse hyperfluorescence on FA. Choroidal lesions are best visualized using ICG angiography. OCT and fundus autofluorescence can be used to monitor the extent and progression of outer retinal atrophy.

The disease is chronic, progressive, and prone to recurrent episodes of inflammation. Vision loss may be caused by CME, epiretinal membrane formation, and/or outer retinal atrophy, which can be extensive and associated with optic atrophy in advanced cases. Virtually all patients with birdshot uveitis are white and HLA-A29 positive; indeed, the diagnosis should be questioned if a patient with suspected birdshot uveitis is either nonwhite or HLA-A29 negative. Disease activity and progression may be assessed in the office using multimodal imaging (FA, ICG angiography, spectral-domain OCT, and fundus autofluorescence) and through periodic electrophysiologic, color vision, and visual field testing—each of which may show a degree of dysfunction far greater than that suggested by routine Snellen visual acuity assessments. Standard autoimmune disease treatment options are employed, although the disease is difficult to control.

Levinson RD, Monnet D. Imaging in birdshot chorioretinopathy. *Int Ophthalmol Clin.* 2012; 52(4):191–198.

Shah KH, Levinson RD, Yu F, et al. Birdshot chorioretinopathy. *Surv Ophthamol.* 2005;50(6): 519–541.

Multifocal choroiditis

Use of the terms *idiopathic multifocal choroiditis, multifocal choroiditis with panuveitis* (MFCPU), *recurrent multifocal choroiditis* (RMC), *punctate inner choroiditis* or

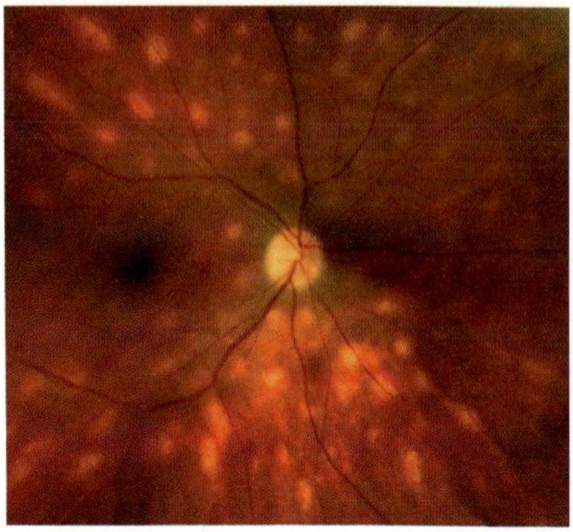

Figure 10-4 Color fundus photograph showing multiple yellow choroiditis spots in birdshot uveitis. *(Courtesy of Richard F. Spaide, MD.)*

choroidopathy (PIC), and *pseudo-presumed ocular histoplasmosis syndrome* (pseudo-POHS), among others, is both inconsistent and confusing in the literature. Recent recommendations suggest that *multifocal choroiditis* (MFC) alone should be used to refer to the occurrence of discrete chorioretinitis lesions in the absence of an identifiable underlying infection (such as tuberculosis or histoplasmosis) or systemic inflammation (such as sarcoidosis). In MFC, lesions are commonly clustered in the macula and around the disc, although they can also occur in the mid- and far periphery, frequently aligned in a curvilinear manner—configurations that are sometimes referred to as *Schlaegel lines.* Patients are typically young and female. Clinical examination usually reveals little or no anterior chamber or vitreous inflammation, although patients can have mild to moderate vitreous inflammation—a presentation some clinicians mean by the use of *MFCPU.* Blurred or decreased vision and scotomas are the most common symptoms. Decreased central vision results most frequently from direct central macular involvement or from the development of CNV, which occurs in one-third of patients. Subretinal fibrosis can occur in and around lesions and, when the central macula is involved, can also limit vision (Fig 10-5). Standard treatment options for autoimmune disease are employed.

Essex RW, Wong J, Jampol LM, Dowler J, Bird AC. Idiopathic multifocal choroiditis: a comment on present and past nomenclature. *Retina.* 2013;33(1):1–4.

Fung AT, Pal S, Yannuzzi NA, et al. Multifocal choroiditis without panuveitis: clinical characteristics and progression. *Retina.* 2014;34(1):98–107.

Jung JJ, Khan S, Mrejen S, et al. Idiopathic multifocal choroiditis with outer retinal or chorioretinal atrophy. *Retina.* 2014;34(7):1439–1450.

Acute zonal occult outer retinopathy

Acute zonal occult outer retinopathy (AZOOR), a presumed inflammatory disorder, damages broad zones of the outer retina in 1 or both eyes. Typically, AZOOR occurs in young women with myopia, and onset is acute and unilateral. Three-fourths of cases progress to bilateral involvement. Initial symptoms include photopsia, nasal visual field loss, and sometimes an enlarged blind spot; visual acuity is rarely affected. On initial presentation, the fundus may appear normal or show evidence of mild vitritis (Fig 10-6). Nearly 25%

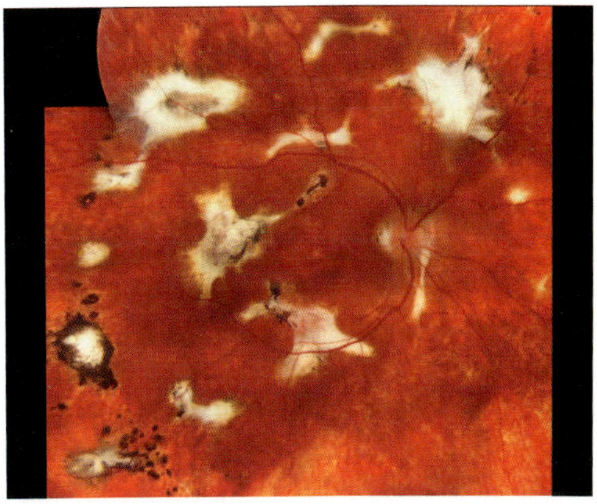

Figure 10-5 Color fundus photograph of multifocal choroiditis with subretinal fibrosis. *(Courtesy of Richard F. Spaide, MD.)*

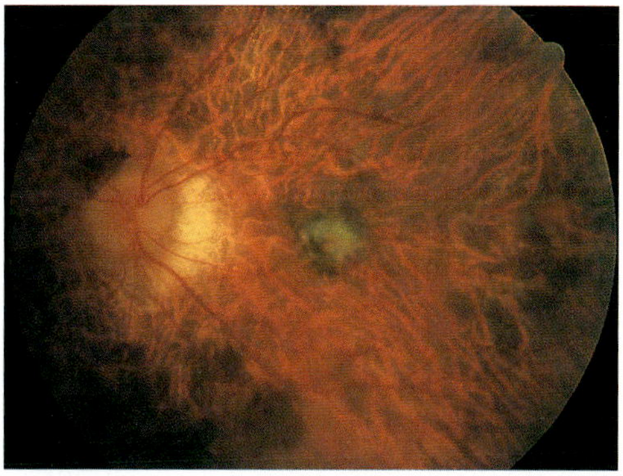

Figure 10-6 Color fundus photograph of advanced acute zonal occult outer retinopathy. *(Courtesy of J. Donald M. Gass, MD.)*

of patients have an afferent pupillary defect. Angiographic findings may include retinal and optic nerve head capillary leakage, especially in patients with evidence of vitritis. On ERG, delayed 30-Hz flicker response is common. Visual field testing may show scotomata, which can enlarge over weeks or months. Outcomes are generally favorable.

Some patients recover from AZOOR, whereas others have persistent, large visual field defects, which tend to stabilize over 6 months. Permanent visual field loss is often associated with late development of fundus changes. Depigmentation of large zones of RPE usually corresponds to scotomata; narrowed retinal vessels may be visible within these areas. The late fundus appearance in some patients may resemble cancer-associated retinopathy or retinitis pigmentosa. Fluorescein angiography images tend to appear normal early on but become expectedly abnormal in eyes with RPE alterations. ICG angiography has been reported to show areas of late hypofluorescence. OCT typically reveals outer retinal atrophy, including disruption of the ellipsoid zone (also known as the *inner-outer segment junction*) and the outer nuclear layer in involved areas. Autofluorescence is typically decreased in areas of involvement and is occasionally associated with either punctate or a peripheral rim of hyperautofluorescence. Immunosuppression does not alter the course of the disease.

The term *AZOOR complex* has been introduced to encompass MFC, MEWDS, and AZOOR, as these conditions may have overlapping clinical features in some patients and may be part of a continuum. This concept is controversial, and the diseases may best be considered separate entities for now.

Gass JD, Agarwal A, Scott IU. Acute zonal occult outer retinopathy: a long-term follow-up study. *Am J Ophthalmol.* 2002;134(3):329–339.

Monson DM, Smith JR. Acute zonal occult outer retinopathy. *Surv Ophthalmol.* 2011;56(1): 23–35.

Acute macular neuroretinopathy

Acute macular neuroretinopathy (AMN) is a rare condition characterized by the acute onset of paracentral scotomas in 1 or both eyes in young, otherwise healthy patients. Women outnumber men nearly 6 to 1. Clinically, reddish-brown teardrop or wedge-shaped lesions are observed around the fovea with the tips of the lesions pointing centrally; they correspond in size and location to the subjective paracentral scotomas. The lesions can be difficult to see on fundus examination or with color photography but are readily apparent on near-infrared imaging. The retinal vessels and optic nerve are unaffected, and there is no vitreous inflammation. High-resolution OCT is particularly helpful and has revealed 2 patterns: (1) type 1, which has involvement of the middle retina or inner nuclear layer; and (2) type 2, which has involvement of the outer retina—including both the outer nuclear layer and the hyperreflective bands associated with the photoreceptors of the ellipsoid zone. Both patterns are believed to result from ischemia of the deep capillary plexus of the central retina.

The lesions typically resolve over several weeks to months with corresponding visual recovery, except in rare cases that remain symptomatic for years. The pathogenesis of AMN is unclear. Several associations have been noted, however, including a preceding flulike illness, the use of oral contraceptives or caffeine, and injection of adrenaline or epinephrine. Lesions resembling AMN can occur following mild to moderate, blunt, or whiplash-type trauma. Whether these lesions are AMN or traumatic maculopathy is controversial.

Bos PJ, Deutman AF. Acute macular neuroretinopathy. *Am J Ophthalmol.* 1975;80(4): 573–584.

Fawzi AA, Pappuru RR, Sarraf D, et al. Acute macular neuroretinopathy: long-term insights revealed by multimodal imaging. *Retina.* 2012;32(8):1500–1513.

Sarraf D, Rahimy E, Fawzi AA, et al. Paracentral acute middle maculopathy: a new variant of acute macular neuroretinopathy associated with retinal capillary ischemia. *JAMA Ophthalmol.* 2013;131(10):1275–1287.

Acute idiopathic maculopathy

Acute idiopathic maculopathy (AIM) is a rare disorder that presents with sudden, severe central or paracentral vision loss, typically in younger individuals following a flulike illness. Men and women are affected equally. Central unilateral lesions were described initially, but both bilateral and eccentric macular lesions have since been added to the spectrum. The main clinical finding is an exudative neurosensory macular detachment with little or no vitreous inflammation and variable discoloration of the underlying RPE. Mild disc swelling, retinal hemorrhages, vasculitis, and subretinal infiltrates occur infrequently. Fluorescein angiography typically shows progressive irregular hyperfluorescence at the level of the RPE, followed in the late stages by pooling in the detachment space. ICG angiography shows early and persistent hypofluorescence. High-resolution OCT imaging documents the size and extent of the detachment space and shows loss of the hyperreflective outer retinal bands associated with the photoreceptors and RPE. The lesions resolve spontaneously but leave a bull's-eye pattern of RPE alteration, which on FA shows central hypofluorescence and surrounding hyperfluorescence. There is typically near-complete recovery of vision over weeks to months. The cause is unknown, although isolated cases have been associated with coxsackievirus infection.

Hoang QV, Strauss DS, Pappas A, Freund KB. Imaging in the diagnosis and management of acute idiopathic maculopathy. *Int Ophthlamol Clin.* 2012;52(4):263–268.

Yannuzzi LA, Jampol LM, Rabb MF, Sorenson JA, Beyrer C, Wilcox LM Jr. Unilateral acute idiopathic maculopathy. *Arch Ophthalmol.* 1991;109(10):1411–1416.

Chorioretinal Autoimmune Conditions

The following sections detail selected autoimmune diseases affecting the retina and choroid. These conditions are generally treated using standard autoimmune treatment options. Specific treatment considerations are mentioned when applicable.

Inflammatory vasculitis

Behçet disease Behçet disease is a complex systemic disorder characterized by recurrent attacks of inflammation and vascular occlusion involving multiple organ systems. Recurrent oral ulceration affects nearly all patients, and cutaneous lesions such as erythema nodosum are common. Central nervous system involvement may develop in more than 50% of patients and should be suspected in any patient with neurologic signs. Other systemic manifestations include arthritis, epididymitis, and intestinal ulcers. Behçet disease tends to affect men more than women and is particularly common in Japan, Southeast Asia, the Middle East, and the Mediterranean region. The etiology is unknown.

Uveitis is common and may be anterior, posterior, or diffuse (panuveitis). Posterior segment involvement may include vitritis, an occlusive retinal vasculitis, intraretinal hemorrhages, macular edema, focal areas of retinal necrosis, and ischemic optic neuropathy. Recurrent episodes of retinal vasculitis may lead to severe ischemia and retinal neovascularization, which should be treated with panretinal photocoagulation. Despite treatment, the visual prognosis is often poor because of progressive retinal ischemia from recurrent episodes of occlusive vasculitis. Use of biologic agents, such as inhibitors of tumor necrosis factor alpha as well as interferon, has shown promise.

Tugal-Tutkun I. Imaging in the diagnosis and management of Behçet disease. *Int Ophthalmol Clin.* 2012;52(4):183–190.

Tugal-Tutkun I, Gupta V, Cunningham ET Jr. Differential diagnosis of Behçet uveitis. *Ocul Immunol Inflamm.* 2013;21(5):337–350.

Lupus vasculitis *Systemic lupus erythematosus* (SLE) is a systemic autoimmune disorder most commonly affecting women of childbearing age. Black and Hispanic women are at higher risk than are white women. As a multisystem disease, SLE can involve almost every ocular and periocular structure. Approximately 3%–10% of patients with SLE have retinal disease ranging from asymptomatic cotton-wool spots and intraretinal hemorrhages to macular infarction with severe central vision loss (Fig 10-7). Lupus choroidopathy is less common and presents as multifocal serous retinal detachments. The retinal and choroidal pathology is vascular and thought to be autoimmune in nature.

The presence of retinal vascular occlusion, including cotton-wool spots, is indicative of active systemic inflammation and should prompt treatment. Sarcoidosis can cause retinal vasculitis (Fig 10-8) and should be evaluated as a possible cause.

Read RW. Clinical mini-review: systemic lupus erythematosus and the eye. *Ocul Immunol Inflamm.* 2004;12(2):87–99.

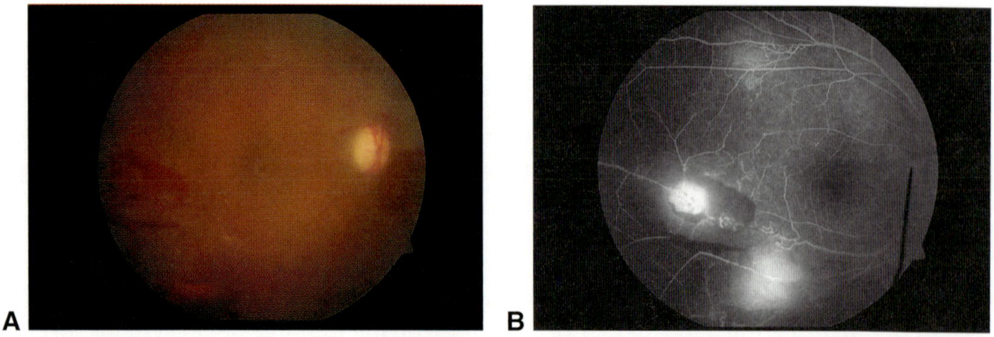

Figure 10-7 Vasculitis secondary to systemic lupus erythematosus. **A,** Color fundus photograph showing vitreous hemorrhage secondary to neovascularization. **B,** Late-phase fluorescein angiography image revealing choroidal and retinal nonperfusion, perivascular staining, and leakage due to neovascularization. *(Courtesy of Matthew A. Thomas, MD.)*

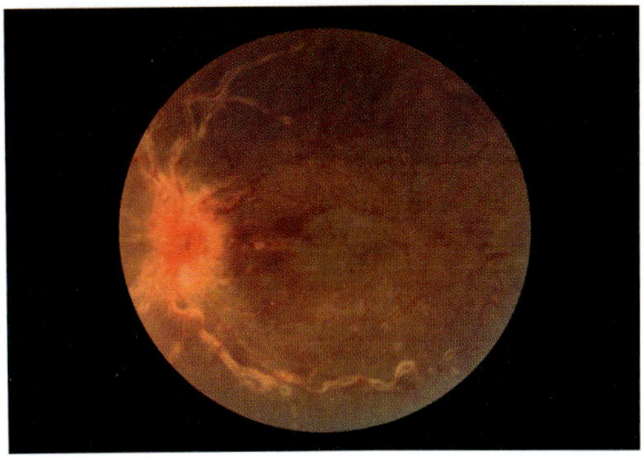

Figure 10-8 Sarcoidosis. Color fundus photograph showing retinal vascular sheathing. *(Courtesy of Ramin Schadlu, MD.)*

Intermediate uveitis

Intermediate uveitis refers to posterior segment inflammation that primarily involves the vitreous cavity. Eighty percent of intermediate uveitis cases are idiopathic. The most commonly identified causes in North America and Europe include sarcoidosis and multiple sclerosis. Use of the term *pars planitis* is variable and inconsistent but often is used to describe inflammatory debris overlying the pars plana ("snowbanking"), regardless of cause. It is best to state precisely whether a snowbank is present and whether the cause of the intermediate uveitis is known, as in, for example, "idiopathic intermediate uveitis with snowbanking," or "intermediate uveitis without snowbanking in the setting of sarcoidosis."

Intermediate uveitis is typically bilateral and can occur in children, adolescents, or adults. Common symptoms include floaters and decreased vision. Characteristic ocular manifestations include vitreous inflammation, snowbanking, and aggregates of vitreous cells ("snowballs"). Both snowbanking and snowballs are most often observed inferiorly. Peripheral neovascularization may form along the inferior snowbank in 5%–10% of cases and can lead to vitreous hemorrhage with tractional or rhegmatogenous retinal detachment. When active, segmental phlebitis, optic disc leakage, and CME are common. Epiretinal membrane formation also occurs.

Vitreous cells or segmental phlebitis in the absence of decreased vision can be observed without treatment. Active CME is best treated with corticosteroids.

de Boer J, Berendschot TT, van der Does P, Rothova A. Long-term follow-up of intermediate uveitis in children. *Am J Ophthalmol.* 2006;141(4):616–621.

Vidovic-Valentincic N, Kraut A, Hawlina M, Stunf S, Rothova A. Intermediate uveitis: long-term course and visual outcome. *Br J Ophthalmol.* 2009;93(4):477–480.

Vogt-Koyanagi-Harada disease

Vogt-Koyanagi-Harada (VKH) disease (or syndrome) is a systemic autoimmune disorder directed against melanocytes in the eye, auditory system, meninges, and skin. VKH disease most commonly affects people of Asian, American Indian, Asian Indian, Mediterranean, and Middle Eastern descent. Patients with the disorder who are Hispanic or African American often have some American Indian ancestry. Ocular findings are typically bilateral and include vitreous inflammation associated with serous retinal detachment. Disc hyperemia and edema are common. Fluorescein angiography studies can be particularly helpful and often show multiple RPE leaks in the areas of detachment, a finding referred to as the "starry night" or "Milky Way" sign (Fig 10-9).

The diagnosis of VKH disease can be made only in patients who have not had penetrating ocular injury or ocular surgery. VKH disease is termed *probable* when characteristic ocular inflammation occurs in the absence of skin or neurologic findings; it is termed *incomplete* if either skin or neurologic findings, but not both, are present; and it is termed *complete* when both skin and neurologic findings develop.

The clinical course of VKH disease can be divided into 3 phases:

1. *prodromal phase:* characterized by a flulike illness with symptoms that can include headache, meningismus, tinnitus, and dysacusis
2. *acute uveitic phase:* closely follows the prodromal phase; characterized by pain, photophobia, and vision loss accompanied by the onset of bilateral panuveitis with serous retinal detachments
3. *chronic (convalescent) phase:* the uveitis subsides, but depigmentation of the skin and uvea can occur; ocular depigmentation may develop at the limbus ("Sugiura" sign), the trabecular meshwork ("Ohno" sign), or within the choroid ("sunset glow" sign)

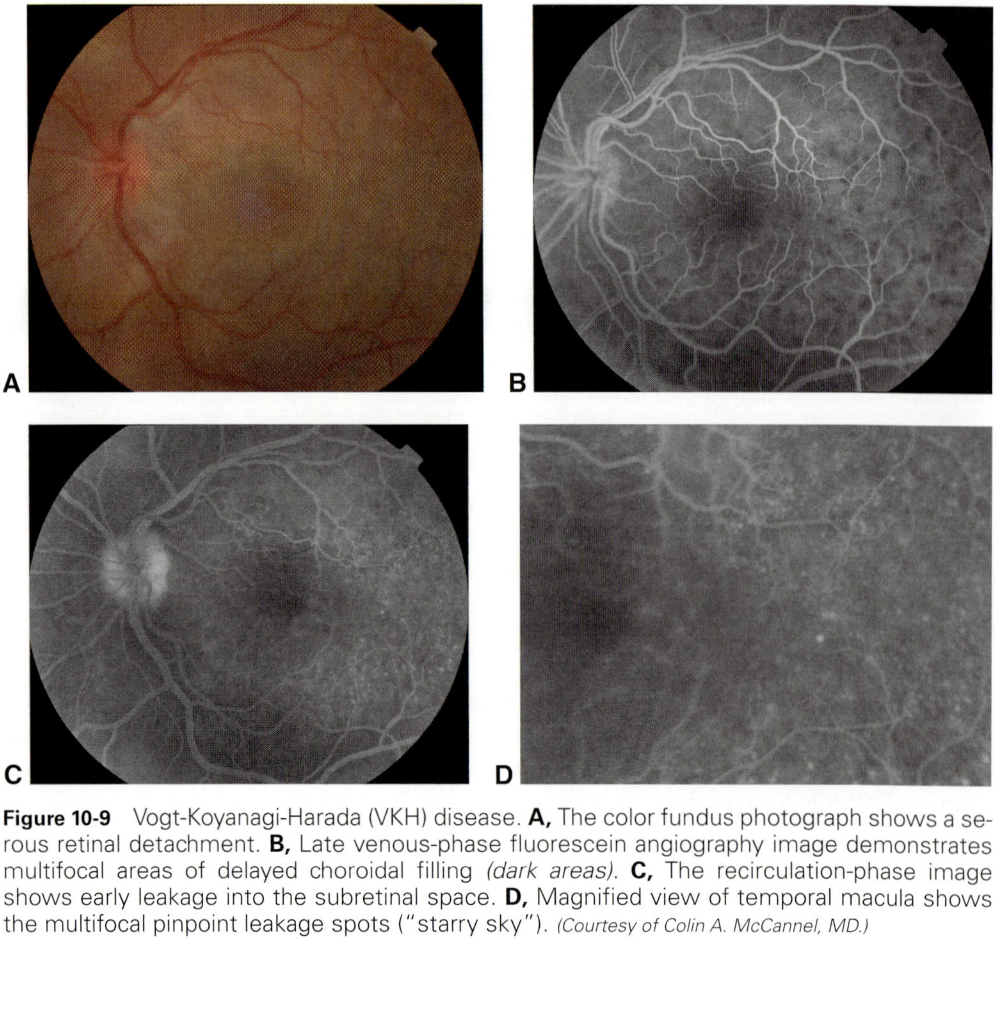

Figure 10-9 Vogt-Koyanagi-Harada (VKH) disease. **A,** The color fundus photograph shows a serous retinal detachment. **B,** Late venous-phase fluorescein angiography image demonstrates multifocal areas of delayed choroidal filling *(dark areas).* **C,** The recirculation-phase image shows early leakage into the subretinal space. **D,** Magnified view of temporal macula shows the multifocal pinpoint leakage spots ("starry sky"). *(Courtesy of Colin A. McCannel, MD.)*

VKH disease tends to respond to standard treatment options. A delay in diagnosis and treatment is associated with an increased risk of depigmentation of the skin and eye and with an increased rate of ocular complications, including cataract, glaucoma, and subretinal fibrosis.

Rao NA, Gupta A, Dustin L, et al. Frequency of distinguishing clinical features in Vogt-Koyanagi-Harada disease. *Ophthalmology.* 2010;117(3):591–599.

Read RW, Holland GN, Rao NA, et al. Revised diagnostic criteria for Vogt-Koyanagi-Harada disease: report of an international committee on nomenclature. *Am J Ophthalmol.* 2001; 131(5):647–652.

Sympathetic Ophthalmia

Sympathetic ophthalmia is a rare condition that is clinically and histologically indistinguishable from ocular findings in VKH disease, except that it occurs only after a penetrating ocular injury or ocular surgery. Inflammation of the exciting (injured or operated) and sympathizing (fellow) eye may occur days to decades after the initial insult. As in VKH disease, the inflammation is bilateral and characterized by the presence of panuveitis, often associated with areas of serous retinal detachment and focal choroiditis (nummular chorioretinal lesions). Nonocular complications, such as vitiligo or poliosis, can occur but are much less common than in VKH disease. Moreover, in the rare instances when sympathetic ophthalmia does follow either injury or surgery, standard treatment approaches almost always control the inflammation. Therefore, enucleation of an injured eye to minimize risk of sympathetic ophthalmia should be undertaken only when the eye is structurally disorganized and has no light perception (NLP).

Castiblanco CP, Adelman RA. Sympathetic ophthalmia. *Graefes Arch Clin Exp Ophthalmol.* 2009;247(3):289–302.

Uveitis Masquerade: Intraocular Lymphoma

Primary vitreoretinal lymphoma was previously referred to as *reticulum cell sarcoma, histiocytic lymphoma,* and *non-Hodgkin lymphoma of the central nervous system.* Most cases are aggressive B-cell tumors. Half of all cases of *primary vitreoretinal lymphoma* occur after 60 years of age. Approximately 80% of patients with primary vitreoretinal lymphoma develop central nervous system (CNS) involvement. Conversely, of patients who present with CNS involvement, approximately 20% will have eye involvement. HIV infection is associated with an increased risk of lymphoma that ranges from 50-fold (with potent antiretroviral therapy) to more than 500-fold (prior to—or without access to—potent antiretroviral therapy). Suggestive clinical features include an incomplete or transient response to corticosteroid treatment, the presence of atypical vitreous cells—which may be uncharacteristically white and/or occur in sheets—and the presence of subretinal infiltrates, which can be transient and/or shift location over time (Fig 10-10). Disc edema and serous retinal detachment can also occur. Patients with suspected primary vitreoretinal lymphoma should undergo magnetic resonance imaging (MRI) of the brain with contrast as well as a spinal tap for cytologic studies to evaluate for CNS involvement. Confirmatory CNS or vitreoretinal biopsy is usually performed. It is notoriously difficult to arrive

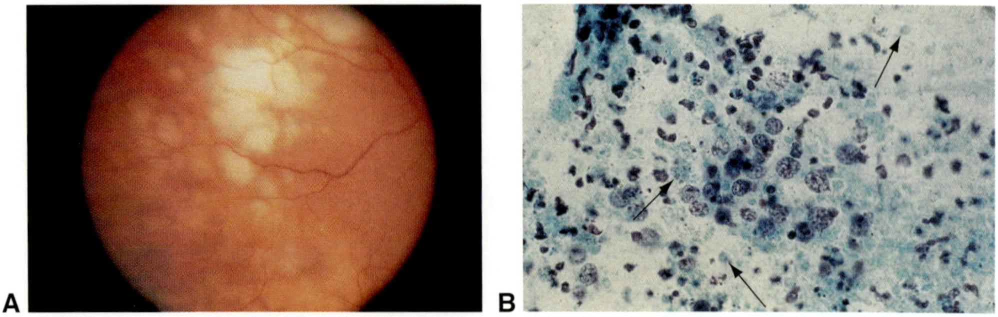

Figure 10-10 Intraocular lymphoma. **A,** Color fundus photograph showing sub–retinal pigment epithelial infiltrates. **B,** Cytologic preparation of vitreous cells reveals many atypical cells with large nuclei and multiple nucleoli. Cell ghosts *(arrows)* are also present. *(Courtesy of David J. Wilson, MD.)*

at a diagnosis from tests on a vitreous specimen because of the low cell concentrations and the propensity of lymphoma cells to undergo autolysis. Best results are achieved with rapid processing and analysis by cytology, immunoglobulin or T-cell receptor gene rearrangement studies, flow cytometry, and cytokine analyses. Current management practices involve both chemotherapy and radiation treatment, but the recurrence rate is high and long-term prognosis guarded.

Uveal lymphoma, in contrast, is usually more indolent and is associated with systemic lymphoma in up to one-third of cases. Characteristic clinical findings include uveal thickening, which often produces a birdshot uveitis–like fundus picture with or without serous retinal detachment. Episcleral involvement may manifest anteriorly as salmon-colored conjunctival infiltration or posteriorly as a juxtascleral mass on ultrasound. Biopsy of affected tissues can confirm the diagnosis. Evaluation for systemic involvement includes use of computed tomography (CT) or combined CT and positron emission tomography (PET) imaging of the thorax, abdomen, and pelvis.

Chan CC, Sen HN. Current concepts in diagnosing and managing primary vitreoretinal (intraocular) lymphoma. *Discov Med.* 2013;15(81):93–100.

Infectious Retinal and Choroidal Inflammation

The following sections provide brief descriptions of selected infectious diseases that can cause retinal and choroidal inflammation.

Cytomegalovirus Retinitis

Cytomegalovirus (CMV) *retinitis* is the most common ocular opportunistic infection in patients with advanced AIDS and usually occurs when CD4+ T-cell counts are less than 50/µL. Patients with CMV retinitis typically present with floaters or decreased visual acuity. Clinically, CMV retinitis has a characteristic appearance that consists of opacification of the necrotic retina, typically along retinal vessels and often with areas of hemorrhage (Fig 10-11). Periphlebitis and even "frosted branch" angiitis may be prominent features.

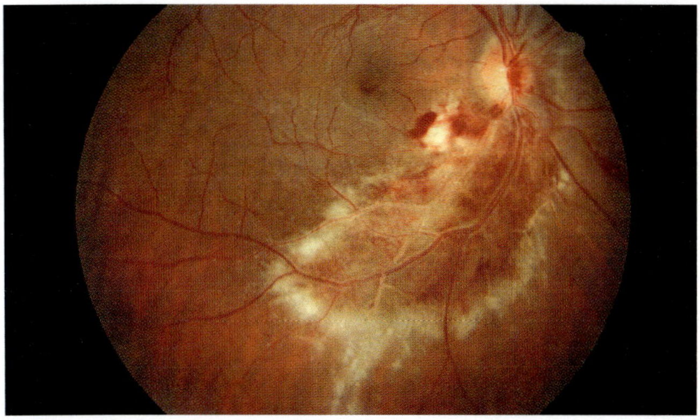

Figure 10-11 Color fundus photograph showing the perivascular distribution of cytomegalovirus retinitis. *(Courtesy of Mark W. Johnson, MD.)*

The degree of vitreous inflammation is highly variable. Early CMV retinitis may resemble the cotton-wool spots of HIV-related retinopathy. Although the diagnosis is often made clinically, polymerase chain reaction (PCR)–based analysis of ocular fluids may be useful in atypical cases.

CMV retinitis can be treated with ganciclovir or foscarnet, administered systemically or intravitreally. High-dose induction therapy is typically given for 2–3 weeks, after which maintenance therapy is continued until immune reconstitution results in restoration of anti-CMV T-cell immunity—usually at $CD4^+$ T-cell counts greater than 200/μL. Immune recovery uveitis and its complications, most notably CME and epiretinal membrane formation, occurs in approximately 20% of HIV-seropositive patients following immune reconstitution. Up to 50% of eyes with CMV retinitis eventually develop a rhegmatogenous retinal detachment.

CMV retinitis can occur in the absence of HIV infection. This scenario is uncommon, however, and is almost always associated with relative immune suppression, such as that which occurs with use of systemic corticosteroids, noncorticosteroid immunosuppressive agents, or chemotherapeutics; with an underlying cancer or non–HIV-related immune deficiency (such as Good syndrome); or with advanced age.

Takakura A, Tessler HH, Goldstein DA, et al. Viral retinitis following intraocular or periocular corticosteroid administration: a case series and comprehensive review of the literature. *Ocul Immunol Inflamm.* 2014;22(3):175–182.

Non-CMV Necrotizing Herpetic Retinitis

Both varicella-zoster virus (VZV) and herpes simplex virus (HSV) can cause necrotizing retinitis in patients whether immunocompromised or not. Unlike CMV, these infections can progress rapidly and therefore should be treated aggressively. Two distinct clinical syndromes have been described: (1) *acute retinal necrosis* (ARN) syndrome and (2) *progressive outer retinal necrosis* (PORN) syndrome. ARN does not require that a patient be severely immunocompromised in order to occur. Characteristic features include the presence of one—or more typically, multiple—foci of retinitis, which usually occur in the periphery and are associated with occlusive retinal vasculitis and moderate to severe anterior chamber and vitreous inflammation (Fig 10-12). ARN tends to occur in older patients as VZV-related immunity wanes, whereas HSV retinitis typically affects younger patients, some of whom have a history of herpetic encephalitis.

PORN occurs in patients who are severely immunocompromised, usually as the result of AIDS, and consists of rapidly progressive, multifocal necrotizing retinitis with little or no anterior chamber or vitreous inflammation. Initial involvement of the peripheral retina is most common (Fig 10-13), although the macula can be involved at presentation

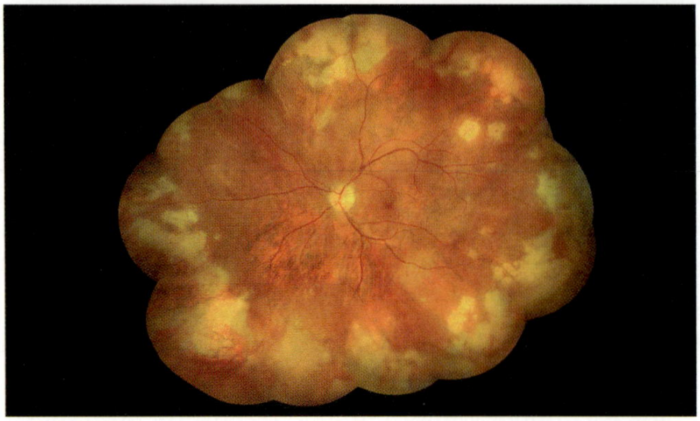

Figure 10-12 Peripheral necrotizing herpetic retinitis (acute retinal necrosis). Color fundus photograph montage showing intraretinal hemorrhage and full-thickness opacification of the retina. *(Courtesy of Mark W. Johnson, MD, and Richard Hackel, CRA. Used with permission from Aizman A, Johnson MW, Elner SG. Treatment of acute retinal necrosis syndrome with oral antiviral medications.* Ophthalmology. *2007;114(2):307–312.)*

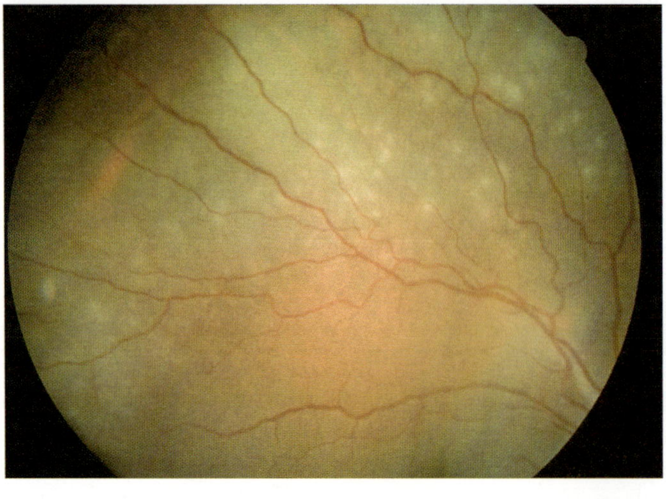

Figure 10-13 Progressive outer retinal necrosis syndrome. Fundus photograph of the superotemporal fundus shows many round, white lesions with little confluence at the advancing posterior aspect of the infection, which is characteristic of this condition. The lesions have an appearance that suggests they are affecting the outer retina. In fundus areas not visualized, similar lesions are present throughout the midperiphery and are confluent in the most anterior retina. *(Courtesy of Colin A. McCannel, MD.)*

as well. In fact, although the inflammation in eyes with necrotizing herpetic retinitis appears to decrease in patients with relative immune compromise, either VZV or HSV retinitis can initially involve any portion of the retina independent of immune status.

Evaluation should include serologic testing for syphilis as well as intraocular fluid aspiration for use in PCR analysis for identification of DNA from VZV, HSV, CMV, and *Toxoplasma gondii*. Because ARN and PORN progress rapidly, treatment should commence immediately upon suspicion of either. Some specialists initiate therapy with intraocular injection of ganciclovir or foscarnet, particularly when the macula or optic nerve is threatened. High-dose antiviral therapy, using either intravenous acyclovir or oral valacyclovir for a minimum of 7 days, should be administered. Thereafter, immunocompetent patients should be treated with oral suppressive therapy for 3–4 months, and patients with HIV/AIDS should be treated at least until the $CD4^+$ cell count exceeds 200/µL, or perhaps indefinitely (Table 10-1). Once antiviral therapy is initiated, systemic corticosteroids can be added and then tapered over 3–6 weeks.

Wong RW, Jumper JM, McDonald HR, et al. Emerging concepts in the management of acute retinal necrosis. *Br J Ophthalmol.* 2013;97(5):545–552.

Endogenous Bacterial Endophthalmitis

Endogenous bacterial endophthalmitis results from hematogenous seeding of the eye, typically during transient bacteremia. Although decreased vision and eye pain are common symptoms, many patients do not have constitutional symptoms. A wide range of

Table 10-1 Treatment Options for Herpetic Retinitis Caused by Cytomegalovirus (CMV), Varicella-Zoster Virus (VZV), or Herpes Simplex Virus (HSV)

Intraocular treatments

CMV, VZV, HSV

- Ganciclovir, 2 mg
- Foscarnet, 1.2–2.4 mg
- Ganciclovir intraocular implant (for long-term treatment)

Systemic treatments

	Drug	Induction/high dose	Maintenance/suppression
CMV			
	Ganciclovir*	5 mg/kg, intravenously, every 12 hours for 2 weeks	Valganciclovir, 900 mg, once or twice per day or Ganciclovir intraocular implant
	Foscarnet*†	90 mg/kg, intravenously, every 12 hours for 2 weeks	
VZV/HSV			
	Acyclovir*	15 mg/kg/day, intravenously, in 3 divided doses	800 mg, orally, 5 times per day
	Valacyclovir*	2 g, orally, 3 times per day	1 g, orally, 3 times per day
	Prednisone (optional)	0.5 mg/kg/day for 3–6 weeks‡	

*Standard adult dosages. Monitoring of kidney function is required, as kidney toxicity can occur.
†Monitoring of bone marrow function is required, as suppression can occur.
‡After antiviral therapy is initiated.

bacteria can cause endogenous bacterial endophthalmitis. In North America, 40% of cases occur in patients with endocarditis, most typically caused by either *Staphylococcus* or *Streptococcus* species. In contrast, 60% of endogenous endophthalmitis cases in Asia occur in patients with liver abscesses caused by *Klebsiella pneumoniae.* Nearly one-third of cases occur in patients who have urinary tract infections, most often caused by *Escherichia coli.* Other cases can be associated with intravenous drug use or with procedures known to produce bacteremia, particularly placement of indwelling catheters.

Clinical presentation can vary and depends on both the size of the inoculum and the virulence of the organism; it ranges from a focal chorioretinitis (Fig 10-14) with little vitreous inflammation to a dense panophthalmitis that offers limited view of the posterior segment. The patient should undergo systemic evaluation for the source of infection and initiate treatment with systemic antibiotics. Additionally, intravitreal injection of broad-spectrum antibiotics should be considered.

Binder MI, Chua J, Kaiser PK, Procop GW, Isada CM. Endogenous endophthalmitis: an 18-year review of culture-positive cases at a tertiary care center. *Medicine (Baltimore).* 2003;82(2):97–105.

Durand ML. Endophthalmitis. *Clin Microbiol Infect.* 2013;19(3):227–234.

Fungal Endophthalmitis

Endophthalmitis caused by fungal infections may be either endogenous or exogenous. *Exogenous fungal endophthalmitis* is uncommon in North America and Europe. In contrast, in tropical regions such as India, fungi account for up to one-fifth of culture-positive cases following surgery or trauma. *Endogenous fungal endophthalmitis* is rare regardless of setting and typically occurs in either severely immunocompromised patients with persistent fungemia or otherwise healthy intravenous drug users following transient fungemia. Clinical presentation is often subacute and the diagnosis typically delayed for weeks. *Aspergillus* (Fig 10-15) and *Fusarium* are the most commonly identified causative species. Fungal keratitis may also progress to endophthalmitis, most typically when caused by *Fusarium.* Treatment is frequently difficult and typically involves vitrectomy, intravitreous injection of amphotericin B and/or voriconazole, and systemic antifungal therapy. Two-thirds of patients with fungal endophthalmitis lose useful vision.

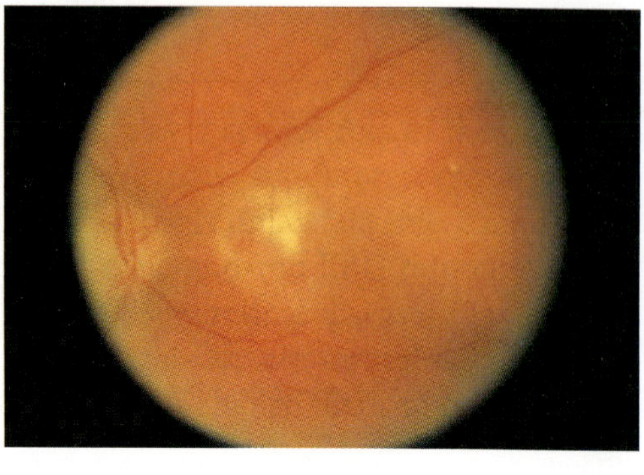

Figure 10-14 Color fundus photograph of focal endogenous bacterial endophthalmitis. *(Courtesy of Janet L. Davis, MD.)*

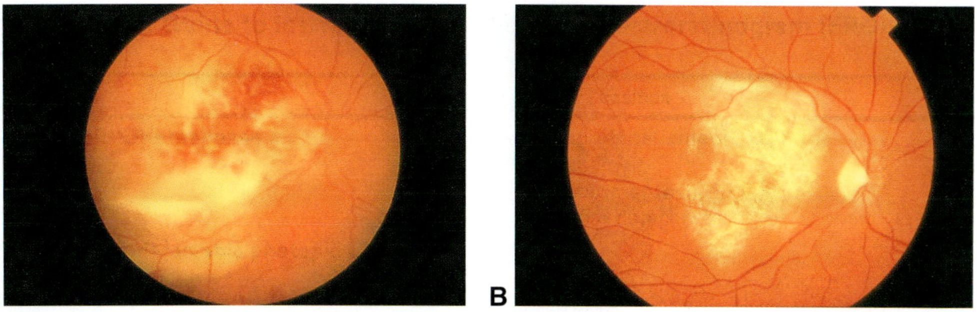

A B

Figure 10-15 Color fundus photograph of endophthalmitis caused by infection with *Aspergillus* species. **A,** Features present include mild vitritis, a diffuse macular chorioretinal lesion with subretinal and subhyaloid hypopyon, intraretinal hemorrhage, and papillitis. **B,** Same eye 2 months after treatment shows macular scar, preserved overlying retinal vessels, and temporal disc pallor. Final visual acuity was 20/400. *(From Weishaar PD, Flynn HW Jr, Murray TG, et al. Endogenous* Aspergillus *endophthalmitis. Clinical features and treatment outcomes.* Ophthalmology. *1998;105(1):60.)*

Rao NA, Hidayat AA. Endogenous mycotic endophthalmitis: variations in clinical and histopathologic changes in candidiasis compared with aspergillosis. *Am J Ophthalmol.* 2001;132(2):244–251.

Wykoff CC, Flynn HW Jr, Miller D, Scott IU, Alfonso EC. Exogenous fungal endophthalmitis: microbiology and clinical outcomes. *Ophthalmology.* 2008;115(9):1501–1507.

Yeast (Candida) *endophthalmitis*

Endogenous yeast endophthalmitis is most frequently caused by *Candida* species. Affected patients frequently have had prior use of indwelling catheters, long-term antibiotic treatment, or immunosuppressive therapy. Many also have a history of hyperalimentation, recent abdominal surgery, or diabetes mellitus. The initial intraocular inflammation is usually mild to moderate, and yellow-white choroidal or chorioretinal lesions may be single or multiple (Fig 10-16). Subretinal infiltrates may coalesce into a mushroom-shaped white nodule that projects through the retina into the vitreous. Exogenous *Candida* endophthalmitis is rare.

The diagnosis of *Candida* endophthalmitis is usually made according to the history, clinical setting, and presence of characteristic fundus features. Intraocular culture specimens are best obtained during pars plana vitrectomy, as it is difficult to culture the localized vitreous clusters of fungus from specimens taken via diagnostic vitreous tap. After completion of the vitrectomy, intravitreal amphotericin B or voriconazole is usually injected.

The ophthalmologist should seek consultation with a specialist in infectious diseases to evaluate the patient for systemic disease and assist with treatment planning. If the macula is not involved, visual prognosis after treatment is generally good. Focal chorioretinal lesions are often successfully treated with systemic medications alone. Intravenous fluconazole and voriconazole penetrate the eye well and have been used to treat focal lesions.

Oude Lashof AM, Rothova A, Sobel JD, et al. Ocular manifestations of candidemia. *Clin Infect Dis.* 2011;53(3):262–268.

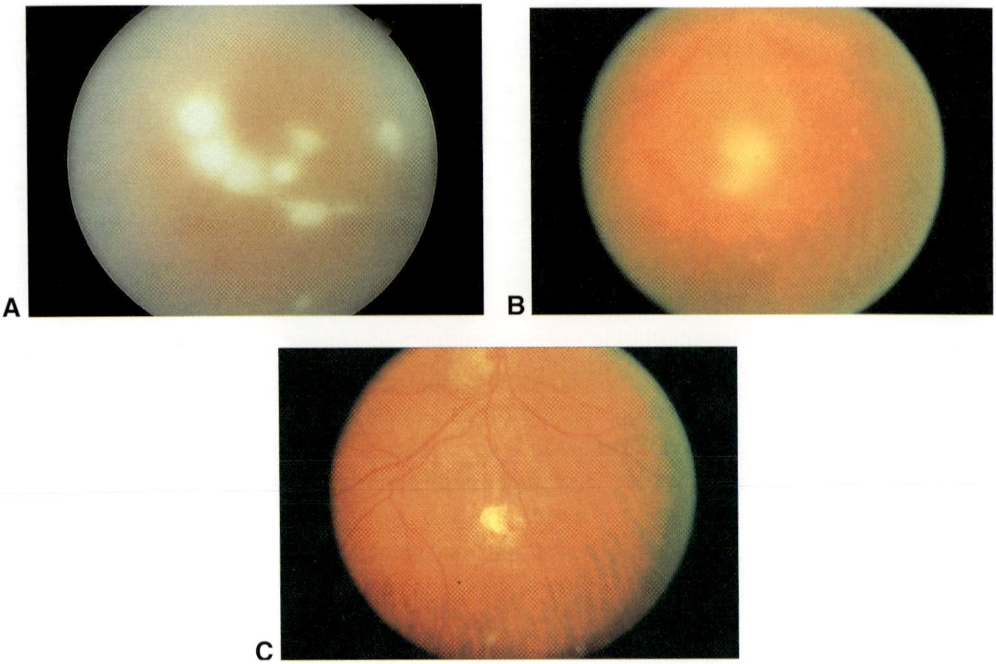

Figure 10-16 Endogenous yeast *(Candida)* endophthalmitis. **A,** Color fundus photograph of vitreous infiltrates in a "string-of-pearls" configuration. **B,** Color fundus photograph of endogenous endophthalmitis before treatment. **C,** Color fundus photograph of endogenous endophthalmitis resolved after treatment with vitrectomy and intravitreal amphotericin B. *(Courtesy of Harry W. Flynn, Jr, MD.)*

Tuberculosis

Even though one-third of the world's population has been exposed to *Mycobacterium tuberculosis,* active *M tuberculosis* uveitis is uncommon, even in endemic areas. Suggestive clinical findings include solitary (Fig 10-17) or multifocal choroiditis, serpiginous-like chorioretinitis, and Eales disease–like peripheral nonperfusion in association with uveitis. Patients suspected of having tuberculous uveitis should undergo testing for prior *M tuberculosis* exposure, including a chest X-ray and either purified protein derivative (PPD) skin testing or a blood-based interferon-gamma release assay.

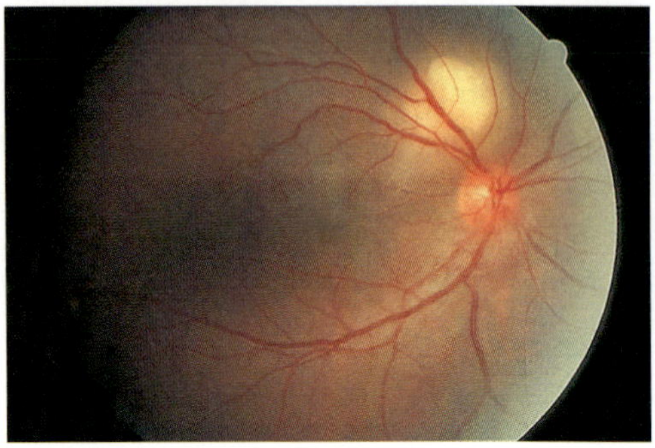

Figure 10-17 Ocular tuberculosis. Color fundus photograph showing a choroidal granuloma superotemporal to the optic disc. *(Courtesy of Janet L. Davis, MD.)*

Once the diagnosis of ocular tuberculosis is either confirmed or strongly suggested, the patient should be treated for extrapulmonary tuberculosis as recommended by either the US Centers for Disease Control and Prevention or the World Health Organization.

Abouammoh M, Abu El-Asrar AM. Imaging in the diagnosis and management of ocular tuberculosis. *Int Ophthalmol Clin.* 2012;52(4):97–112.

Gupta A, Bansal R, Gupta V, Sharma A, Bambery P. Ocular signs predictive of tubercular uveitis. *Am J Ophthalmol.* 2010;149(4):562–570.

Syphilitic Chorioretinitis

Uveitis is often the presenting sign of syphilis but can occur at any stage of the infection. Syphilitic uveitis is confirmed through serologic testing with both the specific and sensitive fluorescent treponemal antibody absorption (FTA-ABS) test and the nonspecific VDRL or rapid plasma reagin (RPR) tests, which are complementary to each other. Patients with uveitis who test positive for syphilis on serologic tests should also have measures taken of their cerebrospinal fluid anti–treponemal antibody titers before and, when present, after completion of therapy to document a complete response to treatment.

Many patients with syphilitic uveitis present with a fairly nondescript panuveitis, which supports the need for routine syphilis testing in all sexually active adults with uveitis. Specifically suggestive clinical findings include inflammatory ocular hypertensive syndrome, iris roseola, and retinochoroiditis (Fig 10-18). The retinochoroiditis is often

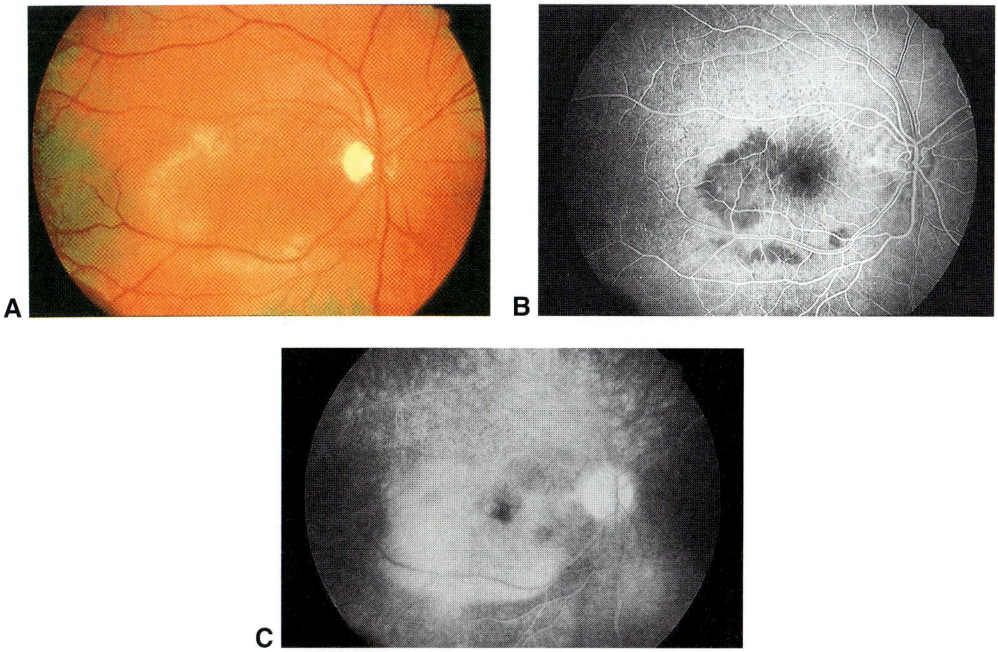

A B C

Figure 10-18 Syphilitic retinochoroiditis. **A,** Color fundus photograph of a placoid yellow lesion involving the macula. **B,** Early-phase angiography image shows hypofluorescence. **C,** Late-phase angiography image shows diffuse hyperfluorescence. *(Courtesy of J. Donald M. Gass, MD.)*

diaphanous—appearing less opaque than either herpetic or toxoplasmic necrotizing retinitis—and is accompanied by overlying inflammatory accumulations termed *retinal precipitates.* A distinctive form of syphilitic outer retinitis termed *acute syphilitic posterior placoid chorioretinitis* (ASPPC) is characterized by the presence of a placoid, round or oval, yellow-white lesion that involves or is near the macula. HIV coinfection is common. Patients with syphilitic uveitis should be treated for neurosyphilis.

Cunningham ET Jr, Eandi CM, Pichi F. Syphilitic uveitis. *Ocul Immunol Inflamm.* 2014;22(1): 2–3.

Cat-Scratch Disease

Cat-scratch disease is associated with 2 ocular syndromes: (1) Parinaud oculoglandular syndrome, which consists of conjunctival inflammation with preauricular adenopathy, and (2) Leber stellate neuroretinitis, which includes macular star formation and optic disc swelling, often associated with a peripapillary serous macular detachment (Fig 10-19). Small, focal areas of retinitis or chorioretinitis occur frequently in patients with neuroretinitis. Immunocompetent adults with cat-scratch disease are treated with doxycycline, 100 mg twice daily for 4–6 weeks. Oral erythromycin can be used in children. Prolonged treatment with doxycycline and rifampin can be used in immunocompromised adults or in patients with persistent infection.

McClintic J, Srivastava SK. Imaging in the diagnosis and management of ocular cat scratch disease. *Int Ophthalmol Clin.* 2012;52(4):155–161.
Roe RH, Jumper JM, Fu AD, Johnson RN, McDonald HR, Cunningham ET Jr. Ocular bartonella infections. *Int Ophthalmol Clin.* 2008;48(3):93–105.

Toxoplasmic Retinochoroiditis

Toxoplasmic retinochoroiditis is the most common cause of posterior segment infection worldwide. The causative organism, *Toxoplasma gondii,* is an obligate, intracellular parasitic protozoan. Seropositivity for *T gondii* is very common and therefore alone does not confirm that uveitis is related to toxoplasmosis. Congenital disease occurs via acquisition of the organism by a pregnant woman exposed to tissue cysts or oocytes in uncooked meat or substances contaminated with cat feces (see also BCSC Section 6, *Pediatric Ophthalmology and Strabismus,* Chapter 28). The typical ocular finding in congenital toxoplasmosis is a chorioretinal scar, usually in the macula and often bilateral. Most cases of toxoplasmosis

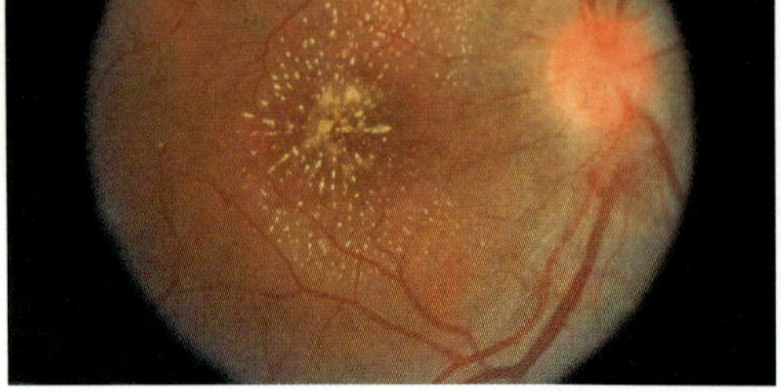

Figure 10-19 Color fundus photograph of neuroretinitis showing optic disc swelling and macular star formation resulting from cat-scratch disease *(Bartonella henselae). (Courtesy of George Alexandrakis, MD.)*

are currently assumed to be acquired postnatally, although proving this assumption can be difficult. A positive serologic test result for immunoglobulin (Ig) M anti–*T gondii* antibodies supports the diagnosis of an acquired disease.

Decreased vision and floaters are the most common presenting symptoms of toxoplasmic retinochoroiditis. Clinically, the disorder consists of a focal area of intense, necrotizing retinochoroiditis, typically with moderate to severe overlying vitreous inflammation (Fig 10-20). Recurrent disease is indicated by an adjacent or nearby retinochoroidal scar. Multiple active lesions are rare and should prompt HIV testing. HIV-seropositive patients with ocular toxoplasmosis have a high risk of CNS involvement and so should undergo magnetic resonance imaging with contrast.

Several approaches have been used to treat active ocular toxoplasmosis. The simplest approach is treatment with trimethoprim-sulfamethoxazole. Classic therapy utilizes sulfadiazine with pyrimethamine and prednisone; the addition of clindamycin results in so-called quadruple therapy. None of these approaches has been shown to be superior to another with regard to final vision outcome, lesion size, or recurrence rate. Treatment

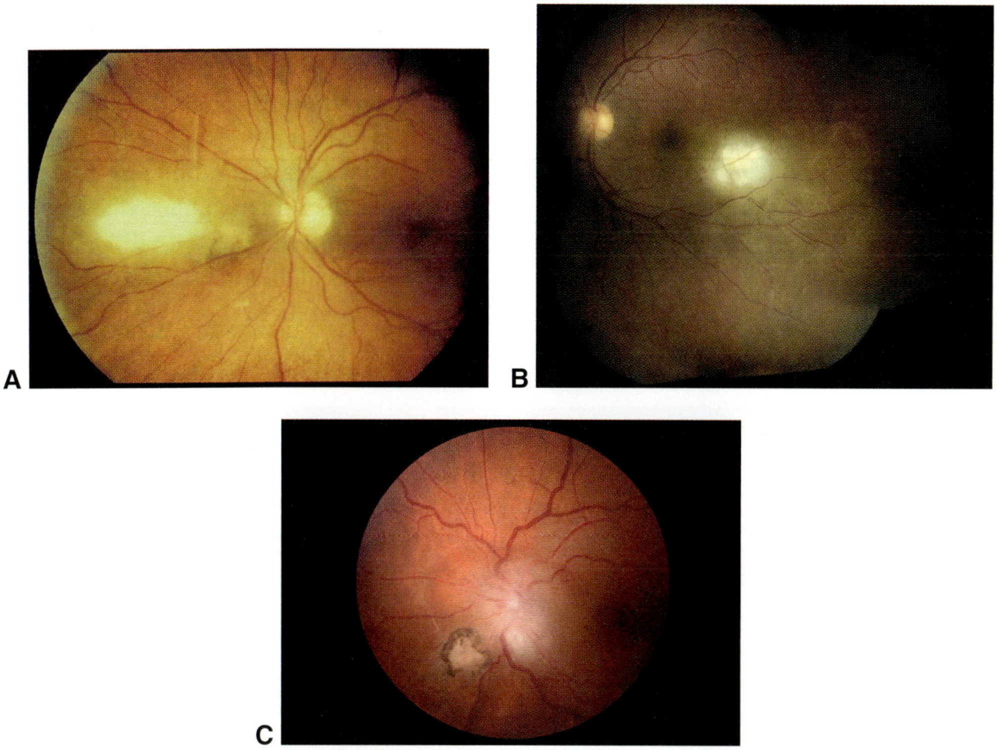

Figure 10-20 Toxoplasmic retinochoroiditis. **A,** Color fundus photograph of the nasal retina shows an ovoid area of retinal opacification with a hyperpigmented retinochoroidal scar at the inferotemporal border of the lesion, which is the result of reactivated toxoplasmic retinochoroiditis. **B,** Color fundus photographic montage shows primary toxoplasmic retinochoroiditis in an immunocompetent patient, with minimal vitreous reaction and the superficial retina seemingly minimally affected. This appearance is sometimes referred to as *outer retinal toxoplasmosis.* **C,** Color fundus photograph shows active peripapillary toxoplasmic retinochoroiditis and an adjacent, inactive retinochoroidal scar. Optic disc edema and a peripapillary serous retinal detachment are also present. *(Parts A and B courtesy of Colin A. McCannel, MD; part C courtesy of Nancy M. Holekamp, MD.)*

typically lasts 4–6 weeks, and complete healing of active lesions occurs over 4–6 months. When used, systemic corticosteroids should be given under antibiotic cover. Use of long-acting, depot periocular or intraocular corticosteroid injections should be avoided. Long-term, maintenance treatment with trimethoprim-sulfamethoxazole has been used to decrease the attack rate in patients experiencing frequent recurrences or in severely immunosuppressed patients. Intravitreal clindamycin with or without dexamethasone has been used to treat vision-threatening lesions or for patients who are intolerant of or fail to respond to systemic therapy.

Holland GN. Ocular toxoplasmosis: a global reassessment. Part I: epidemiology and course of disease. *Am J Ophthalmol.* 2003;136(6):973–988.

Holland GN. Ocular toxoplasmosis: a global reassessment. Part II: disease manifestations and management. *Am J Ophthalmol.* 2004;137(1):1–17.

Toxocariasis

Toxocariasis is a parasitic infection caused by 1 of 2 roundworms: *Toxocara canis* or *T cati*—common intestinal parasites of dogs and cats, respectively. Humans are infected following ingestion of soil or vegetables contaminated by the ova. Although ocular toxocariasis is part of a systemic infestation by the nematode, systemic manifestations such as visceral larval migrans, fever, and eosinophilia are relatively uncommon. Children and young adults are affected disproportionately. Common symptoms include decreased vision and floaters. The condition is unilateral in most cases and typically has 1 of 3 presentations: (1) a peripheral granuloma, which often produces a traction band that extends toward the macula (Fig 10-21) and occasionally mimics unilateral intermediate uveitis with snowbank formation; (2) a posterior pole granuloma, which can decrease vision dramatically when the central macula is involved; or (3) a moderate to severe panuveitis that can mimic endogenous endophthalmitis. Enzyme-linked immunosorbent assay (ELISA)

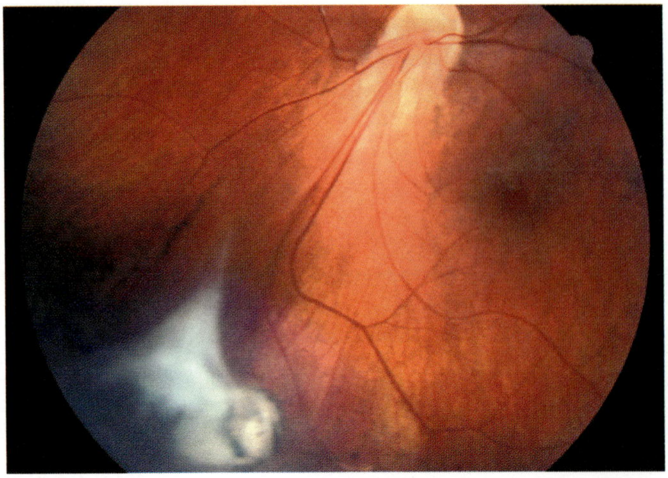

Figure 10-21 Color fundus photograph from a 6-year-old boy with reduced and distorted vision. The image shows a peripheral toxocariasis cyst with associated fibrosis *(bottom left)*. The fibrosis results in considerable traction, and the macula is dragged inferiorly and distorted. *(Courtesy of Colin A. McCannel, MD.)*

analysis of serum or intraocular fluids can help establish the diagnosis in these cases but is relatively insensitive. Vitreous inflammation, CME, and tractional retinal detachment are the most common causes of vision loss. Most specialists assume that the uveitis of toxocariasis represents an immune response to antigens released from a dead or dying worm. Thus, treatment typically involves use of local or systemic corticosteroids, and antihelminthic therapy has little or no therapeutic role.

Arevalo JF, Espinoza JV, Arevalo FA. Ocular toxocariasis. *J Pediatr Ophthalmol Strabismus.* 2013;50(2):76–86.

Stewart JM, Cubillan LD, Cunningham ET Jr. Prevalence, clinical features, and causes of vision loss among patients with ocular toxocariasis. *Retina.* 2005;25(8):1005–1013.

Woodhall D, Starr MC, Montgomery SP, et al. Ocular toxocariasis: epidemiologic, anatomic, and therapeutic variations based on a survey of ophthalmic subspecialists. *Ophthalmology.* 2012;119(6):1211–1217.

Lyme Disease

Lyme disease is caused by the spirochete *Borrelia burgdorferi,* which is transmitted to humans by ticks from animal reservoirs: primarily rodents, deer, birds, cats, and dogs. Early systemic manifestations consist of myalgias, arthralgias, fever, headache, malaise, and a characteristic skin lesion known as *erythema migrans* or a bull's-eye rash, which consists of an annulus of erythema surrounding an area of central clearing. In later stages, as neurologic or musculoskeletal findings manifest, ocular inflammation may develop but is uncommon. Lyme disease–related eye findings include keratitis, scleritis, and uveitis, which may include anterior chamber or vitritis inflammation, retinal vasculitis, papillitis, or optic neuritis. Chronic uveitis in patients who reside in or have traveled to an endemic area or who have had a recent tick bite or an erythema migrans–like skin lesion should suggest the possibility of Lyme disease. Initial serologic testing is performed using a sensitive ELISA. If an ELISA result is positive or equivocal, then separate IgM and IgG immunoblotting should be performed on the same serum sample. Because ELISA and immunoblot specificity is limited in endemic areas, positive test results should be viewed as supportive. Treatment for early disease consists of tetracycline, doxycycline, or penicillin. Advanced disease may require intravenous ceftriaxone or penicillin.

Karma A, Seppälä I, Mikkilä H, Kaakkola S, Viljanen M, Tarkkanen A. Diagnosis and clinical characteristics of ocular Lyme borreliosis. *Am J Ophthalmol.* 1995;119(2):127–135.

Mikkilä HO, Seppälä IJ, Viljanen MK, Peltomaa MP, Karma A. The expanding clinical spectrum of ocular lyme borreliosis. *Ophthalmology.* 2000;107(3):581–587.

Diffuse Unilateral Subacute Neuroretinitis

Diffuse unilateral subacute neuroretinitis (DUSN) is a rare condition that typically occurs in otherwise healthy, young patients and is caused by the presence of a mobile subretinal nematode. Prompt diagnosis and treatment of the condition can help prevent vision loss, which can be severe. The clinical findings in DUSN can be divided into acute and end-stage manifestations. In the acute phase, patients frequently have decreased visual acuity, vitritis, papillitis, and crops of gray-white or yellow-white outer retinal and choroidal lesions. The clustering of the lesions is important because it often helps localize the causative nematode. The degree of vision loss is often greater than might be expected from the clinical examination. Left untreated, late sequelae ultimately develop, which include optic atrophy, retinal arterial narrowing, and diffuse RPE disruption with severe vision loss. The late findings can be misinterpreted as unilateral retinitis pigmentosa.

The causative nematodes in DUSN have yet to be definitively established, although *Toxocara* species, *Baylisascaris procyonis,* and *Ancylostoma caninum* have all been implicated. Raccoon exposure appears to be common in North America. The characteristic lesions are believed to result from a single nematode migrating within the subretinal space. If the nematode can be observed, which occurs in less than half of cases, it should be destroyed using laser photocoagulation. After the worm is killed, vision usually stabilizes.

de Amorim Garcia Filho CA, Gomes AH, de A Garcia Soares AC, de Amorim Garcia CA. Clinical features of 121 patients with diffuse unilateral subacute neuroretinitis. *Am J Ophthalmol.* 2012;153(4):743–749.

West Nile Virus Chorioretinitis

West Nile virus (WNV) infection is transmitted to humans by an infected mosquito of the genus *Culex,* with birds serving as the primary reservoir. Human infection is most often subclinical, although a febrile illness occurs in approximately 20% of cases. Ocular manifestations usually occur in very ill diabetic patients with encephalitis. Most typically observed is a multifocal chorioretinitis that is usually bilateral and includes lesions arranged in distinctive curvilinear clusters that often follow the course of retinal nerve fibers (Fig 10-22). Vision typically remains good unless the lesions involve the central macula.

Khairallah M, Kahloun R. Ocular manifestations of emerging infectious diseases. *Curr Opin Ophthalmol.* 2013;24(6):574–580.

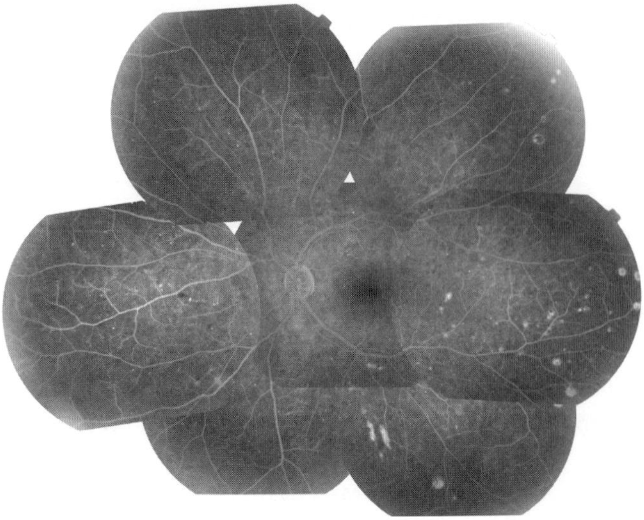

Figure 10-22 West Nile virus chorioretinitis. Collage of fluorescein angiography images showing punched-out lesions that characteristically arrange in almost confluent streaks in some areas. Alterations caused by nonproliferative diabetic retinopathy are also apparent; West Nile virus chorioretinitis typically occurs in diabetic patients. *(Courtesy of Robert Beardsley, MD, and Colin A. McCannel, MD.)*

CHAPTER **11**

Congenital and Stationary Retinal Disease

Color Vision (Cone System) Abnormalities

Color vision defects can be congenital or acquired. Congenital color vision defects are stationary and usually affect both eyes equally, whereas acquired defects may be progressive and may be uniocular, depending on the underlying cause.

Congenital Color Deficiency

Trichromacy

Congenital color vision defects are traditionally classified by an individual's color-matching performance. A person with normal color vision (*trichromatism*, or *trichromacy*) can match any colored light by varying a mixture of 3 different-colored lights, or primary colors (eg, a long-wavelength red, middle-wavelength green, and short-wavelength blue light).

Individuals with *anomalous trichromatism* make up the largest group of color-deficient persons; they include approximately 5%–6% of males. These individuals also can use 3 primary colors to match a given color, but because one of their cone photopigments has an abnormal absorption spectrum, they use different proportions of colors from those used by persons with normal color vision. For approximately 5% of males, the medium-wavelength (M-cone) photopigment has an abnormal absorption spectrum that is closer to that of the long-wavelength (L-cone) photopigment, a condition known as *deuteranomalous trichromatism*. For 1% of males, the L-cone photopigment has an absorption spectrum that is closer to that of the M-cone photopigment, termed *protanomalous trichromatism*. *Congenital tritanomalous* defects are even rarer than tritanopic defects (described in the next section), and some specialists question whether such defects exist.

Anomalous trichromacy ranges in severity. Some individuals have only a mild abnormality and may, for example, fail some of the sensitive Ishihara test plates but have no trouble naming colors or passing the less-sensitive screening tests such as the Farnsworth Panel D-15 test (see Chapter 3). Others have poor color discrimination and may appear to have dichromacy on some of the color vision tests.

Hereditary congenital color vision defects are most frequently X-linked-recessive, red-green abnormalities; they affect 5%–8% of males and 0.5% of females. Acquired defects are more frequently of the blue-yellow, or tritan, variety and affect males and females equally. Table 11-1 shows the traditional classification of color vision deficits on the basis of color-matching test results.

Dichromacy

Individuals who need only 2 primary colors to make a color match have dichromacy. It is assumed that such individuals lack one of the cone photopigments. Approximately 2% of males have dichromacy; 1% are missing the long-wavelength (L-cone) photopigment, a disorder termed *protanopia,* and 1% are missing the medium-wavelength (M-cone) photopigment, called *deuteranopia.* A rare, third form of congenital dichromacy is lack of the short-wavelength (S-cone) photopigment, termed *tritanopia,* which is an autosomal-dominant defect that occurs in approximately 0.001% of the population.

Achromatopsia

An absence of color discrimination, or *achromatopsia,* means that any spectral color can be matched with any other solely by intensity adjustments. The congenital achromatopsias are disorders of photoreceptor function. Essentially, there are 2 forms of achromatopsia: (1) *rod monochromatism,* and (2) *S-cone monochromatism (blue-cone monochromatism).* Both disorders typically present with congenital nystagmus, poor visual acuity, and photophobia. Electroretinography (ERG) enables the distinction from congenital motor nystagmus or ocular albinism, both of which are associated with normal cone ERGs (see Chapter 3, Fig 3-2).

Rod monochromatism (complete achromatopsia) is the most severe form; affected individuals have normal rod function but no detectable cone function and see the world in shades of gray. Patients may have full to partial expression of the disorder, with visual acuity ranging from 20/80 to 20/200. Nystagmus is usually present in childhood and

Table 11-1 Classification and Male-Population Incidence of Color Vision Defects

Color Vision	Inheritance	Incidence in Male Population (%)
Hereditary		
Trichromatism		
Normal	–	92.0
Deuteranomalous	XR	5.0
Protanomalous	XR	1.0
Tritanomalous	AD	0.0001
Dichromatism		
Deuteranomalous	XR	1.0
Protanomalous	XR	1.0
Tritanomalous	AD	0.001
Achromatopsia (monochromatism)		
Typical (rod monochromatism)	AR	0.0001
Atypical (blue-cone monochromatism)	XR	Unknown
Acquired		
Tritanomalous (blue-yellow)	Unknown	Unknown
Protanomalous-deuteranomalous (red-green)	Unknown	Unknown

AD = autosomal dominant; AR = autosomal recessive; XR = X-linked recessive.

may improve with age. Characteristically, the ERG in patients with rod monochromatism shows an absence of cone-derived responses and normal rod responses. Dark adaptometry shows no cone plateau and no cone–rod break. The disorder exhibits autosomal-recessive inheritance.

As of mid-2014, 5 genes had been identified that are associated with the disorder: (1) *CNGA3,* on 2q11, which accounts for 20%–30% of cases and encodes the alpha subunit of the cone photoreceptor cyclic guanosine monophosphate (cGMP)–gated cation channel; (2) *CNGB3,* on 8q21–q22, which accounts for 40%–50% of cases and encodes the beta 3 subunit of the cGMP-gated cation channel; (3) *GNAT2,* on 1p13.3, which encodes the alpha subunit of cone-specific transducin; (4) *PDE6C,* on 10q23.33, which encodes cGMP-specific cone phosphodiesterase 6C alpha protein; and (5) *PDE6H,* on 12p13, which encodes the inhibitory γ subunit of the cone photoreceptor cGMP phosphodiesterase. The latter 3 genes account for less than 5% of cases.

In *S-cone* (or *blue-cone*) *monochromatism,* rods and S cones are normal, but L- and M-cone function is absent. The condition is usually X-linked and can be difficult to distinguish clinically from rod monochromatism in the absence of a family history or results of specialized color or ERG testing. Persons with S-cone monochromatism exhibit preserved S-cone ERG responses, severely reduced cone flicker ERGs, and normal rod ERGs; they typically have a visual acuity of approximately 20/80, which is better than that in typical rod monochromatism.

Dingcai C. Color vision and night vision. In: Ryan SJ, Schachat AP, Wilkinson CP, Hinton DR, Sadda SR, Wiedemann P, eds. *Retina.* Vol 1. 5th ed. Philadelphia: Elsevier/Saunders; 2013: 285–299.

Wu DM, Amani AF. Abnormalities of cone and rod function. In: Ryan SJ, Schachat AP, Wilkinson CP, Hinton DR, Sadda SR, Wiedemann P, eds. *Retina.* Vol 2. 5th ed. Philadelphia: Elsevier/Saunders; 2013:899–906.

Night Vision (Rod System) Abnormalities

Congenital Night-Blinding Disorders With Normal Fundi

Congenital stationary night blindness (CSNB) is a nonprogressive disorder of night vision. Three genetic subtypes have been described:

1. X-linked, the most common
2. autosomal recessive
3. autosomal dominant (rare), typified by the large French Nougaret pedigree

Snellen visual acuities of patients with CSNB range from normal to occasionally as poor as 20/200, but most cases of decreased vision are associated with significant myopia. The fundus is usually normal, with the exception of myopic changes. Difficulty with night vision is the common presenting symptom, but nystagmus and reduced visual acuity may also be presenting symptoms. Although dark-adaptometry curves are typically 2–3 $\log_{10}$ units above normal, some CSNB patients never complain of nyctalopia, perhaps because they have become accustomed to it as a way of life (Fig 11-1).

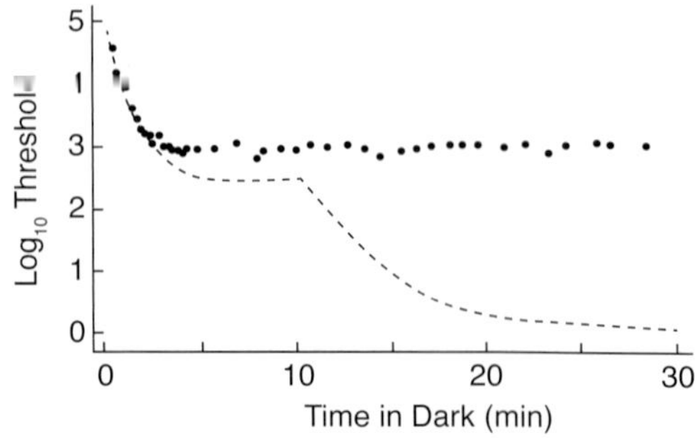

Figure 11-1 Dark-adaptometry curve in congenital stationary night blindness (CSNB). The dark-adaptometry curve of this patient *(dotted curve)* with CSNB shows no rod adaptation. *Dashed curve* indicates normal response. *(Used with permission from Ripps H. Night blindness revisited: from man to molecules. Proctor lecture.* Invest Ophthalmol Vis Sci. *1982;23(5):588–609.)*

Electroretinography is important in the diagnosis of CSNB. The most common ERG pattern is the *negative* ERG (the Schubert-Bornschein form of CSNB), in which the bright-flash, dark-adapted ERG has a normal (or near-normal) a-wave but a markedly reduced b-wave. The normal a-wave excludes significant rod photoreceptor dysfunction, and the result thus facilitates the distinction of CSNB from the potentially blinding disorder retinitis pigmentosa (RP; see Chapter 3).

X-linked CSNB has been categorized into 2 types: "complete" and "incomplete." Patients with the complete type (cCSNB) have an undetectable rod-specific, dim-flash, dark-adapted ERG and psychophysical thresholds that are mediated by cones. Patients with incomplete CSNB (iCSNB) have some detectable rod function on ERG and an elevated dark-adaptation final threshold. Subsequently, advances in molecular biology have shown the 2 forms to be genetically distinct; X-linked cCSNB is associated with a mutation in *NYX* and X-linked iCSNB with a mutation in *CACNA1F*. *NYX* encodes nyctalopin, a protein required for normal synaptic transmission between retinal photoreceptors and depolarizing (on-) bipolar cells. The ERG findings are those of panretinal loss of on-bipolar cell function in rods and in all 3 cone types. Cone off-bipolar cell function is spared (Fig 11-2). *CACNA1F* encodes a transmembrane protein that functions as an alpha-1 subunit of the voltage-dependent calcium channel, and functions of both on- and off-pathways are

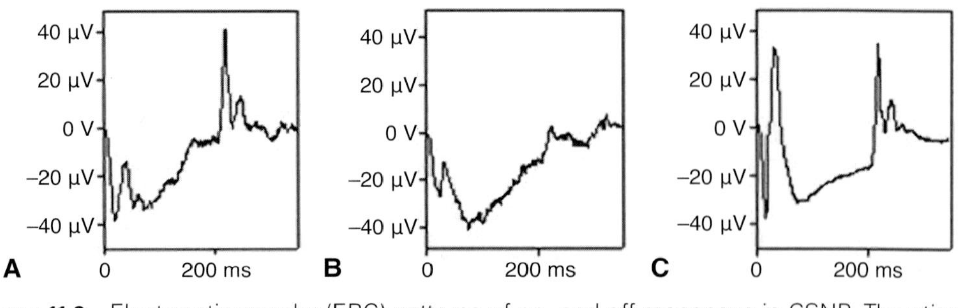

Figure 11-2 Electroretinography (ERG) patterns of on- and off-responses in CSNB. The stimulus has a 200-millisecond (ms) duration to enable independent recording of the ERG responses to onset and offset. **A,** The pattern of a patient with "complete" CNSB shows a negative-waveform on-response but a normal off-response. **B,** A patient with "incomplete" CSNB shows both on- and off-response abnormalities. **C,** Pattern of a normal subject. (See also Chapter 3, Fig 3-2.) *(Courtesy of Graham E. Holder, PhD.)*

affected (see Fig 11-2). Standard cone-system ERGs in iCSNB are therefore more abnormal than those in cCSNB (see Chapter 3, Fig 3-2).

The ERG categories of cCSNB and iCSNB also apply to the autosomal-recessive forms of CSNB. The most common causes of recessive cCSNB are mutations in *GRM6* or *TRPM1*. Other genes implicated in recessive cCSNB include *GPR179* and *LRIT3*. An identical pattern also occurs in melanoma-associated retinopathy (MAR), a paraneoplastic autoimmune retinopathy that can develop in patients with cutaneous malignant melanoma, emphasizing the need always to place ERG responses in their clinical context. MAR patients usually present with an acquired night blindness and shimmering photopsias; CSNB patients are night-blind from birth. In at least some patients, MAR is mediated through TRPM1 (transient receptor protein member 1), which is expressed in melanocytes and retinal on-bipolar cells. A recessive form of iCSNB relates to mutation in *CABP4*.

Congenital Night-Blinding Disorders With Fundus Abnormality

Fundus albipunctatus relates to mutation in *RDH5* (12q13–q14). *RDH5* encodes 11-*cis*-retinol dehydrogenase, a microsomal enzyme in the retinal pigment epithelium (RPE) that converts 11-*cis*-retinol into 11-*cis*-retinal and is therefore involved in the regeneration of rhodopsin. Patients have very delayed rhodopsin regeneration, and although levels eventually normalize, the process may take many hours in the dark. Accordingly, many ERG testing laboratories practice overnight dark adaptation of 1 eye in appropriate patients. Affected individuals are night blind from birth and usually exhibit yellow-white dots in the posterior pole (sparing the fovea) that extend into the midperiphery (Fig 11-3). ERG responses commonly show a cone-isolated retina pattern, with undetectable rod-specific ERG, and a severely reduced bright-flash dark-adapted ERG (arising in dark-adapted cones) that normalizes with sufficiently extended dark adaptation. Patients with a

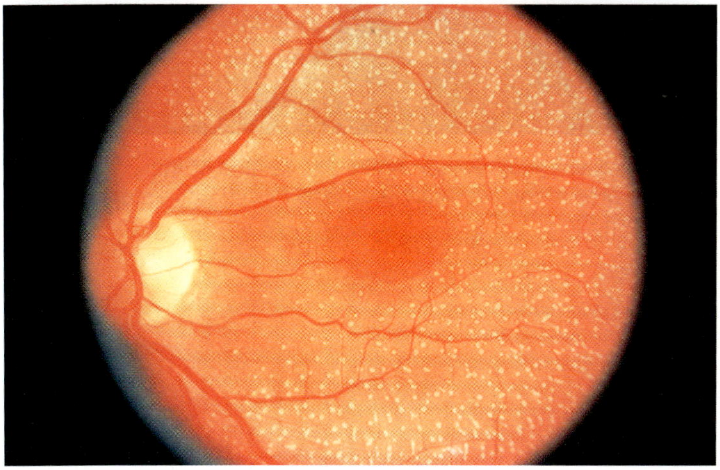

Figure 11-3 Fundus photograph of a patient with fundus albipunctatus, showing multiple spots of unknown material scattered primarily throughout the deep retina. *(From Fishman GA, Birch DG, Holder GE, Brigell MG.* Electrophysiologic Testing in Disorders of the Retina, Optic Nerve, and Visual Pathway. *Ophthalmology Monograph 2. 2nd ed. San Francisco: American Academy of Ophthalmology; 2001:51.)*

normal fundus but characteristic ERG findings and molecular confirmation of the mutation have been described; visual acuity and color vision are usually good.

Fundus albipunctatus must be distinguished from *retinitis punctata albescens,* a disorder related to mutation in *RLBP1,* which encodes cellular retinaldehyde-binding protein. The condition is a progressive rod–cone dystrophy. The white dots may be finer than those of *RDH5* retinopathy, and there may be attenuation of the retinal vessels. ERG responses are usually very abnormal and show some recovery with extended dark adaptation but do not normalize.

Oguchi disease is also associated with night blindness from birth. It results from mutation in the gene *SAG* (2q37), which encodes arrestin, or in *GRK1* (13q34), which encodes rhodopsin kinase. This very rare disorder is most common in Japanese patients. The fundus in Oguchi disease is normal after dark adaptation but shows a peculiar yellow iridescent sheen after even brief light exposure (the *Mizuo-Nakamura phenomenon;* Fig 11-4).

Cukras CA, Zein WM, Caruso RC, Sieving PA. Progressive and "stationary" inherited retinal degenerations. In: Yanoff M, Duker JS, eds. *Ophthalmology.* 4th ed. St. Louis: Elsevier/Saunders; 2013:480–490.

Dryja TP. Molecular genetics of Oguchi disease, fundus albipunctatus, and other forms of stationary night blindness. LVII Edward Jackson Memorial Lecture. *Am J Ophthalmol.* 2000;130(5):547–563.

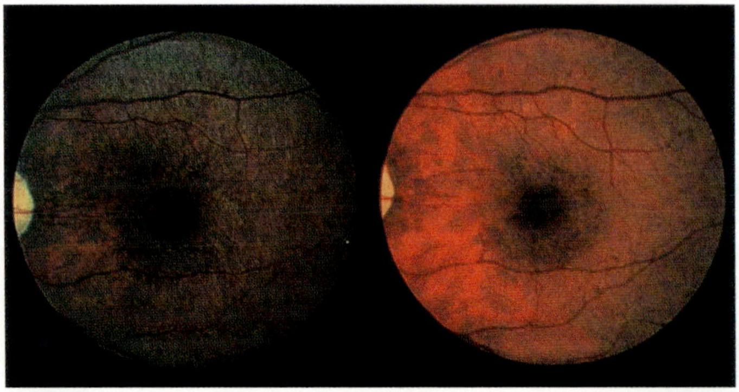

Figure 11-4 The Mizuo-Nakamura phenomenon. The fundus of this patient with X-linked cone dystrophy is unremarkable in the dark-adapted state *(right)* but has a yellow iridescent sheen after exposure to light *(left).*

CHAPTER 12

Hereditary Retinal and Choroidal Dystrophies

The hereditary dystrophies of the posterior segment constitute a large and potentially confusing group of disorders. The *Online Mendelian Inheritance in Man* (OMIM) website lists more than 750 genetic disorders with significant involvement of the retina, choroid, or both. Another excellent online resource, *RetNet,* lists more than 200 different retinal degenerations in which the chromosomal site and often the specific gene defect have been identified. The causative mutations are heterogeneous, and patients with these diseases can present in various ways. Traditionally, anatomical classifications have divided the disorders by apparent topography or layer of involvement, such as retina, macula, retinal pigment epithelium (RPE), choroid, and vitreous/retina. This approach is not sufficient, however, because many dystrophies overlap and may involve multiple layers or areas. A second type of organization, based on the patient's family history, is used to establish the inheritance pattern of the disease. Approximately 60% of thorough pedigrees give useful information. A third approach in diagnostic evaluation is to establish the disease phenotype by clinical examination and electrophysiologic and psychophysical testing. Careful analysis of the information gathered by these 3 approaches allows most conditions to be assigned to a disease group, and many can be given a specific clinical diagnosis that can be confirmed by molecular testing.

Hereditary diseases of the eye, with rare exceptions, have bilateral symmetric involvement. If ocular involvement is unilateral, other causes—such as birth defect, intrauterine or antenatal infection, and inflammatory disease—should be considered before a hereditary dystrophy is diagnosed. Given that retinal degenerations can occur as part of a systemic disorder, obtaining a thorough medical history is crucial, as is ruling out any reversible cause of retinal degeneration or dysfunction, such as vitamin A deficiency (also see Chapter 13).

Obtaining an accurate family history is essential to determining the inheritance pattern. The mendelian patterns of inheritance are well known—namely, autosomal dominant, autosomal recessive, and X-linked recessive. In addition, mitochondrial and X-linked dominant retinal disorders have been described. Patients with retinal degenerative disease may have a negative family history. Such a patient may have a *de novo* mutation; alternatively, the disease may be mild in other family members, making them relatively asymptomatic. For this reason, it may be important to examine relatives, if possible, for any signs of retinal degeneration.

The search for gene defects and pathophysiologic mechanisms underlying retinal dystrophies is ongoing. Perhaps the most important insight gained thus far is that depending on where a mutation lies in a gene, there may be varying expression or even different phenotypes. This phenomenon has been observed for a number of autosomal dominant genes. For example, mutations in the RDS/peripherin gene *(PRPH2)* have been reported to cause cone–rod dystrophy, retinitis pigmentosa (RP), and pattern dystrophy phenotypes; mutations in the rhodopsin gene *(RHO)* can cause stationary night blindness (CSNB) or RP; and mutations in the cone–rod homeobox-containing gene *(CRX)* can give rise to a Leber congenital amaurosis phenotype or a cone–rod dystrophy phenotype. Autosomal recessive genes have also demonstrated varying phenotypes depending on the location and type of mutation within the gene. For example, mutations in *ABCA4* cause Stargardt disease as well as juvenile or adult macular dystrophy, RP, or cone–rod dystrophy that is either mild or severe and progressive.

To aid in clinical identification and management, dystrophies with primary diffuse photoreceptor involvement are classified separately from those with predominantly macular involvement, for which the symptoms and prognoses generally differ. The category of diffuse photoreceptor dystrophy is further subcategorized into rod-dominant and cone-dominant syndromes. The choroidal and vitreoretinal dystrophies are separated for ease in clinical description.

Daiger SP, Sullivan LS, Bowne SJ. Genetic mechanisms of retinal disease. In: Ryan SJ, Schachat AP, Wilkinson CP, Hinton DR, Sadda SR, Wiedemann P, eds. *Retina.* 5th ed. Philadelphia: Elsevier/Saunders; 2013:624–634.

Heckenlively JR, Daiger SP. Hereditary retinal and choroidal degenerations. In: Rimoin DL, Connor JM, Pyeritz RE, Korf BR, eds. *Emery and Rimoin's Principles and Practice of Medical Genetics.* 3 vols. 5th ed. Philadelphia: Churchill Livingstone; 2007:chap 137.

McKusick-Nathans Institute of Genetic Medicine, Johns Hopkins University School of Medicine. Online Mendelian Inheritance in Man website. Available at www.omim.org. Updated daily. Accessed September 5, 2014.

The University of Texas–Houston Health Science Center. RetNet, the Retinal Information Network website. Available at www.sph.uth.edu/retnet. Accessed September 5, 2014.

Diagnostic and Prognostic Testing

The electroretinogram (ERG) and perimetry testing play a central role in the diagnosis and follow-up of chorioretinal degeneration; however, fundus autofluorescence and optical coherence tomography (OCT) are playing an increasingly important role. Comparison between the cone-isolated, rod-isolated, and mixed-cone-and-rod ERG responses shows the diagnostic patterns commonly observed in hereditary retinal diseases (Table 12-1). Perimetry testing, fundus autofluorescence, and spectral-domain optical coherence tomography (SD-OCT) may show characteristic patterns of change that can help establish correct diagnoses.

Table 12-1 Basic Guide to Interpreting Standardized Electroretinogram (ERG) Responses*

ERG Finding	Disease or Condition
Undetectable ERG response	Leber congenital amaurosis Retinal aplasia Retinitis pigmentosa (RP) Total retinal detachment
Abnormal or undetectable photopic ERG response **Often mild rod ERG abnormalities**	Cone degenerations Achromatopsia X-linked blue-cone monochromatism X-linked cone dystrophy with tapetal-like sheen
Barely or undetectable scotopic ERG response **Abnormal photopic b-wave ERG response**	Rod–cone degenerations (RP) Leber congenital amaurosis Choroideremia Chorioretinitis (variable) Secondary RP, including some storage diseases Progressive retinitis punctata albescens
Abnormal cone and rod b-wave amplitudes **Cones relatively more affected than rods**	Cone–rod degenerations/dystrophies Autosomal dominant Autosomal recessive X-linked recessive Postinflammatory degenerations
Negative waveforms: in dark-adapted bright-flash ERG, a-wave is normal to attenuated; b-wave does not return to the isoelectric point	X-linked retinoschisis Congenital stationary night blindness Enhanced S-cone syndrome (Goldmann-Favre syndrome) Some autoimmune retinopathies
Nonspecific abnormalities	Metallic foreign bodies Chorioretinitis (acute or old) Early panretinal degeneration Partial retinal vascular occlusion Low serum taurine levels Vasculitis/diabetic retinopathy

*See also Audo I, Robson AG, Holder GE, Moore AT. The negative ERG: clinical phenotypes and disease mechanisms of inner retinal dysfunction. *Surv Ophthalmol.* 2008;53(1):16–40.

Modified from Rimoin DL, Connor JM, Pyeritz RE, Korf BR, eds. *Emery and Rimoin's Principles and Practice of Medical Genetics*. 4th ed. New York: Churchill Livingstone; 2002:3566. Copyright © 2001, with permission from Elsevier.

Diffuse Photoreceptor Dystrophies

Panretinal degeneration is associated with numerous hereditary retinal conditions, most of which are forms of RP and thus are rod–cone dystrophies. The ERG pattern of loss can also be cone predominant (cone–rod); in advanced cases, the ERG signal may be extinguished.

Visual field testing helps further characterize the diagnosis and assess the patient's level of function. Rod–cone RP degenerations show contracted fields. Partial to full-ring scotomata are common in midequatorial regions but often expand into the periphery, leaving only a small central island of visual field (Fig 12-1). In cone–rod RP degenerations, ring scotomata are closer to fixation. In patients with primary cone degenerations and cone–rod dystrophies, central scotomata are common.

Retinitis Pigmentosa

Panretinal pigmentary disturbances of the RPE and retina are divided into 2 large groups: (1) primary retinitis pigmentosa and (2) secondary pigmentary retinopathy. *Primary retinitis pigmentosa* (RP) refers to hereditary disorders that diffusely involve photoreceptor and pigment epithelial function; these conditions are characterized by progressive visual field loss and abnormal ERG responses. The disease process is confined to the eyes and is not associated with other systemic manifestations. *Secondary pigmentary retinopathy* refers to disorders in which the retinal degeneration is associated with single– or multiple–organ system disease. Secondary forms of pigmentary retinopathy are reviewed in Chapter 13. Occasionally, the term *pigmentary retinopathy* is used purely descriptively, and no associated disease is present. As such, it is important to understand the context in any discussion of pigmentary retinopathy.

Clinical features and diagnosis

Typical fundus findings in RP include arteriolar narrowing, variable waxy pallor of the disc, and variable amounts of bone spicule–like pigment changes (Fig 12-2). The peripheral retina and RPE appear atrophic even if spicules are absent *(RP sine pigmento),* and the macula typically shows a loss of the foveal reflex and irregularity of the vitreoretinal interface. Cystoid macular edema (CME) is occasionally present. Vitreous cells and mild posterior subcapsular cataracts are also commonly observed.

Several photoreceptor dystrophies have typical phenotypes, such as the deep retinal white dots or flecks in *retinitis punctata albescens* (Fig 12-3), choriocapillaris atrophy

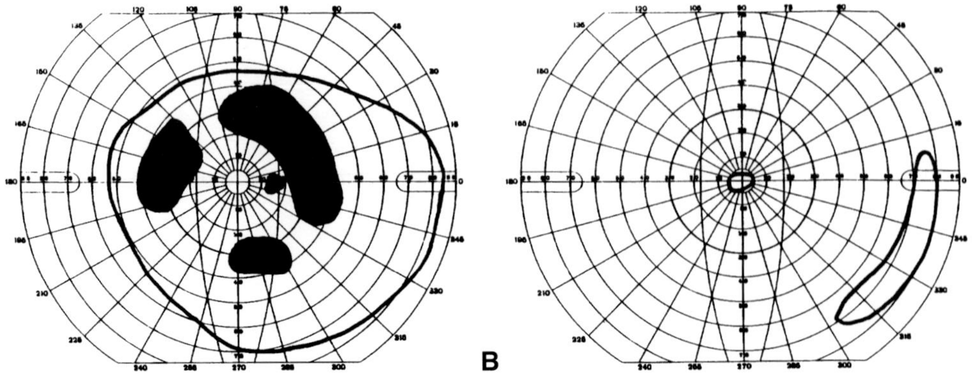

A B

Figure 12-1 Examples of visual fields in retinitis pigmentosa (RP), obtained with a Goldmann III-4 test object. **A,** Early disease: midperipheral scotomata. **B,** Late disease: severe loss, sparing only a central tunnel and a far-peripheral island, which may eventually disappear. *(Courtesy of Michael F. Marmor, MD.)*

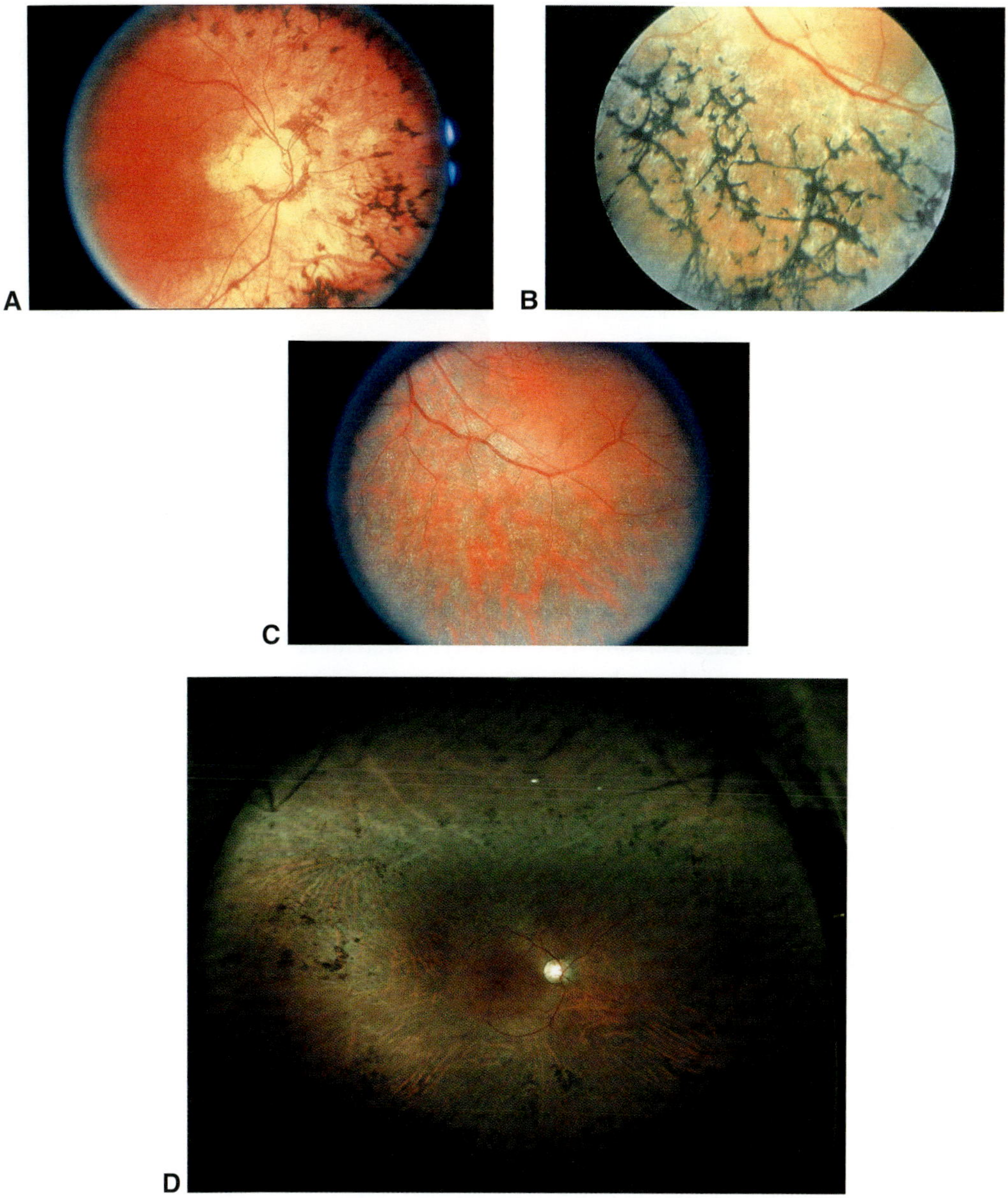

Figure 12-2 Different fundus photographic appearances in RP. **A,** Posterior fundus, showing waxy disc pallor, vascular attenuation, and a dull macula. **B,** Fundus with dense, peripheral, bone spicule–like changes. **C,** Fundus showing peripheral atrophy but virtually no spicules. **D,** Ultra-wide-angle fundus image of a patient with retinitis pigmentosa. Extensive pigmentary abnormalities, including bone spicules, are visible. *(Parts A and C courtesy of Michael F. Marmor, MD; part B courtesy of Carl D. Regillo, MD; part D courtesy of Colin A. McCannel, MD.)*

in choroideremia, macular RPE atrophy in *PRPH2* mutations, or the preserved para-arteriolar RPE in the phenotype RP12. Distinctive phenotypes are the exception, however, and most cases have diffuse pigment epithelial changes that are secondary effects of the diffuse photoreceptor degeneration.

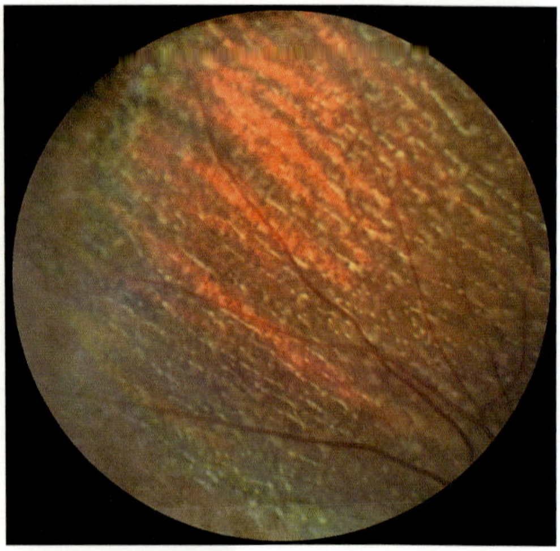

Figure 12-3 Color fundus photograph of a patient with retinitis punctata albescens, showing numerous deep retinal white dots. *(Courtesy of John R. Heckenlively, MD.)*

The ERG response in RP typically shows a loss or marked reduction in rod- more than cone-derived responses. Both a- and b-waves are reduced because the photoreceptors are primarily involved. The b-waves are characteristically prolonged in time as well as diminished in amplitude. Persons with the carrier state of X-linked recessive RP often show a mild reduction or delay in b-wave responses.

Late in the course of many types of RP, the ERG responses may become undetectable with conventional testing. An undetectable ERG signal is not diagnostic of RP but simply documents severe loss of retinal function.

When evaluating suspected RP in a patient with a negative family history *(simplex RP),* the clinician must consider acquired causes of retinal degeneration that can mimic RP, including previous ophthalmic artery occlusion, diffuse uveitis, infections such as syphilis, paraneoplastic syndromes, and retinal drug toxicity. Secondary forms of pigmentary retinopathy associated with metabolic or other organ system disease must also be considered (see Chapter 13).

Gregory-Evans K, Pennesi ME, Weleber RG. Retinitis pigmentosa and allied disorders. In: Ryan SJ, Schachat AP, Wilkinson CP, Hinton DR, Sadda SR, Wiedemann P, eds. *Retina.* Vol 2. 5th ed. Philadelphia: Elsevier/Saunders; 2013:761–835.

Regional variants of retinitis pigmentosa

Several variants of RP present with unusual or regional distribution of the retinal degeneration. Many of these cases show an unusually sharp demarcation between affected and unaffected areas of the retina in contrast to the diffuse damage of more typical RP (Fig 12-4). It is important to recognize these forms because some are either nonprogressive or very slowly progressive.

Sectorial RP refers to disease involving only 1 or 2 sectors of the fundus. This condition is generally symmetric in both eyes, which helps rule out acquired damage (eg, from trauma, vascular insult, or inflammation).

Patients with cone–rod dystrophy, in which cone-derived ERG responses are more abnormal than the rod ERG responses, present with macular involvement or markedly reduced visual acuity very early in the course of disease, which is unusual for RP. Visual

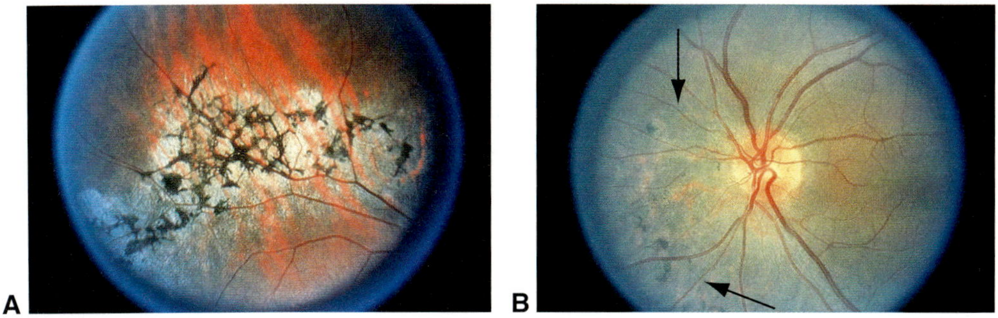

Figure 12-4 Color fundus photographs of delimited forms of RP. Note the sharp demarcation between the areas of degeneration and other regions of the fundus that appear quite healthy. **A,** Fundus with degenerative changes near the arcades. **B,** Fundus with sectorial RP *(between arrows)*, showing vascular narrowing and spicules only in the inferonasal quadrant. *(Courtesy of Michael F. Marmor, MD.)*

field loss may progress outward from the center rather than inward *(central RP)*. Some patients show a tight ring scotoma within the central 20° or 30° *(pericentral RP)*. This group of regional variants is probably heterogeneous because most of the cases appear sporadic and few are well characterized clinically or genetically.

Unilateral RP is rare, and most cases of unexplained unilateral pigmentary retinopathy are probably postinflammatory or posttraumatic. In authentic cases, the clinical presentation and findings in the involved eye are similar to those of typical RP. Before making a diagnosis of unilateral RP, the clinician must first rule out secondary causes, document a normal ERG response in the unaffected eye, and monitor the patient for at least 5 years to rule out bilateral but highly asymmetric disease.

Genetic considerations

Currently, more than 100 different genetic types of RP (or similar degenerations) have been described; more than 50 genes causing RP have been identified; and all inheritance patterns are represented. *Autosomal dominant RP* (ADRP) accounts for 10%–20% of RP cases, depending on the country surveyed. The first mutations discovered to cause RP were in the gene coding for rhodopsin, the visual pigment in rods that mediates night vision. The severity of disease resulting from rhodopsin mutations varies considerably. For example, mild disease (a form of stationary night blindness) is associated with codon 90 mutations, whereas severe forms are associated with mutations that interfere with the attachment of vitamin A to the rhodopsin protein. Mutations in *PRPH2* have particularly wide disease expression, ranging from RP to pattern macular dystrophies (eg, adult vitelliform dystrophy, butterfly dystrophy), but are the most common cause of dominantly inherited maculopathy. The 172 mutation, which is the most common, can result in a range of phenotypes including macular dystrophy, cone dystrophy, and cone–rod dystrophy; functional studies are necessary to enable accurate counseling.

Autosomal recessive RP (ARRP) represents approximately 20% of RP cases, although the percentage increases when the definition includes families with several affected siblings *(multiplex RP)* or consanguinity of parents. *X-linked RP* (XLRP) accounts for approximately 10% of RP cases in the United States and up to 25% in England. This percentage excludes choroideremia, an X-linked, childhood-onset, rod–cone dystrophy, which is characterized by visual field loss similar to that of typical RP.

Up to 40% of cases presenting in the United States have no family history. Most are generally assumed to represent ARRP, although undoubtedly a few are autosomal dominant with reduced penetrance or are X-linked recessive, in which the last affected male was several generations past. Rare cases of mitochondrial and X-linked dominant inheritance have been reported in patients with RP.

Berger W, Kloeckener-Gruissem B, Neidhardt J. The molecular basis of human retinal and vitreoretinal diseases. *Prog Retin Eye Res.* 2010;29(5):335–375.

Management

Patients with newly diagnosed RP are likely to be concerned about the possibility of blindness. The clinician should dispel popular misconceptions about this condition. Patients with RP may fear they will become blind within 1 year, but in fact the disease is a chronic degenerative problem, and most patients retain vision for decades. Total blindness is an infrequent endpoint, and patients who desire to have children but worry about passing on the disorder may benefit from genetic counseling. Many patients with RP benefit from support to adjust to narrowed visual fields and reduced night vision. Low-vision aids frequently help patients with subnormal visual acuity, and patients with advanced disease may need vocational rehabilitation and mobility training.

Management of RP includes ophthalmic evaluations every 1–2 years. Although at present, the death of photoreceptor cells in RP cannot be arrested or reversed, follow-up visits are necessary to address refractive management and monitor for CME, which develops in 10%–20% of RP patients. CME can be managed with use of oral carbonic anhydrase inhibitors, such as acetazolamide (Fig 12-5), or intravitreal injection of triamcinolone acetonide in refractory cases. Treatment-resistant CME is common.

Nutritional supplements have been investigated as therapy for RP. One large study reported that high daily doses of vitamin A palmitate (15,000 IU/day) can slow the decline in ERG response in RP by approximately 20% per year. However, the benefits must be weighed against the risk of long-term liver toxicity and the drug's teratogenicity. Docosahexaenoic acid (DHA), an omega-3 fatty acid found in oily fish and thought to be

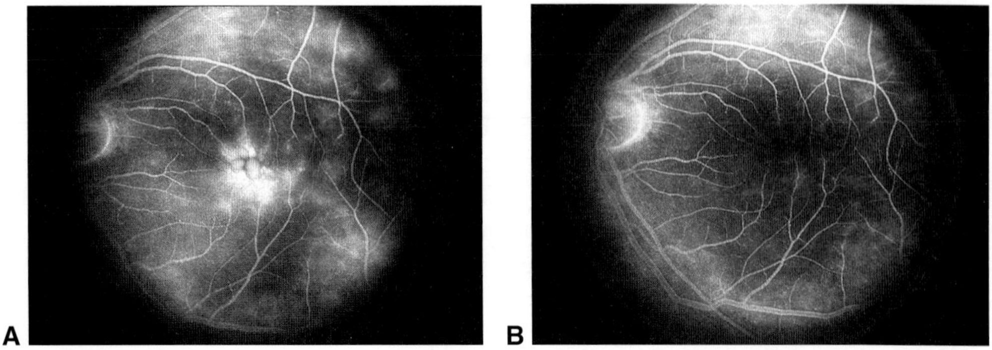

Figure 12-5 Cystoid macular edema responsive to treatment in RP. **A,** Dye leakage, as shown on fluorescein angiography image. **B,** Eye of the same patient after 2 weeks of treatment with oral acetazolamide. *(Courtesy of Michael F. Marmor, MD.)*

important for photoreceptor function, was evaluated in 2 clinical trials for its potential to slow vision loss in RP. Neither study showed a clear benefit.

Excessive light exposure may play a role in retinal degenerations caused by rhodopsin mutations. Recommendations for patients to employ UV-absorbing sunglasses and brimmed hats for protection from high levels of light exposure seem prudent despite the absence of direct evidence of benefit.

Efforts to restore at least some vision in patients rendered completely blind from RP include the use of electronic chips that interface with the remaining retina tissue. One such device, the Argus II Retinal Prosthesis System (Second Sight Medical Products, Sylmar, California), is now commercially available, and others are in development. The device consists of an external camera and a retinal surface chip that stimulates remaining retinal cells, providing minimal rudimentary vision. There is broad optimism that gene therapy and regenerative medicine strategies may lead to treatments to modify the course of RP and/or restore vision in patients with RP.

Berson EL, Rosner B, Sandberg MA, et al. A randomized trial of vitamin A and vitamin E supplementation for retinitis pigmentosa. *Arch Ophthalmol.* 1993;111(6):761–772.

Fishman GA, Gilbert LD, Fiscella RG, Kimura AE, Jampol LM. Acetazolamide for treatment of chronic macular edema in retinitis pigmentosa. *Arch Ophthalmol.* 1989;107(10): 1445–1452.

Hartong DT, Berson EL, Dryja TP. Retinitis pigmentosa. *Lancet.* 2006;368(9549):1795–1809.

Maguire AM, High KA, Auricchio A, et al. Age-dependent effects of RPE65 gene therapy for Leber's congenital amaurosis: a phase 1 dose-escalation trial. *Lancet.* 2009;374(9701): 1597–1605.

Leber Congenital Amaurosis

The early-onset retinal dystrophies are collectively termed *Leber congenital amaurosis* (LCA) (also see BCSC Section 6, *Pediatric Ophthalmology and Strabismus,* Chapter 25). Currently, 3 autosomal dominant and 18 recessive mutations have been identified. LCA is typically characterized by severely reduced vision from birth, associated with wandering nystagmus. Visual acuity may range from 20/200 to no light perception. In the early stages, obvious fundus changes are rare. Later, round, subretinal black-pigmented clumps may develop in some patients. Some infants with LCA rub or poke their eyes (the *oculodigital reflex*), as do other infants with poor vision. Most children with LCA have normal intelligence, and some of the observed psychomotor impairment may be secondary to sensory deprivation. Cataracts and keratoconus may be present in older children.

The ERG response is typically minimal or undetectable. This lack of response differentiates LCA from dystrophic diseases in which the ERG response diminishes with age and from syndromes with similar clinical presentation, such as albinism, achromatopsia, and CSNB.

One form of LCA bearing a mutation in *RPE65* has been treated successfully by gene therapy in clinical trials by use of an adeno-associated virus. The results of a phase 1 trial showed sustained improvement in 12 patients with *RPE65*-associated LCA after gene-replacement therapy.

den Hollander AI, Roepman R, Koenekoop RK, Crèmers FP. Leber congenital amaurosis: genes, proteins and disease mechanisms. *Prog Retin Eye Res.* 2008:27(4):391–419.

Cone Dystrophies

The cone dystrophies should not be confused with congenital color blindness, in which there are color deficits for specific colors but no associated retinal degeneration, or with macular dystrophies, in which the defect is confined largely to the central retinal cones. Patients with congenital color blindness (protanopia, deuteranopia, and tritanopia) have normal visual acuity and do not show signs of progressive disease. Congenital color deficiency and other congenital stationary cone dysfunction syndromes, including rod monochromatism and blue-cone monochromatism, are discussed in Chapter 11.

The progressive cone dystrophies are a heterogeneous group of diseases with onset in the teenage or later adult years. In some patients, secondary rod photoreceptor involvement develops in later life, leading to overlap between progressive cone and cone–rod dystrophies. Cone dystrophies are diagnosed when ERG results indicate an abnormal or undetectable photopic ERG response and a normal or near-normal rod-isolated ERG response. When present, the cone flicker ERG response is almost invariably delayed, in keeping with generalized cone system dysfunction. Peripheral visual fields may remain normal. All 3 mendelian inheritance patterns are associated with cone dystrophies.

A diagnosis of cone dystrophy is suggested by the progressive loss of visual acuity and color discrimination, often accompanied by hemeralopia (day blindness) and photophobia (light intolerance). Ophthalmoscopy may show a symmetric bull's-eye pattern of macular atrophy (Fig 12-6) or more severe atrophy, such as demarcated circular macular lesions. Mild to severe temporal optic atrophy and tapetal retinal reflexes (with a glistening greenish or golden sheen) may also be present. Patients with cone dystrophies may have fundi that appear normal, especially early in the course of their disease, and may be suspected of malingering.

Selected cone dystrophies

Currently, more than 25 gene mutations are known to cause progressive cone and cone–rod dystrophies. Dominant cone dystrophy linked to 6p21.1 is caused by mutations in

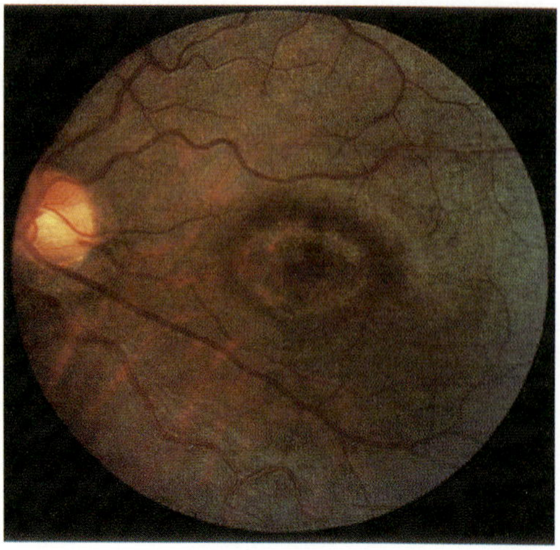

Figure 12-6 Color fundus photograph of cone dystrophy, showing the bull's-eye pattern of central atrophy.

the gene coding for guanylate cyclase activator 1A *(GUCA1A),* a calcium-binding protein expressed in photoreceptor outer segments. Mutations in *GUCY2D* at 17p13.1 have been identified in a family with autosomal dominant progressive cone degeneration. Different mutations of both alleles in the same gene cause autosomal recessive LCA. These patients exhibit foveal atrophy that may be misdiagnosed as Stargardt disease, but ERG studies of these patients show the photopic response is severely abnormal, the scotopic response is maintained, and the Goldmann visual field is full. An adult-onset, X-linked recessive cone dystrophy with a tapetal-like sheen and Mizuo-Nakamura phenomenon (in which the fundus appearance changes with dark adaptation) has been reported in several pedigrees, but the affected gene has not yet been identified.

A specific disorder known as *cone dystrophy with supernormal ERG,* which is related to a mutation in *KCNV2,* has pathognomonic (diagnostic) ERG findings. It was the first disorder of the human visual system known to be related to a potassium channel. The disorder is recessively inherited, and patients usually present with loss of visual acuity. There are no specific fundus features (there are often nonspecific changes at the macula), and the diagnosis is made by ERG.

Robson AG, Webster AR, Michaelides M, et al. "Cone dystrophy with supernormal rod electroretinogram": a comprehensive genotype/phenotype study including fundus autofluorescence and extensive electrophysiology. *Retina.* 2010;30(1):51–62.

Vincent A, Robson AG, Holder GE. Pathognomonic (diagnostic) ERGs. A review and update. *Retina.* 2013;33(1):5–12.

Cone–rod dystrophies

The term *cone–rod* comes from electroretinographic testing, in which cone-derived ERG signals are more affected than rod-derived signals and both are abnormal. Numerous entities can yield this ERG pattern. Molecular genetics helps differentiate the specific causes among the members of this group. Recently, it has become apparent that some of the mutations that result in the severe phenotype of LCA cause a cone–rod dystrophy if there is a different mutation in the same gene or if there is a mutation in only 1 allele. Important genes in which mutations are associated with cone–rod degenerations are those for Stargardt disease *(ABCA4),* Alström disease *(ALMS1),* and dominant spinocerebellar ataxia *(SCA7).* Dominant cone–rod dystrophy may result from mutations in *GUCY2D,* whereas recessive mutations cause LCA. Similarly, various mutations in *CRX* can cause RP, LCA, or cone–rod dystrophy.

Patients with progressive cone–rod dystrophy demonstrate expanding central scotomata over time. Ophthalmoscopy at later stages may show bone spicule–like (intraretinal) hyperpigmentation and atrophy in the fundus periphery, and patients may report night blindness, poor central visual acuity, and symptoms of dyschromatopsia. The expression of these disorders varies widely, and patients must be monitored over time to determine the disease course.

Hamel CP. Cone rod dystrophies. *Orphanet J Rare Dis.* 2007;2:7.

Michaelides M, Hardcastle AJ, Hunt DM, Moore AT. Progressive cone and cone-rod dystrophies: phenotypes and underlying molecular genetic basis. *Surv Ophthalmol.* 2006;51(3):232–258.

Macular Dystrophies

The macular dystrophies can be difficult to manage. The differential diagnosis is sometimes challenging, and several of the conditions cause vision loss to the level of 20/200 or worse at a relatively young age. These diseases cannot currently be arrested or reversed, yet patients can be reassured that the condition progresses slowly.

Stargardt Disease

Stargardt disease is the most common juvenile macular dystrophy and a common cause of central vision loss in adults younger than 50 years. The vast majority of cases are autosomal recessive. The visual acuity in Stargardt disease typically ranges from 20/50 to 20/200. Most patients retain fair visual acuity (eg, 20/70–20/100) in at least 1 eye.

The classic Stargardt phenotype is characterized by a juvenile-onset foveal atrophy surrounded by discrete, yellowish, round or pisciform flecks at the level of the RPE (Fig 12-7A). If the flecks are widely scattered throughout the fundus, the condition is commonly referred to as *fundus flavimaculatus.* A clinical diagnosis of Stargardt disease may be confirmed by the finding of a "dark choroid" on fluorescein angiography. This phenomenon—in which the retinal circulation is highlighted against a hypofluorescent background because of blocking of choroidal fluorescence—is present in at least 80% of patients with the disorder (Fig 12-7B). Fundus autofluorescence imaging may show characteristic findings: peripapillary sparing of the RPE changes; central macular hypoautofluorescence; and, over time, a radially outward expanding pattern of hyperautofluorescent flecks, which leave hypoautofluorescent flecks in their wake. The exact findings appear to vary by genotype.

The age of onset and presenting clinical features in Stargardt disease are quite variable, sometimes even among individuals within the same family. In most patients, the condition is slowly progressive with the accumulation of lipofuscin-like material in the RPE (Fig 12-8). The differential diagnosis of Stargardt disease includes conditions that may

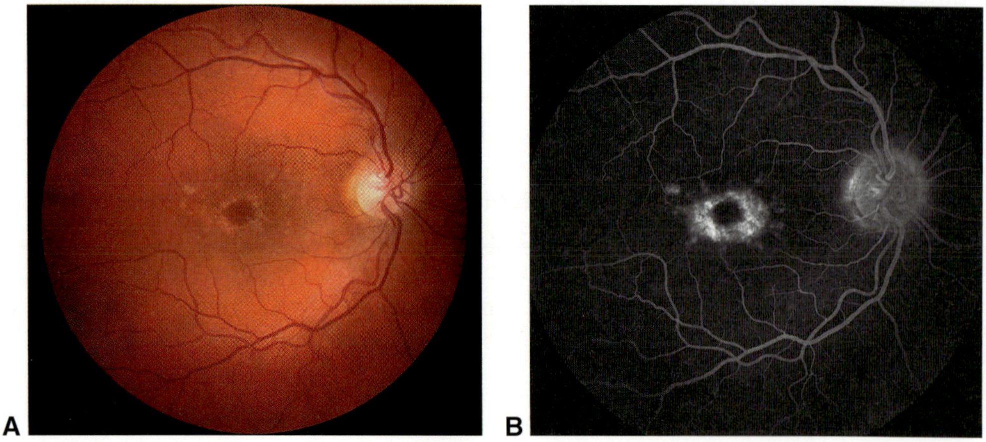

Figure 12-7 Stargardt disease. **A,** Color fundus photograph showing paramacular yellowish flecks and "beaten-bronze" central macular atrophy. **B,** Fluorescein angiography image of the same eye showing a dark choroid, hyperfluorescence associated with flecks, and bull's-eye pattern of macular transmission defect. *(Courtesy of Mark W. Johnson, MD.)*

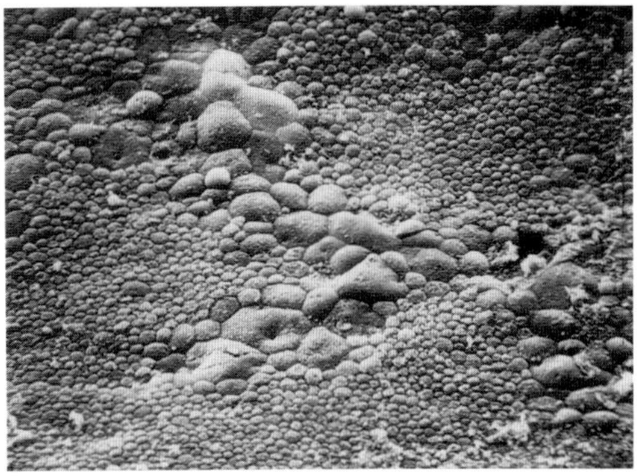

Figure 12-8 Scanning electron micrograph of the retinal pigment epithelium (RPE) in Stargardt disease. The flecks represent regions of RPE cells engorged with abnormal lipofuscin-like material. *(From Eagle RC Jr, Lucier AC, Bernardino VB Jr, Yanoff M. Retinal pigment epithelial abnormalities in fundus flavimaculatus: a light and electron microscopic study.* Ophthalmology. *1980;87(12):1189–1200.)*

Table 12-2 Differential Diagnosis of Bull's-Eye Maculopathy

Stargardt disease
Cone and cone–rod dystrophies
Hydroxychloroquine/chloroquine retinal toxicity
Age-related macular degeneration
Chronic macular hole
Central areolar choroidal dystrophy
Olivopontocerebellar atrophy
Ceroid lipofuscinosis

cause a bull's-eye atrophic maculopathy (Table 12-2). Vitamin A supplementation accelerates the accumulation of lipofuscin pigments in the RPE and should be avoided in patients with Stargardt disease. Recent evidence has shown that ERG recordings play a useful role in prognosis.

Stargardt disease is caused by mutations in the *ABCA4* gene, which encodes an ATP-binding cassette (ABC) transporter protein expressed by rod outer segments. The gene is very large (50 exons) and has many polymorphisms, and as of 2014 more than 650 disease-causing variants have been identified. Other, less frequent causes of a similar phenotype include mutations in the dominant genes *STGD4* and *ELOVL4* (the latter of which encodes a photoreceptor-specific component of the fatty acid elongation system) and mutations in *PRPH2.*

American Academy of Ophthalmology. SmartSight website. Available at http://one.aao.org/smart-sight-low-vision. Accessed September 15, 2014.

Koenekoop RK, Lopez I, den Hollander AI, Allikmets R, Cremers FP. Genetic testing for retinal dystrophies and dysfunctions: benefits, dilemmas and solutions. *Clin Experiment Ophthalmol.* 2007;35(5):473–485.

Walia S, Fishman GA. Natural history of phenotypic changes in Stargardt macular dystrophy. *Ophthalmic Genet.* 2009;30(2):63–68.

Vitelliform Degenerations

Best disease or Best vitelliform dystrophy

Best disease is an autosomal dominant maculopathy caused by mutations in the *BEST1* (or *VMD2*) gene, which is located on the long arm of chromosome 11 and encodes the protein bestrophin. Bestrophin localizes to the basolateral plasma membrane of the RPE and functions as a transmembrane chloride channel (see the RetNet website). The resulting lipofuscin accumulation may be secondary to abnormal ion flux.

Affected individuals frequently show a yellow, egg yolk–like (vitelliform) macular lesion in childhood, which eventually breaks down, leaving a mottled geographic atrophic appearance (Fig 12-9). Late in the course of the disease, the geographic atrophy may be difficult to distinguish from other types of macular degeneration or dystrophy. Some patients (up to 30% in some series) have extrafoveal vitelliform lesions in the fundus. However, the macular appearance in all stages is deceptive, as most patients maintain relatively good vision throughout the course of the disease. Even patients with "scrambled-egg" macular lesions typically have 20/30 visual acuity. In approximately 20% of patients, a choroidal neovascular membrane develops in 1 eye during the course of the disease and, if untreated, may result in poor vision.

The ERG response is characteristically normal, and the electro-oculogram (EOG) result is always abnormal. The light rise of the EOG (see Chapter 3) is typically severely reduced or absent. The EOG abnormality is always present in Best disease and serves as a marker for the disease, even in individuals who are asymptomatic and have normal fundi. Rather than attempt an EOG recording in a child with vitelliform lesions, many clinicians perform EOG recordings of the parents to identify the carrier. The EOG may be useful in evaluating poorly defined central macular lesions.

Autosomal recessive bestrophinopathy

A recently described recessive disorder, autosomal recessive bestrophinopathy (ARB), also related to mutation in *BEST1,* is associated with severe loss of the EOG light rise as well but shows progressive retinal dysfunction on ERG. Patients with ARB usually present with loss of visual acuity and show diffuse irregularity of the RPE and dispersed punctate flecks, which are distinct from extramacular vitelliform lesions.

Agarwal A. *Gass' Atlas of Macular Diseases.* 5th ed. Philadelphia: Saunders; 2012:278–280.

Boon CJ, Klevering BJ, Leroy BP, Hoyng CB, Keunen JE, den Hollander AI. The spectrum of ocular phenotypes caused by mutations in the BEST1 gene. *Prog Retin Eye Res.* 2009;28(3): 187–205.

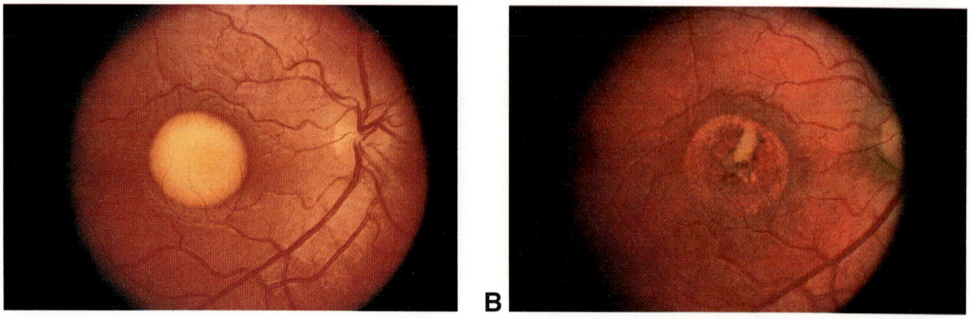

A B

Figure 12-9 Color fundus photographs of Best vitelliform dystrophy. **A,** Characteristic "yolk" stage, during which visual acuity is typically good. **B,** Atrophy and scarring after the yolk breaks down. *(Courtesy of Mark W. Johnson, MD.)*

Adult-onset vitelliform lesions

Several types of symmetric yellow deposits that resemble Best disease may develop in the macula of older adults. The most common disorder, *adult-onset foveomacular vitelliform dystrophy,* is one of the *pattern dystrophies* (discussed later in this chapter), which are usually caused by mutations in *PRPH2.* This disorder is characterized by yellow subfoveal lesions that are bilateral, round or oval, and typically one-third disc diameter in size; they often contain a central pigmented spot (Fig 12-10). Occasionally, the lesions may be larger and misdiagnosed as Best disease or even as age-related macular degeneration. This dystrophy generally appears in the fourth to sixth decades in patients who either are visually

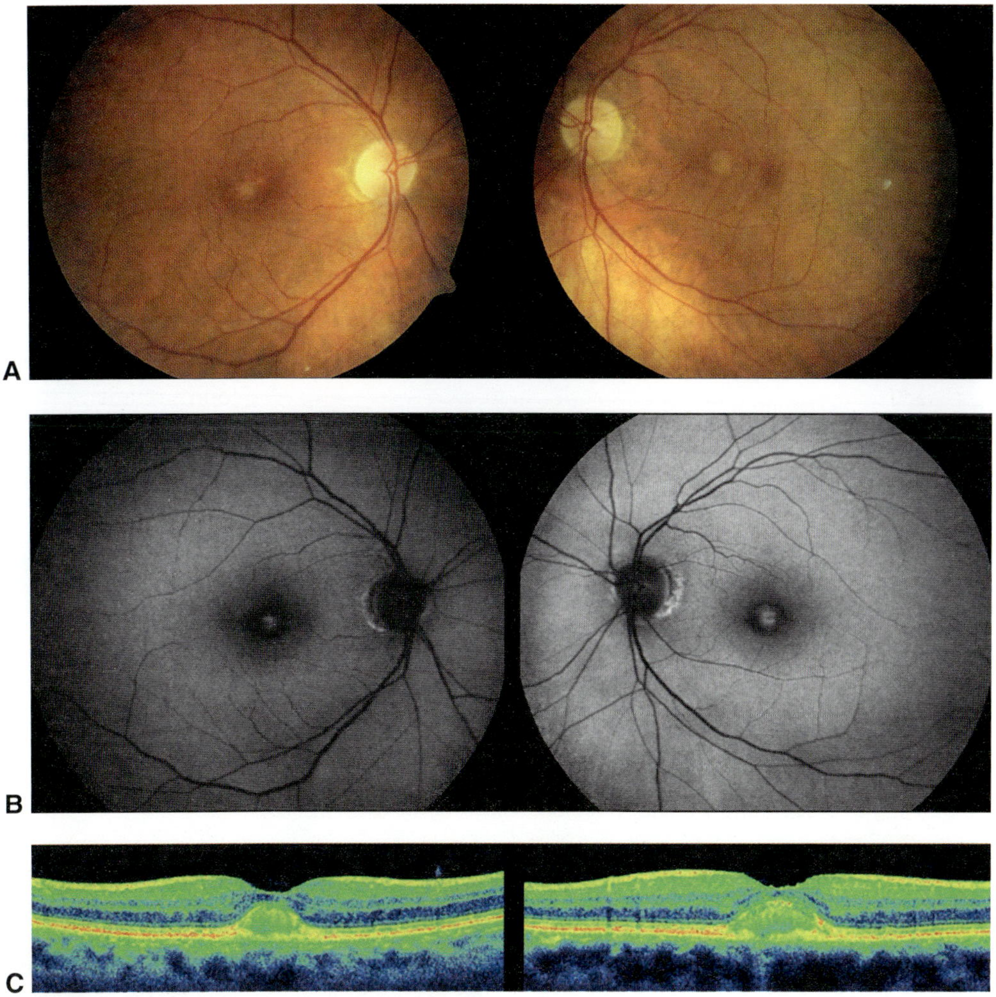

Figure 12-10 Adult vitelliform pattern dystrophy. *Left panels* in each part are images of the left eye, and *right panels,* of the right eye of the same patient. **A,** Color fundus photographs demonstrate small, round, yellow subfoveal lesions, which show hyperautofluorescence on autofluorescence imaging **(B). C,** Spectral-domain optical coherence tomography images show the reflective, dome-shaped subfoveal material elevating the overlying neurosensory retina. *(Courtesy of Stephen J. Kim, MD.)*

asymptomatic or have mild blurring and metamorphopsia. Eventually, the lesions may fade, leaving an area of RPE atrophy, but most patients retain reading vision in at least 1 eye throughout their lives. The EOG patterns in these individuals tend to be normal or only mildly subnormal. Autosomal dominant inheritance has been recognized in some families.

Patients with numerous basal laminar (cuticular) drusen may develop an unusual *vitelliform exudative macular detachment* (Fig 12-11). The yellowish subretinal fluid blocks background fluorescence early, often stains late in the angiogram study, and may be mistaken for choroidal neovascularization. Patients with yellowish macular detachments often maintain good visual acuity for many months but may eventually lose central vision because of geographic atrophy or choroidal neovascularization and disciform scarring.

In some patients with large, soft drusen, there is a large, central coalescence of drusen, or *drusenoid RPE detachment,* which may occasionally mimic a macular vitelliform lesion (Fig 12-12). Such lesions often have pigment mottling on their surface and are surrounded by numerous other individual or confluent soft drusen. They may remain stable (and allow for good vision) for many years, but eventually they tend to flatten and evolve into geographic atrophy.

Agarwal A. *Gass' Atlas of Macular Diseases.* 5th ed. Philadelphia: Saunders; 2012:278–280.

Early-Onset Drusen

Early-onset (or familial) drusen typically manifests at younger ages than do those in most cases of age-related macular degeneration. Drusen are usually numerous and vary in size,

A

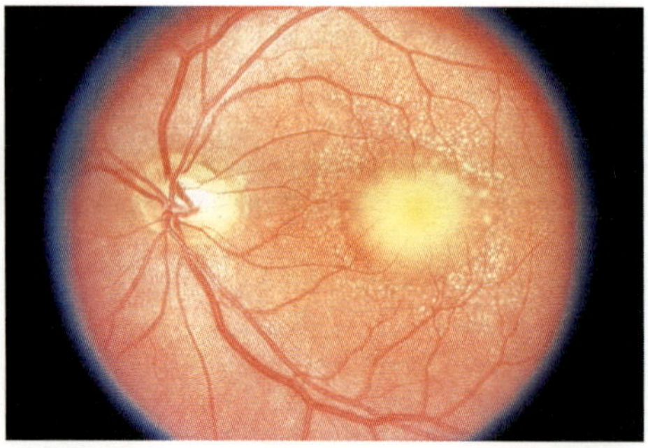

B

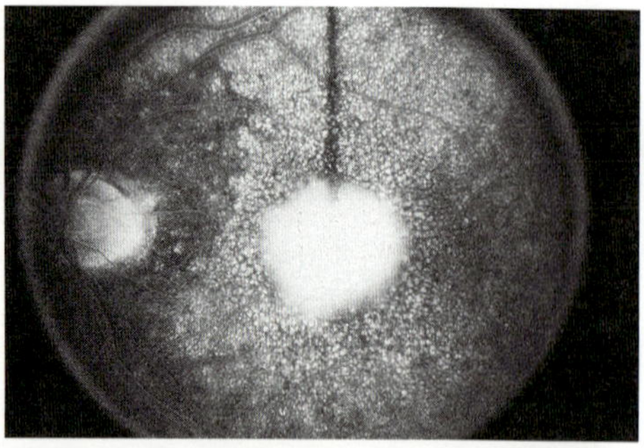

Figure 12-11 **A,** Color fundus photograph of vitelliform lesion in the setting of numerous cuticular (basal laminar) drusen. **B,** Corresponding late-phase fluorescein angiography image showing staining of drusen and vitelliform lesion. *(Courtesy of Michael F. Marmor, MD.)*

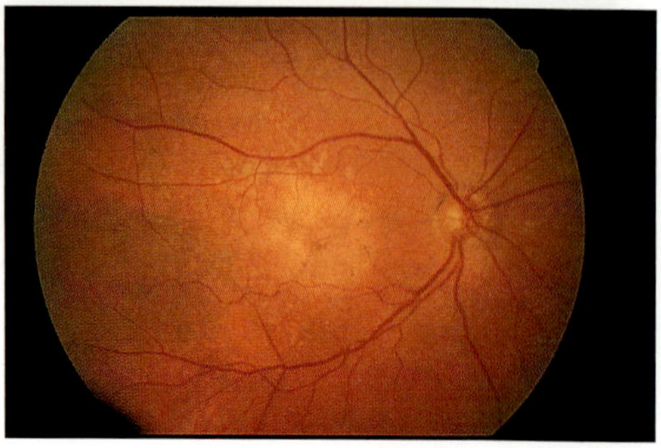

Figure 12-12 Color fundus photograph showing central coalescence of large drusen simulating a macular vitelliform lesion. *(Courtesy of Mark W. Johnson, MD.)*

typically extending beyond the vascular arcades and nasal to the optic disc (Fig 12-13). Although early-onset drusen are presumed to be genetically determined, the inheritance pattern in the vast majority of young patients is never established. Nonetheless, early-onset drusen have been classified into 3 entities: (1) large colloid drusen, (2) Malattia leventinese, and (3) cuticular drusen. On fundus examination, *large colloid drusen* appear as large, yellowish, and bilateral lesions located in the macula and/or the periphery of the retina. They are hyperautofluorescent.

Malattia leventinese and *Doyne honeycomb dystrophy* are 2 phenotypes of the same condition and are the classic autosomal dominant drusen. The condition is caused by an autosomal dominant mutation in the gene *EFEMP1,* which is located on chromosome 2 and codes for fibulin 3 (also known as *epidermal growth factor–containing fibulin-like extracellular matrix protein 1*). The phenotype is distinctive because the drusen often develop in a radiating pattern from the fovea.

The *cuticular* or *basal laminar drusen* phenotype is a clinical syndrome that may occur in middle age (Fig 12-14). Patients with this phenotype may be at greater risk of macular degeneration as they age. The syndrome involves innumerable, homogeneous, round

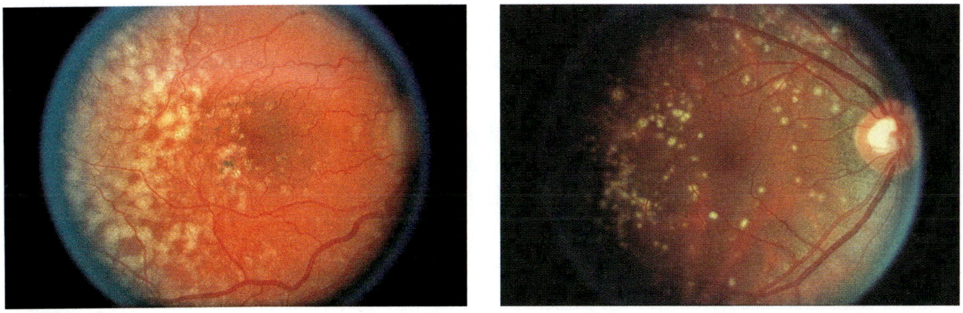

Figure 12-13 Color fundus photographs of different manifestations of early-onset drusen. Variable size and distribution of the drusen are evident. *(Courtesy of Michael F. Marmor, MD.)*

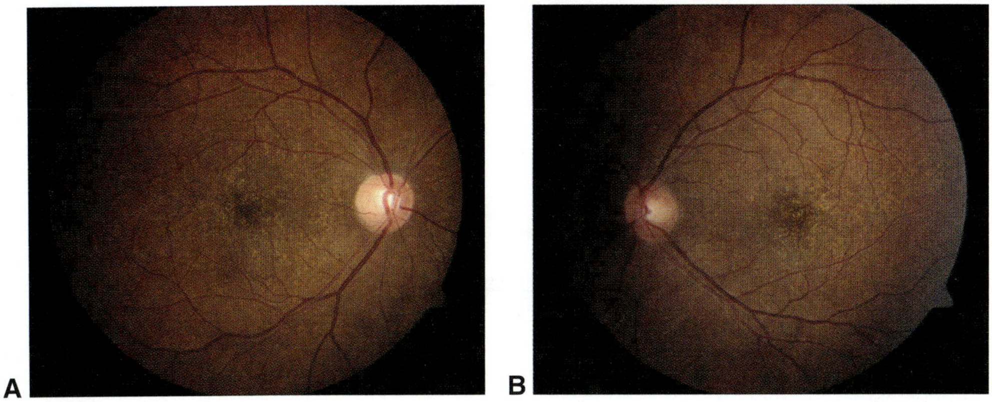

Figure 12-14 Basal laminar (cuticular) drusen. Color fundus photographs of the left **(A)** and right **(B)** eyes of a 38-year-old man with numerous round, yellow drusen scattered in the macula. Basal laminar (cuticular) drusen result from nodular thickening of the basement membrane of the RPE and are more easily seen angiographically and in young patients with brunette fundi. *(Courtesy of Stephen J. Kim, MD.)*

drusen that are more apparent on angiography than on biomicroscopy and impart a "starry-sky" appearance. These drusen are associated with a vitelliform macular detachment. SD-OCT imaging reveals that these sub-RPE drusen have a pointed or conical appearance. The phenotype is strongly associated with the Tyr402His mutation of the *CFH* gene.

Other drusenlike deposits that manifest before age 50 include deposits associated with some hereditary renal disorders that involve basement membrane abnormalities. These disorders include Alport syndrome and membranoproliferative glomerulonephritis type II.

Grassi MA, Folk JC, Scheetz TE, Taylor CM, Sheffield VC, Stone EM. Complement factor H polymorphism p. Tyr402His and cuticular drusen. *Arch Ophthalmol.* 2007;125(1):93–97.

Kim DD, Mieler WF, Wolf MD. Posterior segment changes in membranoproliferative glomerulonephritis. *Am J Ophthalmol.* 1992;114(5):593–599.

Stone EM, Lotery AJ, Munier FL, et al. A single *EFEMP1* mutation associated with both Malattia Leventinese and Doyne honeycomb retinal dystrophy. *Nat Genet.* 1999;22(2): 199–202.

Pattern Dystrophies

The pattern dystrophies are a group of disorders characterized by the development, typically in midlife, of various patterns of yellow, orange, or gray pigment deposition at the level of the RPE in the macular area. The inheritance is typically autosomal dominant. These dystrophies may be subdivided into 4 major patterns according to the distribution of pigment deposits: (1) *adult-onset foveomacular vitelliform dystrophy* (discussed earlier in this chapter), (2) *butterfly-type pattern dystrophy* (Fig 12-15), (3) *reticular-type pattern dystrophy* (Fig 12-16), and (4) *fundus pulverulentus* (coarse pigment mottling). Note, however, that considerable variation in clinical presentation exists.

The clinical pattern may vary among affected family members, or even between the 2 eyes of a given patient, and it can evolve from 1 pattern to another over time. The

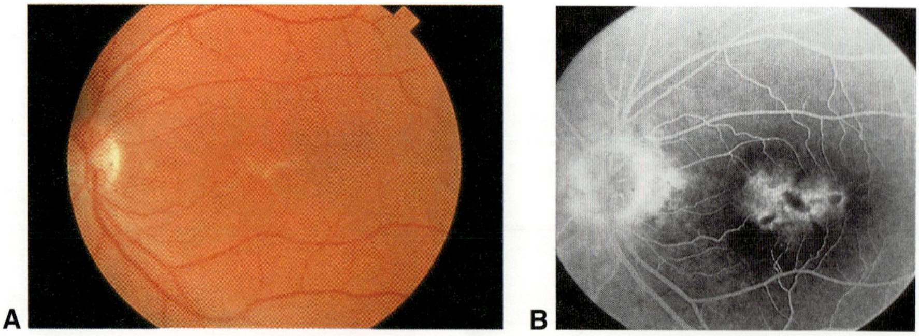

Figure 12-15 Butterfly-type pattern dystrophy. **A,** Color fundus photograph from a 56-year-old woman showing a typical yellow macular pigment pattern. **B,** Fluorescein angiography image shows blocked fluorescence of the pigment lesion itself and a rim of hyperfluorescence from surrounding retinal pigment epithelial atrophy. *(Used with permission from Song M-K, Small KW. Macular dystrophies. In: Regillo CD, Brown GC, Flynn HW Jr, eds.* Vitreoretinal Disease: The Essentials. *New York: Thieme; 1999:297. © Thieme.)*

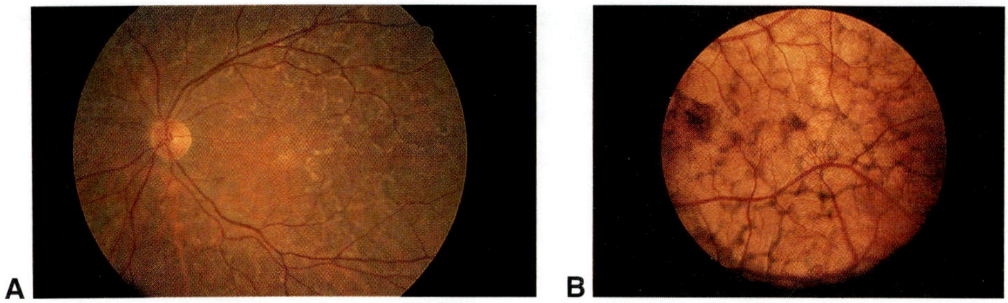

Figure 12-16 Color fundus photographs showing 2 examples of reticular-type pattern dystrophy, characterized by a "fishnet" pattern of yellowish-orange **(A)** or brown **(B)** pigment deposition in the posterior fundus. *(Courtesy of Mark W. Johnson, MD.)*

overlapping ophthalmoscopic features of these patterns and their similar clinical implications suggest that they are either closely related or variable expressions of the same genetic defect. Most forms of autosomal dominant pattern dystrophy have been associated with mutations in *PRPH2.* Mistaking pattern dystrophies for age-related macular degeneration can lead to unnecessary use of Age-Related Eye Disease Study (AREDs) formula vitamins by patients.

The most common presenting symptom of the pattern dystrophies is slightly diminished visual acuity or mild metamorphopsia. Patients are often asymptomatic, however, and the conditions are identified only upon the discovery of unusual macular lesions during routine ophthalmoscopy. Results of functional and electrophysiologic testing are generally normal, except for a borderline or mildly reduced EOG consistent with a diffuse RPE disorder. The risk of choroidal neovascularization is low, and geographic macular atrophy may develop progressively.

Agarwal A. *Gass' Atlas of Macular Diseases.* 5th ed. Philadelphia: Saunders; 2012:278–280.

Marmor MF. The pattern dystrophies. In: Heckenlively JR, Arden GB, eds. *Principles and Practice of Clinical Electrophysiology of Vision.* 2nd ed. Cambridge, MA: MIT Press; 2006:757–761.

Sorsby Macular Dystrophy

Sorsby macular dystrophy, a dominantly inherited disease, involves the development of bilateral, subfoveal, choroidal neovascular lesions at approximately 40 years of age (Fig 12-17). As the macular lesions evolve, they take on the appearance of geographic atrophy, with pronounced clumps of black pigmentation around the central ischemic and atrophic zone (a *pseudoinflammatory* appearance). An early sign of the disease is the presence of numerous fine drusenlike deposits or a confluent plaque of faintly yellow material beneath the RPE of the posterior pole. Histologic specimens show a lipid-containing deposit between the basement membrane of the RPE and the inner collagenous layers of the Bruch membrane that may impede transport and contribute to the pathogenesis. The gene for Sorsby dystrophy, *TIMP3* (on chromosome 22), codes for a tissue inhibitor of metalloproteinase, which is involved in extracellular matrix remodeling.

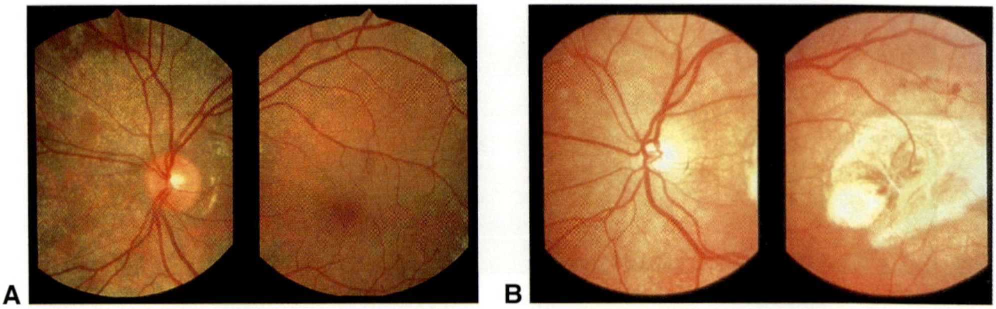

Figure 12-17 Color fundus photographs of Sorsby macular dystrophy. **A,** Characteristic pale drusen. **B,** Late disciform scarring after the development of choroidal neovascularization. *(Courtesy of Alan Bird, MD.)*

Choroidal Dystrophies

In several conditions, a primary retinal or RPE disease causes atrophy of the choriocapillaris. Historically, these conditions were named according to the clinically obvious choroidal involvement, but those names do not reflect current molecular knowledge.

Diffuse Degenerations

Choroideremia

Choroideremia is an X-linked chorioretinal dystrophy characterized by diffuse and progressive degeneration of the RPE and choriocapillaris (Fig 12-18). In affected males, the degeneration initially manifests as mottled areas of pigmentation in the anterior equatorial region and macula. The anterior areas gradually degenerate to confluent scalloped areas of RPE and choriocapillaris loss; larger choroidal vessels are preserved. Furthermore, the retinal vessels appear normal, and there is no optic atrophy. Patients have night blindness and show progressive peripheral visual field loss over 3–5 decades. Most patients maintain good visual acuity.

The fluorescein angiographic changes are pronounced; the scalloped areas of missing choriocapillaris appear hypofluorescent next to brightly hyperfluorescent areas of perfused choriocapillaris. Fundus autofluorescence shows hypoautofluorescence in the areas of atrophy, as well as a characteristic speckled pattern of autofluorescence in the nonatrophic areas. The ERG response is abnormal early in the course of the disease and is generally extinguished by midlife. The differential diagnosis of choroideremia includes gyrate atrophy (discussed in the next section), thioridazine hydrochloride retinal toxicity, and Bietti crystalline dystrophy.

The disease is caused by mutations in *CHM,* which is located at Xq21.2 and encodes for a geranylgeranyl transferase Rab escort protein. Histologic studies of choroideremia and studies of the localization of the *CHM* protein place the basic defect in the RPE, not in the choroid. Initial results from a phase 1/2 trial have demonstrated vision improvement in 5 of 6 patients treated with gene therapy. Carriers of X-linked choroideremia often show patches of subretinal black mottled pigment, and on occasion, older female carriers

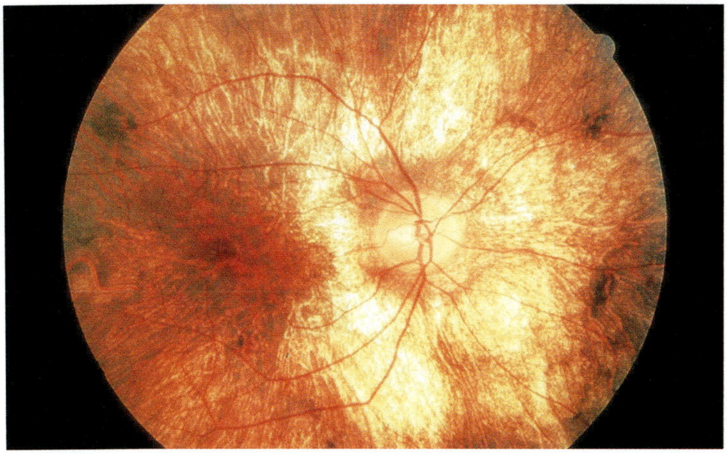

Figure 12-18 Fundus photograph of a patient with choroideremia. *(From Fishman GA, Birch DG, Holder GE, Brigell MG.* Electrophysiologic Testing in Disorders of the Retina, Optic Nerve, and Visual Pathways. *2nd ed. Ophthalmology Monograph 2. San Francisco: American Academy of Ophthalmology; 2001:67.)*

show a lobular pattern of choriocapillaris and RPE loss. Carriers of choroideremia are usually asymptomatic and have normal ERG signals.

MacLaren RE, Groppe M, Barnard AR, et al. Retinal gene therapy in patients with choroideremia: initial findings from a phase 1/2 clinical trial. *Lancet.* 2014;383(9923): 1129–1137.

Gyrate atrophy

Gyrate atrophy is an autosomal recessive dystrophy caused by mutations in the gene for ornithine aminotransferase *(OAT),* located on chromosome 10. The disorder is the result of a tenfold elevation in plasma levels of ornithine, which is toxic to the RPE and choroid. Patients with gyrate atrophy have hyperpigmented fundi, accompanied by lobular loss of the RPE and choroid. The finding of generalized hyperpigmentation of the remaining RPE helps distinguish gyrate atrophy clinically from choroideremia. In the early stages of the disease, patients have large, geographic, peripheral paving-stone–like areas of atrophy of the RPE and choriocapillaris, which gradually coalesce to form a characteristic scalloped border at the junction of normal and abnormal RPE (Fig 12-19). Night blindness usually develops during the first decade of life, and patients experience progressive loss of visual field and visual acuity later in the course of the disease. The clinical diagnosis can be confirmed by findings of elevated serum or plasma ornithine levels; molecular confirmation can be obtained by mutational analysis of *OAT.*

Regional and Central Choroidal Dystrophies

Several dystrophies show macular or regional choroidal degeneration. Most distinctive ophthalmoscopically are the central atrophies, which include *central areolar choroidal dystrophy* (CACD) and *North Carolina macular dystrophy,* both autosomal dominant disorders. Several genetic types of central choroidal dystrophy probably exist, with overlapping

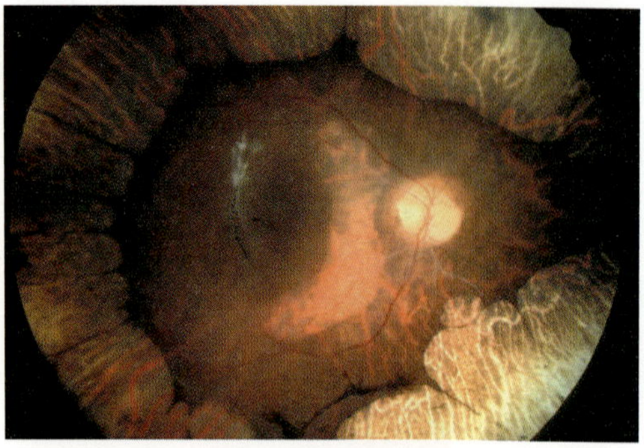

Figure 12-19 Gyrate atrophy. Wide-angle color fundus photograph showing scalloped edges of remaining posterior retina, as is typically seen in gyrate atrophy. A crescent of nasal macular atrophy is also present. *(Courtesy of Colin A. McCannel, MD.)*

clinical features. All are characterized by demarcated atrophy of the RPE and choriocapillaris in the macula and normal full-field ERG signals; however, there may be differences in onset and progression. The central atrophic lesions must be distinguished from those of acquired diseases such as toxoplasmosis and, in older patients, from age-related macular degeneration or late stages of other macular dystrophies that may cause a central round or bull's-eye pattern of RPE atrophy (see Table 12-2).

Young patients with CACD exhibit nonspecific mottled depigmentation within the macula that, over time, develops into a round or oval area of sharply demarcated geographic atrophy (Fig 12-20). Visual acuity typically stabilizes at approximately 20/200. Associated choroidal neovascularization rarely develops. Several mutations in *PRPH2,* each affecting an arginine residue, and a mutation in *GUCY2D* have been reported to cause autosomal dominant CACD.

North Carolina macular dystrophy begins in infancy with a cluster of peculiar yellowish-white lesions at the level of the RPE in the macula. These lesions tend to increase in number and become confluent; in some patients, they progress to severely atrophic macular lesions that can appear excavated or staphylomatous (Fig 12-21). Disease progression appears to stabilize in most patients by the early teenage years, and visual acuity is usually better than anticipated from the ophthalmoscopic appearance, typically ranging from 20/20 to 20/200. The gene responsible for this disease has been mapped to the long arm of chromosome 6.

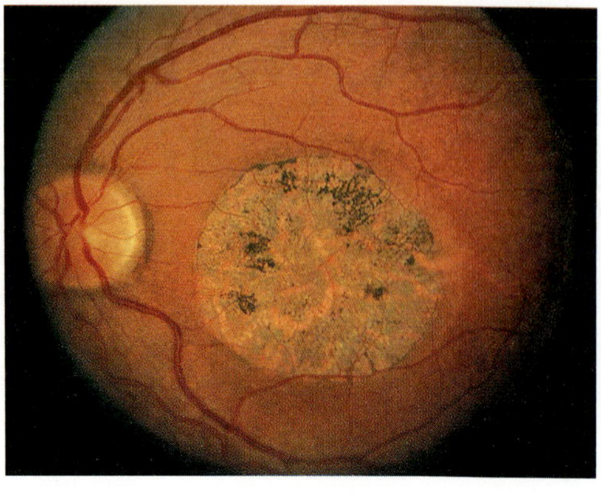

Figure 12-20 Color fundus photograph of central areolar choroidal dystrophy in a patient with autosomal dominant inheritance pattern. *(Courtesy of Mark W. Johnson, MD.)*

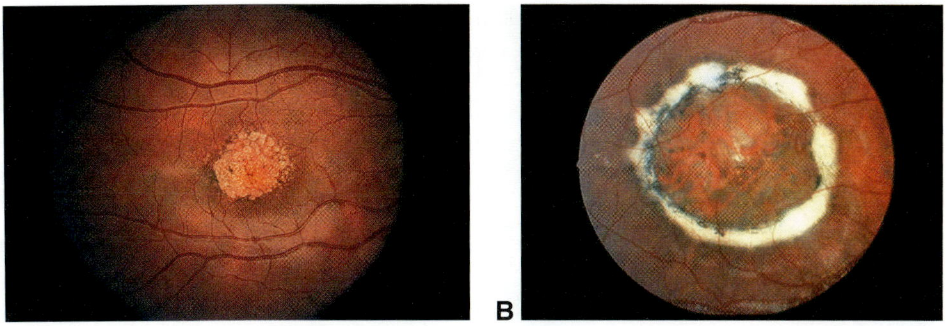

Figure 12-21 Color fundus photographs showing clinical variation in North Carolina macular dystrophy. **A,** Fundus of a 7-year-old patient with a cluster of peculiar yellowish-white atrophic lesions in the macula. **B,** Example of a severe, almost colobomatous, macular defect. *(Part A courtesy of Mark W. Johnson, MD; part B courtesy of Kent Small, MD.)*

Inner Retinal and Vitreoretinal Dystrophies

X-Linked Retinoschisis

Retinoschisis refers to a splitting of the neurosensory retina. The phenotype of *congenital X-linked retinoschisis* (XLRS) is somewhat variable, even within families. A common diagnostic feature, easily observed in pediatric patients, is foveal schisis, which appears as small, cystoid spaces and fine radial striae in the central macula (Fig 12-22), and is often best observed on fundus autofluorescence imaging. In severe cases with peripheral schisis, there may be extensive areas of inner retinal elevation resembling total or subtotal retinal detachment. A recent genotype–phenotype correlation study, the largest to date, identified other presenting signs, such as parafoveal white dots, and showed that schisis is occasionally absent on OCT imaging, even in molecularly confirmed disease. Central vision may initially be quite good, but with time, degeneration occurs and the visual acuity typically decreases to 20/200. Peripheral retinoschisis is not a constant feature and may occur in up to 50% of affected males. Histologic studies have shown that the splitting in peripheral XLRS occurs in the nerve fiber layer, whereas in degenerative retinoschisis, the level of splitting is variable and usually deeper within the retina (see Chapter 15). Pigmentary deposits may develop in peripheral areas destroyed by the disease process, so advanced cases of XLRS can be mistaken for RP. Boys with XLRS frequently present with vitreous hemorrhages from torn retinal vessels in areas of retinoschisis.

The panretinal involvement and inner retinal location of the disease are reflected in the ERG response, which has a negative waveform such that the a-wave is normal or near normal, but the b-wave is reduced (see Chapter 3, Fig 3-2). Negative waveforms of the dark-adapted, bright-flash ERG occur in diseases in which the inner retina is affected and the photoreceptors are generally unaffected (see Table 12-1).

The gene associated with XLRS, *RS1,* encodes an adhesion protein called *retinoschisin,* which localizes to all retinal neurons, beginning with ganglion cells in embryonic development. Presumably, retinoschisin is essential for Müller cell health because mutations in its coding cause Müller cell degeneration. Müller cells span the layers of the retina; their end plates form the inner limiting membrane, and their distal ends form the outer limiting

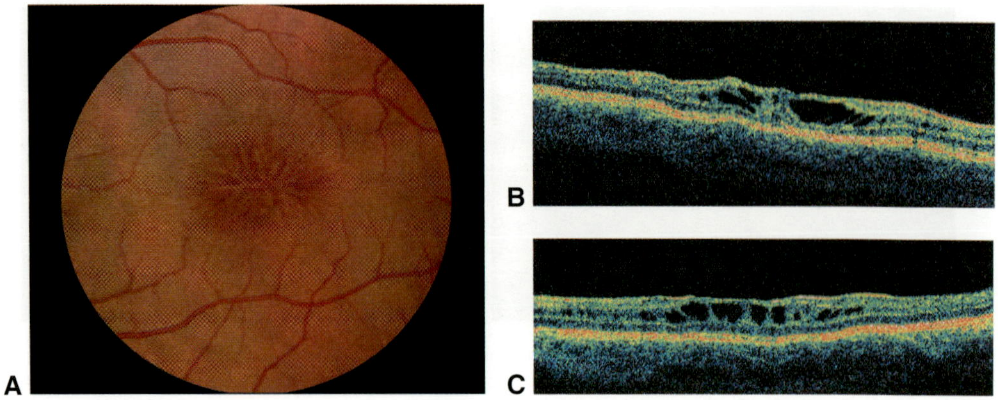

Figure 12-22 Juvenile retinoschisis. **A,** Color fundus photograph showing a characteristic pattern of macular schisis that is a more consistent finding than peripheral changes. Vertical **(B)** and horizontal **(C)** optical coherence tomography scans show schisis spaces in the middle layers of the macula. *(Courtesy of Mark W. Johnson, MD.)*

membrane between inner segments. Loss of this bridging cellular matrix protein appears to be key to the pathologic changes present in congenital retinoschisis.

American Academy of Ophthalmology. SmartSight website. Available at http://one.aao.org/smart-sight-low-vision. Accessed September 15, 2014.

Vincent A, Robson AG, Neveu MM, et al. A phenotype-genotype correlation study of X-linked retinoschisis. *Ophthalmology.* 2013;120(7):1454–1464.

Enhanced S-Cone Syndrome

Initially described in 1990, enhanced S-cone (or blue-cone) syndrome (ESCS, where "S" refers to short wavelength) is related to the Goldmann-Favre syndrome. Its most prominent features include night blindness, increased sensitivity to blue light, pigmentary retinal degeneration, an optically empty vitreous, pathognomonic ERG abnormalities, and varying degrees of peripheral to midperipheral visual field loss. The posterior pole may show round, yellow, sheenlike lesions along the arcades, accompanied by areas of diffuse degeneration. Deep nummular pigmentary deposition is usually observed at the level of the RPE around the vascular arcades; their presence may lead to an incorrect diagnosis of "atypical" RP. Macular (and sometimes peripheral) schisis may be present. The ERG response includes no detectable dim-flash, rod-specific signal; delayed and simplified responses to a brighter flash that have the same waveform under both dark-adapted and light-adapted conditions; and a flicker ERG response of lower amplitude than that of the single-flash photopic a-wave.

This autosomal recessive disorder results from mutations in *NR2E3,* which codes for a ligand-dependent transcription factor. There is evidence that the disorder is the result of abnormal cell-fate determination, leading to excess S cones at the expense of other photoreceptor subtypes.

Marmor MF, Jacobson SG, Foerster MH, Kellner U, Weleber RG. Diagnostic clinical findings of a new syndrome with night blindness, maculopathy, and enhanced S cone sensitivity. *Am J Ophthalmol.* 1990;110(2):124–134.

CHAPTER 13

Retinal Degenerations Associated With Systemic Disease

The retina is a highly complex neural tissue with large metabolic and oxidative demands. It can be affected by a host of systemic diseases and metabolic disorders. Important diagnostic and prognostic questions that arise in evaluating a patient who presents with retinal degeneration include the following:

- Is the degeneration hereditary or acquired?
- Is the condition stable or progressive?
- Can a precise diagnosis be made?

Optimal management, including genetic and other counseling, adequate support, and local and systemic therapy, is guided by an accurate diagnosis.

Retinal Degeneration With Systemic Involvement

Pigmentary retinopathy and retinal degenerations may be associated with a wide spectrum of genetic or acquired diseases. The term *pigmentary retinopathy* refers broadly to a panretinal disturbance of the retina and retinal pigment epithelium (RPE). Pigment deposits define most pigmentary retinopathies and typically present in the form of pigment clumps or spicules, but some diseases have a generalized depigmentation characterized by atrophy and little or no pigment deposition. This section summarizes some important examples of these disorders (Table 13-1).

Infantile-Onset to Early Childhood–Onset Syndromes

Any infant suspected of poor or declining vision when the eyes have clear media should be evaluated for retinal disease. If a severely diminished or extinguished electroretinogram (ERG) signal is present at birth, the clinician should first consider *Leber congenital amaurosis* (LCA) (also see Chapter 12). If the ERG signal is diminished and the changes are progressive, evaluation should include careful screening for congenital syndromes and metabolic disorders that affect the retina. Many of the metabolic syndromes and degenerations affecting the retina early in life show progressive vision deterioration from birth, and many are associated with pigmentary changes. Among the conditions that must be considered are the neuronal ceroid lipofuscinoses (Batten disease), peroxisome disorders such as Refsum disease, Zellweger (cerebrohepatorenal) syndrome, and neonatal

Table 13-1 Selected Systemic Diseases With Pigmentary Retinopathies

Disorder	Features
Autosomal dominant disorders	
Arteriohepatic dysplasia (Alagille syndrome)	Intrahepatic cholestatic syndrome, posterior embryotoxon, Axenfeld anomaly, congenital heart disease, flattened facies and bridge of nose, bony abnormalities, myopia, pigmentary retinopathy
Charcot-Marie-Tooth disease	Pigmentary retinopathy, degeneration of lateral horn of spinal cord, optic atrophy
Myotonic dystrophy (Steinert disease)	Muscle wasting, "Christmas tree" cataract, retinal degeneration, pattern dystrophy or reticular degeneration; ERG subnormal to abnormal
Oculodentodigital dysplasia syndrome	Thin nose with hypoplastic alae, narrow nostrils, abnormality of fourth and fifth fingers, hypoplastic dental enamel, congenital cataract, colobomas
Olivopontocerebellar atrophy	Retinal degeneration (peripheral and/or macular), cerebellar ataxia, possible external ophthalmoplegia
Stickler syndrome (arthro-ophthalmopathy)	Progressive myopia with myopic retinal degeneration, arthropathy including joint hypermobility and arthritis, midfacial hypoplasia, high arched or cleft palate, bifid uvula; retinal detachment common; ERG subnormal to abnormal
Waardenburg syndrome	Hypertelorism, wide bridge of nose, cochlear deafness, white forelock, heterochromia iridis, poliosis, pigment disturbance of RPE, choroidal vitiligo; ERG normal to subnormal
Wagner hereditary vitreoretinal degeneration	Narrowed and sheathed retinal vessels, pigmented spots in the retinal periphery and along retinal vessels, choroidal atrophy and optic atrophy, extensive liquefaction and membranous condensation of vitreous body; subnormal ERG; overlapping features with Stickler syndrome
Autosomal recessive disorders	
Bardet-Biedl syndrome	Pigmentary retinopathy, bull's-eye maculopathy, mild cognitive disabilities, polydactyly, obesity, hypogenitalism, progressive visual field loss; ERG severely diminished to undetectable
Bietti crystalline dystrophy	Yellow-white crystals scattered in posterior pole, round subretinal pigment deposits, confluent loss of RPE and choriocapillaris on fluorescein angiogram, possible crystals in limbal cornea
Spinocerebellar degeneration	Ataxia, limb incoordination, nerve deafness, maculopathy, retinal degeneration, optic atrophy
Homocystinuria	Fine pigmentary or cystic degeneration of retina, marfanoid appearance, myopia, lens subluxation or dislocation, cardiovascular abnormalities (thromboses), glaucoma, cognitive disabilities
Mannosidosis	Macroglossia, flat nose, large head and ears, skeletal abnormalities, possible hepatosplenomegaly, storage material in retina; resembles Hurler syndrome
Mucopolysaccharidosis type I H (Hurler syndrome)	Early corneal clouding, gargoyle facies, deafness, cognitive disabilities, dwarfism, skeletal abnormalities, hepatosplenomegaly, optic atrophy; subnormal ERG

Disorder	Features
Mucopolysaccharidosis type I S (Scheie syndrome)	Coarse facies, aortic regurgitation, stiff joints, early clouding of the cornea, normal life span, normal intellect, pigmentary retinopathy
Mucopolysaccharidosis type III (Sanfilippo syndrome)	Milder somatic stigmata than in Hurler syndrome, but severe pigmentary retinopathy
Neonatal adrenoleukodystrophy	Pigmentary retinopathy, optic atrophy, seizures, hypotonia, adrenal cortical atrophy, psychomotor impairment; extinguished ERG
Neuronal ceroid lipofuscinoses (Batten disease)	Haltia-Santavuori, onset 8–18 months with rapid deterioration, fine granular inclusions Jansky-Bielschowsky, onset 2–4 years, rapid CNS deterioration, curvilinear body inclusions Lake-Cavanagh, onset 4–6 years, ataxia, dementia, curvilinear and fingerprint inclusions Spielmeyer-Vogt-Batten, onset 6–8 years, slowly progressive, fingerprint inclusions, bull's-eye maculopathy
Refsum disease	Elevations of phytanic acid, pigmentary retinopathy, optic atrophy, partial deafness, cerebellar ataxia, ichthyosis
Usher syndrome	Congenital deafness (profound or partial), pigmentary retinopathy
Zellweger (cerebrohepatorenal) syndrome	Muscular hypotonia, high forehead and hypertelorism, hepatomegaly, deficient cerebral myelination, nystagmus, cataract, microphthalmia, retinal degeneration; undetectable ERG
X-linked recessive pigmentary retinopathies	
Incontinentia pigmenti (Bloch-Sulzberger syndrome)	Skin pigmentation in lines and whorls, alopecia, dental anomalies, optic atrophy, falciform folds, cataract, nystagmus, strabismus, patchy mottling of fundi, conjunctival pigmentation
Mucopolysaccharidosis type II (Hunter syndrome)	Little corneal clouding, mild clinical course; onset of signs age 2–4 years: full lips, large rounded cheeks, broad nose, enlarged tongue (macroglossia), cognitive disabilities, pigmentary retinopathy; subnormal ERG; over time, voice changes from vocal cord enlargement; possible airway obstruction from airway narrowing
Pelizaeus-Merzbacher disease	Infantile progressive leukodystrophy, cerebellar ataxia, limb spasticity, cognitive impairment, possible pigmentary retinopathy with absent foveal reflex
Mitochondrial disorders	
Kearns-Sayre syndrome; maternally inherited diabetes and deafness (MIDD); mitochondrial encephalopathy, lactic acidosis, strokelike episodes (MELAS)	Progressive external ophthalmoplegia, ptosis, pigmentary retinopathy and/or macular atrophy, heart block (Kearns-Sayre syndrome); ERG normal to abnormal

CNS = central nervous system; ERG = electroretinogram; RPE = retinal pigment epithelium.

Data from Rimoin DL, Connor JM, Pyeritz RE, Korf BR, eds. *Emery and Rimoin's Principles and Practice of Medical Genetics*. 3 vols. 4th ed. New York: Churchill Livingstone; 2002:chap 137.

adrenoleukodystrophy. The presence or development of seizures and a deterioration of neurologic and mental function may suggest systemic syndromes. Commonly, poor eyesight is initially blamed for the declining cognitive and neuromuscular skills until the metabolic disorder is eventually diagnosed.

den Hollander AI, Roepman R, Koenekoop RK, Cremers FP. Leber congenital amaurosis: genes, proteins and disease mechanisms. *Prog Retin Eye Res.* 2008:27(4):391–419.

Bardet-Biedl Syndrome

The *Bardet-Biedl syndrome* comprises several different diseases with a similar constellation of findings, including pigmentary retinopathy (with or without pigment deposits), obesity, polydactyly, hypogonadism, and cognitive disability. These disorders were previously classified as autosomal recessive, but molecular studies strongly suggest that many are multigenic, with 2 or even 3 different mutations contributing to the phenotype. Studies have identified at least 18 causative genes, which are present in approximately 75% of affected families. Increasing evidence suggests that the primary functions of the proteins affected in Bardet-Biedl syndrome are to mediate and regulate microtubule-based intracellular transport processes; therefore, the syndrome is a ciliopathy. Other retinal ciliopathies resulting from genetic mutations causing retinal and systemic ciliary dysfunction include Alström, Senior-Løken, Joubert, Jeune, and the various Usher syndromes.

Patients with Bardet-Biedl syndrome typically demonstrate a severe form of rod–cone dystrophy, usually sine pigmento, with a bull's-eye atrophic maculopathy (Fig 13-1); however, a wide spectrum of retinal disease severity is observed, even within a single genotype. Affected patients are most easily recognized by obesity and a history or presence of

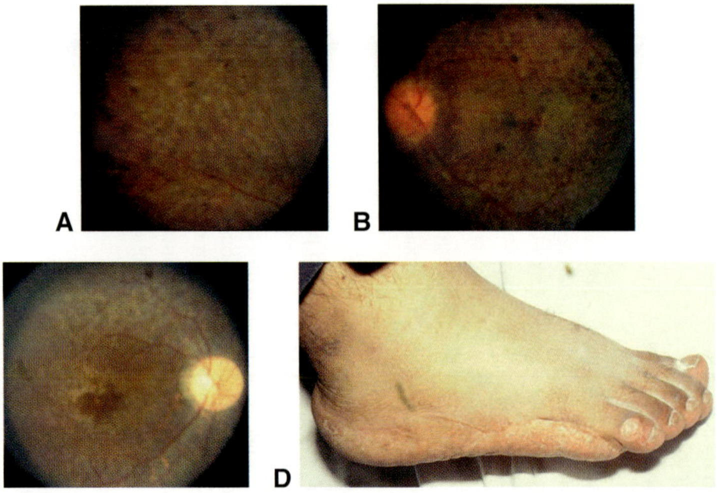

Figure 13-1 Bardet-Biedl syndrome. **A, B,** Color fundus photographs showing pigmentary alterations in the periphery and macula. **C,** Color fundus photograph of the sibling, demonstrating similar macular changes. **D,** Clinical photograph of a patient's foot with 6 toes (polydactyly). *(Courtesy of David Sarraf, MD.)*

polydactyly. It may be necessary to inspect feet or hands for evidence of extra digit excision. The hands often appear puffy, making knuckles indistinct. Because these patients tend to have severe retinopathy and cognitive disabilities, clinicians should devote extra attention to supporting the parents in their efforts to obtain special educational support.

Blacque OE, Leroux MR. Bardet-Biedl syndrome: an emerging pathomechanism of intracellular transport. *Cell Mol Life Sci.* 2006;63(18):2145–2161.

M'hamdi O, Ouertani I, Chaabouni-Bouhamed H. Update on the genetics of Bardet-Biedl syndrome. *Mol Syndromol.* 2014;5(2):51–56.

Hearing Loss and Pigmentary Retinopathy: Usher Syndrome

Usher syndrome is the most common name used to describe the association of retinitis pigmentosa (RP) with congenital sensorineural hearing loss, whether partial or profound. This disease was first described in 1906 by Charles Usher, a British ophthalmologist. Although some patients with RP become deaf in later adult years, this acquired deafness is not classified as Usher syndrome. Both the profound (type 1) and partial (type 2) forms show autosomal recessive inheritance and tend to be stable throughout adult life. Ophthalmologists should recognize patients with RP who present with nasal speech or wear hearing aids; these traits are suggestive of Usher syndrome type 2. Slowly progressive deafness has been identified in one subgroup of patients with Usher syndrome; these patients have mutations in *USH3A,* which is a gene encoding clarin-1, a transmembrane protein with a possible role in hair cell and photoreceptor synapses. The hearing level of most Usher patients is typically stable over time, however.

Currently, there are 11 subtypes of Usher types 1 and 2 for which the chromosome location is known; of these, 9 have cloned genes. The proteins encoded by these genes are part of a dynamic protein complex present in the cilia of the inner ear and in the cone outer segments of the photoreceptor cells of the retina. For example, Usher type 2A is caused by mutations in the gene for *usherin* (at 1q41), which encodes a basement-membrane protein found in many tissues, including structural basement membranes in the retina and inner ear. Usher type 1B is caused by defective myosin, a common component of cilia and microvilli. This finding is intriguing because photoreceptors are modified ciliated cells, and cilia are also sensory structures for otologic function. Usher type 1C is caused by mutations in the *harmonin* gene, which encodes a protein expressed in inner ear sensory hair cells.

The exact incidence of Usher syndrome has been difficult to determine, but surveys of patients with RP suggest that approximately 10% have profound deafness, and ophthalmic examinations of children in schools for the deaf reveal that approximately 6% have RP. The prevalence of Usher syndrome is thought to be 3 cases per 100,000 persons.

In addition to Usher syndrome, other genetic conditions and environmental insults may lead to pigmentary retinopathy and hearing loss; these include Alport, Alström, Cockayne, and Hurler syndromes; dysplasia spondyloepiphysaria congenita; Refsum disease; and congenital rubella. By careful study of individual patients and families, clinicians can diagnose Usher syndrome with relative certainty. Molecular testing for specific forms of Usher syndrome can help confirm the diagnosis.

Kremer H, van Wijk E, Märker T, Wolfrum U, Roepman R. Usher syndrome: molecular links of pathogenesis, proteins and pathways. *Hum Mol Genet.* 2006;15(Spec No 2):R262–R270.

Neuromuscular Disorders

Pigmentary retinopathy associated with complex neuromuscular pathology is present in a variety of disorders, including some spinocerebellar degenerations, some forms of olivopontocerebellar atrophies, Charcot-Marie-Tooth disease, myotonic dystrophy, neuronal ceroid lipofuscinoses (Batten disease), progressive external ophthalmoplegia syndromes, and peroxisome disorders (Zellweger syndrome, Refsum disease, and neonatal adrenoleukodystrophy) (see Table 13-1). Mitochondrial, autosomal dominant, and autosomal recessive inheritance patterns are all found in this group of disorders. These neurologic conditions vary widely in age of onset and retinal findings, and the ophthalmologist normally makes the diagnosis in collaboration with a neurologist or medical geneticist. The roles of the ophthalmologist are to confirm the pigmentary retinopathy and assist in the visual rehabilitation of the patient. The ERG abnormalities found in these neurologic disorders only confirm the presence of retinopathy but are not diagnostic for any one disorder.

Although *Duchenne muscular dystrophy* does not cause a pigmentary retinopathy, it deserves mention because the ERG signal shows a negative waveform similar to that found in patients with congenital stationary night blindness (CSNB)—specifically, a normal a-wave but a reduced b-wave (see Chapters 3 and 11). This ERG response suggests a defective "on-response" pathway, but patients with this disorder do not have night blindness. Interestingly, Duchenne muscular dystrophy is caused by mutations in the gene for *dystrophin,* a protein that is abundant in muscle but also found in neural synaptic regions and in the retina. Rarely, Duchenne muscular dystrophy can be associated with a proliferative retinopathy similar to proliferative diabetic retinopathy.

Barboni MT, Nagy BV, de Araújo Moura AL, et al. ON and OFF electroretinography and contrast sensitivity in Duchenne muscular dystrophy. *Invest Ophthalmol Vis Sci.* 2013;54(5):3195–3204.

Other Organ System Disorders

Most retinopathies associated with other organ systems are rare and genetic, and clinicians may find the Online Mendelian Inheritance in Man website (www.omim.org) useful in recognizing them. Collaboration with pediatric and medical geneticists is often required to identify rare candidate diseases.

Renal diseases

Several forms of congenital renal disease may be associated with retinal degeneration. *Familial juvenile nephronophthisis* is one of the family of renal-retinal dysplasia (and ciliopathy) characterized by autosomal recessive inheritance and childhood onset of end-stage renal disease. Senior-Løken and Joubert syndromes can be complicated by an early form of RP with an extinguished ERG signal and severe annular constriction. Joubert syndrome is notable for cerebellar malformation (a characteristic "molar tooth" deformity on magnetic resonance imaging of the brain) and can also be associated with chorioretinal coloboma. Patients with the Bardet-Biedl syndrome commonly have urethral reflux with pyelonephritis and kidney damage, whereas patients with Alström syndrome, another retinal ciliopathy, may demonstrate obesity, short stature, and cardiomyopathy in addition to renal disease. Jeune syndrome is an interesting retinal ciliopathy that is complicated by cystic kidney disease and asphyxiating thoracic dystrophy.

Liver disease

Patients with Alagille syndrome present with hepatorenal abnormalities including cholestatic jaundice and have several characteristic ocular findings, including posterior embryotoxin and pigmentary retinopathy, that can have a peripapillary and macular predilection. There have been 230 different mutations in the *JAG1* gene attributed to this syndrome.

Gastrointestinal disease

Familial adenomatous polyposis (FAP, also known as *Gardner syndrome*) is associated with pigmented lesions that are similar to those in congenital hypertrophy of the RPE. The lesions in FAP, however, are smaller, ovoid, more variegated, and typically multiple and bilateral. More than 4 widely spaced, small (<0.5-disc-diameter) lesions per eye and bilateral involvement suggest FAP. Note that congenital grouped pigmentation ("bear tracks") is not associated with FAP. Caused by mutations in the adenomatous polyposis gene *(APC),* FAP has an autosomal dominant inheritance pattern with incomplete expression. The pigmented retinal lesions constitute an important marker for identifying family members at risk of colonic polyps, which have a high malignant potential.

Dermatologic diseases

Ichthyosis, comprising abnormal scaling, dryness, and tightness of the skin, may be found in conjunction with the pigmentary retinopathy of Refsum disease and the crystalline maculopathy of Sjögren-Larsson syndrome. *Incontinentia pigmenti (Bloch-Sulzberger syndrome)* is a rare, X-linked disorder presenting only in females as the mutation is lethal in males. It is characterized by streaky skin lesions and abnormalities of the teeth and central nervous system (CNS). Ocular involvement occurs in approximately one-third of affected females and includes pigmentary abnormalities as well as peripheral retinal nonperfusion and neovascularization that may cause tractional and cicatricial retinal detachment (also see BCSC Section 6, *Pediatric Ophthalmology and Strabismus*). *Pseudoxanthoma elasticum* is associated with a "plucked-chicken" skin appearance, peripapillary angioid streaks, and a *peau d'orange* fundus appearance (see Chapter 4).

Holmström G, Thorén K. Ocular manifestations of incontinentia pigmenti. *Acta Ophthalmol Scand.* 2000;78(3):348–353.

Traboulsi EI. Ocular manifestations of familial adenomatous polyposis (Gardner syndrome). *Ophthalmol Clin North Am.* 2005;18(1):163–166.

Dental disease

Amelogenesis imperfecta is a genetic disease causing abnormalities in dentition development resulting from defective enamel production. When associated with a cone–rod dystrophy this condition is referred to as *Jalili syndrome* and has a wide range of clinical retinal manifestations, including macular coloboma and pigmentary retinopathy.

Paraneoplastic and Autoimmune Retinopathies

Occasionally, retinal degeneration is a complication of cancer by a paraneoplastic immunologic mechanism. BCSC Section 9, *Intraocular Inflammation and Uveitis,* explains the role of the immune system in this process. The 2 main paraneoplastic retinopathy syndromes are (1) *cancer-associated retinopathy* (CAR) and (2) *melanoma-associated retinopathy* (MAR). A third entity, *autoimmune retinopathy,* refers to an acquired, presumed immunologically mediated, retinal degeneration resembling paraneoplastic retinopathy but without any identifiable systemic malignancy.

The 23-kDa protein recoverin was the first retinal protein for which systemic antibodies were detected in CAR; it is also the most specific for that disease. Studies have since identified antibodies against many other retinal proteins, including enolase, arrestin, transducin, and neurofilament protein.

Patients with CAR and antirecoverin antibodies typically experience rapidly progressive loss of peripheral and central vision, often accompanied by photopsias and a ring scotoma. Fundus examination shows arterial narrowing typically unassociated with significant pigment spiculation (Fig 13-2). Late in the course of disease, pigmentary alterations at the level of the RPE can occur. Whereas the ERG signal is severely reduced (for a- and b-waves) or extinguished in CAR, electronegative waveforms have been associated with MAR. Paraneoplastic and autoimmune retinopathies associated with antienolase antibodies are characterized predominantly by cone dysfunction, a slow progression of central vision loss, and eventual optic disc pallor.

The loss of retinal function may precede clinical recognition of the cancer. Therefore, any late-onset, rapidly progressive retinal dysfunction should raise suspicion of an

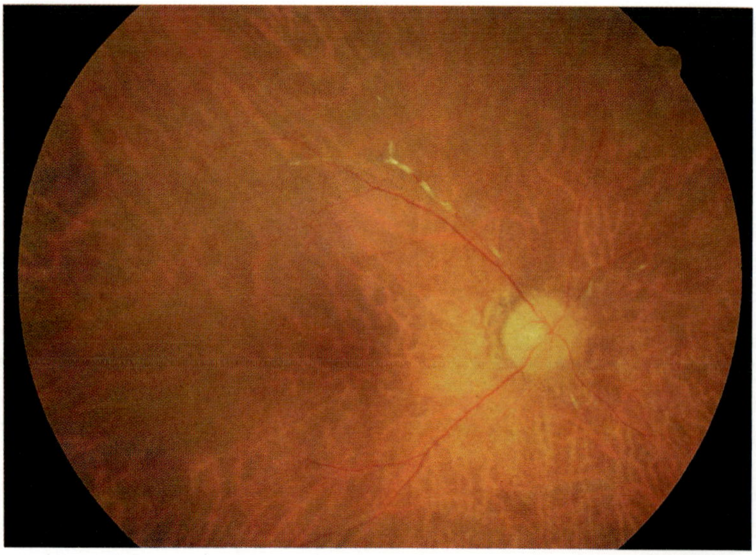

Figure 13-2 Color fundus photograph of cancer-associated retinopathy (CAR) in a patient with ovarian carcinoma. Note the severe vascular attenuation without obvious pigmentary alterations. *(Courtesy of John R. Heckenlively, MD.)*

underlying malignancy causing an autoimmune retinopathy. Management of these disorders involves systemic immunosuppression or local steroid therapy.

Other paraneoplastic syndromes with retinal findings have been reported. *Bilateral diffuse uveal melanocytic proliferation* (BDUMP) is characterized by multiple melanocytic lesions of the choroid that may be associated with rapidly progressive posterior subcapsular cataract, iris and ciliary body cysts, and exudative retinal detachment. BDUMP has been associated with various systemic malignancies (see Chapter 9). *Acute exudative polymorphous vitelliform maculopathy,* characterized by multiple waxing and waning subretinal vitelliform lesions, has been reported in association with metastatic melanoma and other systemic malignancies.

Rahimy E, Sarraf D. Paraneoplastic and non-paraneoplastic retinopathy and optic neuropathy: evaluation and management. *Surv Ophthalmol.* 2013;58(5);430–458.

Weleber RG, Watzke RC, Shults WT, et al. Clinical and electrophysiologic characterization of paraneoplastic and autoimmune retinopathies associated with antienolase antibodies. *Am J Ophthalmol.* 2005;139(5):780–794.

Metabolic Diseases

In evaluating patients with retinal degeneration, it is important to consider metabolic diseases, although detailed descriptions of the many metabolic disorders with retinal manifestations is beyond the scope of this chapter. Some disorders, such as albinism and conditions associated with CNS abnormalities, are covered more fully in BCSC Section 6, *Pediatric Ophthalmology and Strabismus.* Other metabolic disorders, such as abetalipoproteinemia and Refsum disease, are among the differential diagnostic concerns for RP, even though their retinopathy may be granular and atypical.

Albinism

Albinism includes a group of different genetic abnormalities in which the synthesis of melanin is reduced or absent. The current classification scheme is based on the gene mutation, replacing the older terminology of complete versus partial and tyrosinase-positive versus tyrosinase-negative disorders. When the reduction in melanin biosynthesis affects the eyes, skin, and hair follicles, the disease is called *oculocutaneous albinism.* These disorders usually have an autosomal recessive inheritance pattern. If the skin and hair appear normally pigmented and only the ocular pigmentation is clinically affected, the condition is called *ocular albinism.* Ocular albinism typically has an X-linked inheritance pattern. Female carriers of X-linked ocular albinism may show partial iris transillumination and fundus pigment mosaicism. Genetic counseling includes careful determination of the inheritance pattern and molecular testing as appropriate.

Regardless of the type of albinism, ocular involvement generally conforms to 1 of 2 clinical patterns: (1) congenitally subnormal visual acuity (typically 20/100–20/400) and nystagmus or (2) normal or minimally reduced visual acuity without nystagmus. The first pattern is true albinism; the second has been termed *albinoidism* because of its milder visual consequences. Both patterns share the clinical features of photophobia, iris transillumination, and hypopigmented fundi. They differ according to whether or not the fovea develops normally; in true albinism, the fovea is hypoplastic, with no foveal pit or reflex and no evident luteal pigment (Fig 13-3). The gold standard for diagnosis of true albinism is the finding of characteristic abnormalities of the flash and pattern visual evoked potentials (VEPs). Compared with a normal symmetric response, in albinism, a single eye stimulation will result in an asymmetric occipital response because there is a greater number of decussating fibers.

In childhood, all patients with *oculocutaneous albinism* appear similarly hypopigmented. However, with age, patients with tyrosinase-positive forms gradually accumulate more pigment and exhibit a slow darkening of the skin, hair, and irides that occurs over many years. In general, the more pigmentation the patient demonstrates, such as around hair follicles and in the RPE in the posterior pole, the better the visual prognosis. Many patients have improved nystagmus and visual acuity as pigmentation increases.

It is important for the clinician to be aware of 2 forms of oculocutaneous albinism with potentially lethal systemic implications. The first, *Chédiak-Higashi syndrome,* combines albinism with neutropenia and an extreme susceptibility to infections as well as other complications such as bleeding (caused by deficient platelets) that can cause childhood or adolescent mortality. The second, *Hermansky-Pudlak syndrome,* is characterized by a platelet defect that causes easy bruising and bleeding. In the United States, most patients with Hermansky-Pudlak syndrome are of Puerto Rican descent. If either of these 2 types of albinism is suspected, hematologic consultation is imperative.

King RA, Jackson IJ, Oetting WS. Human albinism and mouse models. In: Wright AF, Jay B, eds. *Molecular Genetics of Inherited Eye Disorders.* Chur, Switzerland: Harwood Academic; 1994:89–122.

Central Nervous System Metabolic Abnormalities

A wide range of fundus changes, from pigmentary retinopathy to a cherry-red spot, may be associated with inherited metabolic diseases known to affect the CNS and retina. Although a comprehensive description is beyond the scope of this chapter, the following discussion includes some of the major conditions (see Table 13-1). See BCSC Section 6,

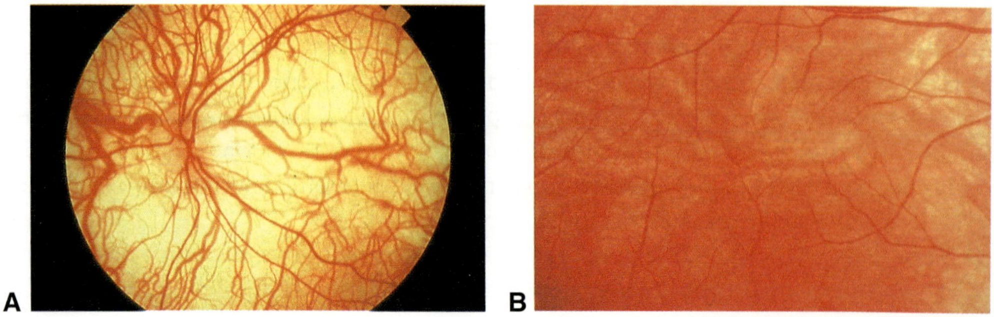

Figure 13-3 Albinism. **A,** Color fundus photograph showing generalized fundus hypopigmentation. **B,** High-magnification color fundus photograph showing foveal hypoplasia. No foveal reflex or luteal pigment is evident. *(Courtesy of Carl D. Regillo, MD.)*

Pediatric Ophthalmology and Strabismus, for a listing of the ocular findings in inborn errors of metabolism.

Neuronal ceroid lipofuscinoses

The neuronal ceroid lipofuscinoses (NCLs) are a group of autosomal recessive diseases caused by the accumulation of waxy lipopigments (eg, ceroid and lipofuscin) within the lysosomes of neurons and other cells, leading to cellular dysfunction and death, possibly by apoptosis. These disorders are characterized by progressive dementia, seizures, and loss of vision associated with a pigmentary retinopathy in early-onset cases. The diagnosis is made clinically and by demonstrating characteristic curvilinear, fingerprint-like, or granular inclusions on electron microscopy of a peripheral blood smear or biopsy of conjunctival or other tissue.

Several types of NCLs have been described, partly on the basis of the age of symptom onset. To date, more than 12 genes and more than 400 mutations underlying human NCLs have been identified, but there remain disease subgroups whose molecular genetics are unknown. The infantile and juvenile types are associated with pigmentary retinopathies (see Table 13-1):

- infantile NCL (Haltia-Santavuori disease), onset between 8 and 18 months of age
- late-infantile NCL (Jansky-Bielschowsky disease), onset between 2 and 4 years of age
- early-juvenile NCL (Lake-Cavanagh disease), onset between 4 and 6 years of age
- juvenile NCL (Spielmeyer-Vogt-Batten disease), onset between 6 and 8 years of age

Ocular findings in infantile NCL include optic atrophy; macular pigmentary changes, including bull's-eye atrophic maculopathy, mottling of the fundus periphery, and retinal vascular attenuation; and reduced or absent ERG signals (Fig 13-4). Retinal changes in the infantile forms may make the disorder difficult to distinguish from LCA. The 2 adult forms of NCL do not have ocular manifestations.

Abetalipoproteinemia and vitamin A deficiency

Abetalipoproteinemia is an autosomal recessive disorder in which apolipoprotein B is not synthesized, which causes fat malabsorption, fat-soluble vitamin deficiencies, and retinal and spinocerebellar degeneration. Red blood cells show acanthocytosis. Supplementation

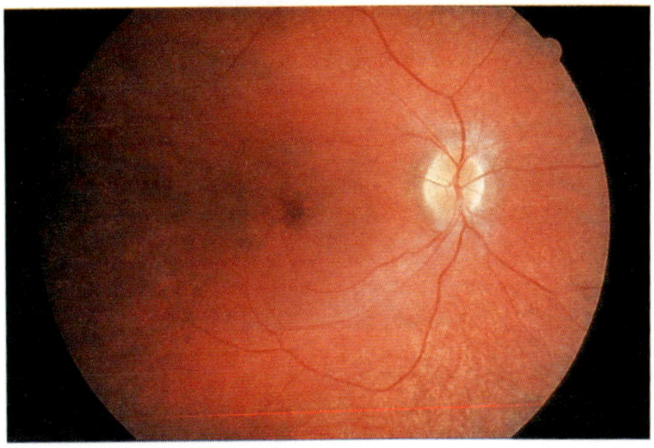

Figure 13-4 Batten disease (juvenile neuronal ceroid lipofuscinosis). Color fundus photograph showing optic atrophy, retinal vascular attenuation, and peripheral pigmentary loss. *(Courtesy of Elias Traboulsi, MD.)*

with vitamins A and E is needed to prevent or ameliorate the retinal degeneration. Testing for vitamin A levels is useful diagnostically in these and other retinopathies.

The most common form of vitamin A deficiency retinopathy occurs in patients who have undergone gastric bypass surgery for obesity or small-bowel resection for Crohn disease. These patients have malabsorption of fat-soluble vitamins and may develop a blind loop syndrome, in which an overgrowth of bacteria consumes vitamin A. Patients experience nyctalopia, and if the condition remains untreated, eventually demonstrate vision loss and diffuse, drusenlike spots similar to those observed in retinitis punctata albescens. Before retinal degeneration develops, the condition can be fully reversed with vitamin A supplementation.

Peroxisomal disorders and Refsum disease

The peroxisomal disorders are mostly autosomal recessive diseases caused by the dysfunction or absence of peroxisomes or peroxisomal enzymes. The biochemical hallmarks are defective oxidation and accumulation of very long chain fatty acids. *Zellweger syndrome* is the prototype of peroxisomal diseases. Severe infantile-onset retinal degeneration is associated with hypotonia, psychomotor impairment, seizures, characteristic facies, renal cysts, and hepatic interstitial fibrosis. Death usually occurs in infancy. Patients with *neonatal adrenoleukodystrophy* also present in infancy but generally survive until age 7–10 years (Fig 13-5).

Similar but less severe findings are present in *infantile Refsum disease,* in which the serum phytanic acid level is elevated. Sometimes not diagnosed until adulthood, Refsum disease is characterized by pigmentary retinopathy with reduced or extinguished ERG signals, cerebellar ataxia, polyneuropathy, anosmia, hearing loss, and cardiomyopathy. Nyctalopia may be an early symptom. Diagnosis is made by demonstrating elevated plasma levels of phytanic acid or reduced phytanic acid oxidase activity in cultured fibroblasts. Dietary restriction of phytanic acid precursors may slow or stabilize the neuropathy but typically not the retinal degeneration.

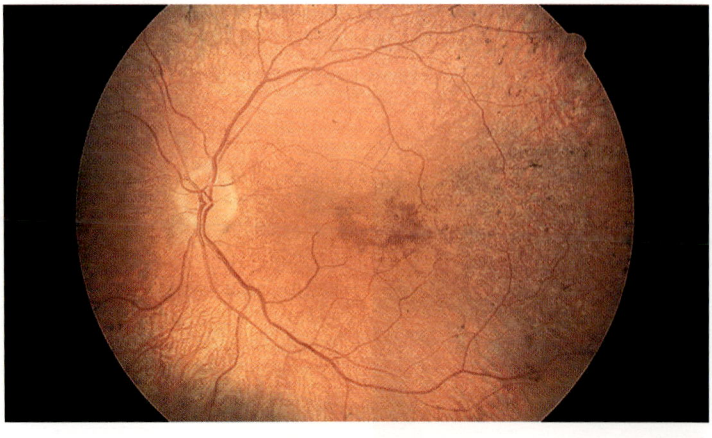

Figure 13-5 Neonatal adrenoleukodystrophy. Color fundus photograph showing retinal arteriolar attenuation, diffuse pigmentary alterations, and mild optic atrophy. *(Courtesy of Mark W. Johnson, MD.)*

Mucopolysaccharidoses

The systemic *mucopolysaccharidoses* (MPSs) are caused by inherited defects in catabolic lysosomal enzymes that degrade the glycosaminoglycans dermatan sulfate, keratan sulfate, and heparan sulfate. Consequently, excessive quantities of incompletely metabolized acid mucopolysaccharides, complex lipids, or both are stored in lysosomes. The MPSs are transmitted as autosomal recessive traits except for type II, an X-linked recessive disorder (see Table 13-1).

Only MPSs in which heparan sulfate is stored are associated with retinal dystrophy. These include MPS type I H *(Hurler syndrome)* and MPS type I S *(Scheie syndrome),* the clinical features of which include coarse facies, cognitive disabilities, corneal clouding, and retinal degeneration. The retinal pigmentary changes may be subtle, but the ERG response is abnormal. MPS type II *(Hunter syndrome)* also features pigmentary retinopathy but not corneal clouding; patients have coarse facies and short stature and may show cognitive disabilities. MPS type III *(Sanfilippo syndrome)* shows mild somatic stigmata but severe pigmentary retinopathy.

Other lysosomal metabolic disorders

Tay-Sachs disease (GM_2 gangliosidosis type I), caused by a deficient subunit A of hexosaminidase A, is the most common ganglioside storage disease. Glycolipid accumulation in the brain and retina causes cognitive disability and blindness, and death generally occurs between the ages of 2 and 5 years. Ganglion cells surrounding the fovea become filled with ganglioside and appear grayish or white, causing a cherry-red spot (Fig 13-6). *Sandhoff disease* (GM_2 gangliosidosis type II) and *generalized gangliosidosis* (GM_1 gangliosidosis type I) can also show cherry-red spots.

The chronic nonneuronopathic adult form of *Gaucher disease* does not have cerebral involvement. This disease is characterized by large accumulations of glucosylceramide in

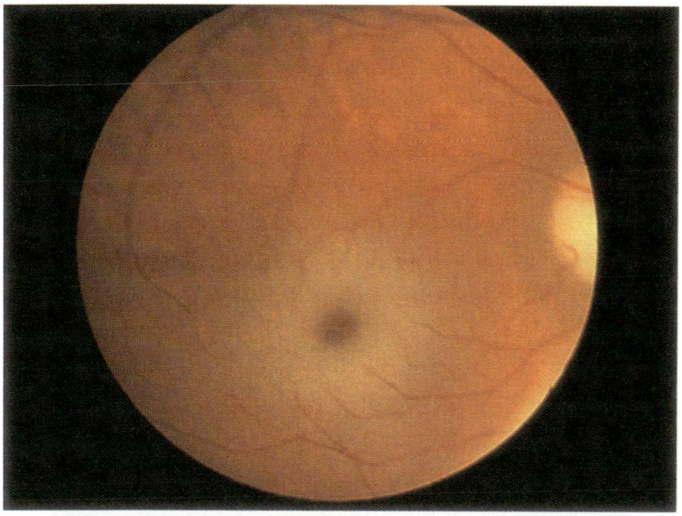

Figure 13-6 Tay-Sachs disease. Color fundus photograph showing a cherry-red spot.

the liver, spleen, lymph nodes, skin, and bone marrow. Some patients have a cherry-red spot; others show whitish superficial lesions in the midperiphery of the fundus. Spectral-domain optical coherence tomography (SD-OCT) analysis demonstrates multiple characteristic hyperreflective lesions located along the retinal surface.

The various types of *Niemann-Pick disease* are caused by the absence of different sphingomyelinase isoenzymes. Type B (chronic) Niemann-Pick disease, also known as *sea-blue histiocyte syndrome,* is the mildest, and although there is no functional involvement of the CNS, patients have a macular halo that is considered diagnostic (Fig 13-7). Type A (acute neuronopathic) Niemann-Pick disease shows a cherry-red spot in about 50% of cases.

Cherry-red spots are also observed in sialidoses and galactosialidoses. These conditions include mucolipidosis type I, the cherry-red spot–myoclonus syndrome, and Goldberg-Cotlier syndrome (GM_1 gangliosidosis type IV). Mucolipidosis type IV causes diffuse retinal degeneration.

Fabry disease (angiokeratoma corporis diffusum) is an X-linked condition caused by mutations in the gene encoding alpha-galactosidase A. Ceramide trihexoside accumulates in the smooth muscle of blood vessels in the kidneys, skin, gastrointestinal tract, CNS, heart, and reticuloendothelial system, leading to various ocular and systemic clinical findings. The first symptom may be burning paresthesias or pain in the extremities in late childhood. Ocular signs include corneal verticillata (whorls), tortuous conjunctival vessels, tortuous and dilated retinal vessels, and lens changes (Fig 13-8). Tortuosity of conjunctival and retinal vessels is also characteristic of fucosidosis.

Haltia M. The neuronal ceroid-lipofuscinoses: from past to present. *Biochim Biophys Acta.* 2006;1762(10):850–856.

Gregory-Evans K, Pennesi ME,Weleber RG. Retinitis pigmentosa and allied disorders. In: Ryan SJ, Schachat AP, Wilkinson CP, Hinton DR, Sadda SR, Wiedemann P, eds. *Retina.* 5th ed. Philadelphia: Elsevier/Saunders; 2013:761–835.

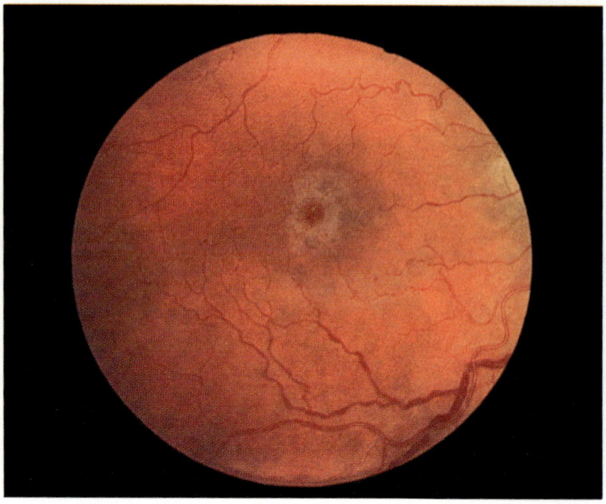

Figure 13-7 Chronic Niemann-Pick disease. Color fundus photograph showing a macular halo. *(Courtesy of Mark W. Johnson, MD.)*

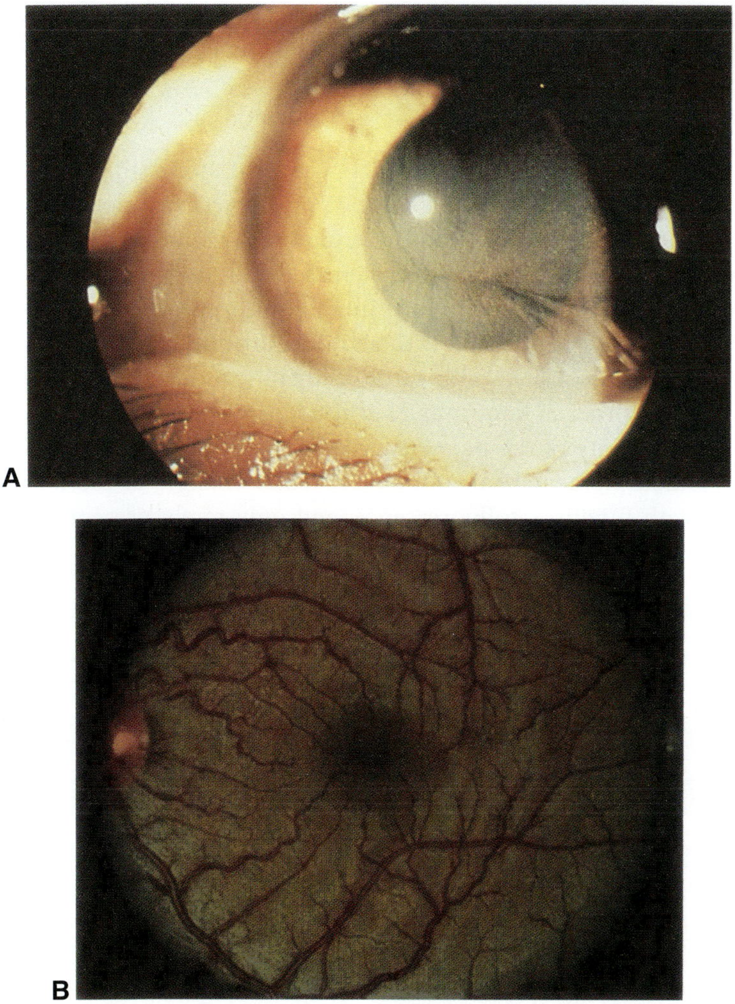

Figure 13-8 Fabry disease. **A,** Slit-lamp biomicroscopic image showing corneal whorls (cornea verticillata). **B,** Color fundus photograph showing retinal vascular tortuosity.

Amino Acid Disorders

In *cystinosis,* intralysosomal cystine accumulates because of a defect in transport out of lysosomes. Three types, all autosomal recessive, are recognized: (1) nephropathic, (2) late-onset (or intermediate), and (3) benign. Cystine crystals accumulate in the cornea and conjunctiva in all 3 types, but retinopathy develops only in patients with the nephropathic type. These patients are asymptomatic until 8–15 months of age, when they present with progressive renal failure, growth delays, renal rickets, and hypothyroidism. The retinopathy is characterized by areas of patchy depigmentation of the RPE alternating with irregularly distributed pigment clumps and associated fine retinal crystals. Despite the abnormal fundus appearance, no significant visual disturbance occurs. Treatment with cysteamine may be beneficial; it reacts with lysosomal cystine to form a mixed disulfide that can exit the lysosome. Bietti crystalline dystrophy may also cause crystalline keratopathy and retinopathy associated with patchy loss of the choriocapillaris and RPE and with associated photoreceptor loss, as observed through SD-OCT analysis.

Mitochondrial Disorders

Mutations and deletions in mitochondrial DNA are associated with several different syndromes, many of which involve myopathy. *Chronic progressive external ophthalmoplegia* belongs to a group of diseases collectively termed *mitochondrial myopathies,* in which mitochondria are abnormally shaped and increased in number. Ragged-red fibers may be evident with muscle biopsy specimens. In addition to progressive external ophthalmoplegia, the syndrome is associated with atypical RP and various systemic abnormalities (Fig 13-9). When associated with cardiomyopathy and cardiac conduction defects (heart block), the disorder is known as *Kearns-Sayre syndrome;* onset is usually before age 10 years. The severity of the pigmentary retinopathy is highly variable; the disease often shows mottled pigmentary or atrophic macular changes at the level of the RPE, well-illustrated with fundus autofluorescence, and only rarely presents with panretinal

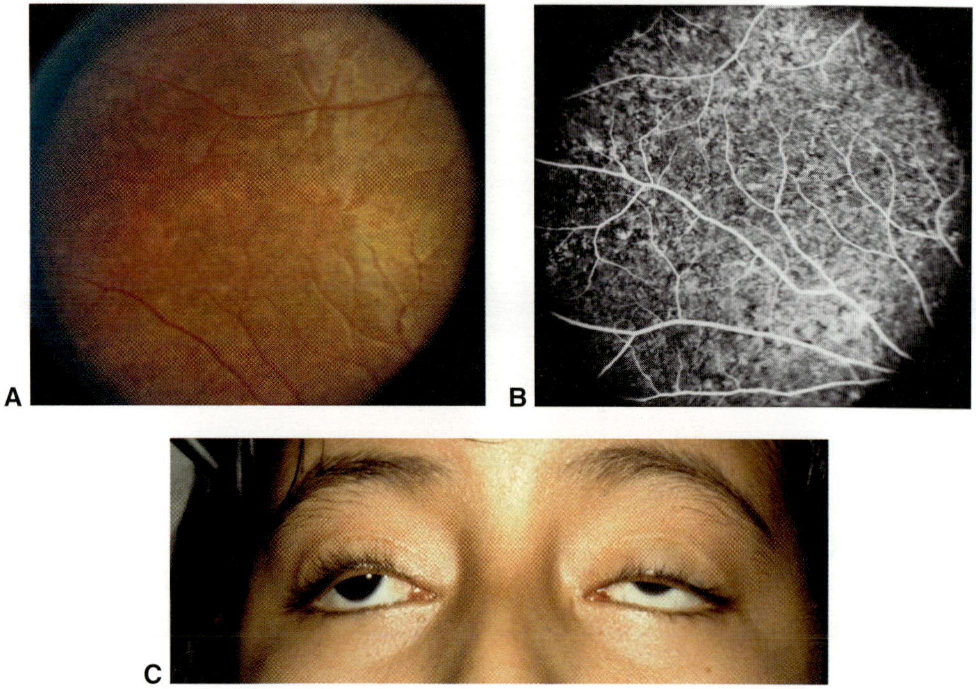

Figure 13-9 Chronic progressive external ophthalmoplegia (CPEO) and mitochondrial associated retinopathy. **A,** Color fundus photograph showing diffuse retinal pigment epithelial mottling. **B,** Corresponding mottled hyper- and hypofluorescence in the arteriovenous-phase fluorescein angiography image. **C,** Color photograph showing bilateral ptotic eyelids, and eyes in a misaligned exotropic position from poor extra-ocular muscle function consistent with CPEO caused by a mitochondrial mutation. *(Courtesy of David Sarraf, MD.)*

degeneration and bone spicules. Many patients retain good visual function and a normal ERG signal. Other mitochondrial myopathies with pigmentary retinopathy include *MIDD* (*m*aternally *i*nherited *d*iabetes and *d*eafness; Fig 13-10), *MELAS* (*m*itochondrial *e*ncephalomyopathy, *l*actic *a*cidosis, and *s*troke), and *NARP* (*n*eurogenic muscle weakness, *a*taxia, and *r*etinitis *p*igmentosa) syndromes.

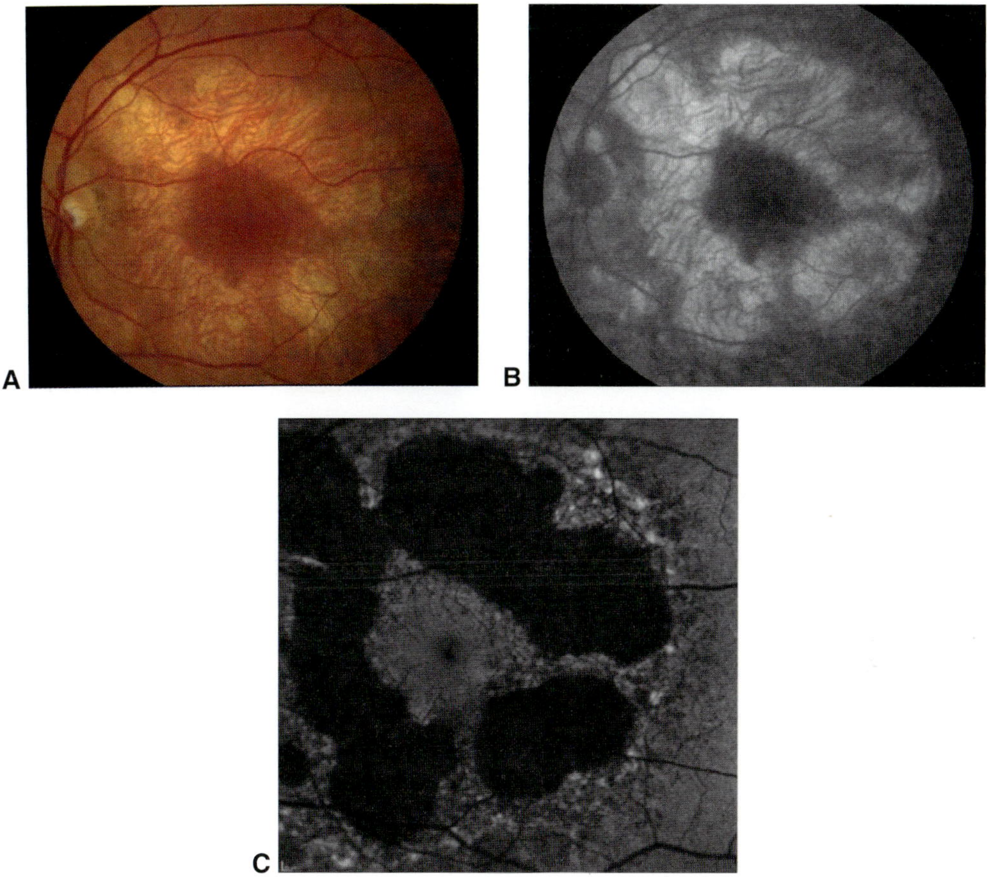

Figure 13-10 Maternally inherited diabetes and deafness (MIDD). Color fundus photograph **(A)**, late fluorescein angiography frame **(B)**, and fundus autofluorescence image **(C)** showing retinal pigment epithelial atrophy in a perifoveal distribution in a patient with MIDD caused by a mitochondrial mutation. These findings were all symmetrically present in the fellow eye. *(Courtesy of Herb Cantrill, MD.)*

CHAPTER 14

Systemic Drug-Induced Retinal Toxicity

Although the retina and retinal pigment epithelium (RPE) are protected from systemic toxic elements by the blood–retina barrier, they remain vulnerable to drug toxicities that can lead to dysfunction and secondary retinal degeneration. Retinal toxicities caused by systemic therapeutics may be categorized according to the level and pattern of toxicity. Broadly, these toxicities consist of (1) abnormalities at the level of the RPE/photoreceptor complex, (2) occlusive retinopathy or microvasculopathy, (3) ganglion cell and optic nerve toxicities, and (4) other manifestations of toxicity that include macular edema, crystalline retinopathy, and alterations in color vision and electroretinogram (ERG) signals.

Drugs Causing Abnormalities of the Retinal Pigment Epithelium/Photoreceptor Complex

Chloroquine Derivatives

Although retinal toxicity from *chloroquine* use remains a problem in many parts of the world, it is rare in the United States, where the medication has largely been replaced by the much safer, related drug *hydroxychloroquine*. These medications are used for the treatment of malaria and of rheumatologic and dermatologic disorders. Both medications bind to melanin in the RPE, which may concentrate or prolong their effects. Although the incidence of toxicity is low, it is of serious concern because associated vision loss rarely recovers and may even progress after the drug is discontinued. Patients and their primary care physicians must be made aware of the ophthalmic risks and the need for regular screening examinations to detect retinal toxicity at an early stage before vision loss occurs. Typical symptoms can include paracentral scotomas, central visual decline and/or reading difficulty.

The earliest signs of toxicity include bilateral paracentral visual field defects and/or inner segment ellipsoid loss in a paracentral location, which can be observed with spectral-domain optical coherence tomography (SD-OCT) imaging as the "flying saucer" sign. With continued drug exposure, progressive pigmentary changes may develop, and a bilateral atrophic bull's-eye maculopathy may ensue (Fig 14-1). End-stage cases of advanced toxicity may show panretinal degeneration simulating retinitis pigmentosa; it can occur from long-term exposure to either drug or acute overdosing of chloroquine. In

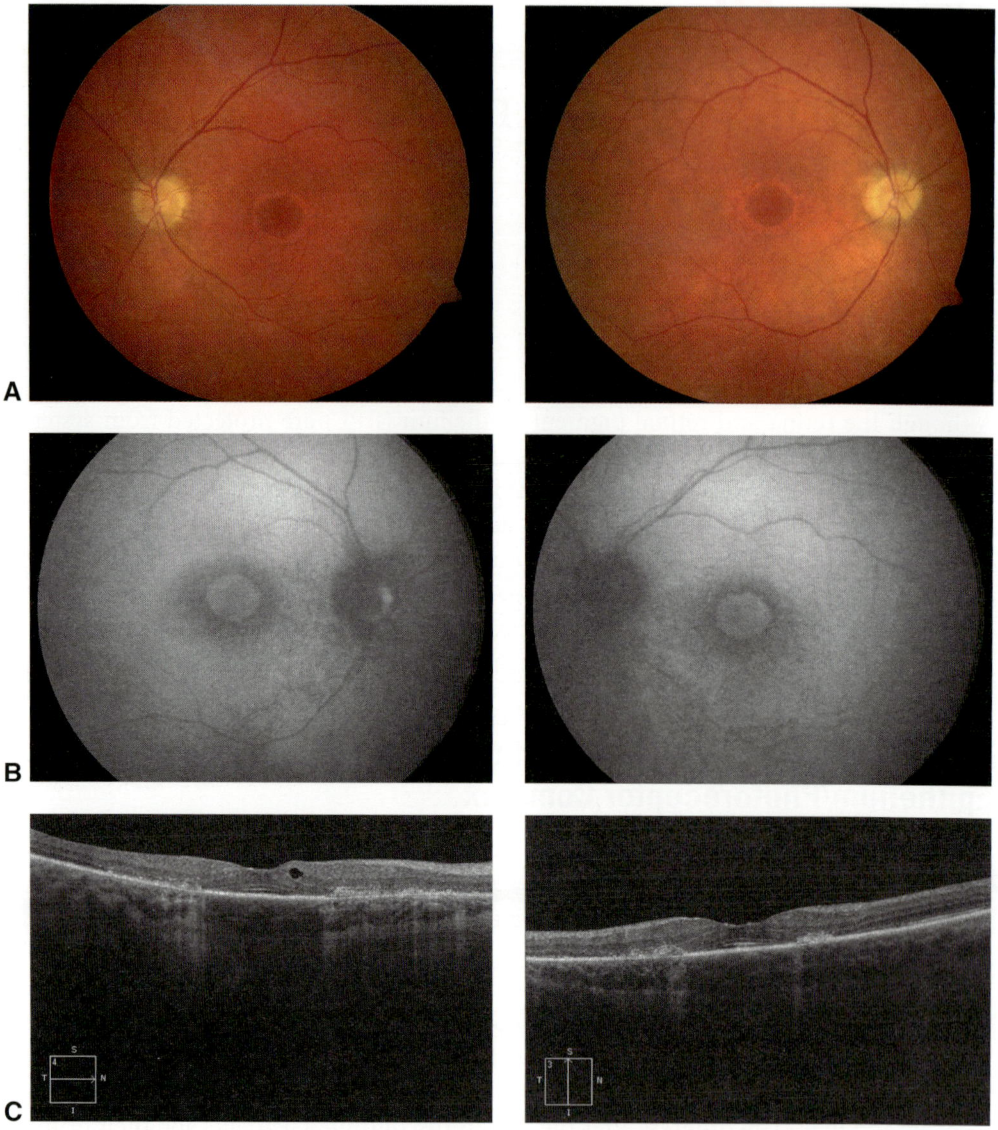

Figure 14-1 Bilateral, symmetric bull's-eye maculopathy in a patient with hydroxychloroquine toxicity. **A,** Color fundus photographs of left and right eyes. **B,** Corresponding fundus autofluorescence images. **C,** Spectral-domain optical coherence tomography (SD-OCT) images demonstrating the characteristic "flying-saucer" sign with inner segment ellipsoid loss in a parafoveal location. *(Courtesy of Stephen J. Kim, MD.)*

some patients, corneal intraepithelial deposits, usually referred to as *corneal verticillata,* may also be observed.

Ophthalmic screening of patients receiving chloroquine or hydroxychloroquine is aimed primarily at early detection and minimization of toxicity. As summarized in a 2011 Clinical Statement from the American Academy of Ophthalmology (http://one.aao.org/clinical-statement/revised-recommendations-on-screening-chloroquine-h), the risk of toxicity is low for individuals who have no complicating conditions and take less than 6.5 mg/kg/day of hydroxychloroquine or 3 mg/kg/day of chloroquine. The most recent data suggest that a hydroxychloroquine dosage of 5.0 mg/kg/day based on the patient's real body weight may be safer across all body mass indexes than the dosage recommendation of 6.5 mg/kg/day using the patient's ideal body weight.

Cumulative total doses greater than 1000 g of hydroxychloroquine and 460 g of chloroquine place patients at high risk of toxicity. Additional risk factors include older age (ie, more than 60 years), obesity, short stature, kidney or liver disease, and concomitant retinal disease such as age-related macular degeneration (AMD). Nevertheless, well-documented cases of hydroxychloroquine maculopathy have occurred with "safe" daily doses and in the absence of other risk factors.

Baseline evaluation for patients beginning treatment with a chloroquine derivative should include a complete ophthalmic examination. For follow-up comparison, the ophthalmologist should employ fundus photography, SD-OCT, and automated threshold field testing with a white pattern (Humphrey white 10-2 protocol), although some clinicians prefer red for its increased sensitivity. Patients who are at risk of toxicity or have unclear symptoms can be further assessed with fundus autofluorescence and multifocal electroretinography (mfERG). Signs of toxicity are a central ring of hyper- or hypoautofluorescence and paracentral mfERG depressions, respectively. However, mfERG testing can yield false-positive results. In contrast to previous teachings, fluorescein angiography, full-field electroretinography, Amsler grid testing, color vision testing, and electro-oculography are considered less effective methods for detecting toxicity. Cessation of the drug at the first sign of toxicity is recommended, although reduction in dosage may also be considered in some circumstances.

Marmor MF, Kellner U, Lai TY, Lyons JS, Mieler WF; American Academy of Ophthalmology. Revised recommendations on screening for chloroquine and hydroxychloroquine retinopathy. *Ophthalmology.* 2011;118(2):415–422.

Melles RB, Marmor MF. Pericentral retinopathy and racial differences in hydroxychloroquine toxicity. *Ophthalmology.* 2015;122(1):110–116.

Melles RB, Marmor MF. The risk of toxic retinopathy in patients on long-term hydroxychloroquine therapy. *JAMA Ophthalmol.* 2014;132(12):1453–1460.

Phenothiazines

Phenothiazines, including *chlorpromazine* and *thioridazine,* are concentrated in uveal tissue and RPE by binding to melanin granules. High-dose chlorpromazine therapy commonly causes abnormal pigmentation of the eyelids, interpalpebral conjunctiva, cornea, and anterior lens capsule. Anterior and posterior subcapsular cataracts may also develop. However, pigmentary retinopathy from chlorpromazine therapy is unusual.

In contrast, high-dose thioridazine treatment can cause development of a severe pigmentary retinopathy within a few weeks or months of dosing initiation (Fig 14-2). Toxicity is rare at doses of 800 mg/day or lower. Initially, patients experience blurred vision, and the fundus shows coarse retinal pigment epithelial stippling in the posterior pole. Eventually, patchy nummular atrophy of the RPE and choriocapillaris may develop. The late

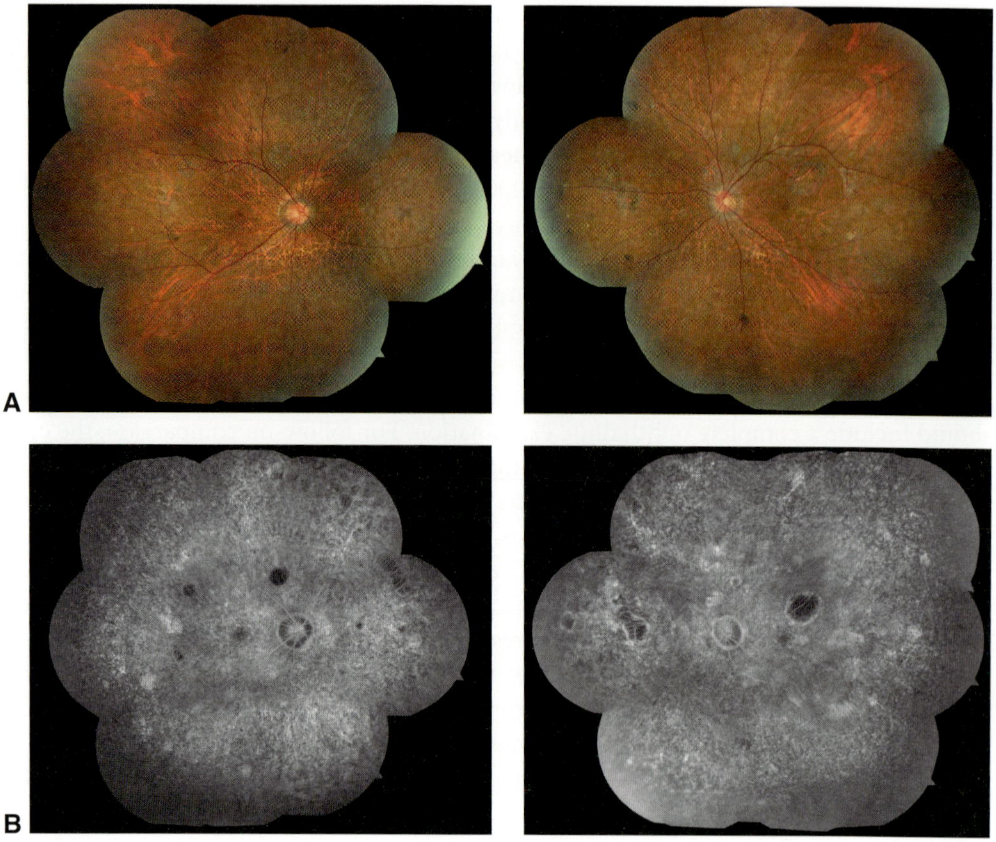

Figure 14-2 Thioridazine toxicity in a patient with schizophrenia. A, Color fundus photograph montages of right and left eyes. B, Corresponding fluorescein angiography montages. Note the diffuse nummular loss of retinal pigment epithelium (RPE) in the posterior pole and periphery of each eye. *(Courtesy of David Sarraf, MD.)*

stages may be mistaken for choroideremia or Bietti crystalline corneoretinal dystrophy; late-stage symptoms include visual field loss and nyctalopia (night blindness).

Vision may initially improve after treatment is discontinued but may deteriorate years later if the chorioretinal atrophy slowly progresses because of continued release of the drug from melanocytes. Generally, patients taking thioridazine are not monitored ophthalmoscopically because toxicity is rare at standard doses. However, symptomatic patients or patients suspected of having toxicity, especially those who have taken high doses of the drug, should undergo a full retinal evaluation.

Miscellaneous Medications

Other systemic medications inducing toxicity of the RPE include *clofazimine* and *deferoxamine. Clofazimine* is a phenazine dye used to treat dapsone-resistant leprosy and various autoimmune disorders, such as psoriasis and lupus. Its toxicity manifests as a bull's-eye maculopathy. *Deferoxamine* is an iron-chelating agent, which can cause reticular or vitelliform retinal pigment epithelial changes in the macula and can be associated with macular edema caused by retinal pigment epithelial pump failure. Nucleoside reverse transcriptase inhibitors (NRTIs) such as *dideoxyinosine* have been used in the systemic treatment of patients infected with human immunodeficiency virus (HIV) because they can inhibit replication of the virus. However, this class of medications can cause mitochondrial toxicity and damage to tissues with high oxygen requirements, such as the optic nerve and RPE. Patients may develop peripheral vision loss associated with a bilateral, symmetric, and midperipheral pattern of concentric mottling and atrophy of the RPE and choriocapillaris. The fundus changes are most readily identified with fundus autofluorescence imaging.

MEK inhibitors, a class of drugs used as chemotherapeutic agents in the treatment of metastatic cancers, can cause a condition similar to central serous chorioretinopathy. This condition is characterized by multifocal serous retinal detachments, one of which almost always involves the fovea (Fig 14-3). The fluid resolves when the medication is discontinued. The use of *sildenafil* has been associated, rarely, with serous macular detachment and central serous chorioretinopathy, presumably caused by choroidal vascular dilation and choroidal congestion manifesting as increased choroidal thickness on enhanced depth imaging (EDI) SD-OCT. *Corticosteroids* are the most common medications to be associated with the development of central serous chorioretinopathy.

The *alkyl nitrites* ("poppers") are a class of recreational drugs that are inhaled to induce a euphoric effect and enhance sexual arousal; in rare cases, these drugs can cause a toxic maculopathy. Patients are typically young and present with central scotoma or photopsia. Fundus examination may demonstrate a yellow spot on the fovea. SD-OCT imaging is essential and may reveal focal disruption of the central inner segment ellipsoid band, indicating an abnormality of the foveal cones (Fig 14-4). This abnormality may or may not improve over time.

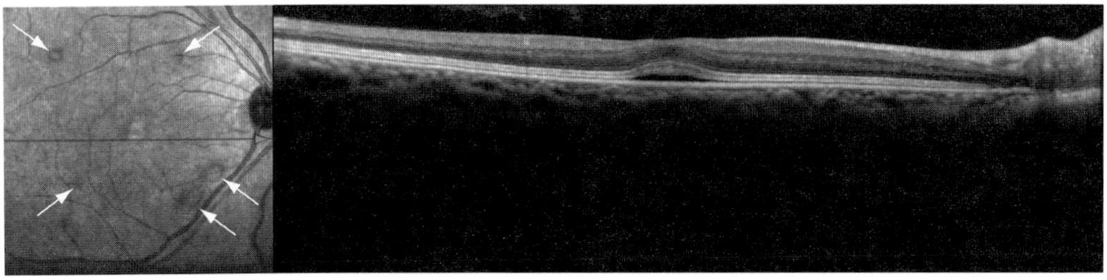

Figure 14-3 SD-OCT scan through the inferior fovea of a patient being treated with an MEK inhibitor for metastatic melanoma. There is a foveal serous detachment and additional, small, serous retinal detachments throughout the macula *(arrows)*. *(Courtesy of Tara A. McCannel, MD, PhD.)*

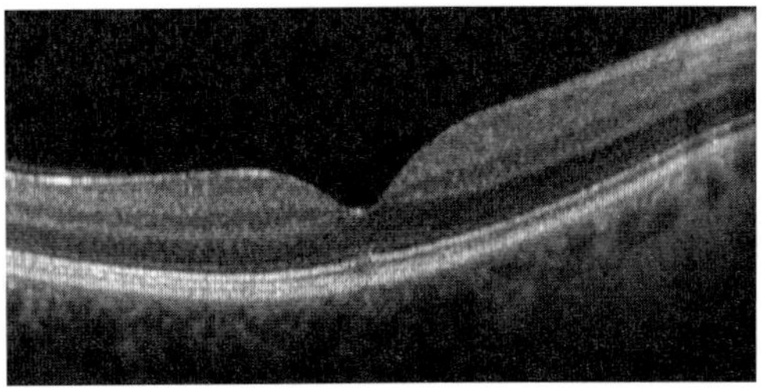

Figure 14-4 SD-OCT image showing maculopathy in the right eye of a patient with a 10-day history of a central white spot that developed after inhalation of an alkyl nitrite ("popper") for recreational purposes. Note the central presence of inner segment ellipsoid disruption. *(Courtesy of Maziar Lalezary, MD.)*

Davies AJ, Kelly SP, Naylor SG, et al. Adverse ophthalmic reaction in poppers users: case series of 'poppers maculopathy'. *Eye (Lond).* 2012;26(11):1479–1486.

Gabrielian A, MacCumber MM, Kukuyev A, Mitsuyasu R, Holland GN, Sarraf D. Didanosine-associated retinal toxicity in adults infected with human immunodeficiency virus. *JAMA Ophthalmol.* 2013;131(2):255–259.

McCannel TA, Chmielowski B, Finn RS, et al. Bilateral subfoveal neurosensory retinal detachment associated with MEK inhibitor use for metastatic cancer. *JAMA Ophthalmol.* 2014;132(8):1005–1009.

Drugs Causing Occlusive Retinopathy or Microvasculopathy

Interferon alfa-2a is an antiviral and immunomodulatory drug used for the treatment of viral hepatitis. This treatment may be complicated by the development of cotton-wool spots and retinal hemorrhages in 2%–3% of children and 20%–29% of adults. Affected patients may experience symptoms such as paracentral visual field defects, but vision loss is rarely significant or permanent. Ergot alkaloids (vasoconstrictors used to treat migraines) and oral contraceptives have been associated with thrombotic complications, including retinal vein and retinal artery occlusions. *Procainamide* can induce systemic lupus erythematosus and cause extensive "pruning" of second-order retinal vessels and infarction of the retina, leading to severe vision loss.

Aminoglycosides—administered intraocularly but not systemically—deserve special mention in the context of medication toxicities. *Amikacin* and especially *gentamicin* can cause macular infarction and severe macular ischemia, leading to irreversible central vision loss. These agents' narrow therapeutic window has caused their use to decline. Other antibiotics are now used to prevent and treat endophthalmitis.

Raza A, Mittal S, Sood GK. Interferon-associated retinopathy during the treatment of chronic hepatitis C: a systematic review. *J Viral Hepat.* 2013;20(9):593–599.

Drugs Causing Ganglion Cell and Optic Nerve Toxicity

Quinine is used as a muscle relaxant for leg cramps and as an antimalarial. It has a narrow therapeutic index that is safe at doses under 2 g, but it causes morbidity at doses greater than 4 g and mortality at doses greater than 8 g. At toxic levels, acute severe vision loss may occur as a result of retinal ganglion cell toxicity, mimicking a central retinal artery occlusion. A cherry-red spot may be observed upon ophthalmoscopic examination, and ganglion cell layer thickening and hyperreflectivity may be demonstrated with SD-OCT examination. Diffuse inner-retinal atrophy will ensue, accompanied by retinal vascular attenuation and optic atrophy. Full-field ERG testing will show a negative waveform signal, similar to that observed with a central retinal artery occlusion (Fig 14-5). Blindness caused by quinine toxicity is permanent.

Methanol toxicity causes acute blindness. Posterior segment manifestations include acute transient optic nerve head and macular edema. In histologic studies of acute methanol toxicity, the retina, RPE, and optic nerve demonstrate vacuolization, a sign of cell death. Eventually, optic atrophy and occasionally retinal vascular attenuation caused by

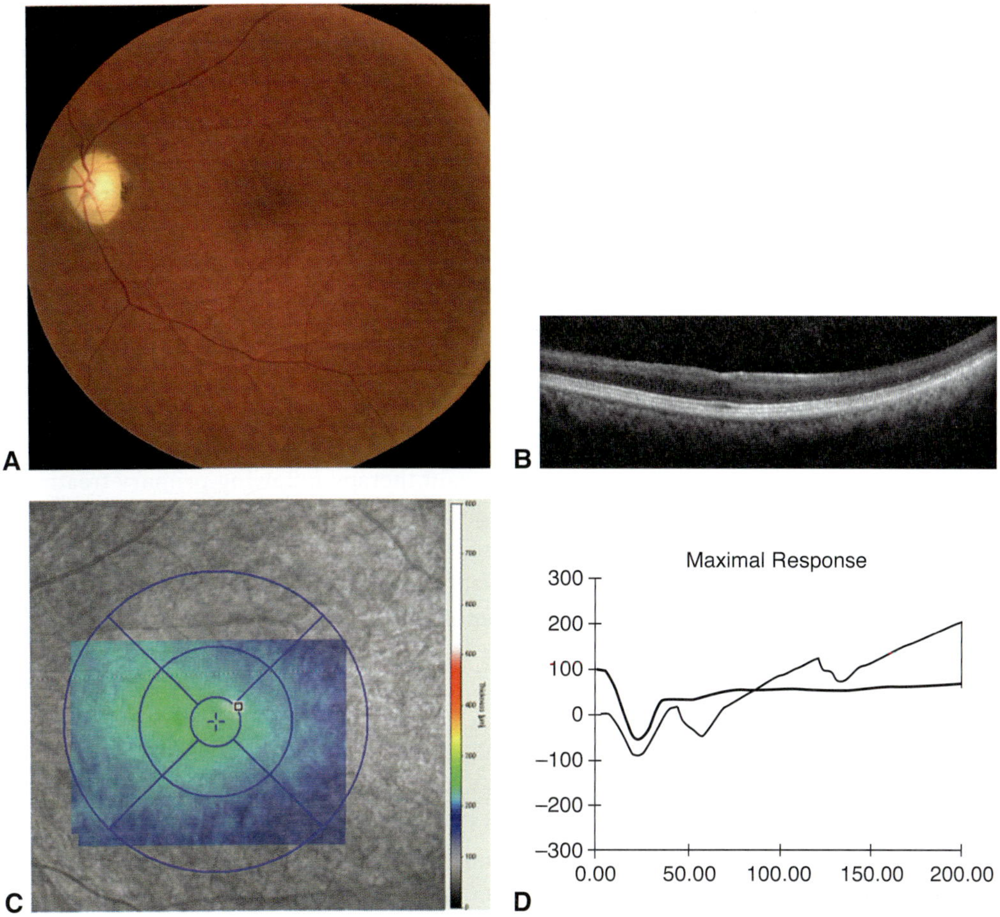

Figure 14-5 Quinine toxicity. **A,** Color fundus photograph showing optic disc pallor and retinal vascular attenuation. **B,** SD-OCT image demonstrating diffuse inner-retinal atrophy. **C,** OCT map analysis showing diffuse retinal thinning. **D,** Full-field electroretinogram showing an electronegative response. *(Courtesy of David Sarraf, MD.)*

diffuse ganglion cell loss may develop. Full-field ERG testing shows an electronegative waveform. The most commonly reported sequela of methanol toxicity is optic atrophy.

Narkewicz MR, Rosenthal P, Schwarz KB, et al; PEDS-C Study Group. Ophthalmologic complications in children with chronic hepatitis C treated with pegylated interferon. *J Pediatr Gastroenterol Nutr.* 2010;51(2):183–186.

Drugs Causing Macular Edema

The *taxanes* are a class of microtubule inhibitors that include *paclitaxel,* albumin-bound paclitaxel, and *docetaxel.* These drugs are employed as chemotherapeutics for the treatment of various cancers, including breast carcinoma. In rare cases, they are associated with cystoid macular edema (CME) that is visible on examination or SD-OCT but not on fluorescein angiography. Similarly, the cholesterol-lowering agent *nicotinic acid* can produce angiographically silent CME. Initially, central vision may be impaired, but full recovery follows discontinuation of the drug and resolution of the cystoid edema.

The glitazones *rosiglitazone* and *pioglitazone* are newer oral hypoglycemics used for the treatment of diabetes mellitus. They can cause severe fluid retention, leading to pulmonary edema, and are occasionally associated with the development or exacerbation of macular edema. Deferoxamine may also cause secondary macular edema caused by RPE toxicity, as mentioned earlier in the chapter.

Drugs Causing Crystalline Retinopathy

Crystalline retinopathies can be caused by systemic medications and other agents and can be associated with ocular and systemic diseases not discussed in this chapter (Table 14-1). *Tamoxifen* is an antiestrogen drug used as adjuvant therapy following primary treatment for breast cancer. Retinopathy is rare at typical doses (20 mg daily), but crystalline retinopathy has been reported in patients receiving high-dose tamoxifen therapy (daily doses greater than 200 mg or cumulative doses greater than 100 g). The maculopathy is characterized by brilliant inner-retinal crystalline deposits clustered around the fovea and may be associated with CME and significant vision loss in severe cases; it may be irreversible. More recently, central loss of the inner segment ellipsoid band in patients receiving low-dose tamoxifen therapy has been observed, rarely, with SD-OCT imaging and without crystals visible on funduscopic examination (Fig 14-6).

A crystalline maculopathy may also occur after ingestion of high doses of *canthaxanthine,* a widely available carotenoid used to simulate tanning. The inner-retinal, glistening canthaxanthine deposits distribute in a doughnut pattern around the macula, with a

Table 14-1 Causes of Crystalline Retinopathy

Systemic diseases
- Primary hereditary hyperoxaluria (primary oxalosis)
- Cystinosis
- Sjögren-Larsson syndrome

Drug-induced causes
- Tamoxifen toxicity
- Canthaxanthine toxicity
- Talc emboli (caused by chronic intravenous drug abuse with methylphenidate)
- Nitrofurantoin toxicity
- Methoxyflurane anesthesia (secondary oxalosis)
- Ethylene glycol ingestion (secondary oxalosis)
- Triamcinolone acetonide injection–associated crystalline maculopathy (caused by intravitreal triamcinolone injection)
- West African crystalline maculopathy (long-term kola nut ingestion)

Ocular diseases
- Bietti crystalline corneoretinal dystrophy
- Calcific drusen
- Gyrate atrophy
- Retinal telangiectasia

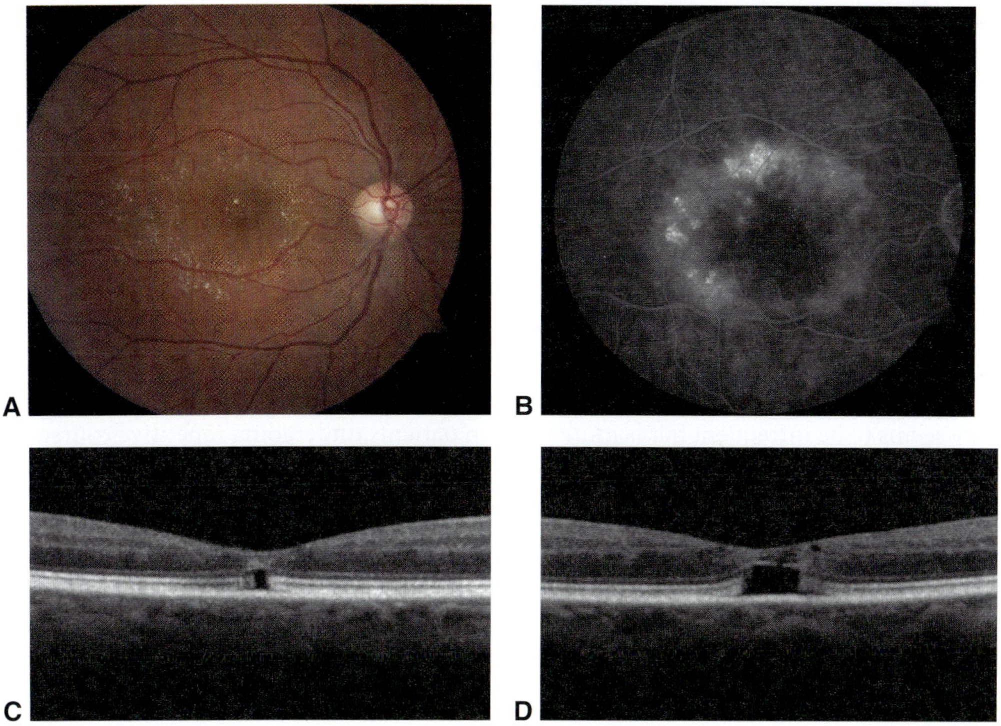

Figure 14-6 Tamoxifen retinopathy. **A,** Color fundus photograph showing tamoxifen retinopathy of the right eye in a male patient who had received high-dose therapy for treatment of glioblastoma of the brain. **B,** Corresponding fluorescein angiography image showing parafoveal cystoid macular edema associated with the extrafoveal tamoxifen deposits. **C, D,** SD-OCT images of left and right eyes from a case of low-dose tamoxifen retinopathy, which caused central disruption and loss of the ellipsoid band in each eye. *(Parts A and B courtesy of David Sarraf, MD; parts C and D, courtesy of Rishi Doshi, MD, and Jorge Fortun, MD.)*

predilection for the juxtapapillary region, but they do not typically cause vision loss and may resolve after the medication is discontinued.

Intravascular crystalline deposits of oxalate have been observed after the ingestion of ethylene glycol and after prolonged administration of *methoxyflurane* anesthesia (an agent that is no longer used in the United States) in patients with renal dysfunction. Other retinal crystals that may be deposited intravascularly include talc emboli, which are injected along with drugs such as methylphenidate in chronic intravenous drug abusers. The refractile talc deposits usually embolize in the smaller-caliber perifoveal retinal arterioles and may rarely cause peripheral retinal neovascularization; they do not typically cause vision loss.

West African crystalline maculopathy was first reported in elderly persons from the Igbo tribe of Nigeria but has been noted in patients from other countries in this region as well. Affected individuals are typically diabetic and demonstrate benign, inert inner-retinal refractile crystals of the fovea that are yellow-green in color. These crystals have been linked to long-term ingestion of kola nuts but are not associated with vision loss.

Drenser K, Sarraf D, Jain A, Small KW. Crystalline retinopathies. *Surv Ophthalmol.* 2006; 51(6):535–549.

Drugs Causing Abnormalities in Color Vision and Electroretinography

Phosphodiesterase 5 (PDE-5) inhibitors such as *sildenafil* and *tadalafil* can also partially inhibit phosphodiesterase 6 (PDE-6), an integral enzyme in the phototransduction cascade. Transient blue tinting of vision and temporarily abnormal ERG responses (including a delayed cone b-wave implicit time) have been observed in patients taking high doses of sildenafil. These changes may occur in up to 50% of patients ingesting doses greater than 100 mg, but no permanent retinal toxic effects have been reported. Reversible yellow tinting of vision, or *xanthopsia,* may be caused by the cardiac glycoside *digitalis.*

Some patients taking *isotretinoin* for the treatment of acne have reported poor night vision and were found to have abnormal dark-adaptation curves and ERG responses. Toxicity seems to be infrequent but is more likely in patients undergoing repetitive courses of therapy. The changes are largely reversible.

The antiepileptic drug *vigabatrin* can cause visual field constriction and ERG abnormalities, including depression of the 30-Hz-cone amplitude.

Marmor MF. Sildenafil (Viagra) and ophthalmology. *Arch Ophthalmol.* 1999;117(4):518–519.

Miscellaneous Drugs Causing Ocular Toxicities

The use of *rifabutin* in patients with HIV infection as prophylaxis against coinfection with *Mycobacterium avium* complex has been associated with vision loss arising from anterior and posterior uveitis with hypopyon and hypotony. The inflammation is reversible following discontinuation of the medication and initiation of steroid drop therapy.

Certain sulfur-derived medications such as *acetazolamide* and *topiramate* can cause medication-induced myopia and associated retinal and choroidal folds and macular edema. Vision loss may be mild (caused by isolated macular folds) or severe (caused by ciliochoroidal effusion, leading to angle-closure glaucoma) and may be reversed with early recognition and prompt discontinuation of the drug.

Historically, and more recently on the Internet, silver has been erroneously claimed to have medicinal benefits. Overingestion can cause slate-gray or blue coloring of the skin, referred to as *argyria.* Ocular argyrosis may develop after colloidal silver ingestion over a period longer than 1 year; this condition manifests as ocular pigmentation, black tears, and a dark choroid. The dark choroid is caused by brown-black granules diffusely deposited in the Bruch membrane, which can lead to "leopard spotting" and drusenlike deposition.

CHAPTER **15**

Retinal Detachment and Predisposing Lesions

Retinal Breaks

A retinal break is any full-thickness defect in the neurosensory retina. Breaks are clinically significant in that they may allow liquid from the vitreous cavity to enter the potential space between the sensory retina and the retinal pigment epithelium (RPE), known as the *epithelioretinal interspace,* thereby causing a rhegmatogenous retinal detachment. Some breaks are caused by atrophy of inner retinal layers (holes); others result from vitreoretinal traction (tears). Breaks resulting from trauma are discussed in the next section. Retinal breaks may be classified as

- flap, or horseshoe, tears
- giant retinal tears
- operculated holes
- dialyses
- atrophic retinal holes

A *flap tear* occurs when a strip of retina is pulled anteriorly by vitreoretinal traction, often in the course of a posterior vitreous detachment or trauma. A tear is considered symptomatic when the patient reports photopsias, floaters, or both. A *giant retinal tear* extends 90° (3 clock-hours) or more circumferentially and usually occurs along the posterior edge of the vitreous base. An *operculated hole* occurs when traction is sufficient to tear a piece of retina completely free from the adjacent retinal surface. A *retinal dialysis* is a circumferential, linear break that occurs at the ora serrata, with vitreous base attached to the retina posterior to the tear's edge; it is commonly a consequence of blunt trauma. An *atrophic hole* is generally not associated with vitreoretinal traction and has not been linked to an increased risk of retinal detachment.

American Academy of Ophthalmology Retina/Vitreous Panel. Preferred Practice Pattern Guidelines. *Posterior Vitreous Detachment, Retinal Breaks, and Lattice Degeneration.* San Francisco: American Academy of Ophthalmology; 2013. Available at: http://one.aao.org/guidelines.

Traumatic Breaks

Blunt or penetrating eye trauma can cause retinal breaks by direct retinal perforation, contusion, or vitreous traction. Fibrocellular proliferation occurring later at the site of an injury may cause vitreoretinal traction and subsequent detachment. Also see Chapter 17.

Blunt trauma can cause retinal breaks by direct contusive injury to the globe through 2 mechanisms: (1) *coup,* adjacent to the point of trauma, and (2) *contrecoup,* opposite the point of trauma. Blunt trauma compresses the eye along its anteroposterior axis and expands it in the equatorial plane. Because the vitreous body is viscoelastic, slow compression of the eye has no deleterious effect on the retina. However, rapid compression of the eye results in severe traction on the vitreous base that may tear the retina.

Contusion injury may cause large, ragged equatorial breaks, dialysis, or a macular hole. Traumatic breaks are often multiple, and they are commonly found in the inferotemporal and superonasal quadrants. The most common injuries are dialyses, which may be as small as 1 ora bay (the distance between 2 retinal dentate processes at the latitude of the ora serrata) or may extend 90° or more. Dialyses are usually located at the posterior border of the vitreous base but can also occur at the anterior border (Fig 15-1). Avulsion of the vitreous base may be associated with dialysis and is considered pathognomonic of ocular contusion. The vitreous base can be avulsed from the underlying retina and nonpigmented epithelium of the pars plana without tearing either one; generally, however, one or both are also torn in the process. Less common types of breaks caused by blunt trauma are horseshoe-shaped tears (which may occur at the posterior margin of the vitreous base, at the posterior end of a meridional fold, or at the equator) and operculated holes.

Trauma in Young Eyes

Although young patients have a higher incidence of eye injury than do other age groups, only in rare instances does the retina detach immediately following blunt trauma because young vitreous has not yet undergone *syneresis,* or liquefaction. The vitreous, therefore, does not provide for fluid movement through the retinal tears or dialyses. With time, however, the vitreous may liquefy over a tear, allowing fluid to pass through the break to detach the retina. The clinical presentation of the retinal detachment is usually delayed:

- 12% of detachments are identified immediately
- 30% are identified within 1 month
- 50% are identified within 8 months
- 80% are identified within 24 months

Traumatic retinal detachments in young patients may be shallow and often show signs of chronicity, including multiple demarcation lines, subretinal deposits, and intraretinal schisis.

When posterior vitreous separation is present or occurs later after trauma, retinal breaks are often associated with abnormal vitreoretinal attachments and may resemble nontraumatic breaks. Retinal detachments may occur acutely in these patients.

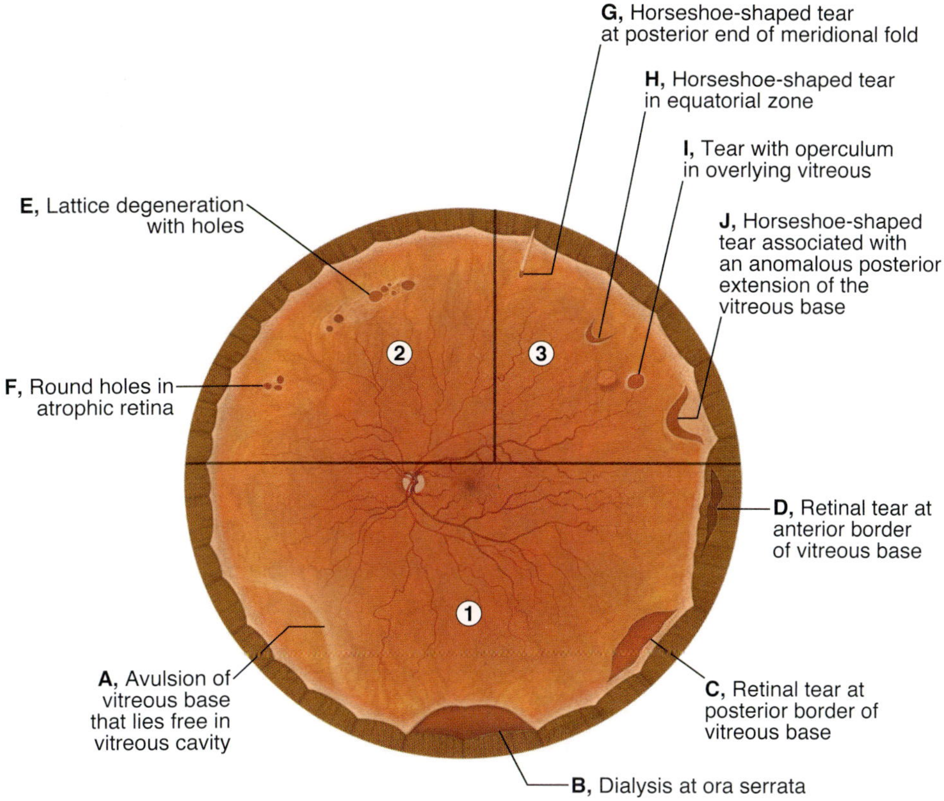

Figure 15-1 Schematic illustration of retinal tears and holes. **Part 1,** Retinal breaks at borders of the vitreous base. **A,** Avulsion of vitreous base that lies free in the vitreous cavity. **B,** Dialysis of the ora serrata. **C,** Retinal tear at the posterior border of the vitreous base. **D,** Retinal tear at the anterior border of the vitreous base. **Part 2,** Retinal breaks with areas of abnormal vitreoretinal interface (lattice degeneration). **E,** Lattice degeneration with holes. **F,** Round holes in atrophic retina. **Part 3,** Retinal breaks associated with abnormal vitreoretinal attachments. **G,** Horseshoe-shaped tear at the posterior end of a meridional fold. **H,** Horseshoe-shaped tear in the equatorial zone. **I,** Tear with operculum in the overlying vitreous. **J,** Horseshoe-shaped tear associated with an anomalous posterior extension of the vitreous base. *(Illustration by Mark M. Miller.)*

Posterior Vitreous Detachment

The vitreous gel is attached most firmly at the *vitreous base,* a circumferential zone straddling the ora serrata that extends approximately 2 mm anterior and 4 mm posterior to the ora. Vitreous collagen fibers at this base are so firmly attached to the retina and pars plana epithelium that the vitreous cannot be separated without tearing these tissues. The vitreous is also firmly attached at the margin of the optic disc, at the macula, along major vessels, at the margins of lattice degeneration, and at chorioretinal scars.

Most retinal tears result from traction caused by spontaneous or traumatic *posterior vitreous detachment* (PVD) (Fig 15-2). The predisposing event is syneresis of the central vitreous. There is increasing evidence that age-related PVD is insidious and slowly

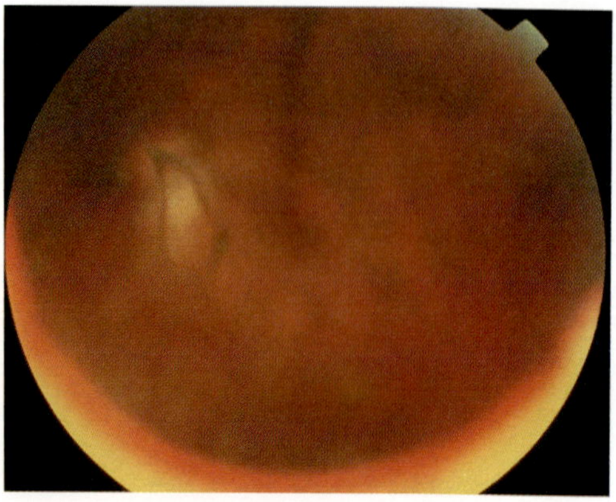

Figure 15-2 Posterior vitreous detachment. Color fundus photograph of a glial floater (Weiss ring) overlying the area of Martegiani of the optic disc. Vitreous hemorrhage is also present. *(Courtesy of Hermann D. Schubert, MD.)*

progressive over many years. A PVD typically begins with a shallow separation in the perifoveal cortical vitreous. Liquid vitreous enters through a cortical tear and detaches the macular vitreous cortex, causing a partial vitreous detachment. The early stages are usually asymptomatic and occult; in most eyes, the evolving PVD remains subclinical for years until separation from the disc margin (the area of Martegiani) occurs. This separation from the disc is often accompanied by symptoms associated with the appearance of a Weiss ring. The vitreous gel remains attached at the vitreous base. Vitreous traction on the retina can produce a retinal break, usually at the posterior edge of the vitreous base (Fig 15-3).

The prevalence of PVD increases with age. Other conditions associated with vitreous syneresis (collapse), synchysis (liquefaction), and PVD include aphakia, pseudophakia with open posterior capsule, inflammatory disease, trauma, vitreous hemorrhage, and axial myopia. Whether the vitreous is attached to or separated from the surface of the retina may be difficult to determine using biomicroscopy. Clinical studies typically reveal a low incidence of PVD in patients younger than 50 years. Autopsy studies demonstrate PVD in fewer than 10% of patients under age 50 years but in 63% of those over age 70 years.

Many patients do not report acute symptoms when a PVD occurs. Symptoms of PVD at the initial examination include the entoptic phenomena of photopsias (flashing lights), multiple floaters, and appearance of a curtain or cloud across the visual field. Patients with these symptoms should be examined promptly, and office staff should be made aware of the urgency of these symptoms. Flashing lights are caused by the physical stimulus of vitreoretinal traction on the retina. Floaters are caused by vitreous opacities such as blood, glial cells torn from the optic disc, or aggregated collagen fibers, all of which can cast shadows on the retina.

Vitreous hemorrhage may arise from avulsion of superficial retinal or prepapillary vessels or from rupture of retinal vessels that cross retinal tears. Important predictors of subsequent new retinal breaks are vitreous hemorrhage at the initial examination and an increase in the number of floaters after the initial examination. Overall, 7%–18% of all patients with acute symptomatic PVD have retinal tears. If vitreous hemorrhage is present, then 50%–70% have retinal tears, versus only 7%–12% without vitreous hemorrhage. Patients with an acute PVD complicated by a retinal tear are 7 times more likely to present with vitreous pigment or granules than are those without a tear.

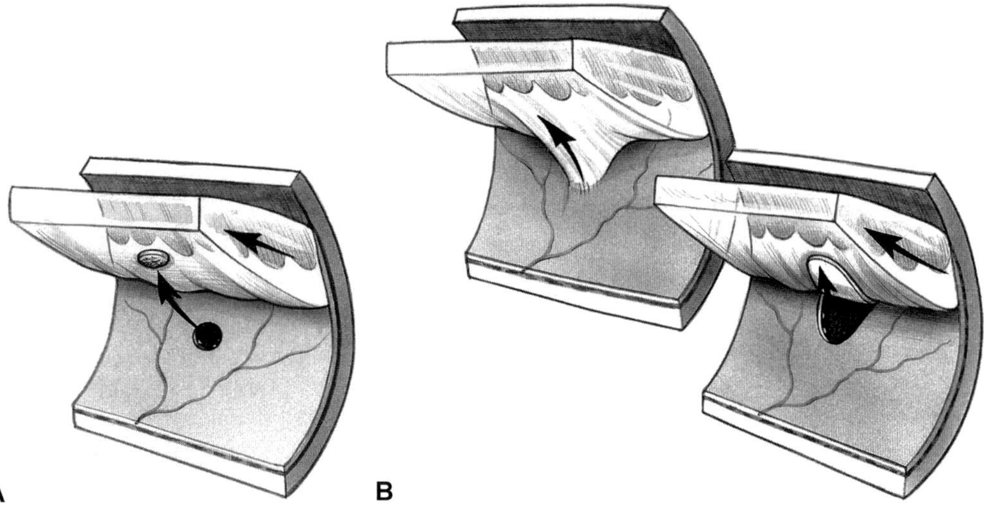

Figure 15-3 Schematic representations of mechanisms of retinal tear formation associated with posterior vitreous separation. **A,** Round or oval hole. **B,** Flap tear: posterior extension of vitreous base with firm vitreoretinal attachment. *(Illustration by Christine Gralapp based on illustrations by Tim Hengst.)*

van Overdam KA, Bettink-Remeijer MW, Klaver CC, Mulder PG, Moll AC, van Meurs JC. Symptoms and findings predictive for the development of new retinal breaks. *Arch Ophthalmol.* 2005;123(4):479–484.

Examination and Management of Posterior Vitreous Detachment

Indirect ophthalmoscopy with scleral depression and slit-lamp biomicroscopy with a 3-mirror lens or indirect contact lens are used to clinically diagnose PVD and rule out retinal breaks or detachment. Reexamination of the patient 2–4 weeks following presentation may be appropriate, as new retinal breaks may occur as the PVD evolves over time. Additional risk factors to consider in follow-up determination include aphakia, myopia, fellow-eye history, family history of retinal detachment, and signs of Stickler syndrome. All patients should be instructed to return to the ophthalmologist immediately if they notice a change in symptoms, such as increasing numbers of floaters or the development of visual field loss.

If a large vitreous hemorrhage precludes a complete examination, bilateral ocular patching and bed rest, with the patient's head elevated 45° or more for a few days, may allow the hemorrhage to settle sufficiently to permit detection of breaks in a superior location. Echography may be performed to find flap tears and rule out retinal detachment and other fundus lesions. If the cause of the hemorrhage cannot be found, the patient should be reexamined at frequent, regular intervals. A vitrectomy may be considered in the search for an etiology of a vitreous hemorrhage.

Byer NE. Natural history of posterior vitreous detachment with early management as the premier line of defense against retinal detachment. *Ophthalmology.* 1994:101(9):1503–1514.

Lesions Predisposing Eyes to Retinal Detachment

Lattice Degeneration

Lattice degeneration, a vitreoretinal interface abnormality, is present in 6%–10% of the general population and is bilateral in one-third to one-half of affected patients. It occurs more commonly in—but is not limited to—myopic eyes; a familial predilection is present.

Lattice degeneration may predispose eyes to retinal breaks and detachment. The most important histologic features include varying degrees of atrophy and irregularity of the inner layers, an overlying pocket of liquefied vitreous, condensation, and adherence of vitreous at the margin of the lesion (Figs 15-4, 15-5, 15-6).

Lattice degeneration is found in approximately 20%–30% of all eyes that present with rhegmatogenous retinal detachments. However, as the lattice degeneration is not necessarily causative, prophylactic laser treatment is not universally recommended. When lattice degeneration is the cause of retinal detachment, a tractional tear at the lateral or

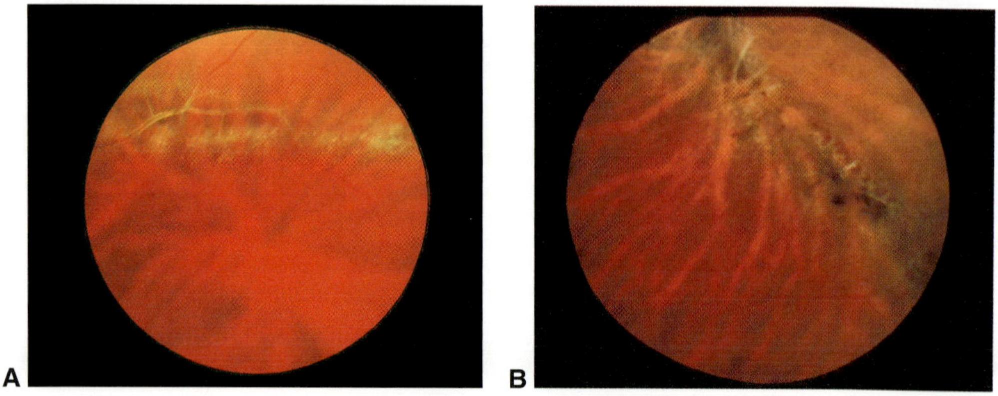

Figure 15-4 **A,** Color fundus photograph of lattice degeneration as viewed without scleral indentation. Vascular sheathing is apparent where the vessel crosses the area of lattice. Characteristic white lattice lines are visible. **B,** Color fundus photograph of another example of lattice degeneration, this case demonstrating associated hyperpigmentation, which is commonly observed. *(Part A used with permission from Byer NE.* Peripheral Retina in Profile: A Stereoscopic Atlas. *Torrance, CA: Criterion Press; 1982.)*

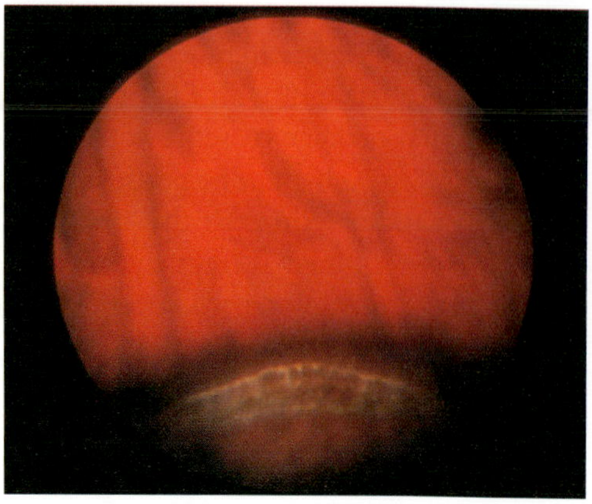

Figure 15-5 Fundus photograph of lattice degeneration as viewed with scleral indentation. *(Reproduced with permission from Byer NE.* Peripheral Retina in Profile: A Stereoscopic Atlas. *Torrance, CA: Criterion Press; 1982.)*

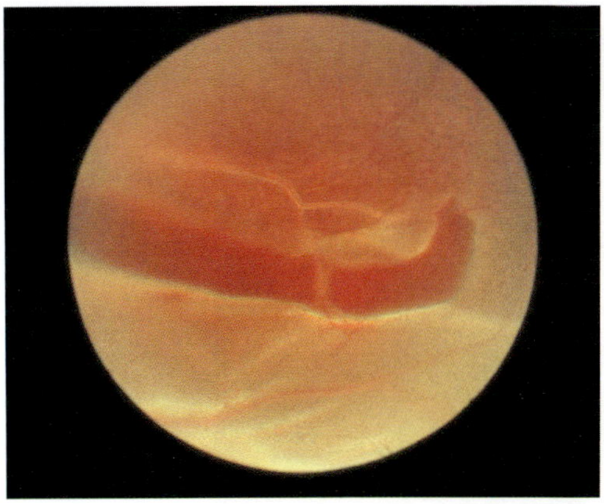

Figure 15-6 Color fundus photograph of lattice degeneration showing a large, posteriorly located flap tear and associated detachment. Note vessel bridging the tear. *(Used with permission from Byer NE.* Peripheral Retina in Profile: A Stereoscopic Atlas. *Torrance, CA: Criterion Press; 1982.)*

posterior margin of the lattice lesion or, less commonly, an atrophic hole within the zone of lattice itself occurs (Fig 15-7). Retinal detachments secondary to atrophic holes typically occur in young patients with myopic eyes and no vitreous detachment; they are typically asymptomatic until fixation is involved.

Byer NE. Lattice degeneration of the retina. *Surv Ophthalmol.* 1979;23(4):213–248.
Byer NE. Long-term natural history of lattice degeneration of the retina. *Ophthalmology.* 1989;96(9):1396–1402.

Vitreoretinal Tufts

Peripheral retinal tufts are small, peripheral, focal areas of elevated glial hyperplasia associated with vitreous or zonular attachment and traction. Tractional tufts are classified according to anatomical, pathogenetic, and clinical distinctions into the following groups:

- noncystic retinal tufts (Fig 15-8)
- cystic retinal tufts
- zonular traction retinal tufts (Fig 15-9)

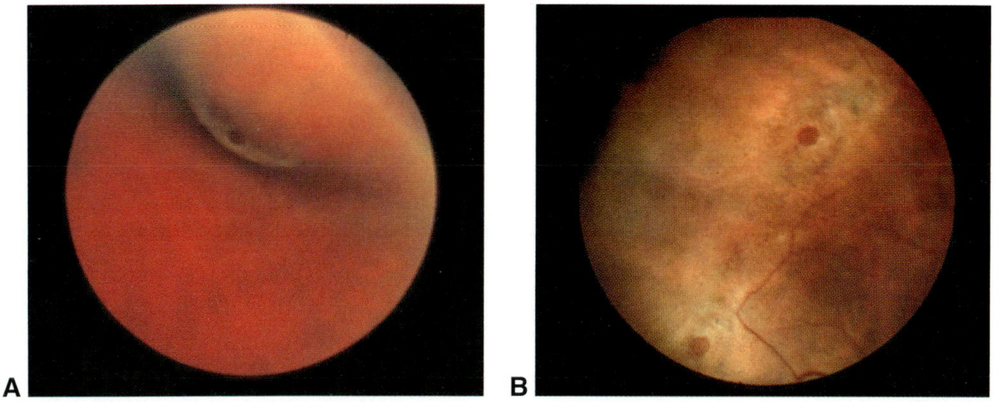

Figure 15-7 **A,** Fundus photograph of lattice degeneration with a small atrophic hole as viewed with scleral depression. **B,** Fundus photograph of an example of an atrophic hole as may be observed in lattice degeneration without scleral depression. *(Part A courtesy of Norman E. Byer, MD.)*

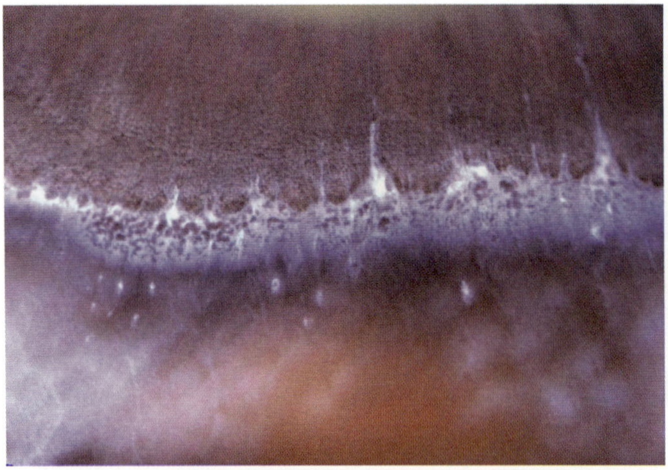

Figure 15-8 Color photograph of a gross eye specimen showing a cluster of white surface nodules with characteristic gross appearance and location of noncystic retinal tufts. *(Used with permission from Foos RY, Silverstein RN, eds.* System of Ocular Pathology. *Vol. 3. Los Angeles: iPATH Press; 2004.)*

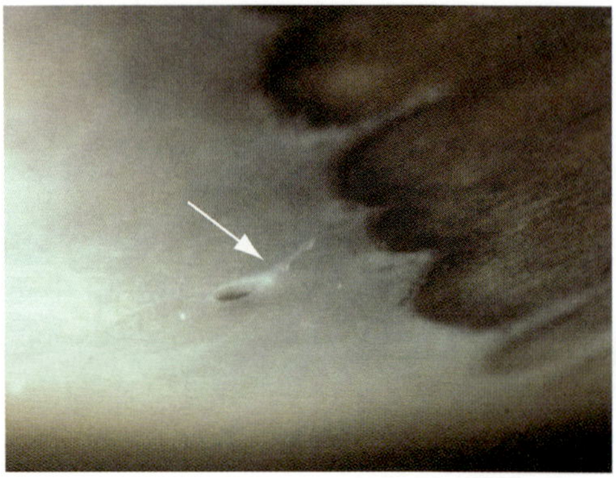

Figure 15-9 Color photograph of a gross eye specimen showing a small zonular traction tuft *(arrow)* with cystic base. Note that the tuft points anteriorly toward the peripheral lens. *(Used with permission from Foos RY, Silverstein RN, eds.* System of Ocular Pathology. *Vol. 3. Los Angeles: iPATH Press; 2004.)*

Retinal pigment epithelial hyperplasia may surround the tuft. Cystic and zonular traction retinal tufts, both with firm vitreoretinal adhesions, may predispose eyes to retinal tears and detachment.

Byer NE. Cystic retinal tufts and their relationship to retinal detachment. *Arch Ophthalmol.* 1981;99(10):1788–1790.

Meridional Folds, Enclosed Ora Bays, and Peripheral Retinal Excavations

Meridional folds are folds of redundant retina, usually located superonasally. They are usually associated with dentate processes but may also extend posteriorly from ora bays. Occasionally, tears associated with PVD occur at the most posterior limit of the folds (see Chapter 1, Fig 1-3). Retinal tears can also occur at or near the posterior margins of enclosed ora bays, which are oval islands of pars plana epithelium located immediately posterior to the ora serrata and completely or almost completely surrounded by peripheral retina (Fig 15-10). Occasionally, tears may occur at the site of peripheral retinal

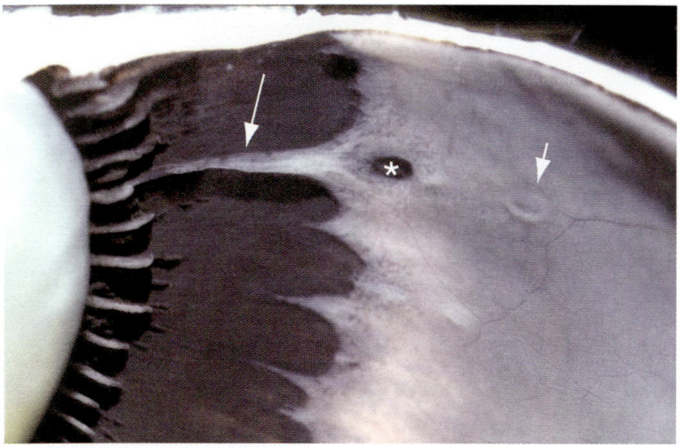

Figure 15-10 Color photograph of a gross eye specimen showing a meridional complex, consisting of an atypical and large dentate process *(arrow)* that is continuous with a ciliary process of the pars plicata and an area of enclosed pars plana and ora bay *(asterisk)*. Slightly posterior to the complex is a small area in the same meridian that appears to be excavated but is in fact a cyst *(small arrow)*. *(Used with permission from Foos RY, Silverstein RN, eds.* System of Ocular Pathology. *Vol. 3. Los Angeles: iPATH Press; 2004.)*

excavations, which represent a mild form of lattice degeneration. The excavations may have firm vitreoretinal adhesions and are found adjacent to, or up to 4 disc diameters posterior to, the ora serrata. They are often aligned with meridional folds.

Engstrom RE Jr, Glasgow BJ, Foos RY, Straatsma BR. Degenerative diseases of the peripheral retina. In: Tasman W, Jaeger EA, eds. *Duane's Clinical Ophthalmology on DVD-ROM.* Vol 3. Philadelphia: Lippincott Williams & Wilkins; 2013:chap 26.

Lesions Not Predisposing Eyes to Retinal Detachment

Paving-Stone Degeneration

Paving-stone (or cobblestone) degeneration is characterized by peripheral, small, discrete areas of atrophy of the outer retina; it appears in 22% of individuals more than 20 years old (Fig 15-11). The atrophic areas may occur singly or in groups and are sometimes confluent. Histologically, these "paving stones" are characterized by atrophy of the RPE and outer retinal layers, attenuation or absence of the choriocapillaris, and adhesions between the remaining neuroepithelial layers and the Bruch membrane. These lesions are most common in the inferior quadrants, anterior to the equator. Ophthalmoscopically, they appear yellowish white and are sometimes surrounded by a rim of hypertrophic RPE. Because the RPE is absent or hypoplastic, large choroidal vessels are visible beneath the lesions.

Retinal Pigment Epithelial Hyperplasia

When stimulated by chronic low-grade traction, retinal pigment epithelial cells proliferate. Diffuse retinal pigment epithelial hyperplasia may be observed straddling the ora

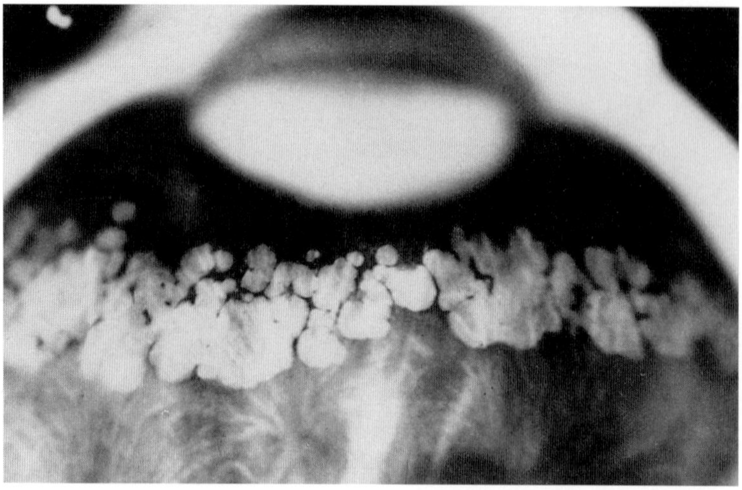

Figure 15-11 Gross appearance of paving-stone degeneration. *(Used with permission from Green WR. Pathology of the retina. In: Frayer WC, ed.* Lancaster Course in Ophthalmic Histopathology, *unit 9, Philadelphia: FA Davis; 1988:181.)*

serrata, in latitudes that correspond roughly to the insertion of the vitreous base, or occurring focally on the pars plana and peripheral retina, especially in areas of focal traction such as vitreoretinal tufts and lattice degeneration. Areas of previous inflammation and trauma may also be sites of retinal pigment epithelial hyperplasia.

Retinal Pigment Epithelial Hypertrophy

Acquired retinal pigment epithelial hypertrophy is a degenerative change associated with aging that commonly occurs in the periphery, often in a reticular pattern. Histologically, it is characterized by large cells and by large, spherical melanin granules. Similar histologic features are present in congenital hypertrophy of the RPE (grouped pigmentation, or "bear tracks").

Peripheral Cystoid Degeneration

Typical peripheral cystoid degeneration, characterized by zones of microcysts in the far-peripheral retina, is present in almost all adults over the age of 20 years. Although retinal holes may form in these areas, they rarely cause retinal detachment. *Reticular peripheral cystoid degeneration* is almost always located posterior to typical peripheral cystoid degeneration. It usually occurs in the inner retina and presents with a linear or reticular pattern following the retinal vessels. This form is found in approximately 20% of adults and may, in some instances, develop into reticular degenerative retinoschisis.

Prophylactic Treatment of Retinal Breaks

Any retinal break can cause a retinal detachment by allowing liquid from the vitreous cavity to pass through it and separate the sensory retina from the RPE. However, the vast majority of retinal holes or breaks do not cause a detachment.

The ophthalmologist may consider prophylactic treatment of breaks in an attempt to reduce the risk of retinal detachment. Treatment does not eliminate the risk of new tears or detachment.

The goal of prophylactic laser treatment or cryotherapy of retinal breaks is to create a chorioretinal adhesion around each break to prevent fluid from entering the subretinal space. If subretinal fluid is present, treatment must be applied so it surrounds the area of subretinal fluid. Similarly, when treating lattice degeneration, the entire lesion needs to be surrounded with treatment applications.

In considering prophylaxis, the ophthalmologist must weigh numerous factors, including symptoms, family history, residual traction, size and location of the break, phakic status, refractive error, status of the fellow eye, presence of subretinal fluid, and availability of follow-up evaluation. Prophylaxis is sometimes contraindicated in eyes with more than 6.00 D of myopia and more than 6 clock-hours of lattice. The following discussion serves only as a broad guideline, as many clinical factors must be considered in a given patient. (Also see the discussion of hereditary vitreoretinopathies with optically empty vitreous in Chapter 16.)

American Academy of Ophthalmology Retina/Vitreous Panel. Preferred Practice Pattern Guidelines. *Posterior Vitreous Detachment, Retinal Breaks, and Lattice Degeneration.* San Francisco: American Academy of Ophthalmology; 2013. Available at: http://one.aao.org/guidelines.

Symptomatic Retinal Breaks

Approximately 20% of eyes with a symptomatic PVD are found to have one or more tractional tears at the time of initial examination. Numerous clinical studies have demonstrated that acute, symptomatic breaks are at greater risk of progressing to retinal detachment, especially if there is associated vitreous hemorrhage. Therefore, *acute symptomatic flap tears* are commonly treated prophylactically.

Acute operculated holes are less likely to cause detachment because there is no residual traction on the adjacent retina, and they usually are not treated. However, if slit-lamp biomicroscopy reveals persistent vitreous traction at the margin of an operculated hole, if the hole is large or located superiorly, or if there is vitreous hemorrhage, prophylaxis should be considered.

Atrophic holes are often incidental findings in a patient who presents with an acute PVD. Generally, they do not require treatment.

Asymptomatic Retinal Breaks

Asymptomatic flap tears progress to retinal detachment in approximately 5% of cases. Because of this low risk, treatment is not universally recommended in emmetropic, phakic eyes. However, asymptomatic flap tears accompanied by lattice degeneration, myopia, subclinical detachment, aphakia, or a history of retinal detachment in the fellow eye have an increased risk of retinal detachment, and treatment may be considered. Asymptomatic operculated holes and atrophic holes rarely cause retinal detachment and are generally not treated.

Byer NE. What happens to untreated asymptomatic retinal breaks, and are they affected by posterior vitreous detachment? *Ophthalmology.* 1998;105(6):1045–1050.

Lattice Degeneration

Although only limited data are available, an 11-year follow-up study of patients with untreated lattice degeneration and no symptomatic tears showed that retinal detachment occurred in approximately 1% of cases. Thus, the presence of lattice, with or without atrophic holes, generally does not require prophylaxis in the absence of other risk factors or symptoms. If lattice degeneration is present in a patient with additional risk factors, such as retinal detachment in the fellow eye, flap tears, or aphakia, then prophylactic treatment can be considered.

Byer NE. Long-term natural history of lattice degeneration of the retina. *Ophthalmology.* 1989;96(9):1396–1402.

Wilkinson CP. Interventions for asymptomatic retinal breaks and lattice degeneration for preventing retinal detachment. *Cochrane Database Syst Rev.* 2014;9:CD003170. [Epub 2014 Sep 5]

Aphakia and Pseudophakia

Because aphakic and pseudophakic eyes have higher risks of retinal detachment (1%–3%) than do phakic eyes, such patients should be warned of potential symptoms and carefully examined if symptoms occur. In a population-based 25-year follow-up study that compared eyes that underwent cataract surgery with eyes that did not, the probability ratio of retinal detachment following cataract surgery was greatest in the first year (an approximately 11-fold difference, compared with approximately 4-fold in years 5 through 20). The cumulative risk of retinal detachment steadily increased to 1.79% at 20 years. Risk factors for the development of retinal detachment following cataract surgery include male sex, younger age, myopia, increased axial length, and posterior capsular tear.

Erie JC, Raecker MA, Baratz KH, Schleck CD, Burke JP, Robertson DM. Risk of retinal detachment after cataract extraction, 1980–2004: a population-based study. *Ophthalmology.* 2006;113(11):2026–2032.

Fellow Eye in Patients With Retinal Detachment

In patients with retinal detachment, the fellow-eye risk of detachment is approximately 10% for phakic retinal detachment and 20%–36% for aphakic or pseudophakic detachment. Prophylactic treatment of flap tears and lattice degeneration is often considered.

Folk JC, Arrindell EL, Klugman MR. The fellow eye of patients with phakic lattice retinal detachment. *Ophthalmology.* 1989;96(1):72–79.

Subclinical Retinal Detachment

The term *subclinical retinal detachment* is used variously. Although it may refer to an asymptomatic retinal detachment, it usually describes a detachment in which subretinal fluid extends more than 1 disc diameter from the break but not more than 2 disc diameters posterior to the equator. Because approximately 30% of such detachments progress, treatment is often recommended. Treatment is advised especially for symptomatic patients or cases involving traction on the break. A demarcation line suggests a lower risk; however, progression may occur through the demarcation line.

Brod RD, Flynn HW Jr, Lightman DA. Asymptomatic rhegmatogenous retinal detachments. *Arch Ophthalmol.* 1995;113(8):1030–1032.

Retinal Detachment

Retinal detachments are classified as

- rhegmatogenous
- tractional
- exudative

The most common are *rhegmatogenous retinal detachments* (RRDs). They are caused by fluid passing from the vitreous cavity through a retinal break into the potential epithelioretinal interspace between the sensory retina and the RPE. The term is derived from the Greek *rhegma,* meaning "break." *Tractional detachments* are caused by proliferative membranes that contract and elevate the retina; they are less common. Combinations of tractional and rhegmatogenous pathophysiologic components may also lead to retinal detachment. *Exudative,* or *secondary, detachments* are caused by retinal or choroidal diseases in which fluid leaks beneath the sensory retina and accumulates.

The differential diagnosis of retinal detachment includes retinoschisis, choroidal tumors, and retinal elevation secondary to detachment of the choroid. Table 15-1 lists diagnostic features of the 3 forms of retinal detachment.

Rhegmatogenous Retinal Detachment

The Rochester epidemiology project, an internationally recognized source of high-quality epidemiology studies, determined that rhegmatogenous retinal detachment has an annual incidence of 12.6 per 100,000 persons. A given individual's risk is affected by the presence or absence of certain factors, including myopia, family history, fellow-eye retinal tear or detachment, recent vitreous detachment, trauma, peripheral high-risk lesions, and vitreoretinal degenerations. Current or recent use of fluoroquinolones may also be a risk factor, but this suggestion is controversial.

In 90%–95% of RRDs, a definite retinal break can be found, often with the help of Lincoff rules (Figs 15-12, 15-13). In the remainder, an occult break is presumed to be present. If no break can be found, the ophthalmologist must rule out all other causes of retinal elevation. Half of patients with RRD have photopsias, or *floaters.* The intraocular pressure is usually lower in the affected eye than in the fellow eye but may occasionally be higher. A Shafer sign, descriptively termed "tobacco dust" for small clumps of pigmented cells, is frequently present in the anterior vitreous. The retina detaches progressively from the periphery to the disc; usually it has convex borders and contours and a corrugated appearance, especially in recent retinal detachments, and undulates with eye movements. In a long-standing RRD, however, the retina may appear smooth and thin. Fixed folds

Table 15-1 Diagnostic Features of the 3 Types of Retinal Detachments

		Nonrhegmatogenous (Secondary)	
	Rhegmatogenous (Primary)	**Tractional**	**Exudative**
History	Aphakia, myopia, blunt trauma, photopsia, floaters, field defect; progressive, generally healthy	Diabetes mellitus, prematurity, penetrating trauma, sickle cell disease, venous occlusions	Systemic factors such as malignant hypertension, eclampsia, renal failure
Retinal break	Identified in 90%–95% of cases	No primary break; may develop secondary break	No break, or coincidental
Extent of detachment	Extends ora to disc early, has convex borders and surfaces; gravity dependent	Frequently does not extend to ora, may be central or peripheral	Volume and gravity dependent; extension to ora is variable, may be central or peripheral
Retinal mobility	Undulating bullae or folds	Taut retina, concave borders and surfaces, peaks to traction points	Smoothly elevated bullae, usually without folds
Evidence of chronicity	Demarcation lines, intraretinal macrocysts, atrophic retina	Demarcation lines	Usually none
Pigment in vitreous	Present in 70% of cases	Present in trauma cases	Not present
Vitreous changes	Frequently syneretic; posterior vitreous detachment, traction on flap of tear	Vitreoretinal traction	Usually clear, except in uveitis
Subretinal fluid	Clear	Clear, no shift	May be turbid and shift rapidly to dependent location with changes in head position
Choroidal mass	None	None	May be present
Intraocular pressure	Frequently low	Usually normal	Varies
Transillumination	Normal	Normal	Normal; however, blocked transillumination if pigmented choroidal lesion present
Examples of conditions causing detachment	Retinal break	Proliferative diabetic retinopathy, retinopathy of prematurity, toxocariasis, sickle cell retinopathy, posttraumatic vitreous traction	Uveitis, metastatic tumor, malignant melanoma, Coats disease, Vogt-Koyanagi-Harada syndrome, retinoblastoma, choroidal hemangioma, senile exudative maculopathy, exudative detachment after cryotherapy or diathermy

Modified from Hilton GF, McLean EB, Brinton DA, eds. *Retinal Detachment: Principles and Practice.* 2nd ed. Ophthalmology Monograph 1. San Francisco: American Academy of Ophthalmology; 1995.

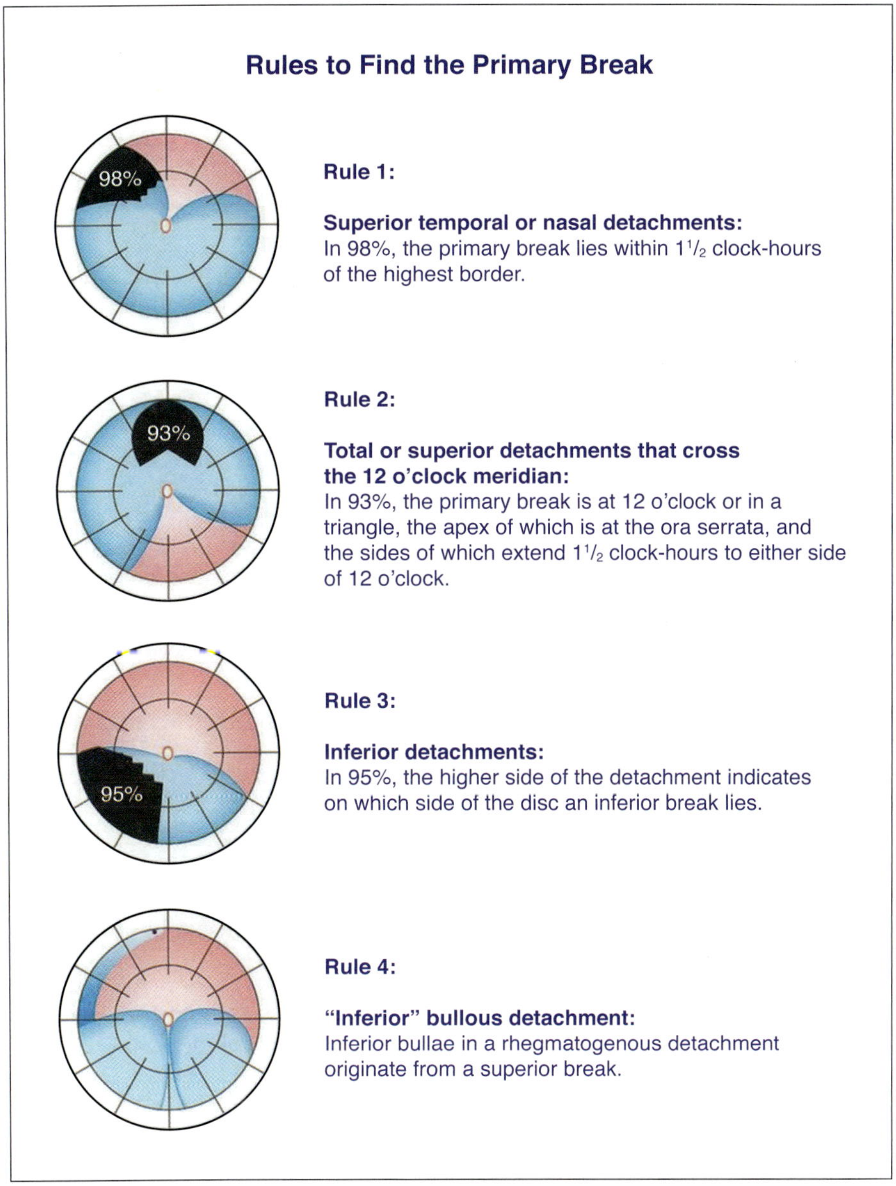

Figure 15-12 Using Lincoff rules to find the primary break. *(Used with permission from Kreissig I.* A Practical Guide to Minimal Surgery for Retinal Detachment. *Vol 1. Stuttgart, New York: Thieme; 2000:13–18. © Thieme.)*

resulting from *proliferative vitreoretinopathy* (PVR) almost always indicate an RRD. Shifting fluid may occur, but it is uncommon and more typical of serous retinal detachments.

PVR is the most common cause of failure following surgical repair of an RRD. In PVR, retinal pigment epithelial, glial, and other cells grow and migrate on both the inner and outer retinal surfaces and on the vitreous face, forming membranes. Contraction of these membranes causes fixed retinal folds, equatorial traction, detachment of the nonpigmented epithelium from the pars plana, and generalized retinal shrinkage (Fig 15-14).

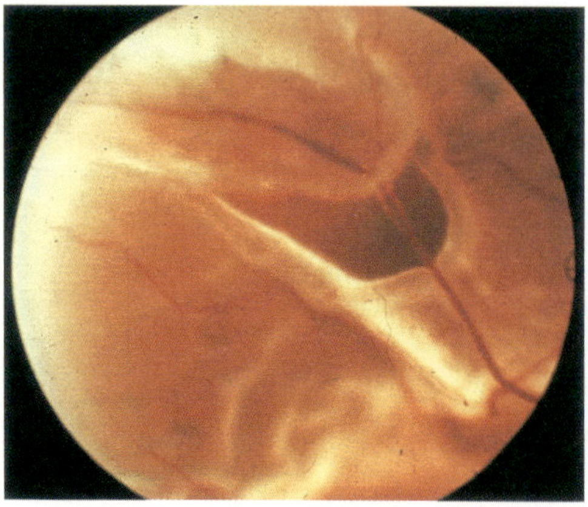

Figure 15-13 Color fundus photograph of a horseshoe retinal tear with a bridging vessel and secondary retinal detachment. Intact retinal vessels can bridge a tear, whereas some vessels crossing a flap tear can rupture and bleed into the vitreous cavity. Along with photopsia, initial symptoms may include black spots from the vitreous hemorrhage.

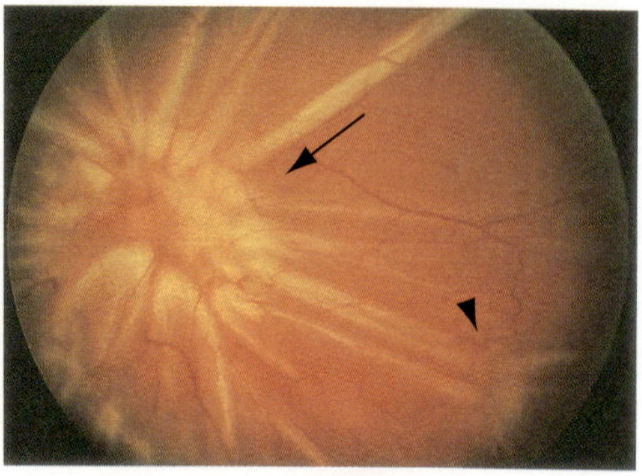

Figure 15-14 Color fundus photograph of a retinal detachment with proliferative vitreoretinopathy. Revised Retina Society classification CP-12 with diffuse retinal contraction in posterior pole *(arrow)* and single midperipheral starfold *(arrowhead)*. See Table 15-2.

As a result, the causative retinal breaks may reopen, new breaks may occur, or a tractional detachment may develop.

To better compare preoperative anatomy with outcomes, researchers developed a generally accepted classification of PVR (Table 15-2). The 1991 classification has 3 grades of PVR (A, B, and C), which correspond to increasing severity of the disease. Anterior and posterior involvement (CA, CP) are distinguished and subclassified into focal, diffuse, subretinal, circumferential, and anterior displacement. The extent of the pathology is described in clock-hours.

Han DP, Lean JS. Proliferative vitreoretinopathy. In: Albert DM, Miller JW, Azar DT, Blodi BA, eds. *Albert & Jakobiec's Principles and Practice of Ophthalmology.* Philadelphia: Saunders; 2008:chap 183.

Rowe JA, Erie JC, Baratz KH, et al. Retinal detachment in Olmsted County, Minnesota, 1976 through 1995. *Ophthalmology.* 1999;106(1):154–159.

Management of rhegmatogenous retinal detachment

The principles of surgery for retinal detachment are as follows:

- Find all retinal breaks.
- Create a chorioretinal irritation around each break.
- Close the retinal breaks.

The most important element in management is a careful retinal examination, first preoperatively and then intraoperatively. Retinal breaks can be closed by several methods, all of which involve bringing the RPE and choroid into contact with the retina long enough to produce a chorioretinal adhesion that will permanently wall off the subretinal space. This

Table 15-2 Classification of Proliferative Vitreoretinopathy, 1991

Grade	Features
A	Vitreous haze, vitreous pigment clumps, pigment clusters on inferior retina
B	Wrinkling of inner retinal surface, retinal stiffness, vessel tortuosity, rolled and irregular edge of retinal break, decreased mobility of vitreous
CP 1–12	Posterior to equator: focal, diffuse, or circumferential full-thickness folds,* subretinal strands*
CA 1–12	Anterior to equator: focal, diffuse, or circumferential full-thickness folds,* subretinal strands,* anterior displacement,* condensed vitreous with strands

*Expressed in number of clock-hours involved.

Used with permission from Machemer R, Aaberg TM, Freeman HM, Irvine AR, Lean JS, Michels RM. An updated classification of retinal detachment with proliferative vitreoretinopathy. *Am J Ophthalmol.* 1991;112(2):159–165.

process usually involves 1 of 3 approaches: (1) *scleral buckling,* (2) *vitrectomy,* or (3) *pneumatic retinopexy.* See Chapter 19 for a more detailed discussion of these techniques and outcomes.

Tractional Retinal Detachment

Vitreous membranes caused by penetrating injuries or by proliferative retinopathies such as diabetic retinopathy can pull the neurosensory retina away from the RPE, causing a tractional retinal detachment. The retina characteristically has smooth concave surfaces and contours and is immobile. The detachment can be central or peripheral and, in rare cases, can extend from the disc to the ora serrata. In most cases, the causative vitreous membrane can be seen biomicroscopically with a 3-mirror contact lens or a 60 D to 90 D indirect lens. If the traction can be released by vitrectomy, the detachment may resolve.

In some cases, traction may tear the retina and cause a combined tractional and rhegmatogenous retinal detachment. Clinically, the tractional retinal detachment loses its concave surface and assumes a shape more reminiscent of an RRD, namely convex. However, the retinal mobility is often limited compared with that of an RRD because of the tethering by proliferative tissue. In addition, corrugations characteristic of an RRD are present, and subretinal fluid, which is more extensive than in tractional retinal detachment, may extend from the disc to the ora. Treatment may require a combination of vitrectomy and a scleral buckling procedure to release the traction and seal the break.

Exudative Retinal Detachment

Recognizing whether a retinal detachment is exudative is crucial because, unlike with other types of retinal detachment, the management of exudative retinal detachment is usually nonsurgical. Exudative detachment occurs when either retinal blood vessels leak or the RPE is damaged, allowing fluid to pass into the subretinal space (Fig 15-15). Neoplasia and inflammatory diseases are the leading causes of large exudative detachments.

The presence of shifting fluid strongly suggests a large exudative retinal detachment. Because the subretinal fluid responds to the force of gravity, it detaches the area of the

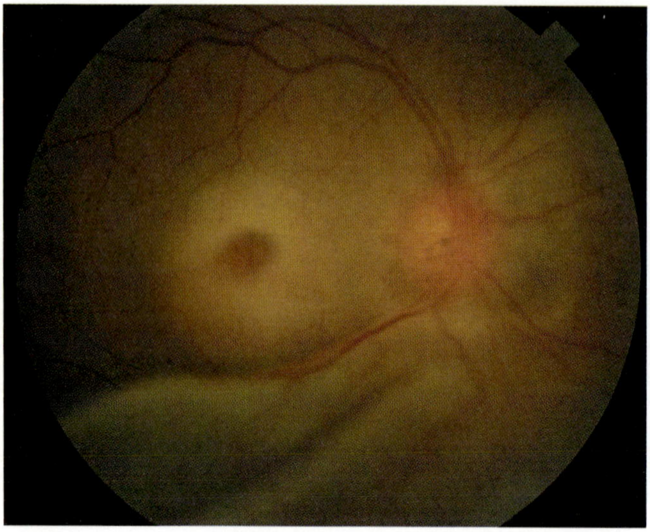

Figure 15-15 Color fundus photograph of an exudative retinal detachment that resulted from metastatic breast carcinoma. *(Courtesy of Hermann D. Schubert, MD.)*

retina in which it accumulates. For example, when the patient is sitting, the inferior retina is detached. However, when the patient becomes supine, the fluid moves posteriorly in a matter of seconds or minutes, detaching the macula. Another characteristic of exudative detachments is the smoothness of the detached retinal surface, in contrast to the corrugated appearance in RRDs. Included in the differential diagnosis is the rhegmatogenous inferior bullous detachment, which may shift and is connected to a small superior tear by a sinus (see Fig 15-12, rule 4). Fixed retinal folds, which usually indicate PVR, are rarely, if ever, present in exudative detachments. Occasionally, the retina is sufficiently elevated in exudative detachments to be visible directly behind the lens (eg, in Coats disease), a rare occurrence in RRDs.

Differential Diagnosis of Retinal Detachment

Retinoschisis

Typical peripheral cystoid degeneration is present in virtually all adults. Contiguous with and extending up to 2–3 mm posterior to the ora serrata, the area of degeneration has a bubbly appearance and is best visualized with scleral depression. The cystoid cavities in the outer plexiform layer contain a hyaluronidase-sensitive mucopolysaccharide. The only known complications of typical cystoid degeneration are coalescence and extension of the cavities and progression to typical degenerative retinoschisis.

Reticular peripheral cystoid degeneration is almost always located posterior to and continuous with typical peripheral cystoid degeneration, but it is considerably less common. It has a linear or reticular pattern that corresponds to the retinal vessels and a finely stippled internal surface. The cystoid spaces are in the nerve fiber layer. This condition may progress to *reticular degenerative retinoschisis* (also known as *bullous retinoschisis*).

Although degenerative retinoschisis is sometimes subdivided into typical and reticular forms, clinical differentiation is difficult. The complications of posterior extension and progression to retinal detachment are associated with the reticular form. Retinoschisis is bilateral in 50%–80% of affected patients, often occurs in the inferotemporal quadrant, and is commonly associated with hyperopia.

In *typical degenerative retinoschisis,* the retina splits in the outer plexiform layer. The outer layer is irregular and appears pockmarked on scleral depression. The inner layer is thin and appears clinically as a smooth, oval elevation, usually in the inferotemporal quadrant but sometimes located superotemporally. Occasionally, small, irregular white dots ("snowflakes") are present; these are footplates of Müller cells and neurons that bridge or formerly bridged the cavity. The retinal vessels may appear sclerotic. In all cases, typical bubbly appearing peripheral cystoid degeneration can be found anterior to the schisis cavity. The schisis may extend posteriorly to the equator, but complications such as hole formation, retinal detachment, or marked posterior extension are rare. The split in the retina almost never extends as far posteriorly as the macula.

In *reticular degenerative retinoschisis,* the splitting occurs in the nerve fiber layer. The very thin inner layer may be markedly elevated. As in typical retinoschisis, the outer layer appears pockmarked and the retinal vessels sclerotic. Posterior extension is more common in reticular than in typical retinoschisis. Approximately 23% of cases have holes in the outer wall that may be large and have rolled edges (Fig 15-16).

Differentiation of Retinoschisis From Rhegmatogenous Retinal Detachment

Retinoschisis must be differentiated from RRD (Table 15-3). Retinoschisis causes an absolute scotoma, whereas RRD causes a relative scotoma. Tobacco dust, hemorrhage, or both are rarely present in the vitreous with retinoschisis, whereas they are commonly observed with RRD. Retinoschisis has a smooth surface and usually appears dome shaped; in contrast, RRD often has a corrugated, irregular surface. In long-standing RRD, however, the retina also may appear smooth and thin, similar to its appearance in retinoschisis. Whereas long-standing RRD may also show atrophy of the underlying RPE, demarcation line(s), and degenerative retinal schisis (macrocysts), the underlying RPE is normal in retinoschisis.

Retinoschisis is associated with approximately 3% of full-thickness retinal detachments. Two types of schisis-related detachments occur. In the first type, if holes are present in the outer but not inner wall of the schisis cavity, the contents of the cavity can migrate through a hole in the outer wall and slowly detach the retina (see Fig 15-16). Demarcation

Table 15-3 Differentiation of Rhegmatogenous Retinal Detachment and Retinoschisis

Clinical Feature	Rhegmatogenous Retinal Detachment	Retinoschisis
Surface	Corrugated	Smooth-domed
Hemorrhage or pigment	Present	Usually absent
Scotoma	Relative	Absolute
Reaction to photocoagulation	Absent	Generally present
Shifting fluid	Usually absent	Absent

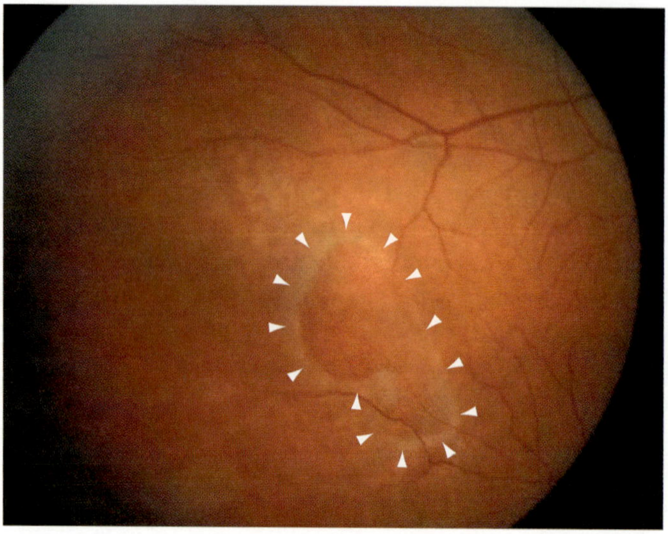

Figure 15-16 Retinoschisis with large, irregular outer-schisis-layer holes *(outlined by arrowheads)* and yellow dots on the inner surface. *(Courtesy of Colin A. McCannel, MD.)*

lines and degeneration of the underlying RPE are common. A demarcation line in an eye with retinoschisis suggests that a full-thickness detachment is present, or was formerly present and has spontaneously regressed. This type of retinoschisis detachment usually does not progress, or it progresses slowly and seldom requires treatment.

In the second type of schisis detachment, holes are present in both the inner and outer layers. The schisis cavity may collapse, and a progressive RRD may result. Such detachments often progress rapidly and usually require treatment. The causative breaks may be located very posteriorly and thus may be difficult to repair with scleral buckling. Vitrectomy may be appropriate.

Byer NE. Long-term natural history study of senile retinoschisis with implications for management. *Ophthalmology.* 1986;93(9):1127–1137.

Macular Lesions Associated With Retinal Detachment

Optic Pit Maculopathy

Optic pits are small, hypopigmented, yellow or whitish, oval or round, excavated colobomatous defects of the optic nerve; they are usually found within the inferior temporal portion of the optic disc margin (Fig 15-17). Most are unilateral and asymptomatic. However, optic pits may lead to serous macular detachments with a poor prognosis if left untreated. The macular retinal thickening and detachment typically extend from the optic pit in an oval shape toward the fovea. The origin of the subretinal fluid is unclear, but liquid vitreous and cerebrospinal fluid have been implicated. Optical coherence tomography reveals macular schisis as well as subretinal fluid. Optic pits are among the few conditions

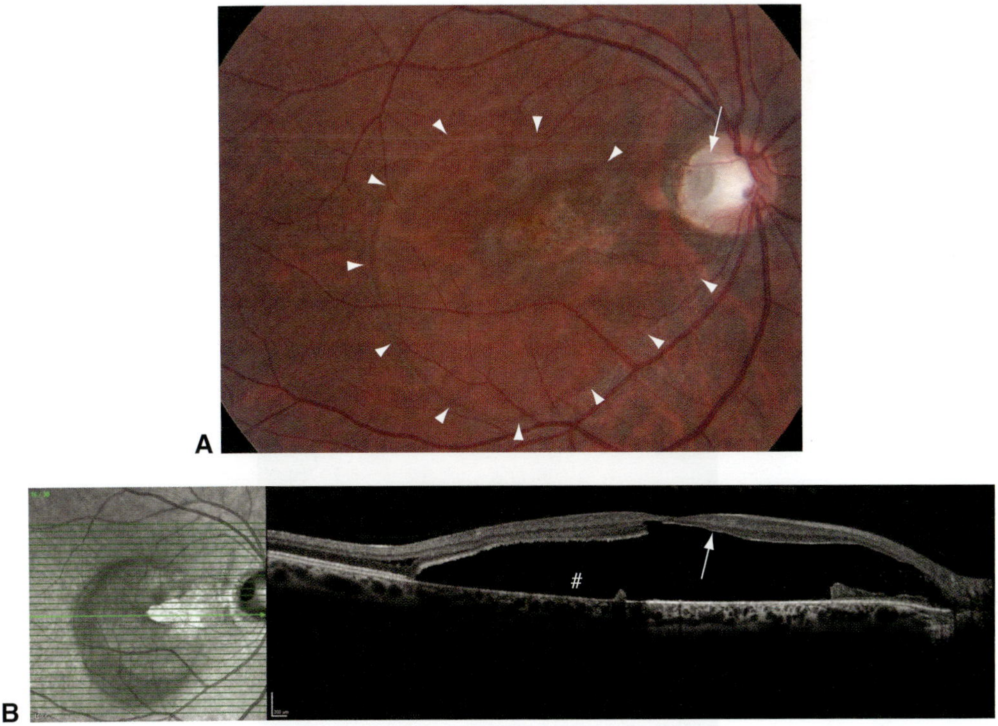

Figure 15-17 Optic nerve pit with macular detachment, retinal thinning, and retinal pigment epithelial atrophy. **A,** Fundus photograph shows an abnormal temporal optic head appearance with an excavation, or pit *(arrow)*. The adjacent retina is thickened and elevated, extending into the macula *(outlined by arrowheads)*. **B,** Optical coherence tomography scan illustrating subretinal fluid *(pound sign)* associated with the optic pit. Note the degenerated outer segments *(arrow)* of the photoreceptors. *(Courtesy of Colin A. McCannel, MD.)*

associated with macular schisis. Various successful treatments have been reported, involving vitrectomy with gas-bubble placement.

The differential diagnosis of optic pits includes glaucomatous nerve damage, such as optic pit–like changes that may occur at the inferior or superior pole of the optic nerve. Optic pits are also included in the differential diagnosis of macular thickening or detachment. Careful examination of the optic nerve margin is important for recognizing this condition.

Macular Holes in High Myopia

A distinct variant of RRD is caused by macular holes, almost always in the setting of a posterior staphyloma of highly myopic eyes (Fig 15-18). Vitreous cavity fluid enters the subretinal space through the macular hole, and the relative recoil forces of the stretched macular retina lining the staphyloma help initiate the detachment. These macular holes with retinal detachment have a far lower success rate for surgical repair than do either macular holes or typical RRDs.

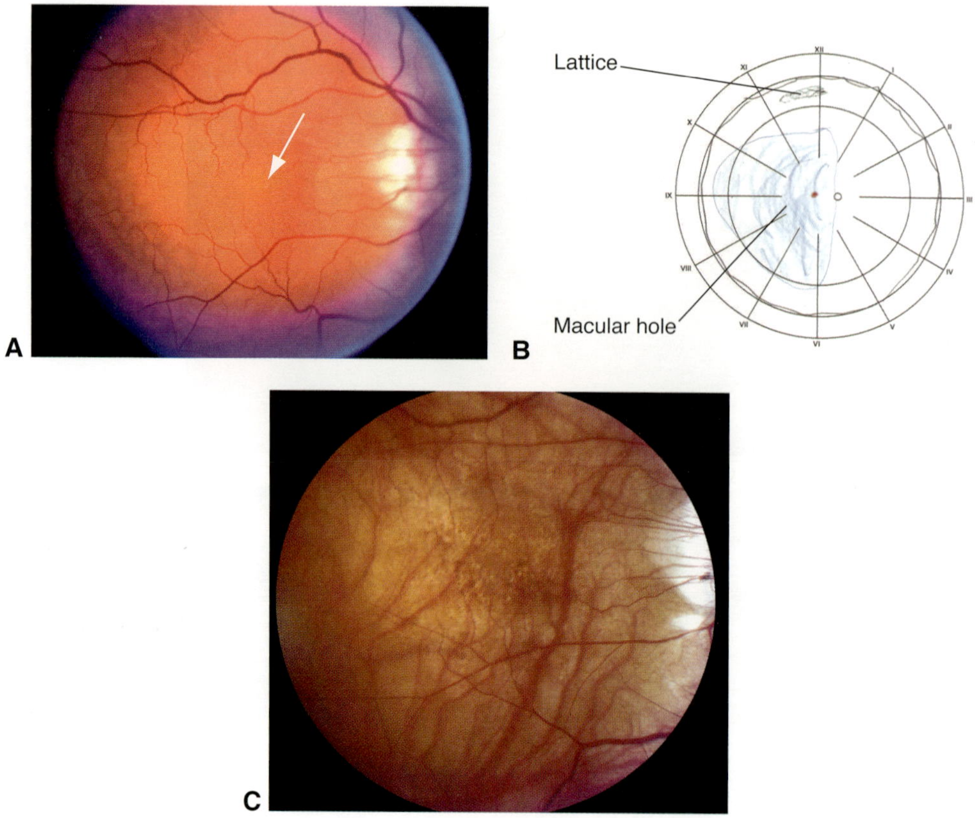

Figure 15-18 A case of rhegmatogenous retinal detachment caused by a macular hole. **A,** Fundus photograph (50-degree camera) of the detached retina with a macular hole visible in the center of the macula *(arrow).* Note the loss of transparency of the detached retina. **B,** A retinal drawing of the extent of the detachment. The area within the blue outline is detached; the *red dot* symbolizes the macular hole. At presentation, the detachment did not extend to the ora serrata; lack of such an extension is uncharacteristic even for a limited rhegmatogenous retinal detachment arising from a peripheral break. A lattice lesion with pigmentation is drawn superiorly. **C,** Fundus photograph (30-degree camera) of the macula after successful retinal reattachment using vitrectomy surgery with gas tamponade. Typical myopic fundus features include retinal pigment epithelial changes from myopic degeneration, fair pigmentation, peripapillary scleral crescent, and prominent large choroidal vessels. *(Courtesy of Colin A. McCannel, MD.)*

CHAPTER **16**

Diseases of the Vitreous and Vitreoretinal Interface

Posterior Vitreous Detachment

The vitreous is a transparent connective tissue composed of collagen and hyaluronan that is attached to the basal lamina of the lens, optic nerve, and retina. Detachment of the anterior cortical gel from the lens and the ligament of Wieger (anterior vitreous detachment) was frequently induced in the past by intracapsular cataract extraction. The more clinically important detachment of the posterior cortical gel from its adhesions at the disc (the area of Martegiani), the macula, and blood vessels is called *posterior vitreous detachment* (PVD). At its base, the vitreous remains firmly attached to the retina—even after severe trauma—sometimes resulting in vitreous base avulsion. Because of this firm attachment, the basal cortical vitreous collagen must be "shaved" during vitrectomy.

With advancing age, there is both liquefaction (synchysis) and collapse (syneresis) of the vitreous gel. The viscous hyaluronan accumulates in lacunae, which are surrounded by displaced collagen fibers. The gel can then contract, possibly because of electrostatic attraction and crosslinking of adjacent collagen fibers in the absence of hyaluronan. With this contraction, the posterior cortical gel detaches toward the firmly attached vitreous base. The prevalence of PVD is increased in patients who have had cataract extractions, particularly if the posterior capsule's integrity has been violated. Prevalence is also increased in individuals with a history of vitritis because of the loss or alteration of hyaluronan. Localized regions of the posterior cortical gel can separate slowly over the course of many years with few if any symptoms, compared with the more acute, symptomatic event.

The diagnosis of PVD is often made with indirect ophthalmoscopy or slit-lamp biomicroscopy, with which the posterior vitreous face may be observed a few millimeters in front of the retinal surface. A translucent ring of fibroglial tissue (the Weiss ring) is frequently torn loose from the surface of the optic nerve head, and its observation helps make the diagnosis of PVD. Although a shallow detachment of the posterior cortical gel may be difficult or impossible to appreciate by biomicroscopy, this type of detachment may be revealed on contact B-scan ultrasonography as a thin, hyperreflective line bounding the posterior vitreous. Optical coherence tomography (OCT) has shown that PVDs often start as a localized detachment of the vitreous over the perifovea, called a *posterior perifoveal vitreous detachment,* later spreading anteriorly to involve larger areas.

Persistent focal attachment of the vitreous to the retina can cause a number of pathologic conditions. Vitreous contraction as well as traction caused by ocular saccades may lead to breaks, particularly at the posterior edge of the vitreous base. Persistent attachment to the macula may lead to vitreomacular traction syndrome. Focal attachment to the foveola can induce foveal cavitation and macular hole formation (Fig 16-1). Remnants of the vitreous often remain on the internal limiting membrane after a posterior vitreous "detachment." For this reason, some authorities state that a presumed PVD often is actually posterior vitreoschisis that is internal or external to the layer of hyalocytes. These vitreous remnants may have a role in epiretinal membrane or macular hole formation and can contribute to tractional detachments in patients with pathologic myopia and to macular edema in patients with diabetes mellitus. Plaques of these adherent remnants of cortical vitreous can often be highlighted during vitreous surgery by applying triamcinolone (Fig 16-2).

Gupta P, Yee KM, Garcia P, et al. Vitreoschisis in macular diseases. *Br J Ophthalmol.* 2011; 95(3):376–380.

Sakamoto T, Ishibashi T. Hyalocytes: essential cells of the vitreous cavity in vitreoretinal pathophysiology? *Retina.* 2011;31(2):222–228.

Epiretinal Membranes

An epiretinal membrane (ERM) is a transparent, avascular, fibrocellular membrane on the inner retinal surface that adheres to and covers the internal limiting membrane (ILM) of the retina. Proliferation of glia, retinal pigment epithelium (RPE), or hyalocytes at the vitreoretinal interface, especially at the posterior pole, results in ERM formation.

Idiopathic ERMs are relatively common; at autopsy, they are discovered in 2% of patients older than 50 years and in 20% older than 75 years. Idiopathic ERMs are most common in persons over age 50 years, and both sexes are equally affected. The incidence

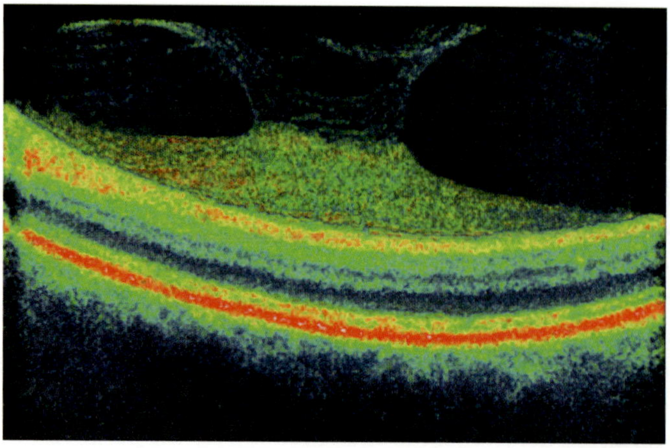

Figure 16-1 A 3-dimensional rendering of spectral-domain optical coherence tomography (SD-OCT) imaging of vitreomacular traction (VMT) syndrome. The cone of vitreous is attached to and elevates the central fovea. *(Courtesy of Richard F. Spaide, MD.)*

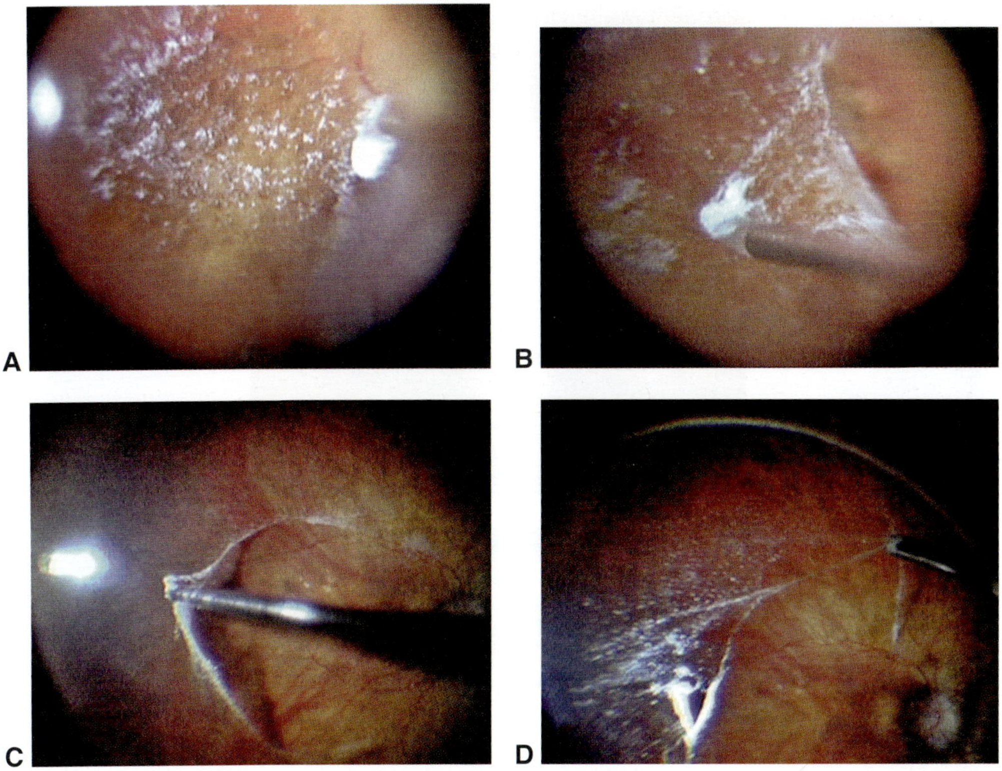

Figure 16-2 Visualization of a thin layer of adherent vitreous during vitrectomy with the use of triamcinolone. This patient appeared to have a posterior vitreous detachment (PVD) and underwent a vitrectomy. **A,** A small amount of triamcinolone was injected into the vitreous cavity; the excess was aspirated from the surface of the retina, leaving a fine distribution of triamcinolone sticking to the adherent vitreous. **B,** The vitreous membrane was elevated using a diamond-dusted silicone scraper. Note that the vitreous is difficult to see; the sheet of triamcinolone is the clue to its presence. **C,** A wide-angle viewing system then was used to visualize the elevation of the adherent vitreous, and the vitrector was set to suction only. **D,** Note the extent of the adherent vitreous sheet, which was removed with the vitrector set to cut. *(Courtesy of Richard F. Spaide, MD.)*

of bilaterality is approximately 10%–20%, and severity is usually asymmetric. Detachment or separation of the posterior vitreous is present in almost all eyes with idiopathic membranes. Schisis of the posterior vitreous may leave variable portions of the posterior cortical vitreous attached to the macula, allowing glial cells from the retina to proliferate along the retinal surface and hyalocytes to proliferate on posterior cortical vitreous remnants on the retinal surface. Secondary ERMs occur regardless of age or sex in association with abnormal vitreoretinal adhesions and areas of inflammation, as well as following retinal detachment or retinal bleeding.

Signs and symptoms

Epiretinal proliferation is generally located in the central macula—over, surrounding, or eccentric to the fovea (Fig 16-3). The membranes usually appear as a mild sheen or

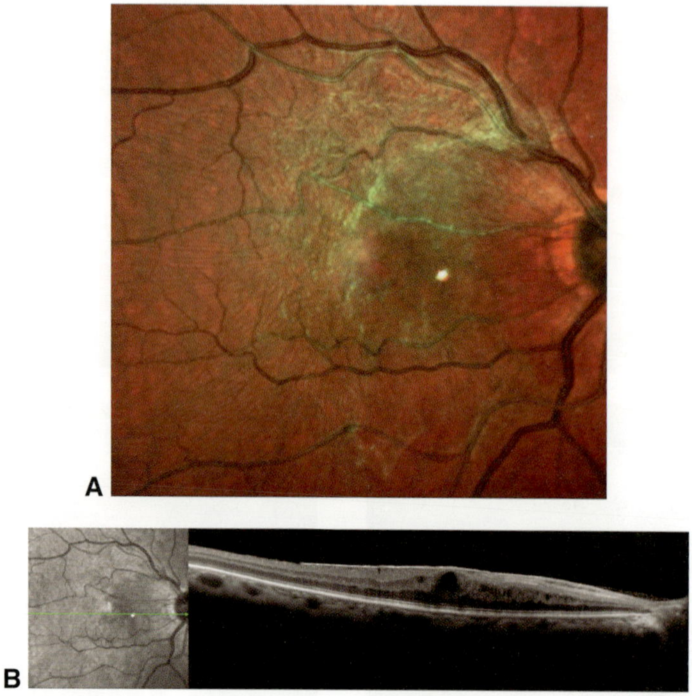

Figure 16-3 Epiretinal membrane (ERM). **A,** Scanning laser ophthalmoscope 30° fundus reflectance multicolor image reveals an ERM in the central macula with radiating striae of the internal limiting membrane (ILM) in the superior, temporal, and inferior macula. The colors in reflectance multicolor images are not exactly true to life. **B,** OCT scan through the fovea shows increased retinal thickening and cystoid edema with a large central cyst. The ERM is distorting the retinal surface temporally, which appears as several small optical voids between the ERM and the retina. *(Courtesy of Colin A. McCannel, MD.)*

glint on the retinal surface. Over time, ERMs become highly reflective and, when thickened, become more opaque, obscuring underlying retinal details. A "pseudohole" may appear if this preretinal membrane has a gap or hole in the central macula. Occasionally, intraretinal hemorrhages or whitened patches of superficial retina representing delayed axoplasmic flow and edema may be present. The cellular origin of ERMs is still under debate. Histologic examination reveals mainly RPE cells and retinal glial cells (astrocytes and Müller cells); however, myofibroblasts, fibroblasts, hyalocytes, and macrophages have also been identified.

Contracture of ERMs produces distortion and wrinkling of the inner surface of the retina, called *cellophane maculopathy* or *preretinal macular fibrosis* when mild, *surface-wrinkling retinopathy* or *retinal striae* when moderate, and *macular pucker* when severe. Increased traction may cause shallow macular detachment, diffuse thickening, or cystic changes. Furthermore, traction on retinal vessels results in increased vascular tortuosity and straightening of the perimacular vessels. Fluorescein angiography may show staining of the optic nerve and capillary leakage in the central macula. The most common OCT findings are an epiretinal reflective layer, loss of the normal retinal contour, and retinal thickening. Additional findings include irregularities of the inner retinal surface and cystic edema.

Treatment

When asymptomatic, intervention is not usually necessary. If the patient is bothered by reduced visual acuity or metamorphopsia, vitrectomy should be considered (see also Chapter 19). The goal of surgery is to optimize visual acuity, reduce metamorphopsia, and restore binocularity if it was affected preoperatively. Asymptomatic ERMs should be monitored periodically, as they will often worsen, sometimes over a relatively short period of time after being stable. In rare cases, an ERM spontaneously detaches from the inner retinal surface, and there is concomitant resolution of the retinal distortion and improvement in symptoms and vision.

Johnson TM, Johnson MW. Epiretinal membrane. In: Yanoff M, Duker J, eds. *Ophthalmology.* 4th ed. St Louis: Mosby; 2013:614–619.

Vitreomacular Traction Diseases

Vitreomacular traction diseases include abnormalities that arise from focal or broad vitreomacular adhesions in the presence of detaching or otherwise detached posterior vitreous. Three categories are recognized: (1) vitreomacular adhesion (VMA), (2) vitreomacular traction (VMT) syndrome, and (3) macular hole. A useful classification system that relies on OCT findings has been developed (Table 16-1).

Vitreomacular adhesions

VMAs in themselves do not necessarily cause visual symptoms. They can be focal or diffuse and can lead to secondary traction disease, that is, VMT and macular hole.

Vitreomacular traction syndrome

In VMT syndrome, the posterior hyaloid is abnormally adherent to the macula (VMA). As the vitreous detaches, the posterior hyaloid remains tethered at the macula, usually the fovea, causing tractional foveal distortion, cystic edema, and in severe cases tractional foveal detachment. These changes lead to decreased visual acuity, metamorphopsia, and often a vague complaint about poor vision in the affected eye out of proportion to the measured visual acuity. Angiography may demonstrate leakage of fluorescein dye from macular vessels as well as from the optic nerve. OCT is useful to demonstrate the

Table 16-1 The International Vitreomacular Traction Study Classification System for Vitreomacular Adhesion, Traction, and Macular Hole

Classification	Subclassification
Vitreomacular adhesion	Size: focal (≤1500 µm) or broad (>1500 µm) Isolated or concurrent
Vitreomacular traction (VMT)	Size: focal (≤1500 µm) or broad (>1500 µm) Isolated or concurrent
Full-thickness macular hole	Size: small (≤250 µm), medium (>250–≤400 µm), or large (>400 µm) Status of vitreous: with or without VMT Cause: primary or secondary

From Duker JS, Kaiser PK, Binder S, et al. The International Vitreomacular Traction Study Group classification of vitreomacular adhesion, traction, and macular hole. *Ophthalmology.* 2013;120(12):2611–2619.

vitreoretinal interface abnormalities and the tractional effects of VMT syndrome on the foveal architecture. Chronic traction is generally understood to be harmful over the long term, particularly when there is cystic edema or vision is affected. Spontaneous separation of the focal vitreoretinal adhesion—with resolution of all clinical features—is rare, particularly when there is an associated epiretinal membrane (Fig 16-4). Intervention should be considered for VMT syndrome and includes pars plana vitrectomy with membrane peeling or intravitreal injection of ocriplasmin (see also Chapter 19).

Ocriplasmin is a recombinant protease with activity against fibronectin and laminin; a multicenter clinical trial found that resolution of vitreomacular traction occurred in 26.5% of ocriplasmin-injected eyes compared with 10.1% of placebo-injected eyes over the same period. In a subset of patients with vitreomacular adhesions smaller than 1500 μm, the rate of resolution increased to 33.6%.

Johnson MW. Tractional cystoid macular edema: a subtle variant of the vitreomacular traction syndrome. *Am J Ophthalmol.* 2005;140(2):184–192.

Stalmans P, Benz MS, Gandorfer A, et al; MIVI-TRUST Study Group. Enzymatic vitreolysis with ocriplasmin for vitreomacular traction and macular holes. *N Engl J Med.* 2012; 367(7):606–615.

Idiopathic Macular Holes

Idiopathic macular holes occur at a rate of approximately 8 per 100,000 persons per year and have a female-to-male ratio of 2 to 1. They occur mostly in the sixth through eighth decades of life and can appear at a younger age in myopic eyes. Idiopathic macular holes are bilateral in approximately 10% of patients. Investigations using OCT suggest that idiopathic macular holes are caused by the same tractional forces as the forces associated with perifoveal vitreous detachment and thus are likely an early stage of age-related PVD. The following description of the stages of macular hole formation is useful in making management decisions (Fig 16-5):

- A stage 0, or premacular, hole occurs when a PVD with persistent foveal attachment develops. Subtle loss of the foveal depression can be observed, and visual acuity is usually unaffected. Most stage 0 holes do not progress to advanced stages. This stage represents a VMA.

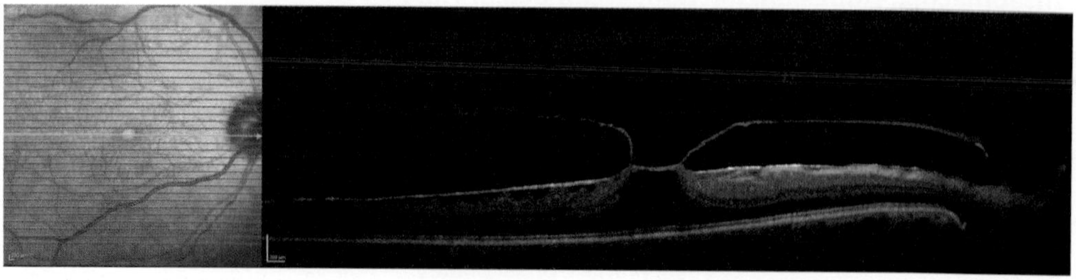

Figure 16-4 Vitreomacular traction syndrome. OCT scan of the macula through the fovea shows vitreomacular traction causing a large foveal cyst and distortion of the inner retina. An ERM is also present. *(Courtesy of Tara A. McCannel, MD, PhD.)*

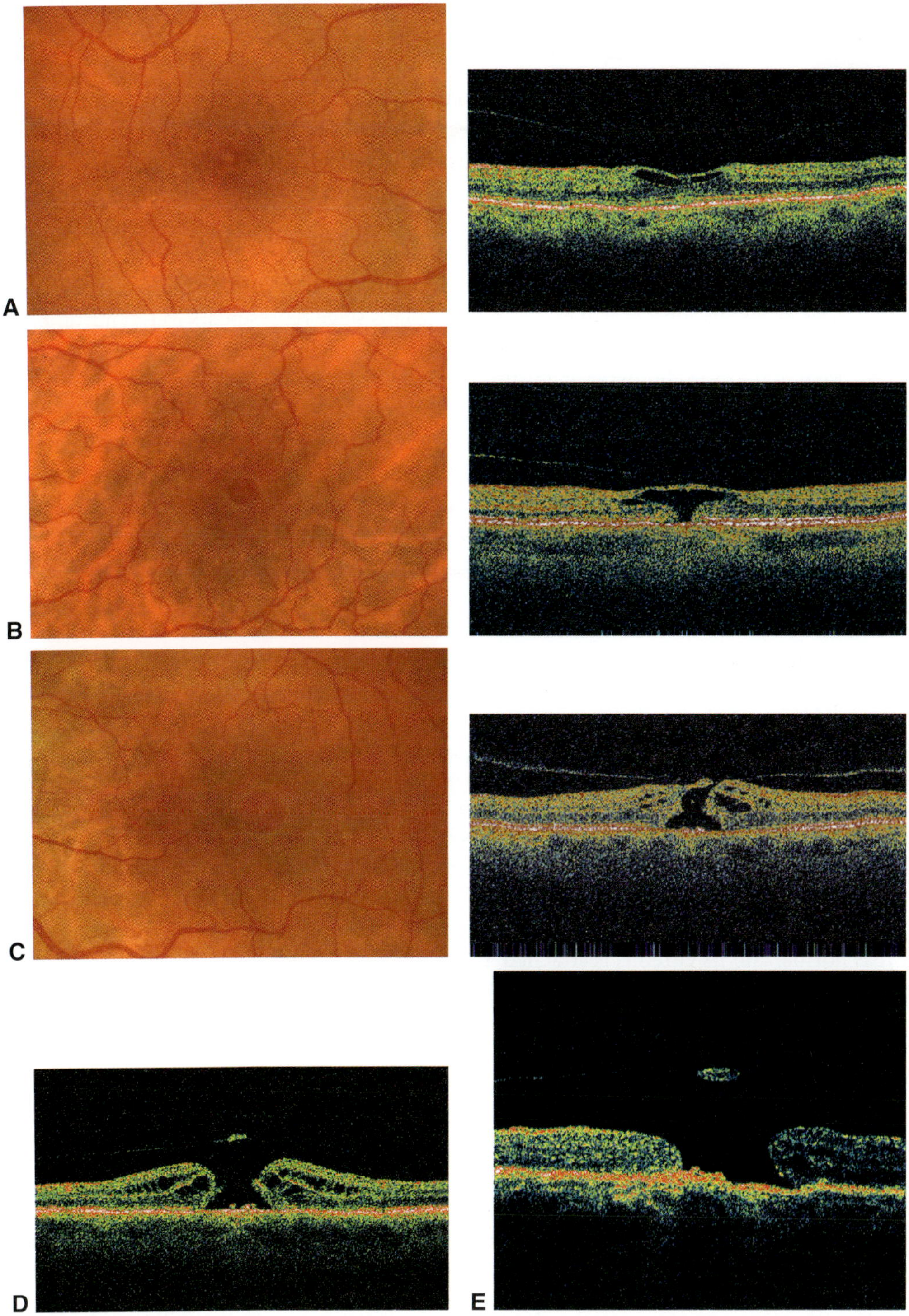

Figure 16-5 Macular holes. **A,** Color fundus photograph of stage 1A hole with horizontal splitting of retinal layers and corresponding OCT scan showing stage 1A hole. **B,** Fundus photograph and corresponding OCT scan of stage 1B hole. **C,** Fundus photograph of stage 2 hole with small opening in inner layer eccentrically and corresponding OCT scan of stage 2 hole. **D,** OCT scan of stage 3 full-thickness hole with elevation of adjacent retinal edges. **E,** OCT scan of stage 4 full-thickness hole with operculum. *(Courtesy of Mark W. Johnson, MD, and Peter K. Kaiser, MD.)*

- A stage 1 macular hole (impending macular hole) typically causes visual symptoms of metamorphopsia and central vision decline, usually to a visual acuity range of 20/25 to 20/60. The characteristic findings are either a small yellow spot (stage 1A) or yellow circle (stage 1B) in the fovea. OCT examination reveals that a stage 1A hole is a foveal "pseudocyst," or horizontal splitting (schisis), associated with vitreous traction to the foveal center. A stage 1B hole indicates a break in the outer fovea, the margins of which constitute the yellow ring noted clinically. Spontaneous resolution of a stage 1 hole occurs in approximately 50% of cases. This stage represents VMT syndrome.
- A stage 2 macular hole represents an early full-thickness macular hole that is less than 400 μm in diameter. It results from the progression of a foveal schisis (pseudocyst) to a full-thickness dehiscence, as a tractional break develops in the "roof" (inner layer) of the pseudocyst. Progression to stage 2 is accompanied by a further decline in visual acuity. OCT demonstrates the full-thickness defect and the posterior hyaloid's continuing attachment to the foveal center. This stage represents VMT syndrome with a small- to medium-sized macular hole.
- A stage 3 macular hole is a fully developed hole (≥400 μm in diameter), typically surrounded by a rim of thickened and detached retina. Visual acuity ranges widely. The posterior hyaloid remains attached to the optic disc but is detached from the fovea. An operculum suspended by the posterior hyaloid may be seen overlying the hole. On OCT, this stage represents a large macular hole with no VMT.
- A stage 4 macular hole is a fully developed hole with a complete posterior vitreous detachment, as evidenced by the presence of a Weiss ring. On OCT, this stage represents a large macular hole with no VMT.

The fellow-eye risk of macular hole development depends on the vitreous attachment status. If a complete vitreous detachment is present in the fellow eye, there is little, if any, risk of macular hole development. If the fellow eye has stage 1A abnormalities, however, there is a substantial risk of progression to a full-thickness macular hole. When the fellow eye is normal and its vitreous is attached, the risk of developing a macular hole in that eye is approximately 10%, the rate of bilaterality.

Management options

For stage 2 or greater macular holes, surgical intervention is recommended—specifically, pars plana vitrectomy with gas tamponade; in most recent series, the success rate for closure and vision improvement was greater than 90% (also see Chapter 19). Stage 1 macular holes have an approximate 50% rate of spontaneous resolution and thus are typically monitored.

An alternative management option is the intravitreal injection of ocriplasmin. Resultant lysis of vitreoretinal adhesions facilitates macular hole closure, or stage 1 hole resolution (see earlier discussion of VMT resolution). This method is most successful for early-stage holes. In the ocriplasmin phase 3 clinical trial, the closure rate of full-thickness macular holes was 40.6% overall and 58.3% for holes of less than 250 μm diameter. Ocriplasmin is most effective in eyes with focal adhesions and much less effective for broad vitreoretinal adhesions or adhesions associated with an ERM.

Duker JS, Kaiser PK, Binder S, et al. The International Vitreomacular Traction Study Group classification of vitreomacular adhesion, traction, and macular hole. *Ophthalmology.* 2013; 120(12):2611–2619.

McCannel CA, Ensminger JL, Diehl NN, Hodge DN. Population-based incidence of macular holes. *Ophthalmology.* 2009;116(7):1136–1139.

Stalmans P, Benz MS, Gandorfer A, et al; MIVI-TRUST Study Group. Enzymatic vitreolysis with ocriplasmin for vitreomacular traction and macular holes. *N Engl J Med.* 2012;367(7): 606–615.

Developmental Abnormalities

Tunica Vasculosa Lentis

Remnants of the tunica vasculosa lentis and hyaloid artery, although commonly observed, are not visually significant. Mittendorf dot, an anterior remnant, is a small, dense, and white round plaque attached to the posterior lens capsule nasally and inferiorly to its posterior pole. A prepapillary remnant known as Bergmeister papilla is a fibroglial tuft of tissue extending into the vitreous for a short distance at the margin of the optic nerve head. The entire hyaloid artery may persist from disc to lens as multilayered fenestrated sheaths forming the Cloquet canal.

Prepapillary Vascular Loops

Initially thought to be remnants of the hyaloid artery, prepapillary vascular loops are normal retinal vessels that have grown into Bergmeister papilla before returning to the retina (Fig 16-6). The loops typically extend less than 5 mm into the vitreous. These vessels may

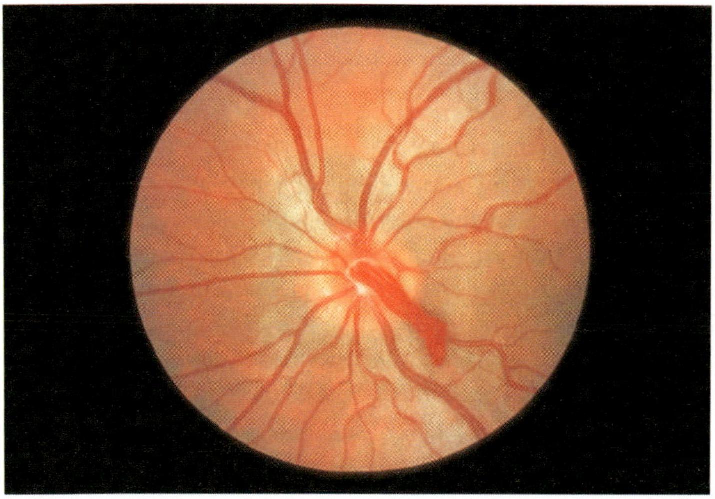

Figure 16-6 Color fundus photograph of a prepapillary vascular loop. *(Courtesy of M. Gilbert Grand, MD.)*

supply one or more quadrants of the retina. Fluorescein angiography (FA) has shown that 95% of these vessels are arterial and 5% are venous. Complications include branch retinal artery obstruction, amaurosis fugax, and vitreous hemorrhage.

Persistent Fetal Vasculature

Persistent fetal vasculature (PFV), previously known as *persistent hyperplastic primary vitreous,* is a congenital anomaly thought to result from failure of the primary vascular vitreous to regress. The disorder is unilateral in 90% of cases and usually has no associated systemic findings. Anterior, posterior, and combined forms of this developmental abnormality have been described.

Anterior persistent fetal vasculature

In anterior PFV, the hyaloid artery remains, and a white vascularized fibrous membrane or mass is present behind the lens. Associated findings include microphthalmos, a shallow anterior chamber, and elongated ciliary processes that are visible around the small lens. Leukocoria is often present at birth. A dehiscence of the posterior lens capsule may, in many cases, cause swelling of the lens and cataract as well as secondary angle-closure glaucoma. In addition, glaucoma may result from incomplete development of the chamber angle.

The natural course of anterior PFV may result in blindness in the most advanced cases. Lensectomy and removal of the fibrovascular retrolental membrane will prevent angle-closure glaucoma; however, growth of a secondary cataract is common. Deprivational and refractive amblyopia is a serious postoperative challenge in these patients.

Anterior PFV should be considered in the differential diagnosis of leukocoria. Differentiating it from retinoblastoma is particularly important. Unlike for PFV, retinoblastoma is usually not obvious at birth, is more often bilateral, and is almost never associated with microphthalmos or cataract. PFV is anterior in the eye at birth; retinoblastomas do not appear in the anterior fundus until well after birth. Ancillary testing, such as diagnostic echography and x-ray techniques to look for calcification within the retinoblastoma, can be helpful in differentiating the 2 disorders.

Posterior persistent fetal vasculature

Posterior PFV may occur in association with anterior PFV or as an isolated finding. The eye may be microphthalmic, but the anterior chamber is usually normal and the lens is typically clear and without a retrolental membrane. A stalk of tissue emanates from the optic disc and courses toward the retrolental region, often running along the apex of a retinal fold that may extend anteriorly from the disc, usually in an inferior quadrant. The stalk fans out circumferentially toward the anterior retina. Posterior PFV should be differentiated from retinopathy of prematurity (ROP), familial exudative vitreoretinopathy, and ocular toxocariasis.

Goldberg MF. Persistent fetal vasculature (PFV): an integrated interpretation of signs and symptoms associated with persistent hyperplastic primary vitreous (PHPV). LIV Edward Jackson Memorial Lecture. *Am J Ophthalmol.* 1997;124(5):587–626.

Hereditary Hyaloideoretinopathies With Optically Empty Vitreous: Wagner and Stickler Syndromes

The hallmark of the group of conditions known as hereditary hyaloideoretinopathies is vitreous liquefaction (synchysis) that results in an optically empty cavity except for a thin layer of cortical vitreous behind the lens and threadlike, avascular membranes that run circumferentially and adhere to the retina. Fundus abnormalities include equatorial and perivascular (radial) lattice degeneration. The electroretinogram response may be subnormal.

In Wagner disease, the optically empty vitreous is accompanied by myopia, strabismus, and cataract but no associated systemic findings. It is not associated with retinal detachment and has an autosomal dominant inheritance pattern.

Stickler syndrome is the most common variety of hereditary hyaloideoretinopathy with associated systemic findings (Fig 16-7) and is transmitted as an autosomal dominant trait. Most patients have a mutation in the gene *COL2A1,* which encodes type II procollagen. Various mutations may produce Stickler syndrome phenotypes of differing severity. Additional ocular abnormalities include myopia, open-angle glaucoma, and cataract. Orofacial findings include midfacial flattening and the Pierre Robin malformation complex of cleft palate, micrognathia, and glossoptosis. These abnormalities may be dramatic at birth, requiring tracheostomy, or they may not be obvious at all. Generalized skeletal abnormalities include joint hyperextensibility and enlargement; arthritis, particularly of the knees; and mild spondyloepiphyseal dysplasia. Early recognition of this syndrome is very important because of the high incidence of retinal detachment. In one series, retinal tears were associated with mutations in *COL2A1* in 91% of cases and retinal detachments in 53%. The detachments may be difficult to repair because of multiple, posterior, or large breaks and a tendency toward proliferative vitreoretinopathy. Patients with this condition typically have cortical vitreous condensations that are firmly

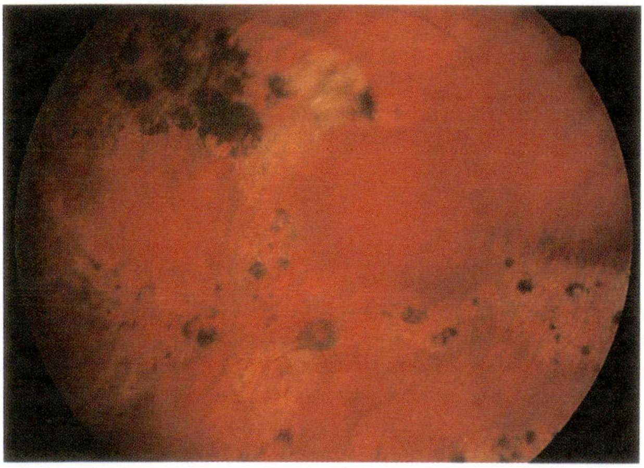

Figure 16-7 Color fundus photograph showing extensive lattice degeneration and pigmentary change in a patient with Stickler syndrome. *(Courtesy of William F. Mieler, MD.)*

adherent to the retina. For this reason, the ophthalmologist should strongly consider prophylactic therapy of retinal breaks. (See Prophylactic Treatment of Retinal Breaks in Chapter 15.)

Other forms of hereditary hyaloideoretinopathy associated with systemic abnormalities include Weill-Marchesani syndrome and some varieties of dwarfism.

Maumenee IH. Vitreoretinal degeneration as a sign of generalized connective tissue diseases. *Am J Ophthalmol.* 1979;88(3 Pt 1):432–449.

Rose PS, Levy HP, Liberfarb RM, et al. Stickler syndrome: clinical characteristics and diagnostic criteria. *Am J Med Genet A.* 2005;138A(3):199–207.

Familial Exudative Vitreoretinopathy

Familial exudative vitreoretinopathy (FEVR) is characterized by failure of the temporal retina to vascularize and is phenotypically similar to ROP. It is usually inherited as an autosomal dominant trait, but X-linked transmission also occurs. Several different gene loci have been associated with the FEVR phenotype: *EVR1, EVR2,* and *EVR4* on chromosome 11 are autosomal dominant, whereas *EVR2* on chromosome arm Xp is X-linked. The *EVR2* gene encodes the Norrie disease protein. Retinal folds, peripheral fibrovascular proliferation, as well as tractional and exudative retinal detachment are often associated with FEVR (Fig 16-8). Temporal dragging of the macula may cause the patient to appear to have exotropia. Late-onset rhegmatogenous retinal detachments may occur. Generally, the earlier the disease presents, the more severe the manifestations.

The condition is frequently bilateral, although the severity of ocular involvement may be asymmetric. Individuals with FEVR, unlike patients with ROP, are born full term and have normal respiratory status. In FEVR, the peripheral retinal vessels form numerous parallel fascicles that end abruptly a variable distance from the ora (brush border). Differentiation of FEVR from ROP is also aided by the family history and a careful examination of all family members. The only finding in some family members with FEVR may be a

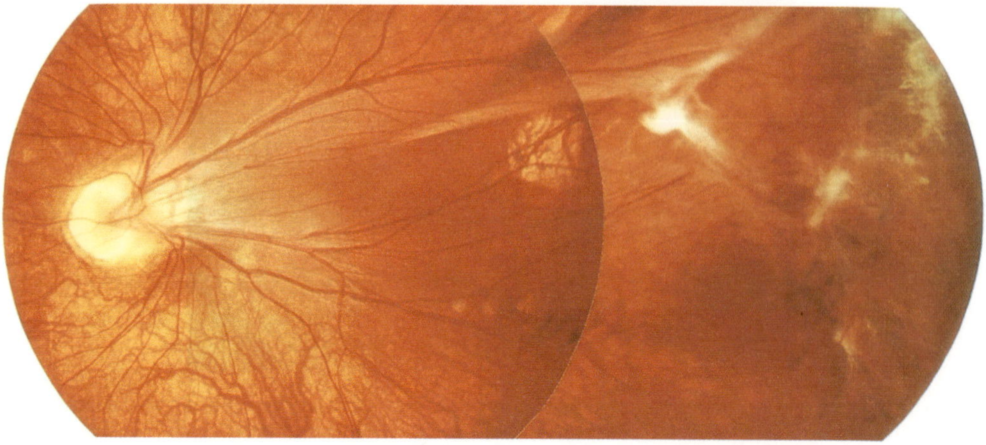

Figure 16-8 Color fundus photograph collage of familial exudative vitreoretinopathy. The temporal zone of nonperfusion is horizontally V-shaped, causing a tractional macular fold.

straightening of vessels and peripheral retinal nonperfusion. Parents of affected children may be mildly affected and asymptomatic. FA with peripheral sweeps is indispensable in examining family members.

Ranchod TM, Ho LY, Drenser KA, Capone A Jr, Trese MT. Clinical presentation of familial exudative vitreoretinopathy. *Ophthalmology.* 2011;118(10):2070–2075.

Vitreous Opacities

Asteroid Hyalosis

Minute white opacities composed of calcium-containing phospholipids are found in the otherwise normal vitreous in asteroid hyalosis (Fig 16-9). Clinical studies have confirmed a relationship between asteroid hyalosis and both diabetes mellitus and hypertension. Asteroid hyalosis has an overall incidence of 1 in 200 persons, most frequently in people older than 50 years. The condition is unilateral in 75% of cases, and significant decreases in visual acuity are rare. When asteroid hyalosis blocks the view of the posterior fundus and retinal pathology is suspected, FA is usually successful in imaging the abnormalities. Occasionally, vitrectomy may be necessary to remove visually significant opacities or to facilitate treatment of underlying retinal abnormalities such as proliferative retinopathy. Many eyes with asteroid hyalosis have an abnormal vitreoretinal interface with unusual vitreoretinal adhesions. These adhesions increase the risk of retinal break formation during vitrectomy surgery.

Mochizuki Y, Hata Y, Kita T, et al. Anatomical findings of vitreoretinal interface in eyes with asteroid hyalosis. *Graefes Arch Clin Exp Ophthalmol.* 2009;247(9):1173–1177.

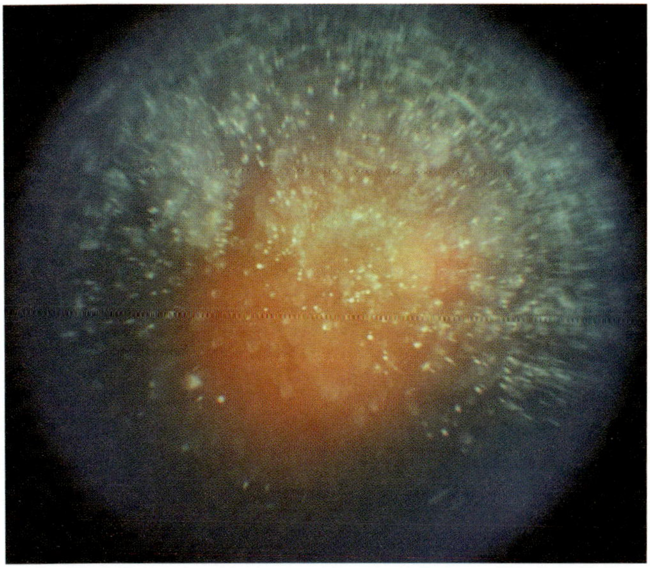

Figure 16-9 Color fundus photograph of asteroid hyalosis. *(Courtesy of Hermann D. Schubert, MD.)*

Vitreous Hemorrhage

A common cause of emergency visits to ophthalmology offices is sudden vision loss due to vitreous hemorrhage not associated with trauma to the eye. In adults, the most common causes include proliferative diabetic retinopathy (see Chapter 5 management discussion), PVD, central retinal vein occlusion, and retinal neovascularization from a variety of causes (see Chapter 7, Table 7-2). In cases of vitreous hemorrhage associated with an acute PVD, retinal tears are found in approximately 50%–70% of eyes and clinical retinal detachment in 8%–12%. In children, X-linked hereditary retinoschisis and pars planitis are common causes of vitreous hemorrhage; however, trauma must always be considered in the differential diagnosis (see Chapter 17).

In most cases of vitreous hemorrhage, the underlying cause can be determined by obtaining a history or on retinal examination. If the hemorrhage is too dense to permit indirect ophthalmoscopy or biomicroscopy, suggestive clues can be obtained from examination of the fellow eye. Diagnostic echography should be performed to detect any tractional tear (often superotemporally) and to rule out retinal detachment or tumor. Bilateral eye patching with bed rest for a few hours to several days, with the head of the bed elevated, may permit the intrahyaloid and retrohyaloid blood to settle, allowing for a better view of the posterior segment. If the etiology still cannot be established, the ophthalmologist should consider frequent reexamination with repeat echography until the cause is found. Alternatively, prompt diagnostic vitrectomy in nondiabetic patients can be considered and may help prevent progression of a retinal tear to retinal detachment. Ghost cell glaucoma can result from long-standing vitreous hemorrhage.

El-Sanhouri AA, Foster RE, Petersen MR, et al. Retinal tears after posterior vitreous detachment and vitreous hemorrhage in patients on systemic anticoagulants. *Eye (Lond).* 2011;25(8): 1016–1019.

Sarrafizadeh R, Hassan TS, Ruby AJ, et al. Incidence of retinal detachment and visual outcome in eyes presenting with posterior vitreous separation and dense fundus-obscuring vitreous hemorrhage. *Ophthalmology.* 2001;108(12):2273–2278.

Witmer MT, Cohen SM. Oral anticoagulation and the risk of vitreous hemorrhage and retinal tears in eyes with acute posterior vitreous detachment. *Retina.* 2013;33(3):621–626.

Pigment Granules

In a patient without uveitis, retinitis pigmentosa, or a history of surgical or accidental eye trauma, the presence of pigmented cells in the anterior vitreous ("tobacco dust"), known as a *Shafer sign,* is highly suggestive of a retinal break (see Chapter 15).

Cholesterolosis

Numerous yellow-white, gold, or multicolored cholesterol crystals are present in the vitreous and anterior chamber in cholesterolosis, also known as *synchysis scintillans.* This condition appears almost exclusively in eyes that have undergone repeated or severe accidental or surgical trauma causing large intravitreal hemorrhages. The descriptive term *synchysis scintillans* refers to the highly refractile appearance of the cholesterol-containing crystals. In contrast to eyes with asteroid hyalosis, in which the opacities are evenly distributed throughout the vitreous cavity, eyes with cholesterolosis frequently have a PVD, which allows the crystals to settle inferiorly.

Amyloidosis

Bilateral vitreous opacification can occur as an early manifestation of the dominantly inherited form of familial amyloidosis, which is most commonly associated with a transthyretin mutation (Fig 16-10). Amyloid infiltration of the vitreous is rare in nonfamilial cases. In addition to the vitreous, amyloid can be deposited in the retinal vasculature, the choroid, and the trabecular meshwork.

Retinal findings include hemorrhages, exudates, cotton-wool spots, and peripheral retinal neovascularization. In addition, infiltrations may be present in the orbit, extraocular muscles, eyelids, conjunctiva, cornea, and iris. Nonocular manifestations of amyloidosis

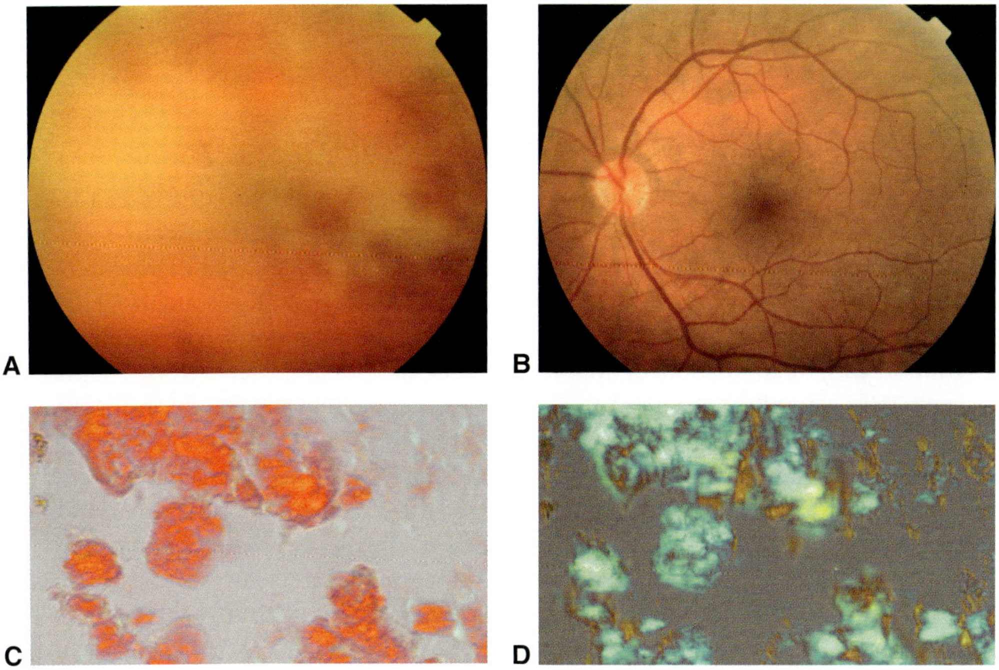

Figure 16-10 Amyloidosis. Images from a 57-year-old woman with a history of vitrectomy for floaters in the right eye. A cataract subsequently developed in the right eye and was extracted. Her vision then decreased in the left eye, which she ascribed to a cataract. **A,** Color fundus photograph of the left eye showed a dense vitreous infiltration; there was no cataract, and intraocular pressure was markedly elevated. Review of systems revealed carpal tunnel syndrome in both wrists. **B,** After vitrectomy surgery on the left eye, the color fundus photograph revealed retinal hemorrhages along the inferotemporal vascular arcade. **C,** The removed vitreous material, stained with Congo red, demonstrated birefringence **(D).** The patient was found to have a mutation affecting transthyretin. Glaucoma commonly develops in patients with transthyretin-related familial amyloidotic polyneuropathy. *(Courtesy of Richard F. Spaide, MD.)*

include upper- and lower-extremity polyneuropathy and central nervous system abnormalities. Amyloid can be deposited in several organs, including the heart and skin, and in the gastrointestinal tract.

Initially, the extracellular vitreous opacities appear to lie adjacent to retinal vessels posteriorly; they later develop anteriorly. At first, the opacities appear granular and have wispy fringes, but as they enlarge and aggregate, the vitreous takes on a "glass-wool" appearance. With vitreous liquefaction or PVD, the opacities may be displaced into the visual axis, causing reduced vision and photophobia.

The differential diagnosis includes chronic (dehemoglobinized) vitreous hemorrhage, lymphoma, sarcoidosis, and Whipple disease. Vitrectomy may be indicated for vitreous opacities when symptoms warrant intervention, but recurrent opacities may develop in residual vitreous. Histologic examination of removed vitreous shows material with a fibrillar appearance and a staining reaction characteristic of amyloid. Birefringence and electron microscopic studies are confirmatory. Immunocytochemical studies have shown the major amyloid constituent to be a protein resembling prealbumin.

Sandgren O. Ocular amyloidosis, with special reference to the hereditary forms with vitreous involvement. *Surv Ophthalmol.* 1995;40(3):173–196.

Vitreous Abnormalities Secondary to Surgery

Incarceration of vitreous in the wound during cataract or vitreous surgery can lead to many postoperative complications. Following cataract surgery with vitreous incarceration, there is an increased risk of infectious endophthalmitis, epithelial ingrowth, hypotony, shallow anterior chamber, peripheral anterior synechiae, and secondary glaucoma. Incarcerated vitreous in the wound and iridovitreal adhesions may cause chronic ocular discomfort with inflammation, cystoid macular edema, and disc edema (Irvine-Gass syndrome). These complications may be reduced by disconnecting any vitreous from anterior adhesions and incarcerations through vitrectomy.

Retinal detachment can be caused by contraction of vitreous incarcerated in cataract or vitrectomy incisions. Such detachments may be rhegmatogenous or tractional and may require treatment with vitrectomy and/or scleral buckling surgery (see Chapter 19).

The risk of complications from vitreous loss during cataract surgery can be sharply reduced by careful anterior vitrectomy followed by meticulous closure of all wounds. For further discussion of the complications of cataract surgery and their management, see BCSC Section 11, *Lens and Cataract.* For information about postoperative endophthalmitis, see BCSC Section 9, *Intraocular Inflammation and Uveitis.*

Harbour JW, Smiddy WE, Rubsamen PE, Murray TG, Davis JL, Flynn HW Jr. Pars plana vitrectomy for chronic pseudophakic cystoid macular edema. *Am J Ophthalmol.* 1995; 120(3):302–307.

CHAPTER 17

Posterior Segment Manifestations of Trauma

This chapter includes a related video, which can be accessed by scanning the QR code provided in the text or going to www.aao.org/bcscvideo_section12.

Ocular trauma is an important cause of visual impairment worldwide. Posterior segment injuries can be classified as follows:

- blunt trauma (with or without break in eyewall)
- penetrating trauma (entrance break; no exit break in eyewall)
- perforating trauma (both entrance and exit breaks in eyewall)
- intraocular foreign bodies, penetrating or perforating

Microsurgical techniques have improved the ability to repair corneal and scleral lacerations, and vitrectomy techniques allow management of severe intraocular injuries (see Chapter 19). Ocular trauma is also discussed in BCSC Section 6, *Pediatric Ophthalmology and Strabismus;* Section 7, *Orbit, Eyelids, and Lacrimal System;* and Section 8, *External Disease and Cornea.*

Evaluation of the Patient After Ocular Trauma

Obtaining a complete history, or as complete as possible under the circumstances, is crucial before a patient with ocular trauma is examined. The following important information is needed:

- How and when was the patient injured?
- Was the injury work related?
- What emergency measures were taken (eg, tetanus shot given, antibiotics administered)?
- Are there concomitant systemic injuries?
- When was the patient's last oral intake (in case surgery is required)?
- What was the health status of the eye before the injury?
- Has the patient had previous ocular surgery, including laser in situ keratomileusis (LASIK)?
- Is the presence of an intraocular foreign body a possibility?
- Was the patient hammering metal on metal or working near machinery that could have caused a projectile to enter the eye?

- Was the patient wearing spectacles or was he or she close to shattered glass?
- How forceful was the injury?
- Was the patient wearing eye protection?

Caution is required to avoid causing more damage to the eye when examining it. The physician should avoid prying open the eye of an uncooperative patient. Initial evaluation should try to determine whether the injury is closed globe or open globe. In an open-globe injury, the eyewall has a full-thickness defect that may be caused by rupture, which is mechanical failure resulting from too much pressure, or by a laceration, which is caused by a sharp object cutting the eyewall. In a suspected open-globe injury, the eye should be covered with a shield. If severe chemosis, ecchymosis, or eyelid edema prevents a thorough examination, the examination is best postponed until the time of surgery. Anesthesia should be considered when examining children or anyone unable to cooperate.

If possible, the clinician should measure the visual acuity of each eye separately and evaluate the pupils for an afferent pupillary defect. Slit-lamp examination can reveal an entrance wound, hyphema, iris damage or incarceration, cataract, or other anterior segment pathology, although a scleral entrance wound is sometimes obscured by ecchymosis. Intraocular pressure (IOP) should be checked. Reduced IOP may suggest a posterior scleral rupture; however, normal IOP does not exclude an occult penetration of the globe.

The eye should be examined with the indirect ophthalmoscope as soon as feasible. A posterior penetration or an intraocular foreign body may be detected before synechiae, cataract, dispersed vitreous hemorrhage, or infection obscures it. Intraocular foreign bodies are discussed later in this chapter.

Ultrasound examination may be necessary for eyes with opaque media after trauma. It might be deferred until after wound repair if the injured eye is collapsed or to prevent expression of intraocular content if there is an unstable or large wound. The use of copious amounts of sterile gel allows the examiner to use minimal pressure on the closed lid. Intraocular air may cause artifacts that complicate the interpretation of ultrasonography. Computed tomography (CT) is very helpful in evaluating patients suspected of having intraocular foreign bodies. Metal foreign bodies may introduce artifacts that make them appear larger than they really are, making exact localization difficult. Wood and plastic may be difficult to detect by CT but may be identified and localized with magnetic resonance imaging (MRI). However, MRI should be used only after the presence of ferromagnetic foreign bodies has been definitively ruled out because of the possibility that such foreign bodies may be moved by the magnetic field, causing additional damage.

Blunt Trauma

In blunt trauma, the object does not penetrate the eye but may cause rupture of the eyewall. Blunt trauma can have numerous serious sequelae:

- angle recession
- hemorrhage into the anterior chamber (hyphema) or vitreous
- retinal tears or detachment
- subluxated or dislocated lens

- commotio retinae
- choroidal rupture
- macular hole
- avulsed optic nerve
- scleral rupture

See Chapter 15 for discussion of traumatic retinal breaks and retinal detachment and BCSC Section 11, *Lens and Cataract,* for discussion of dislocated lenses.

A complete ophthalmic examination is essential after blunt trauma. An eye with minimal or no anterior segment damage may still harbor severe posterior segment injury.

Vitreous Hemorrhage

Vitreous hemorrhage can result from damage to blood vessels of the iris, ciliary body, retina, or choroid and can also be caused by retinal tears. A search for the cause of the vitreous hemorrhage should always be undertaken as soon as possible, as a hemorrhage that is loculated at presentation can later become diffuse. If the posterior segment cannot be visualized because of vitreous hemorrhage, ultrasound examination is indicated. Retinal or choroidal detachment, retinal tears, and posterior vitreous detachment can be detected by ultrasound techniques. Ultrasound signs of an occult scleral rupture include entrapment of vitreous strands into the rupture site.

Bed rest with elevation of the head may enable the hemorrhage to settle sufficiently to allow for more detailed ophthalmoscopic examination. If the source of the hemorrhage still cannot be determined, frequent monitoring and repeat ultrasound examinations are indicated until the hemorrhage clears. In the absence of glaucoma, hypotony, retinal detachment, or endophthalmitis, a unilateral hemorrhage can be monitored until it clears. Macular hole, choroidal rupture in the macula, traumatic maculopathy, retinal detachment, or other injuries can limit recovery of vision.

Commotio Retinae

The term *commotio retinae* refers to damage to the outer retinal layers caused by shock waves that traverse the eye from the site of impact following blunt trauma. Ophthalmoscopic examination shows a sheenlike retinal whitening that appears some hours postinjury (Fig 17-1). The retinal whitening occurs most commonly in the posterior pole but may also be found peripherally. Possible mechanisms for the retinal opacification include extracellular edema, glial swelling, and photoreceptor outer segment disruption. With foveal involvement, a cherry-red spot may appear because the cells involved in the whitening are not present in the foveola. Commotio retinae in the posterior pole may decrease visual acuity to as low as 20/200. Gradual visual recovery may occur if there is no associated macular pigment epitheliopathy, choroidal rupture, or macular hole formation.

Choroidal Rupture

When the eye is compressed along its anterior–posterior axis, tears may occur in the Bruch membrane, which has little elasticity, as well as in the overlying retinal pigment

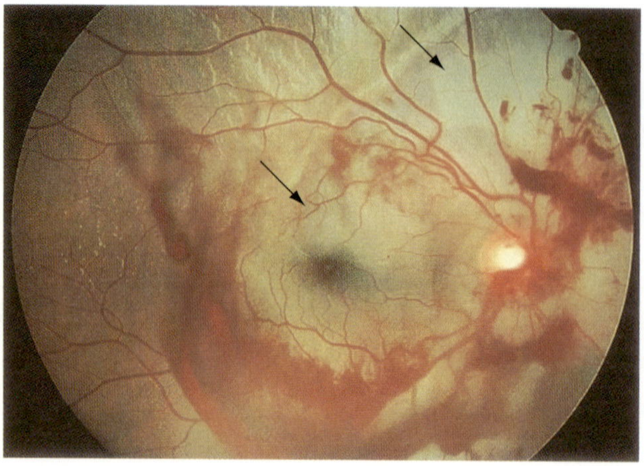

Figure 17-1 Color fundus photograph revealing commotio retinae *(arrows)* and vitreous hemorrhage after blunt trauma.

epithelium (RPE) and fibrous tissue investing the choriocapillaris. Adjacent subretinal hemorrhage is common. Choroidal ruptures may be single or multiple and occur typically in the periphery and concentric to the optic disc (Fig 17-2). Ruptures that extend through the fovea may cause permanent vision loss. There is no effective treatment.

Occasionally, choroidal neovascularization (CNV) develops as a late complication after damage to the Bruch membrane (Fig 17-3). A patient with choroidal rupture near the macula should be alerted to the risk of CNV. Subfoveal CNV, if present, is generally treated

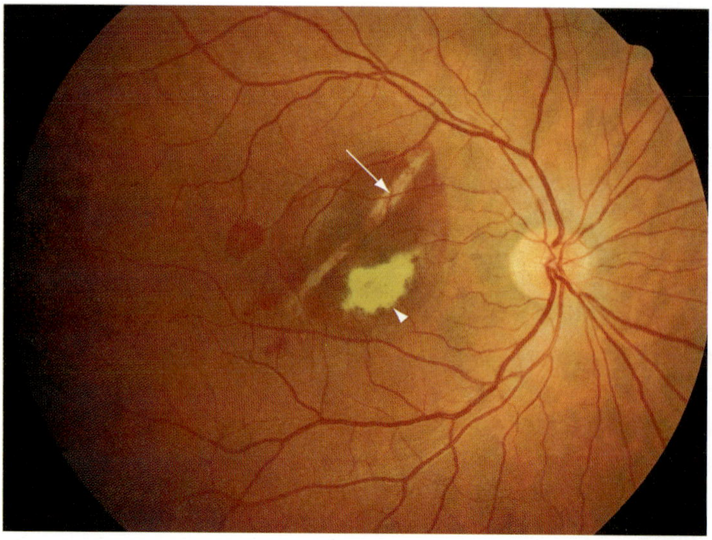

Figure 17-2 Color fundus photograph in a patient with a posttraumatic submacular hemorrhage. The hemorrhage started to clear, revealing a choroidal rupture *(arrow)*. The yellow material located at the inferonasal portion of the macula *(arrowhead)* is dehemoglobinized blood. *(Courtesy of Mark Johnson, MD.)*

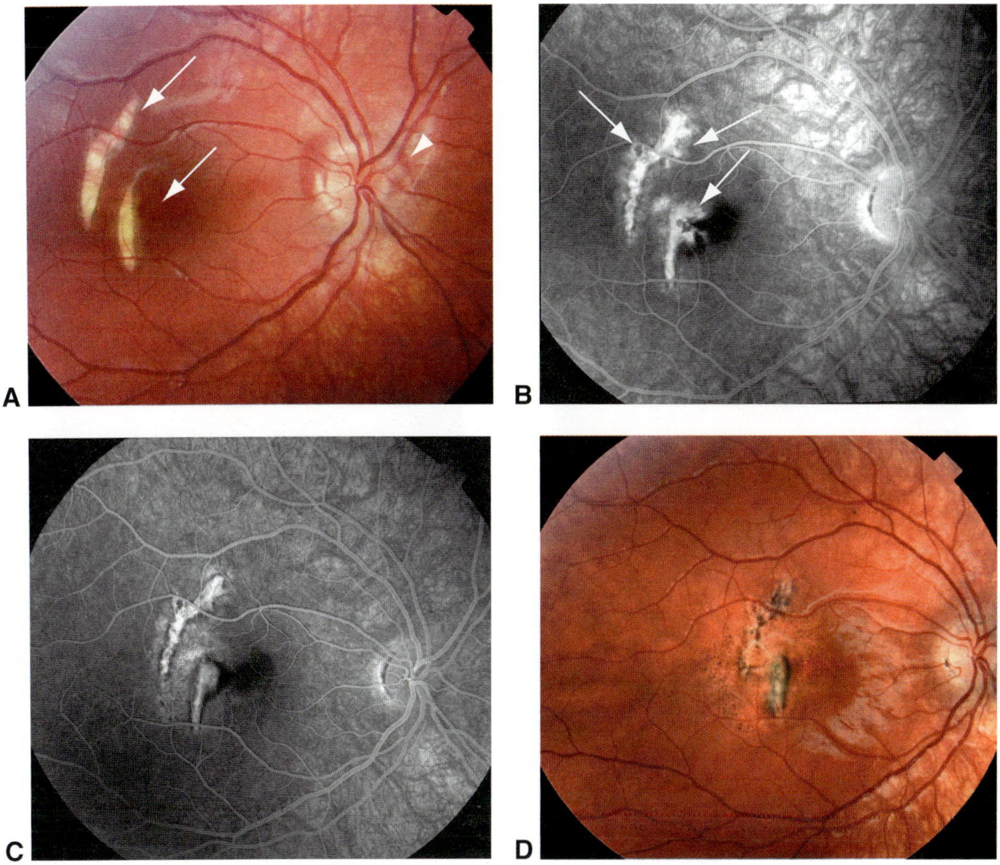

Figure 17-3 Images from a 10-year-old hit in the eye with a tennis ball. **A,** Color fundus photograph reveals choroidal ruptures *(arrows)*. A subretinal hemorrhage is present around the nerve head *(arrowhead)*. The visual acuity was 20/30. **B,** Six weeks later, visual acuity decreased to 20/400. Late-phase fluorescein angiography image shows multiple fronds of choroidal neovascularization (CNV) arising from the choroidal ruptures *(arrows)*. **C,** Late-phase fluorescein angiography image 2 weeks after treatment with corticosteroids and photodynamic therapy shows the CNV has regressed dramatically. **D,** Color fundus photograph taken 6 months after treatment. The scarring around the choroidal ruptures obscures their characteristic appearance. Some pigmentary changes have occurred in the macula as well, but visual acuity is 20/25. *(Courtesy of Richard F. Spaide, MD.)*

with a vascular endothelial growth factor (VEGF) inhibitor. See Chapter 4 for information on the management of CNV.

Posttraumatic Macular Hole

The foveola is extremely thin (130 μm), and blunt trauma may cause a full-thickness macular hole by various mechanisms, including contusion necrosis and vitreous traction. Holes may be observed immediately after blunt trauma that causes severe commotio retinae, following a submacular hemorrhage caused by a choroidal rupture (Fig 17-4), after severe cystoid macular edema, or after a whiplash separation of the vitreous from the retina. In addition, central depressions, or macular pits (similar to those observed in patients after sun gazing),

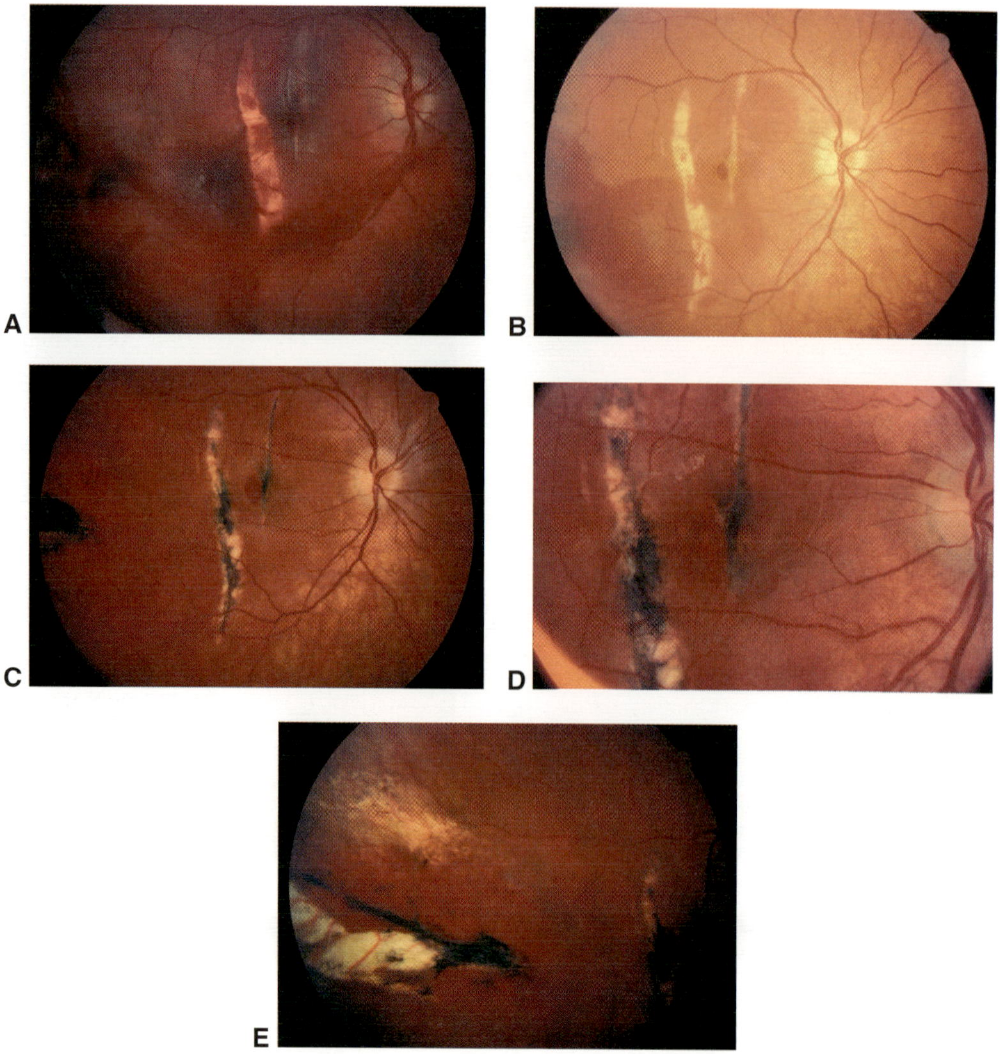

Figure 17-4 Blunt ocular trauma with traumatic choroidal rupture, subretinal hemorrhage, macular hole, and retinal sclopetaria. **A,** Fundus photograph obtained shortly after the 14-year-old boy's right eye was struck by a coin thrown forcefully at him. Choroidal rupture in the macula, submacular hemorrhage, and vitreous hemorrhage emanating from the temporal periphery are apparent. **B,** Several days later, a macular hole developed. **C,** After several weeks, the choroidal rupture was healed, leaving pigment hypertrophy and the macular hole. **D,** Fundus photograph shows a closed macular hole following vitrectomy with internal limiting membrane peeling, gas-bubble placement, and face-down positioning. Visual acuity eventually recovered to 20/60. **E,** Fundus photograph of the temporal periphery shows the sequelae of mild to moderate retinal sclopetaria, the source of the vitreous hemorrhage observed immediately after the injury. *(Courtesy of Colin A. McCannel, MD.)*

have been described following blunt trauma to the eye and whiplash injuries. Lightning and electrical injury can also cause macular holes; patients with these injuries usually have signs of cataract and can have acute peripapillary retinal whitening. Posttraumatic macular holes may close spontaneously or may be successfully closed surgically. Depending on the degree of collateral damage to the fovea, visual acuity recovery varies greatly.

Traumatic Chorioretinal Disruption (Retinal Sclopetaria)

An unusual retinal pathology can be produced by high-speed projectile injuries to the orbit. Large areas of choroidal and retinal rupture and necrosis combine with extensive subretinal and retinal hemorrhage, often involving 2 quadrants of the retina. As the blood resorbs, the injured area is repaired by extensive scar formation and widespread pigmentary alteration (Fig 17-5, see also Fig 17-4). The macula is often involved, with significant associated loss of vision; curiously, however, secondary retinal detachment rarely develops. The pattern of damage is ascribed to shock waves generated by the deceleration of the projectile passing close to the sclera. Blunt trauma from paintball injuries may produce a similar fundus appearance.

Scleral Rupture

Severe blunt injuries can rupture the globe. The 2 most common locations for rupture are the limbus, particularly through previous surgical wounds, or through areas of

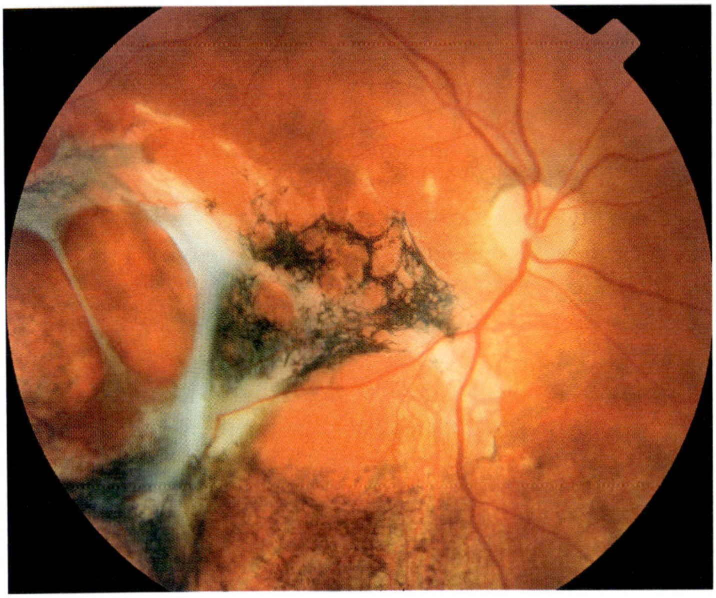

Figure 17-5 A color fundus photograph from a patient shot 2 months earlier in the right inferotemporal orbit with a bullet, causing the sequelae of retinal sclopetaria. The bullet's path missed the globe by several millimeters, and the patient acutely lost visual acuity. The image shows large areas of subretinal proliferation and retinal pigment epithelial hyperplasia, consistent with moderate to severe retinal sclopetaria. Visual acuity returned to 20/70. *(Courtesy of Richard F. Spaide, MD.)*

physiological scleral thinning parallel to and under the insertions of the rectus muscles. Important diagnostic signs of rupture include a marked decrease in ocular ductions, very boggy conjunctival chemosis with hemorrhage (ecchymosis), deepened anterior chamber, and severe vitreous hemorrhage. The IOP is usually reduced but may be normal or even elevated. Presence of an intraocular foreign body must be ruled out in all cases of ruptured globe. The principles of surgical management of ruptured and lacerated globes are discussed in the following section.

Lacerating and Penetrating Injuries

Lacerating injuries result from cutting or tearing of the eyewall by objects of varying sharpness. A penetrating injury of the globe is a laceration of the eyewall at a single entry site. The prognosis is related to the location and extent of the wound, as well as the associated damage and degree of hemorrhage. Any corneal laceration that crosses the limbus must be explored until its posterior extent has been located (see also BCSC Section 8, *External Disease and Cornea*). If a more posterior rupture is suspected, a meticulous, gentle 360° peritomy and scleral exploration, including underneath the rectus muscles, should be performed. If the rupture is very posterior and cannot be accessed and visualized well enough for surgical repair without expression of intraocular content, then the site should be left to heal without suturing.

The principles of initial management of a penetrating injury include careful, gentle microsurgical corneoscleral wound repair, in which incarcerated uvea is reposited or excised. Corneal lacerations may be closed with 10-0 nylon interrupted sutures, and scleral wounds may be closed with stronger 7-0, 8-0, or 9-0 nonabsorbable sutures. Vitreous should be excised from the wound and the anterior chamber re-formed. Any uvea or retina that protrudes should be amputated if contaminated or gently reposited in appropriate circumstances. BCSC Section 4, *Ophthalmic Pathology and Intraocular Tumors,* discusses wound healing in detail in Chapter 2.

Delayed complications of a penetrating injury (eg, tractional retinal detachment, cyclitic membrane formation, and phthisis bulbi) result from intraocular cellular proliferation and membrane formation. Cautious dissection of vitreous and posterior vitreous face may reduce the risk of late tractional retinal detachment by eliminating the scaffold on which the contractile membranes grow. The optimal timing of vitrectomy after penetrating injuries is unknown. Some surgeons favor immediate vitrectomy before cellular proliferation can begin; however, most prefer initially performing a primary repair of the wound to restore the globe and IOP and decrease the risk of endophthalmitis. Depending on the circumstances, vitrectomy may be postponed 2–14 days for the following reasons:

- to decrease the risk of intraoperative hemorrhage in acutely inflamed and congested eyes
- to allow the cornea to clear and improve intraoperative visualization
- to permit spontaneous separation of the vitreous from the retina, which facilitates a safer and more complete vitrectomy

Although there are some theoretical reasons for early vitrectomy, the overruling priority at the time of the acute injury is to close the globe. Primary wound closure should not be delayed by the uncertainty of whether an early vitrectomy should be performed. Immediate vitrectomy may be necessary in some circumstances—for example, if examination or history suggests the possibility of infectious endophthalmitis or a retained intraocular foreign body at the time of primary repair. Also see Chapter 19.

Kuhn F. The timing of reconstruction in severe mechanical trauma. *Ophthalmic Res.* 2014; 51(2):67–72.

Mieler WF, Mittra RA. The role and timing of pars plana vitrectomy in penetrating ocular trauma. *Arch Ophthalmol.* 1997;115(9):1191–1192.

Perforating Injuries

A perforating injury has both entrance and exit wounds. Perforating injuries may be caused by objects of varying sharpness such as needles, knives, high-velocity pellets, or small fragments of metal. An important iatrogenic cause is needle perforation during retrobulbar or peribulbar anesthesia for intraocular surgery. Studies have shown that, after perforating injuries, fibrous proliferation occurs along the scaffold of damaged vitreous between the entrance and exit wounds. The wounds are often closed by fibrosis within 7 days after the injury, with the time depending on wound size. Small-gauge injuries with only a small amount of hemorrhage and no significant collateral damage often heal without serious sequelae. Anterior wounds are usually cleared of incarcerated vitreous and closed with sutures, but small, very posterior wounds are sometimes left unrepaired to avoid vitreous extrusion through the wound during attempted closure.

Vitrectomy may be considered in the following situations:

- the presence of moderate to severe vitreous hemorrhage
- other tissue damage requiring repair
- phacoanaphylactic uveitis, which may occur if the lens is damaged
- signs of developing transvitreal traction

Definitive vitrectomy is usually delayed 7–10 days to allow for preoperative medical management of the traumatic ocular inflammatory response.

During vitrectomy, an attempt should be made to separate the posterior cortical gel to prevent later proliferation and contraction that could lead to retinal detachment. Separating the posterior cortical vitreous from the retina may be difficult, however, in children, in young adults, and in eyes with retinal breaks, a retinal detachment, or both. Retinal detachment is frequently caused by the primary injury or by traction resulting from proliferative vitreoretinopathy (PVR). A prophylactic encircling scleral buckle may be placed at the time of surgery, according to the surgeon's preference.

Intraocular Foreign Bodies

An intraocular foreign body (IOFB) should always be suspected and ruled out in cases of ocular or orbital trauma. In most cases, an IOFB is either observed or suggested by the presence of an entry site. A detailed history also helps the clinician assess the likelihood an IOFB is present. On examination, small IOFBs, such as high-velocity pieces of steel generated by hammering steel on steel or thrown by high-speed machinery, may be overlooked. The possibility of multiple foreign bodies should always be considered.

The composition of the IOFB has implications for imaging. If a sample is available of the suspected IOFB's material, it may be used to determine whether the IOFB is magnetic, radiopaque, or both. If the IOFB is known or suspected to be metallic or the material is unknown, MRI is contraindicated because the magnetic force may move a metallic foreign body, causing further ocular damage. For radiopaque materials, CT is superior to other imaging modalities for visualizing and localizing the IOFB, particularly if it is small or less radiopaque (Fig 17-6). In the absence of CT, however, bone-free x-ray studies may be helpful when such IOFBs are suspected. IOFBs may also be identified and

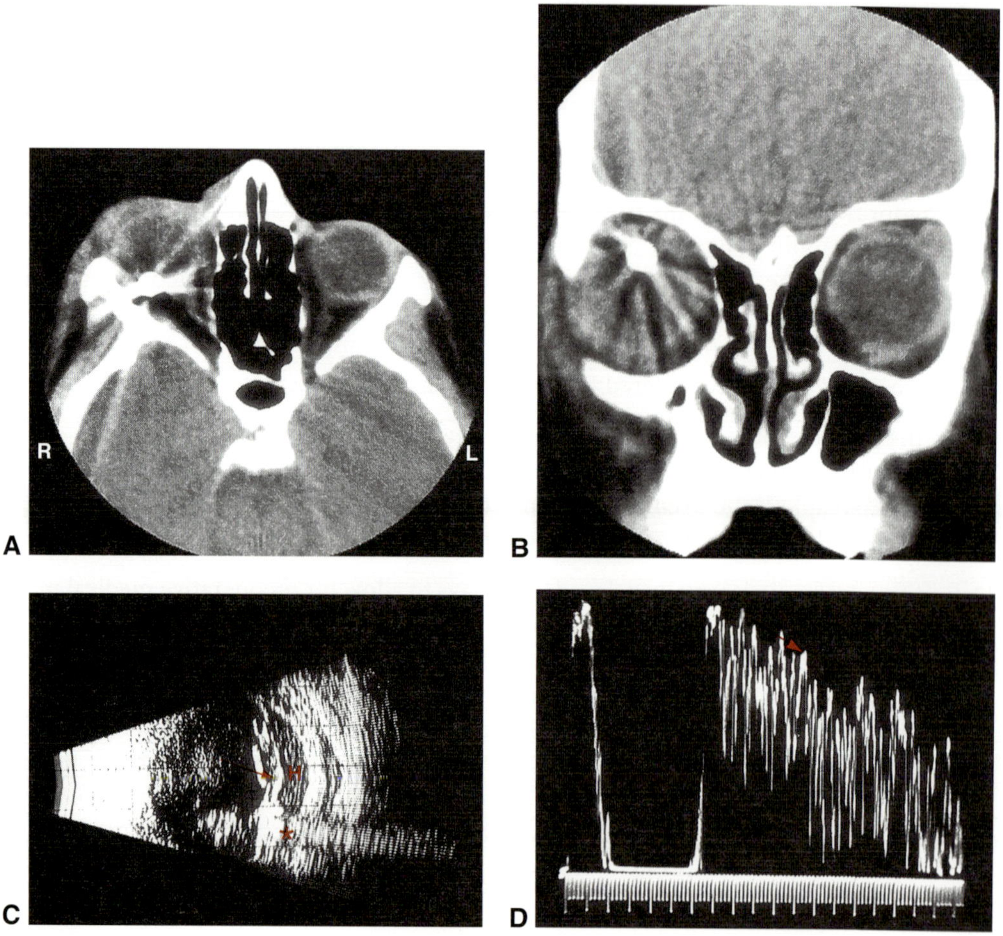

Figure 17-6 Images from a patient with an intraocular BB pellet. Axial **(A)** and coronal **(B)** computed tomography views show the pellet to be in the superior and posterior globe. B-scan echography **(C)** shows retinal detachment *(arrow)* and subretinal hemorrhage *(H)*. A characteristic reverberation of echoes between the front and back surfaces of the round pellet gives a "trail of echoes" artifact that extends posterior to the foreign body on B-scan *(asterisk)* and on A-scan **(D)** *(arrow)*.

localized by an experienced ultrasonographer, which is particularly useful for nonradiopaque materials.

Surgical Techniques for Removal of Intraocular Foreign Bodies

In the case of a magnetic IOFB, surgical planning should address the following issues:

- location of the foreign body in the eye
- surgeon's ability to visualize and localize the foreign body
- size and shape of the foreign body
- composition of the foreign body (ferromagnetic vs nonferromagnetic)
- encapsulation of the foreign body

Pars plana vitrectomy allows removal of traumatized vitreous and facilitates controlled microsurgical extraction of IOFBs as well as media opacities such as cataract and hemorrhage (Video 17-1). Before forceps extraction is attempted, the IOFB should be freed of all attachments. A small rare-earth magnet may be used to engage and separate the foreign body from the retinal surface. Although small foreign bodies can be removed through enlargement of the pars plana sclerotomy site, some large foreign bodies may be extracted more safely through the corneoscleral limbus or the initial wound to minimize collateral damage.

VIDEO 17-1 Removal of large metallic intraocular foreign body (02:15).
Courtesy of Nur Acar, MD.
Scan the QR code or access the video at www.aao.org/bcscvideo_section12.

Retained Intraocular Foreign Bodies

The reaction of the eye to a retained foreign body varies widely and depends on the object's chemical composition, sterility, and location. Inert, sterile foreign bodies such as stone, sand, glass, porcelain, plastic, and cilia are generally well tolerated. If such material is found several days after the injury and does not appear to create an inflammatory reaction, it may be left in place, provided it is not obstructing vision.

Evaluation for retinal toxicity using electroretinography may be helpful in some cases. Zinc, aluminum, copper, and iron are metals that are commonly reactive in the eye. Of these, zinc and aluminum tend to cause minimal inflammation and may become encapsulated. However, any very large foreign body may incite inflammation and thereby cause anterior and posterior proliferative vitreoretinopathy. Epiretinal proliferations, tractional retinal detachment, and phthisis bulbi may result in complete loss of vision. Migration of the foreign body also can occur, especially if it contains copper.

Pure copper is especially toxic, and prompt removal is required. Copper causes acute *chalcosis,* which manifests as severe inflammation and may lead to loss of the eye. If copper is alloyed with another metal so that the material has a final copper content of less than 85% (eg, brass, bronze), chronic chalcosis may occur. Typical findings in chronic chalcosis are deposits in the Descemet membrane (a sign similar to the Kayser-Fleischer ring in Wilson disease and the result of copper's affinity for basement membranes), greenish aqueous particles, green discoloration of the iris, lens capsule ("sunflower" cataract), brownish-red vitreous opacities and strand formation, and metallic flecks on retinal

Table 17-1 Symptoms and Signs of Siderosis

Symptoms
Nyctalopia
Concentrically constricted visual field
Decreased vision
Signs
Rust-colored corneal stromal staining
Iris heterochromia
Pupillary mydriasis and poor reactivity
Brown deposits on the anterior lens
Cataract
Vitreous opacities
Peripheral retinal pigmentation (early)
Diffuse retinal pigmentation (late)
Narrowed retinal vessels
Optic disc discoloration and atrophy
Secondary open-angle glaucoma from iron accumulation in the trabecular meshwork

vessels and the internal limiting membrane in the macular region. Late removal of copper may not cure the chalcosis; in fact, dissemination of the metal during surgery may worsen the inflammatory response.

In *siderosis,* iron-form IOFBs are deposited primarily in neuroepithelial tissues such as the iris sphincter and dilator muscles, the nonpigmented ciliary epithelium, the lens epithelium (see BCSC Section 11, *Lens and Cataract,* Chapter 5, Fig 5-14), the retina, and the RPE. Retinal photoreceptors and RPE cells are especially susceptible to damage from iron (Table 17-1). Electroretinography (ERG) changes in siderosis include an increased a-wave and normal b-wave during the very early phase of toxicity and diminishing b-wave amplitude in later phases. Eventually, the ERG response may become undetectable. Serial ERGs can be helpful in monitoring eyes with small retained foreign bodies. If the b-wave amplitude decreases, removal of the foreign body generally is recommended.

Posttraumatic Endophthalmitis

Endophthalmitis occurs following 2%–7% of penetrating injuries; the incidence is higher in association with intraocular foreign bodies and in rural settings. Posttraumatic endophthalmitis can progress rapidly; its clinical signs include marked inflammation featuring fibrin, hypopyon, vitreous infiltration, and corneal opacification. The risk of endophthalmitis after penetrating ocular injury may be reduced by prompt wound closure and early removal of IOFBs. Use of prophylactic subconjunctival, intravenous, or intravitreal antibiotics is often recommended. Aminoglycoside antibiotics should be avoided because of their narrow therapeutic window and high risk of retinal infarction.

Bacillus cereus, which rarely causes endophthalmitis in other settings, accounts for almost 25% of cases of posttraumatic endophthalmitis. Endophthalmitis caused by *B cereus* has a rapid and severe course and, once established, leads to profound vision loss and often loss of the eye. Most commonly, *B cereus* endophthalmitis is associated with soil-contaminated injuries, especially those involving foreign bodies. Anterior chamber and vitreous cultures should be obtained, and antibiotics should be injected if endophthalmitis is suspected. *Bacillus cereus* is sensitive to vancomycin or clindamycin injected intravitreally.

Gram-negative organisms are frequent pathogens in posttraumatic endophthalmitis; ceftazidime may be an effective therapy that avoids the toxicities associated with aminoglycosides. Because recommendations for antibiotic selection can change, ophthalmologists should consult a recent reference or an infectious disease specialist.

Jindal A, Pathengay A, Mithal K, et al. Endophthalmitis after open globe injuries: changes in microbiological spectrum and isolate susceptibility patterns over 14 years. *J Ophthalmic Inflamm Infect.* 2014;4(1):5.

Sympathetic Ophthalmia

Sympathetic ophthalmia is a rare complication of penetrating ocular trauma in which the fellow, uninjured eye develops a severe autoimmune inflammatory reaction. Although removing an injured eye is thought to reduce the risk of sympathetic ophthalmia, the disorder is treatable with other therapeutic choices that often provide better cosmetic and psychological outcomes. Sympathetic ophthalmia is discussed in more detail in BCSC Section 9, *Intraocular Inflammation and Uveitis.*

Abusive Head Trauma

Severe shaking of infants, a form of nonaccidental trauma, is the cause of abusive head trauma (formerly known as *shaken baby syndrome*). The typical baby is almost always less than 1 year of age and frequently less than 6 months old. The presenting sign of child abuse involves the eye in approximately 5% of cases. Systemic signs and symptoms include

- bradycardia, apnea, and hypothermia
- lethargy, irritability, seizures, hypotonia
- signs of failure to thrive
- full or bulging fontanelles and increased head size
- skin bruises, particularly on the upper arms, chest, or thighs
- spiral fractures of the long bones
- subdural and subarachnoid hemorrhages

Ocular signs include

- retinal hemorrhages and cotton-wool spots (Fig 17-7)
- retinal folds
- hemorrhagic schisis cavities

The retinal hemorrhages in abusive head trauma often have a hemispheric contour. They can begin to resolve very rapidly, so it is important to examine suspected cases on

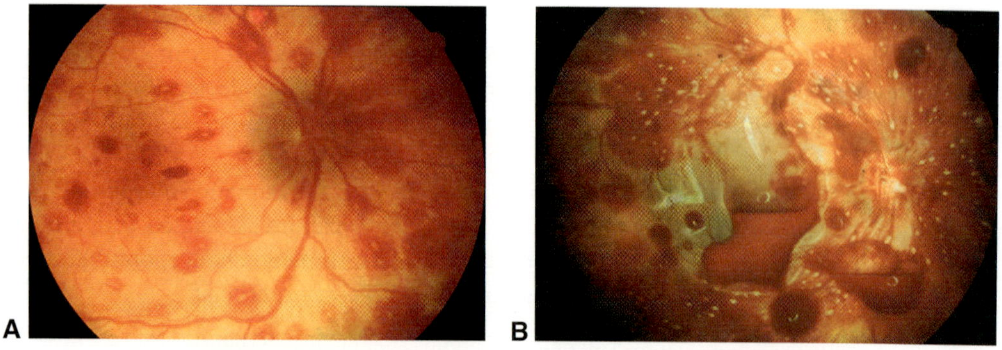

Figure 17-7 Color fundus photographs from a patient with abusive head trauma causing preretinal and retinal hemorrhages. **A,** Image taken several days after hospital admission, by which time many of the smaller hemorrhages had started to resorb. **B,** Numerous hemorrhages are located on and within the retina, and regions of hemorrhagic retinoschisis are observed centrally. Because the baby was upright, the red blood cells sank down into a dependent position within the larger regions of hemorrhagic retinoschisis. Some of the hemorrhages were white centered, whereas others had reflections of the flash from the fundus camera on them. *(Used with permission from Spaide RF, Swengel RM, Scharre DW, Mein CE. Shaken baby syndrome.* Am Fam Physician. *1990;41(4):1145–1152.)*

presentation. The retinopathy may resemble that observed in Terson syndrome or central retinal vein occlusion, neither of which is common in infants. Retinal hemorrhages may be caused by trauma, but they are not usually associated with typical accidents, such as falls at home. Any physician who suspects that child abuse might have occurred is required by law in every US state and Canadian province to report the incident to a designated government agency. Vitrectomy for vitreous hemorrhage should be considered if amblyopia is likely to occur but may be deferred if a bright-flash ERG response shows loss of the b-wave, indicative of extensive retinal damage. See also BCSC Section 6, *Pediatric Ophthalmology and Strabismus.*

Matthews GP, Das A. Dense vitreous hemorrhages predict poor visual and neurological prognosis in infants with shaken baby syndrome. *J Pediatr Ophthalmol Strabismus.* 1996; 33(4):260–265.

Pierre-Kahn V, Roche O, Dureau P, et al. Ophthalmologic findings in suspected child abuse victims with subdural hematomas. *Ophthalmology.* 2003;110(9):1718–1723.

Avulsion of the Optic Disc

A forceful backward dislocation of the optic nerve from the scleral canal can occur under several circumstances, including

- extreme rotation and forward displacement of the globe
- penetrating orbital injury, causing a backward pull on the optic nerve
- sudden increase in IOP, causing rupture of the lamina cribrosa

Total loss of vision characteristically occurs. Findings may vary from a pitlike depression of the optic nerve head to posterior hemorrhage and contusion necrosis (Fig 17-8); however, hemorrhage is usually present acutely.

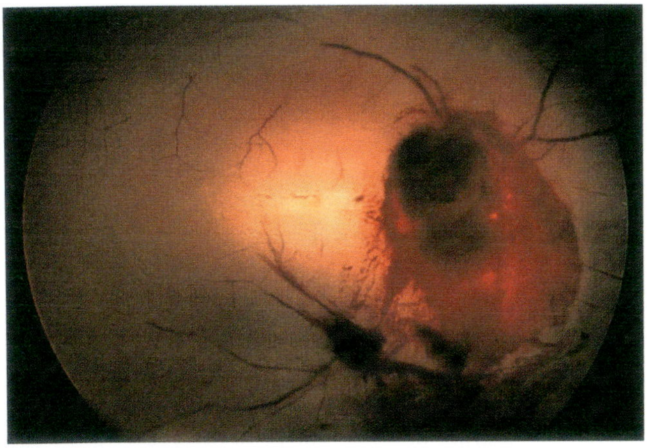

Figure 17-8 Avulsion of the optic nerve. In this color fundus photograph, the nerve is obscured by hemorrhage, and a mixed vascular occlusion is present.

Photic Damage

The eye has several mechanisms to protect itself against light damage, including pupil constriction, light absorption by melanin in the RPE, and the presence of antioxidants, such as lutein and zeaxanthin, in the macula. Light injures the retina by 3 basic mechanisms: (1) mechanical, (2) thermal, and (3) photochemical. *Mechanical injury* occurs when the power of the absorbed light is high enough to form gas or water vapor or to produce acoustic shock waves that mechanically disrupt retinal tissues. The absorbed energy may be enough to strip electrons from molecules in the target tissue, producing a collection of ions and electrons referred to as *plasma.* For example, a Q-switched Nd:YAG laser produces its therapeutic effect through mechanical light damage and uses this effect to disrupt a cloudy posterior capsule behind an intraocular lens.

Thermal injury occurs when excessive light absorption by the RPE and surrounding structures causes local elevation of the tissue temperature, leading to coagulation, inflammation, and scarring of the RPE and the surrounding neurosensory retina and choroid. The end result of the temperature elevation is protein denaturation and scar formation. A therapeutic application of thermal light injury is the retinal burn caused by laser photocoagulation. See Chapter 18 for discussion of photocoagulation.

Photochemical injury results from biochemical reactions that cause retinal tissue destruction without elevation of temperature. It is the result of the transfer of light energy to a molecule; the excess energy initiates reactions that cause tissue damage. For photochemical reactions to occur, the energy of the photon must exceed a certain threshold. Damaging reactions can include oxidation, photoisomerization, photochemical cleavage, and electrocyclic reactions. Each type may cause damage directly or indirectly through formation of reactive molecules, such as lipofuscin, that are photoreactive. Such changes occur primarily at the level of the outer segments of the photoreceptors, which are more sensitive than the inner segments. Examples of photochemical injury are solar retinopathy and photic retinopathy that occurs after excessive exposure to illumination from an operating microscope.

Mainster MA, Turner PL. Photic retinal injuries: mechanisms, hazards, and prevention. In: Ryan SJ, Schachat AP, Wilkinson CP, Hinton DR, Sadda SR, Wiedemann P, eds. *Retina.* Vol 2. 5th ed. Philadelphia: Elsevier/Saunders; 2013:1555–1563.

Solar Retinopathy

Solar retinopathy, also known as *foveomacular retinitis, eclipse retinopathy,* or *solar retinitis,* is a thermally enhanced photochemical retinal injury caused by direct or indirect viewing of the sun; it usually occurs after viewing a solar eclipse or gazing directly at the sun. The damage is thought to result from exposure to visible blue light and shorter wavelengths of ultraviolet A or near-UV radiation, and the extent of the damage depends on the duration of the exposure. Younger patients with clearer lenses and patients who are taking drugs that photosensitize the eye, including tetracycline and psoralens, have a higher risk of solar retinopathy. Patients with uncorrected high refractive errors and dark fundus pigmentation have a slightly lower risk. Symptoms include decreased vision, central scotomas, dyschromatopsia, metamorphopsia, micropsia, and frontal or temporal headache within hours of exposure. Visual acuity is typically reduced to 20/25–20/100 but may be worse depending on degree of exposure. Most patients recover within 3–6 months, with visual acuity returning to the level of 20/20–20/40, but there may be residual metamorphopsia and paracentral scotomata.

The fundus findings are variable and usually bilateral. The characteristic finding in the first few days after exposure is a yellow-white spot in the fovea, which changes after several days into a reddish dot, often surrounded by a pigment halo. Mild cases often have no biomicroscopic fundus changes. After approximately 2 weeks, a small (100–200 μm), reddish, well-circumscribed lamellar hole or depression may evolve that is more apparent on optical coherence tomography. This lesion may lie at or adjacent to the fovea and is usually permanent. Fluorescein angiography reveals leakage in the early stages and window defects in the late stages. Histologic studies have shown RPE damage. No known beneficial treatment exists, and therefore prevention through education is critically important.

Phototoxicity From Ophthalmic Instrumentation

The potential for photochemical damage from exposure to modern ophthalmic instruments has been studied extensively. Injuries have been reported from operating microscopes and from fiber-optic endoilluminating probes used in vitrectomies. The prevalence of photic retinopathy after cataract surgery has been estimated to be 3%–7.4%. The incidence increases with prolonged operating times but can occur even with surgery times as short as 30 minutes. In retinal surgery, photic injury is more likely to occur with prolonged, focal exposure, especially when the light probe is held in close proximity to the retina, as in macular hole and epiretinal membrane procedures. Most affected patients are asymptomatic, but some will notice a paracentral scotoma on the first postoperative day. In general, vision returns to normal after a few months. Acutely affected patients may have a deep, irregular, oval-shaped, yellow-white retinal lesion adjacent to the fovea that resembles the shape of the light source. The lesion typically evolves to become a zone of mottled RPE that transmits hyperfluorescence on fluorescein angiography. Although animal studies generally exaggerate clinical exposures, reports of photic macular lesions occurring after intraocular surgery underscore the need for prevention. During ocular surgery, the risk of photic retinopathy may be reduced by minimizing exposure time, avoiding the use of intense illumination, using oblique illumination when possible during parts of the surgery, filtering out short-wavelength blue light and UV light, and using shielding. BCSC Section 11, *Lens and Cataract,* lists several precautions for minimizing retinal light toxicity. See also BCSC Section 3, *Clinical Optics.*

Youssef PN, Sheibani N, Albert DM. Retinal light toxicity. *Eye.* 2011;25(1):1–14.

Occupational Light Toxicity

Occupational exposure to bright lights can lead to retinal damage. A common cause of occupational injury is arc welding without the use of protective goggles. The damage from the visible blue light of the arc welder leads to photochemical damage similar to that observed in solar retinopathy. Occupational injury from stray laser exposure is also a serious concern.

Handheld Laser-Pointer Injury

The availability of high-power green and blue handheld laser devices has created a serious emerging source of immediate accidental or purposeful sight-threatening macular injury. These devices are easily obtainable via the Internet and resemble the much safer, ubiquitous low-power red laser pointers. They also present the risk of causing secondary harmful effects by visually incapacitating people undertaking visually demanding functions, such as firefighters and airline pilots.

Alsulaiman SM, Alrushood AA, Almasaud J, et al; King Khaled Eye Specialist Hospital Collaborative Retina Study Group. High-power handheld blue laser-induced maculopathy: the results of the King Khaled Eye Specialist Hospital Collaborative Retina Study Group. *Ophthalmology.* 2014;121(2):566–572.

PART III

Selected Therapeutic Topics

CHAPTER 18

Laser Therapy for Posterior Segment Diseases

Basic Principles of Photocoagulation

Photocoagulation uses light energy to coagulate tissue. After light energy is applied to the target tissue, it converts into thermal energy and the tissue temperature rises above 65°C, which causes denaturation of tissue proteins and coagulative necrosis.

Current posterior segment laser delivery systems span the visible light spectrum of 400–700 nm (green, yellow, red) and venture into the infrared wavelengths (>700 nm). Delivery systems may employ a transpupillary approach with slit-lamp or indirect ophthalmoscopic delivery, endophotocoagulation during vitrectomy, or transscleral application with a contact probe.

The effectiveness of photocoagulation depends on the transmission of light through ocular media and the absorption of that light by pigment in the target tissue. Light is absorbed principally by ocular tissues that contain melanin, xanthophyll, or hemoglobin. Figure 18-1 illustrates the absorption spectra of the key pigments found in ocular tissues:

- *Melanin* is an effective absorber of green, yellow, red, and infrared wavelengths.
- Macular *xanthophyll* readily absorbs blue but minimally absorbs yellow and red wavelengths.
- *Hemoglobin* easily absorbs blue, green, and yellow but has minimal absorption of red wavelengths.

Choice of Laser Wavelength

Laser wavelength selection depends on the specific goals of treatment and the degree to which the photocoagulation must be targeted to the particular tissue while sparing adjacent normal tissue. The *area* (depth and diameter) of effective coagulation is directly related to the *intensity* and *duration* of irradiation. For a specific set of laser parameters (spot size, duration, and power), the intensity of the burn obtained depends on the clarity of the ocular media and the degree of pigmentation.

The *green laser* produces light that is absorbed well by melanin and hemoglobin and less completely by xanthophyll. Because of these characteristics and the absence of undesirable short (blue) wavelengths, the green laser has replaced the blue-green laser for treatment of retinal vascular abnormalities and choroidal neovascularization (CNV).

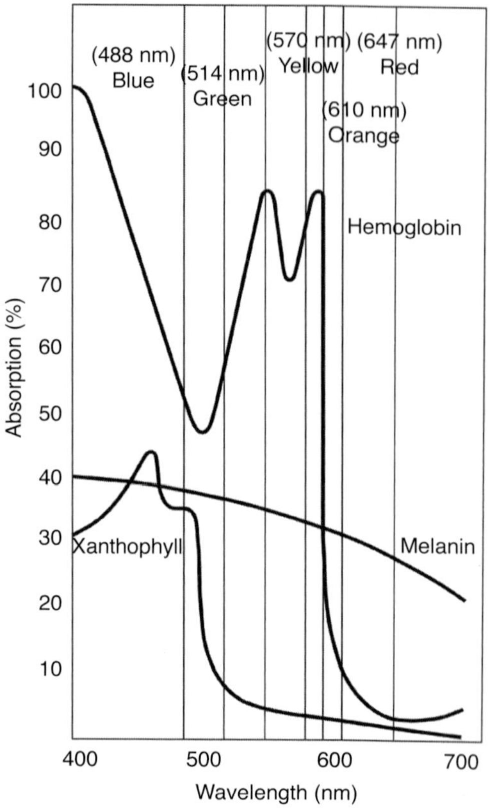

Figure 18-1 Absorption spectra of xanthophyll, hemoglobin, and melanin. *(From Folk JC, Pulido JS.* Laser Photocoagulation of the Retina and Choroid. *Ophthalmology Monograph 11. San Francisco: American Academy of Ophthalmology; 1997:9.)*

The *red laser* penetrates through nuclear sclerotic cataracts and moderate vitreous hemorrhages better than lasers with other wavelengths do. In addition, it is minimally absorbed by xanthophyll and thus may be useful in treatments near the fovea. The red laser causes deeper burns with a higher rate of patient discomfort and inhomogeneous absorption at the level of the choroid. The *infrared laser* has characteristics similar to those of the red laser with even deeper tissue penetration.

The *yellow laser* has, among its advantages, minimal scatter through nuclear sclerotic lenses, low xanthophyll absorption, and little potential for photochemical damage. It appears to be useful for destroying vascular structures while causing minimal damage to adjacent pigmented tissue; thus, it may be valuable for treating retinal vascular and choroidal neovascular lesions. For typical laser wavelengths of specific lasers, see BCSC 3, *Clinical Optics,* Chapter 8.

Laser effects on posterior segment tissues include photochemical and thermal effects and vaporization. Photochemical reactions can be induced by ultraviolet or visible light that is absorbed by tissue molecules or by molecules of a photosensitizing medication (eg, verteporfin), producing cytotoxic reactive oxygen species (eg, free radicals). Absorption of laser energy by pigment results in a 10°C–20°C temperature rise and subsequent protein denaturation. Vaporization is generated by the rise in water temperature above the boiling point, which causes microexplosions, as can occur in overly intense burns. For further discussion of laser light characteristics and light–tissue interactions, see BCSC Section 3, *Clinical Optics.*

Atebara NH, Thall EH. Principles of lasers. In: Yanoff M, Duker JS, eds. *Ophthalmology.* 4th ed. Philadelphia: Elsevier/Saunders; 2014:32–37.

Palanker D, Blumenkranz MS. Retinal laser therapy: biophysical basis and applications. In: Ryan SJ, Schachat AP, Wilkinson CP, Hinton DR, Sadda SR, Wiedemann P, eds. *Retina.* Vol 1. 5th ed. Philadelphia: Elsevier/Saunders; 2013:chap 39.

Practical Aspects of Laser Photocoagulation

Anesthesia

Topical, peribulbar, or retrobulbar anesthesia may be needed to facilitate delivery of laser photocoagulation. The risks of peribulbar and retrobulbar injection should be considered when choosing among these forms of anesthesia.

Lenses

Two types of contact lenses are available to assist in slit-lamp delivery of photocoagulation:

1. negative-power planoconcave lenses
2. high-plus-power lenses

The planoconcave lenses provide an upright image with superior resolution of a small retinal area. Most clinicians favor use of these lenses for macular treatments. Mirrored planoconcave lenses allow for viewing and photocoagulation of more peripheral retina, with the exact location in view depending on the angle of the mirror in use. Planoconcave lenses generally provide the same retinal spot size as that selected on the slit-lamp setting.

High-plus-power lenses provide an inverted image with some loss of fine resolution, but they offer a wide field of view, which facilitates efficient treatment over a broad area. The macula may be kept in view while the midperiphery of the retina is being treated, making these lenses ideal for panretinal photocoagulation. High-plus-power lenses provide a spot size that is magnified over the laser setting size; the magnification factor depends on the lens used (Table 18-1).

Parameters and indications

Selection of laser setting parameters depends on the intent of the treatment, the clarity of the ocular media, and the fundus pigmentation. As a general rule, smaller spot sizes require less energy than larger spot sizes, and longer-duration exposures require less energy than shorter-duration exposures to achieve the same intensity effects. Following are guidelines for conventional laser treatments.

Macular laser Laser photocoagulation still has a role in the management of some forms of macular edema, extrafoveal CNV, and focal retinal pigment epithelium (RPE) abnormalities with leakage, such as those seen in central serous chorioretinopathy. To avoid causing central scotomas and perifoveal capillary dropout, treatment should not be administered within 500 µm of the foveal center. Macular laser treatment for edema generally relies on smaller spot size (100–200 µm) and shorter duration (≤0.1 second) to

Table 18-1 Magnification Factors for Common Laser Lenses

Lens	Magnification	Laser Spot Magnification
Panretinal photocoagulation lenses		
Ocular Mainster PRP 165	0.51×	1.96×
Ocular Mainster Wide Field PDT	0.68×	1.50×
Ocular Pro Retina	0.5×	2.0×
Rodenstock Panfunduscope	0.7×	1.43×
Volk Equator Plus	0.44×	2.27×
Volk HR Wide Field	0.50×	2.0×
Volk QuadrAspheric	0.51×	1.97×
Volk SuperQuad 160	0.5×	2.0×
Focal laser lenses		
Goldmann 3-mirror (central)	0.93×	1.08×
Ocular Fundus Laser	0.93×	1.08×
Ocular Mainster High Magnification	1.25×	0.80×
Ocular PDT 1.6×	0.63×	1.6×
Ocular Reichel-Mainster 1× Retina	0.95×	1.05×
Ocular Reichel-Mainster 2× Retina	0.5×	2.0×
Ocular Yannuzzi Fundus	0.93×	1.08×
Volk Area Centralis	1.06×	0.94×
Volk Centralis Direct	0.9×	1.11×
Volk Fundus 20	1.44×	0.7×
Volk Fundus Laser	1.25×	0.8×
Volk HR Centralis	1.08×	0.93×
Volk HR Wide Field	0.50×	2.0×
Volk PDT Lens	0.66×	1.5×
Volk SuperMacula 2.2	1.49×	0.67×

achieve smaller, less-intense burns. For diabetic macular edema, green or yellow direct laser therapy should be applied to all leaking microaneurysms located between 500 µm and 3000 µm from the center of the macula. For more diffuse leakage or zones of capillary nonperfusion, a light-intensity grid pattern using a green or yellow laser is applied to all areas of diffuse leakage more than 500 µm from the center of the macula and 500 µm from the temporal margin of the optic disc. A similar strategy is employed in treating macular edema caused by branch retinal vein occlusion. If CNV or RPE leakage spots are treated, the aim is to achieve a more intense burn of the entire lesion or area of leakage.

Peripheral retinal photocoagulation Peripheral retinal photocoagulation may be delivered with a slit-lamp or indirect ophthalmoscopic delivery system. The latter system affords less control over precise spot size or burn intensity. For panretinal photocoagulation (PRP) or laser retinopexy, the aim is to achieve somewhat intense, larger laser burns. For PRP, laser spot size typically is 200–500 µm, and laser power is adjusted to achieve cream-colored burns. Applications, or burns, are usually one-half to one burn width apart (see Chapter 5, Fig 5-13) and should spare the macula. For initial PRP treatment, some practitioners leave approximately 1–2 disc diameters of retina outside of the macula and optic nerve head untreated, whereas others treat up to the arcade vessels and up to the optic nerve (Fig 18-2). The initial treatment pattern can be concentrated more densely in the

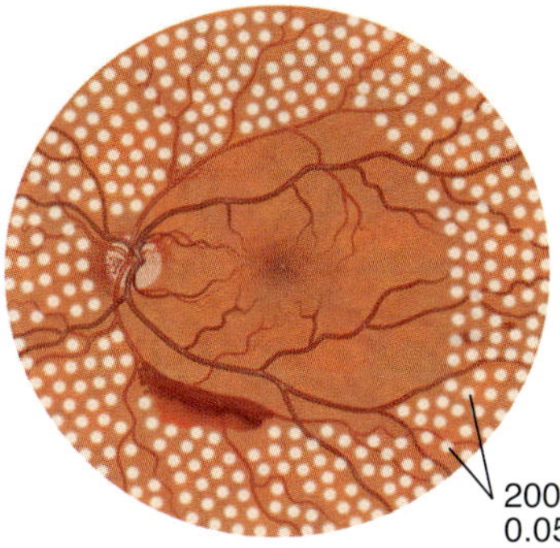

Figure 18-2 Illustration of the posterior extent of full panretinal photocoagulation (peripheral treatment not shown). *(Illustration by Mark Miller.)*

inferior retina to help minimize temporal and inferior visual field loss and to facilitate retreatment in the case of vitreous hemorrhage. The long ciliary nerves in the 3 and 9 o'clock meridians should be avoided, if possible, and any coexisting macular edema should be treated beforehand to avoid its exacerbation after PRP. Typically, 1200–1400 laser applications of 500-µm spot size—the equivalent of smaller burns—are placed. Laser retinopexy achieves a chorioretinal adhesion around retinal tears or is used for demarcation of a (small) retinal detachment; it utilizes spot sizes of 200–500 µm with the goal of creating whitish, but not snow-white, burns. Usually, 2–3 rows of photocoagulation around the break are considered appropriate to achieve the desired adhesion.

Laser ablation of retinal vascular lesions Vascular lesions are often treated using large spot size (≥500 µm), lower power, and long duration so each lesion slowly heats up and coagulates "from the inside out." High-intensity burns whiten the surface of the lesions, after which visible-light laser does not penetrate well, making it difficult to achieve the treatment goal.

Alternative laser delivery systems and strategies

New technologies and concepts have led to novel treatment systems and strategies. Among more recent innovations of slit-lamp delivery systems are pattern scanners that deliver an entire array of laser applications with each foot-pedal depression. Delivery is accomplished by using ultrashort (20–50 millisecond) laser pulses at high intensity in rapid succession. This approach possibly increases the efficiency of treatment, but it may not achieve an effect equivalent to traditional laser treatment on a spot-number-to-spot-number comparison.

Some systems incorporate real-time retinal image overlay and registration with the laser delivery system. This configuration allows for computer-assisted planning and precise targeting of the retinal lesions during treatments.

Delivery systems that apply subthreshold (barely visible to invisible) laser spots administer laser in micropulses (≤0.1 millisecond) that can confine heat conduction to the RPE while limiting thermal damage to the photoreceptors and choriocapillaris. These systems have been shown to be effective in treating diabetic macular edema and have the potential to reduce the number and size of scotomas. However, use of nonvisible laser spots makes titrating and determining the extent of treatment difficult.

Baumal CR, Ip M, Puliafito CA. Light and laser injury. In: Yanoff M, Duker JS, eds. *Ophthalmology.* 4th ed. Philadelphia: Saunders/Elsevier; 2013:461–466.

Chappelow AV, Tan K, Waheed NK, Kaiser PK. Panretinal photocoagulation for proliferative diabetic retinopathy: pattern scan laser versus argon laser. *Am J Ophthalmol.* 2012;153(1): 137–142.e2.

Folk JC, Pulido JS. *Laser Photocoagulation of the Retina and Choroid.* Ophthalmology Monograph 11. San Francisco: American Academy of Ophthalmology; 1997.

Complications of Photocoagulation

The most serious complications of photocoagulation are caused by the use of excessive energy or misdirected light. Among the complications that may be associated with photocoagulation are inadvertent corneal burns, which can lead to opacities. Treatment of the iris may cause iritis and create zones of atrophy. Pupillary abnormalities may arise from thermal damage to the long ciliary nerves in the suprachoroidal space or the iris sphincter muscle. Absorption by lens pigments may create lenticular burns and resultant opacities. Optic neuropathy may occur from treatment directly to or adjacent to the disc, and nerve fiber damage may follow intense absorption in zones of increased pigmentation or retinal thinning. Chorioretinal complications include foveal burns, Bruch membrane ruptures, creation of retinal or choroidal lesions, and exudative choroidal or retinal detachment.

Accidental foveal burns

Great care should be taken to identify the fovea by means of biomicroscopy; this step may be aided by comparing the appearance with recent fluorescein angiography images. Frequent reference to the foveal center throughout the procedure is helpful to maintain orientation. In some instances, the risk of foveal burns may be reduced by immobilizing the globe with peribulbar or retrobulbar anesthesia, especially when juxtafoveal treatment is being performed.

Bruch membrane ruptures

Small spot size, high power, and short duration of applications all increase the risk of a rupture in the Bruch membrane, which may subsequently give rise to hemorrhage from the choriocapillaris and development of CNV.

Retinal lesions

Intense photocoagulation may cause full-thickness retinal holes. Similarly, intense treatment may create fibrous proliferation, striae, and foveal distortion, with resultant metamorphopsia or diplopia. Focal treatment with small-diameter, high-intensity burns may cause vascular occlusion or perforate blood vessels, leading to preretinal or vitreous hemorrhage. In addition, extensive panretinal treatment may induce or exacerbate macular edema, particularly in diabetic patients.

Choroidal lesions

Treatment of CNV may be complicated by subretinal hemorrhage, choroidal ischemia, and additional CNV or chorioretinal anastomosis. Active subretinal hemorrhage that occurs during treatment should be addressed immediately by increasing digital pressure on the contact lens while continuing to treat the remaining portions of the CNV lesion in order to minimize obscuration of landmarks by hemorrhage. Progressive atrophy of the RPE may develop at the margin of photocoagulation scars, resulting in enlarged scotomata. Also, tears of the pigment epithelium may be precipitated by photocoagulation.

Exudative retinal and choroidal detachment

Extensive, intense photocoagulation may lead to massive chorioretinal edema and resultant serous retinal and choroidal detachment (Fig 18-3). The latter, in turn, can lead to narrowing of the anterior chamber angle from forward rotation of the ciliary body, resultant elevated intraocular pressure, and, rarely, aqueous misdirection. This reaction peaks 1–3 days after treatment and resolves spontaneously within a few weeks. Corticosteroids may be helpful to treat massive exudation.

Avoiding laser photocoagulation complications

Awareness and avoidance of the fovea during laser treatment is paramount. Selection of proper wavelength, power, exposure time, and spot size is important. Proper titration of laser power and exposure time may be necessary to achieve the desired tissue effect. Waiting for proper pupillary dilation can help limit iris damage. Careful preoperative explanation of the laser procedure to the patient and comfortable positioning of the patient will facilitate cooperation, steady fixation, and improve safety.

Palanker D, Lavinsky D, Blumenkranz MS, Marcellino G. The impact of pulse duration and burn grade on size of retinal photocoagulation lesion: implications for pattern density. *Retina.* 2011;31(8):1664–1669.

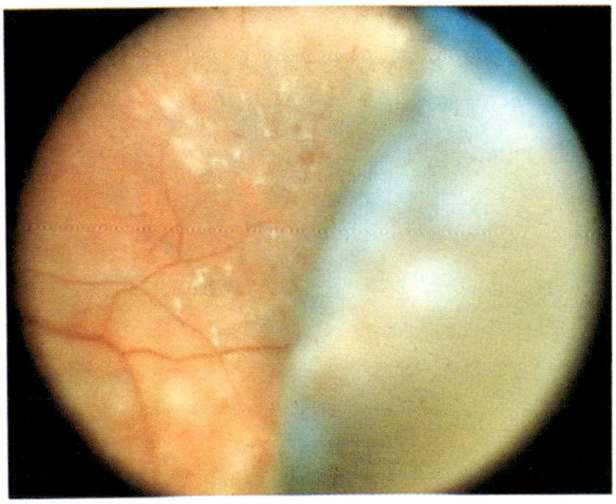

Figure 18-3 Color fundus photograph showing choroidal detachment that occurred following panretinal scatter photocoagulation for diabetic retinopathy. *(Courtesy of M. Gilbert Grand, MD.)*

Transpupillary Thermotherapy

Transpupillary thermotherapy (TTT) acts in a subthreshold manner by slightly raising the choroidal temperature and thus causing minimal thermal damage to the RPE and overlying retina. TTT is administered with an infrared laser (810 nm) using beam sizes from 0.8 mm to 3.0 mm, power settings between 250 mW and 750 mW, and a 1-minute exposure time. For choroidal melanoma, TTT may be considered as a stand-alone treatment for flat tumors, but for thicker tumors, a combination of TTT and plaque radiotherapy results in better local tumor control than TTT alone.

Photodynamic Therapy

Photodynamic therapy (PDT) using the photosensitizing drug verteporfin is approved by the US Food and Drug Administration for treating certain types of subfoveal CNV in age-related macular degeneration and subfoveal CNV secondary to ocular histoplasmosis syndrome and myopia. PDT has generally fallen out of favor for the management of CNV because more effective treatments have become available. However, PDT continues to be a valuable option for the management of some ocular tumors and central serous chorioretinopathy.

PDT is a 2-step procedure:

1. intravenous administration of the photosensitizing drug that localizes to endothelial cells of vessels present in CNV and tumors
2. local activation of the drug by a laser wavelength preferentially absorbed by the sensitizing drug

The low-intensity laser energy produces a photochemical reaction, leading to the formation of reactive oxygen species and free radicals. These radicals cause endothelial cell damage, platelet adherence, vascular thrombosis, and capillary closure.

Complications of Photodynamic Therapy

The most serious adverse effects of PDT are photosensitivity reactions that range from mild to second-degree burns of sun-exposed skin. Such burning can be avoided by having the patient minimize exposure to sunlight for 5 days after treatment. In the Treatment of Age-Related Macular Degeneration with Photodynamic Therapy (TAP) Study Group report, severe vision loss occurred in 0.7%–2.2% of patients within 7 days of PDT treatment of subfoveal lesions. Additionally, verteporfin infusion–related transient lower-back, side, and chest pain were reported in 2.0%–2.5% of patients. In efforts to minimize choriocapillaris nonperfusion and ischemia, treatment using half-fluence PDT (25 J/cm^2 energy; 300 mW/cm^2 light intensity) has become more common and may be as effective as standard-fluence PDT.

CHAPTER 19

Vitreoretinal Surgery and Intravitreal Injections

This chapter includes related videos, which can be accessed by scanning the QR codes provided in the text or going to www.aao.org/bcscvideo_section12.

Pars Plana Vitrectomy

Pars plana vitrectomy is a vitreoretinal surgical technique that is typically used for removing vitreous opacities (vitreous hemorrhage), relieving vitreoretinal traction, restoring the normal anatomical relationship of the retina and retinal pigment epithelium (RPE), and accessing the subretinal space. It involves a closed-system approach that usually requires placement of 3 ports 3–4 mm posterior to the surgical limbus. One port is typically dedicated to infusion of balanced salt solution into the vitreous cavity, by which intraocular pressure (IOP) can be maintained at a desired level. Epinephrine can be added to the infusion solution for mydriasis and to reduce intraoperative bleeding by vasoconstriction, but it may promote ischemia and increase inflammation. Dextrose is often added in phakic diabetic patients to reduce cataractogenesis. The remaining ports are used to access the vitreous cavity with tools such as a fiber-optic endoilluminator to visualize the posterior segment and other instruments to manipulate, dissect, or remove intraocular tissues, fluids, and objects.

Vitrectomy is performed using an operating microscope in conjunction with a contact lens or noncontact viewing system. Direct and indirect visualization are possible, the latter requiring an inverting system to orient the image. The advantages of indirect visualization include a wider viewing angle as well as better visualization through media opacities, miotic pupils, and gas tamponades. Direct viewing systems allow for greater magnification and enhanced stereopsis at the expense of a smaller field of view. Many vitreoretinal surgeons utilize both types of viewing systems and make their selection according to the task.

Vitreoretinal surgery is facilitated by various instruments, visualization aids, and vitreous substitutes. Advanced instrumentation includes the high-speed vitreous cutter, retinal forceps, endolaser probe, micro-pic, retinal scissors, extrusion cannula, and fragmatome, among others. Examples of visualization aids include indocyanine green (ICG) dye to stain the internal limiting membrane (ILM) and triamcinolone suspension to help identify cortical vitreous. Tamponade of the retina can be achieved using air, gas, or silicone oil as a vitreous substitute. Commonly used gases include sulfur hexafluoride (SF_6) and perfluoropropane (C_3F_8), which last approximately 2 and 8 weeks, respectively, at nonexpansile (isovolemic) concentrations. Perfluorocarbon liquids are heavier than water and can be used to temporarily stabilize the retina during dissection and allow for anterior drainage of subretinal fluid during retinal detachment repair.

The development of smaller-gauge vitrectomy instrumentation has facilitated transconjunctival, sutureless vitrectomy techniques. With these systems, 23-, 25-, or 27-gauge trocar cannulas are placed to align conjunctival and scleral openings and to allow instrument insertions. These cannulas avoid the need for a conjunctival cutdown procedure, including cautery, and the wounds generally do not require suture closure because of their self-sealing architecture. A 20-gauge sclerotomy is typically 1 mm in diameter compared with diameters of 0.7 mm, 0.5 mm, and 0.4 mm for the 23-, 25-, and 27-gauge techniques, respectively. Potential advantages of small-gauge vitrectomy include shortened operative time, increased postoperative patient comfort, faster visual recovery, and reduced conjunctival scarring.

Fujii GY, de Juan E Jr, Humayun MS, et al. Initial experience using the transconjunctival sutureless vitrectomy system for vitreoretinal surgery. *Ophthalmology.* 2002;109(10): 1814–1820.

Kim SJ, Martin DF, Hubbard GB 3rd, et al. Incidence of postvitrectomy macular edema using optical coherence tomography. *Ophthalmology.* 2009;116(8):1531–1537.

Vitrectomy for Selected Macular Diseases

Macular Epiretinal Membranes

Epiretinal membranes (ERMs) have a variable clinical course. Indications for surgery are generally twofold: for reduced vision or for distortion causing dysfunction of binocularity. In general, epiretinal membrane peel (Video 19-1) is advised if visual acuity is reduced to 20/40–20/60 or worse. Separately, dysfunction of binocularity that involves difficulty with fusion of 1 distorted and 1 normal-vision image is an indication for surgery, even when the visual acuity is still good (Fig 19-1).

VIDEO 19-1 Vitrectomy for epiretinal membrane peel (03:06).
Courtesy of Colin A. McCannel, MD.
Scan the QR code or access the video at www.aao.org/bcscvideo_section12.

After surgery, approximately two-thirds of patients achieve an improvement in visual acuity of 2 or more lines. Maximal improvement may take up to 6–12 months (Fig 19-2).

Vitreomacular Traction Diseases

Vitreomacular traction syndrome

Vitreomacular traction (VMT) syndrome is a distinct vitreoretinal interface disorder that is differentiated clinically from typical ERM. Whereas ERM formation is generally associated with complete posterior vitreous detachment, VMT syndrome stems from anomalous, incomplete posterior vitreous separation at the macula. The disorder may create focal

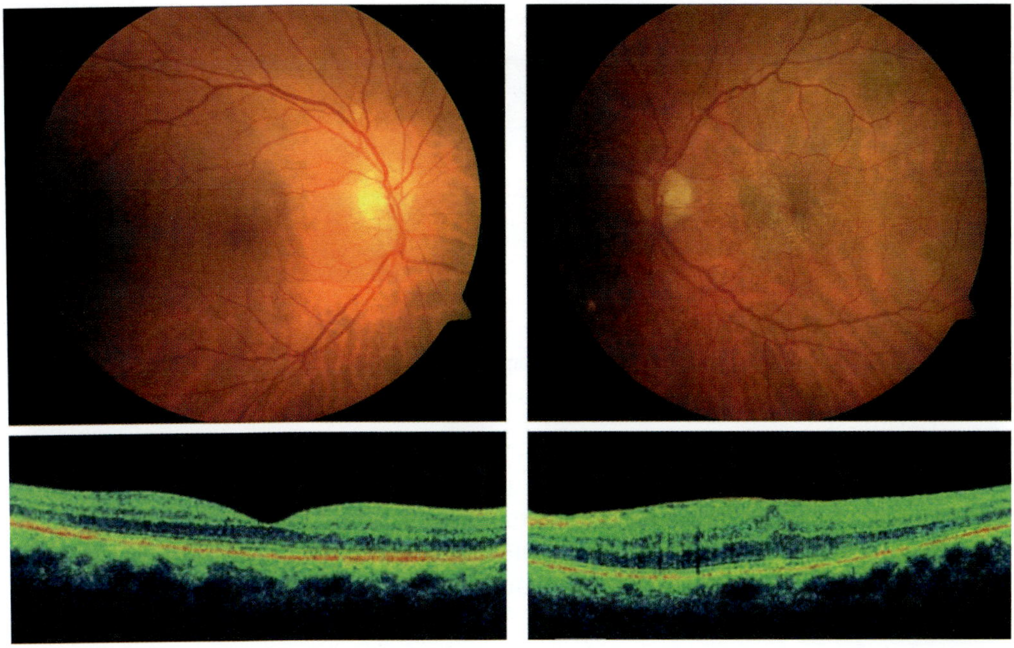

Figure 19-1 Epiretinal membrane (ERM). *Top row,* color fundus photographs of a normal right eye and a left eye with a macular ERM showing distortion of the foveal architecture and retinal striae. *Bottom row,* corresponding optical coherence tomography (OCT) images confirm preretinal traction from the ERM, associated loss of foveal contour, and macular thickening in the left eye. Visual acuity was 20/50 in the left eye with central distortion. This patient was a candidate for pars plana vitrectomy surgery. *(Courtesy of Stephen J. Kim, MD.)*

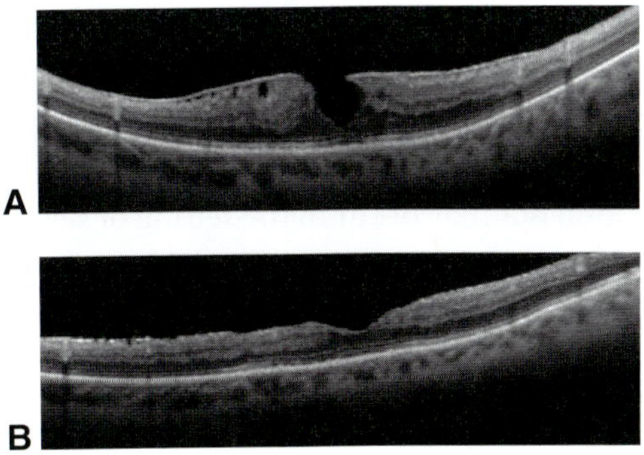

Figure 19-2 ERM forming a pseudohole in a patient with visual distortion and reduced visual acuity (20/50). **A,** OCT image corroborates a preretinal membrane distorting the retinal contour and intraretinal edema. **B,** OCT image at 2 months after surgery shows continued restoration of normal macular contour and absence of preretinal membrane and traction; visual acuity had improved to 20/25. *(Courtesy of Edward F. Cherney, MD.)*

elevation of the fovea (Fig 19-3) and, occasionally, a shallow retinal detachment. VMT syndrome is best diagnosed and differentiated from ERMs with the aid of optical coherence tomography (OCT), which classically shows the hyaloid inserting onto tractionally elevated retina. Symptoms include decreased vision and distortion. VMT syndrome is often progressive and is associated with a greater loss of vision than are ERMs alone. Surgical treatment consists of a standard pars plana vitrectomy and peeling of the cortical vitreous from the surface of the retina. Intraoperative use of triamcinolone may aid visualization of the cortical vitreous. See Chapter 16 for further discussion of VMT syndrome.

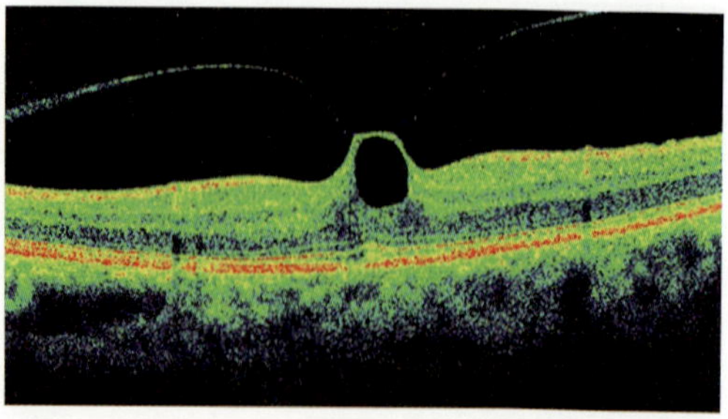

Figure 19-3 Vitreomacular traction syndrome in a patient with visual acuity of 20/60 and mild ophthalmoscopic findings. OCT scan shows a partial posterior detachment with persistent hyaloidal insertion at the center of the macula. Note the elevated fovea with complete loss of contour and inner schisis cavity. Pars plana vitrectomy with membrane peeling led to an improved visual acuity of 20/25 and resolution of symptomatic distortion. *(Courtesy of Stephen J. Kim, MD.)*

Voo I, Mavrofrides EC, Puliafito CA. Clinical applications of optical coherence tomography for the diagnosis and management of macular diseases. *Ophthalmol Clin North Am.* 2004; 17(1):21–31.

Idiopathic macular holes

Vitrectomy is indicated for all recent full-thickness macular holes (stages 2, 3, and 4). Vitrectomy surgery is not generally recommended for stage 1 macular holes because approximately 50% of them will resolve spontaneously. However, early intervention for holes at stage 2 or higher is important, as shorter time intervals between the development and the closure of macular holes have been associated with improved anatomical and functional outcomes.

Surgery for full-thickness macular holes typically consists of a standard pars plana vitrectomy, separation and removal of the posterior cortical vitreous, removal of the ILM, and use of an intraocular air or gas tamponade with face-down positioning (Video 19-2). ILM peeling has been demonstrated in numerous studies to improve the rate of hole closure, particularly for larger stage 3 or 4 holes, and reduced re-opening rates. The intraoperative use of dyes (ICG, trypan blue, brilliant blue G) or other visualization techniques (eg, triamcinolone) to aid in peeling the ILM is widely practiced, despite potential toxicity. Timing of face-down positioning ranges from a few hours to 2 or more weeks. The success rate of macular hole closure is greater than 90% in most recent series (Fig 19-4). Reopening of the hole after successful closure is uncommon but may occur in the setting of severe cystoid macular edema.

VIDEO 19-2 Vitrectomy for macular hole repair with ILM peeling (02:49).
Courtesy of Colin A. McCannel, MD.
Scan the QR code or access the video at www.aao.org/bcscvideo_section12.

Pharmacologic therapy administered by intravitreal injection is now available for vitreomacular traction and macular holes (<400 µm in diameter) with use of ocriplasmin, a recombinant protease that has activity against fibronectin and laminin (see Chapter 16 for discussion of ocriplasmin).

Kelly NE, Wendel RT. Vitreous surgery for idiopathic macular holes. Results of a pilot study. *Arch Ophthalmol.* 1991;109(5):654–659.

Kumagai K, Furukawa M, Ogino N, Uemura A, Demizu S, Larson E. Vitreous surgery with and without internal limiting membrane peeling for macular hole repair. *Retina.* 2004; 24(5):721–727.

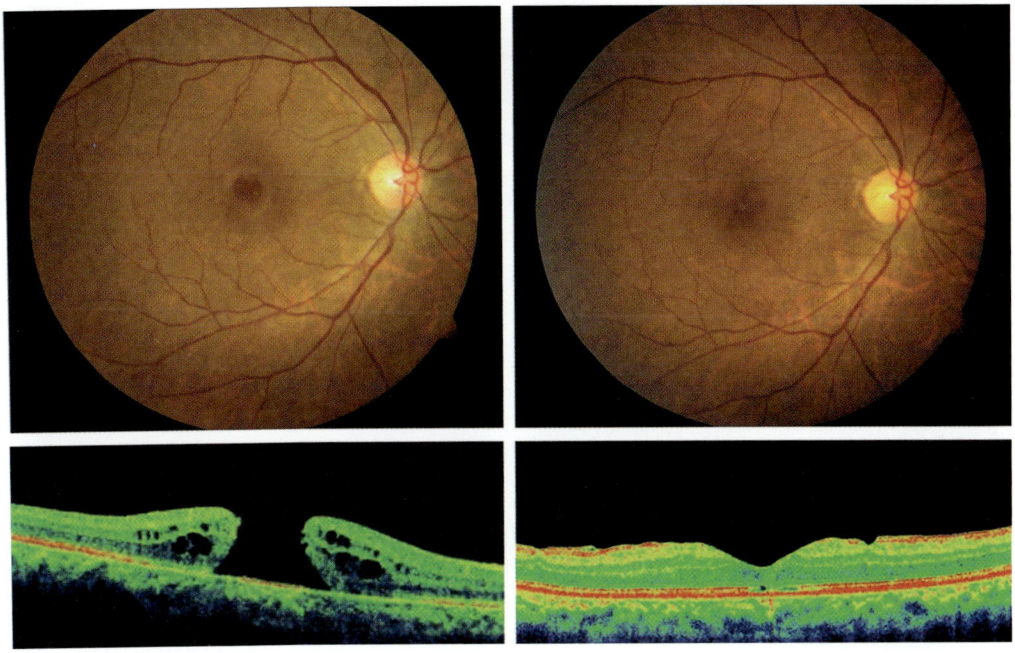

Figure 19-4 Idiopathic macular hole. *Left,* color fundus photograph and corresponding OCT image of a patient with full-thickness macular hole and reduced visual acuity (20/100) for 3 months. *Right,* after vitrectomy, membrane peeling, and fluid–gas exchange, the macular hole closed and visual acuity improved to 20/25. Postoperative color fundus photograph and OCT image show restoration of normal foveal anatomy. *(Courtesy of Stephen J. Kim, MD.)*

Submacular Hemorrhage

Vitrectomy for submacular hemorrhage remains unproven and controversial. The clinical course of submacular hemorrhages is variable. Patients with neovascular age-related macular degeneration (AMD) and larger submacular hemorrhages generally have poor visual outcomes. For removal of thick submacular hemorrhages, pars plana vitrectomy techniques can be considered. In the era prior to availability of anti–vascular endothelial growth factor (VEGF) agents, the Submacular Surgery Trials (SST) Protocol H—a randomized, prospective study—evaluated the outcomes of observation versus vitrectomy for eyes with submacular hemorrhage caused by AMD. The study found that vitrectomy surgery in which the hemorrhage was removed from the subretinal space did not improve or stabilize visual acuity and thus recommended against this surgery. An alternate vitrectomy technique was developed subsequently; it involves pneumatic displacement of subretinal blood away from the macular center without attempting to remove the hemorrhage. This technique can be performed with a standard vitrectomy, subretinal injection of tissue plasminogen activator (tPA) via a 39- to 41-gauge cannula, and air–fluid exchange. Postoperative face-down positioning can result in substantial inferior extramacular displacement of blood (Fig 19-5). Office-based intravitreal injection of expansile gas (eg, SF_6 or C_3F_8) and face-down positioning, with or without adjunctive intravitreal tPA administration, has also been reported. Finally, successful resolution of submacular hemorrhage with

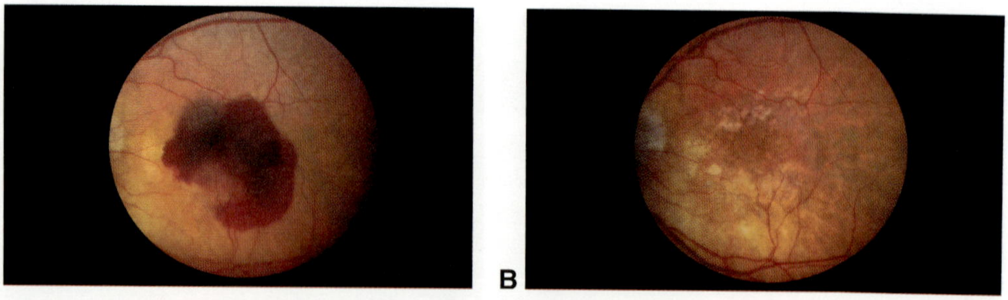

Figure 19-5 Submacular hemorrhage in age-related macular degeneration. **A,** Fundus photograph of a patient who had a submacular hemorrhage for 5 days and counting fingers vision. **B,** After vitrectomy with subretinal infusion of tissue plasminogen activator and pneumatic displacement, dry atrophic changes are apparent. Visual acuity improved to 20/100. *(Courtesy of Nancy M. Holekamp, MD.)*

improvement of visual acuity has been reported with administration of anti-VEGF agents alone; this approach may be a viable alternative to vitrectomy surgery in cases for which maintaining the intraocular half-life of anti-VEGF agents for future treatment is important.

Bressler NM, Bressler SB, Childs AL, et al; Submacular Surgery Trials (SST) Research Group. Surgery for hemorrhagic choroidal neovascular lesions of age-related macular degeneration: ophthalmic findings. SST report no. 13. *Ophthalmology.* 2004;111(11):1993–2006.

Vitrectomy for Complications of Diabetic Retinopathy

Vitreous Hemorrhage

Vitreous hemorrhage is a common complication of proliferative diabetic retinopathy. Vitrectomy is indicated when a vitreous hemorrhage fails to clear spontaneously after approximately 4 weeks to 3 months; timing of the surgery is determined by surgeon preference and patient visual requirements. Possible indications for more prompt intervention include bilateral vitreous hemorrhages or ultrasonic evidence of retinal tear, underlying rhegmatogenous retinal detachment, or tractional retinal detachment that threatens the macula. Serial ultrasonography is recommended to assess the anatomical condition of the retina in the absence of ophthalmoscopic visualization. If surgery is indicated, treatment involves a standard pars plana vitrectomy with removal of vitreous hemorrhage (Video 19-3) and release of the hyaloid from fronds of retinal neovascular ingrowth. Vitreoretinal traction at the disc and along the arcade vessels, if present, is addressed at the time of surgery, along with any macular ERMs. Complete panretinal photocoagulation and hemostasis are generally achieved during the procedure. Preoperative injection of an anti-VEGF agent may improve the safety of surgery by reducing intraoperative bleeding, but it should be performed within 10 days before surgery to reduce the risk of retinal tears that may result from regression of tractional neovascular membranes.

VIDEO 19-3 Vitrectomy for vitreous hemorrhage (03:04).
Courtesy of Colin A. McCannel, MD.
Scan the QR code or access the video at www.aao.org/bcscvideo_section12.

Diabetic Tractional Retinal Detachment

Tractional retinal detachment (TRD) occurs when the hyaloid contracts but is prevented from separating from the retinal interface by fronds of neovascular ingrowth. The tractional forces are transmitted to full-thickness retina and, in the absence of a retinal break, cause schisis and/or detachment of the underlying retina from its corresponding RPE (Fig 19-6). Vitrectomy is indicated when progression of a TRD threatens or involves the macula. In certain complex cases, spontaneous breaks also occur in atrophic retina under traction, resulting in combined traction and rhegmatogenous detachments; this variety of TRD is also a strong indication for surgical intervention. Whenever possible, panretinal photocoagulation should precede vitrectomy but is sometimes more difficult to accomplish in the presence of vitreous hemorrhage. Some surgeons utilize adjunctive intravitreal injection of an anti-VEGF agent preoperatively. The goal is to induce regression of neovascularization to facilitate dissection and minimize intraoperative bleeding.

Vitrectomy for TRD is performed to relieve vitreoretinal traction that interferes with retinal reattachment. Surgery involves peeling cortical vitreous and posterior hyaloid from the retinal surface, particularly in areas of neovascular ingrowth. Point adhesions of cortical vitreous to surface retinal neovascularization can be relieved using various instruments and unimanual or bimanual techniques; current vitrectomy probes can now supplant these instruments in many cases and give surgeons control of flow, cut rate, and duty cycle. Various surgical methods to remove fibrovascular tissue have been described, including segmentation, delamination, and en bloc and modified en bloc excision.

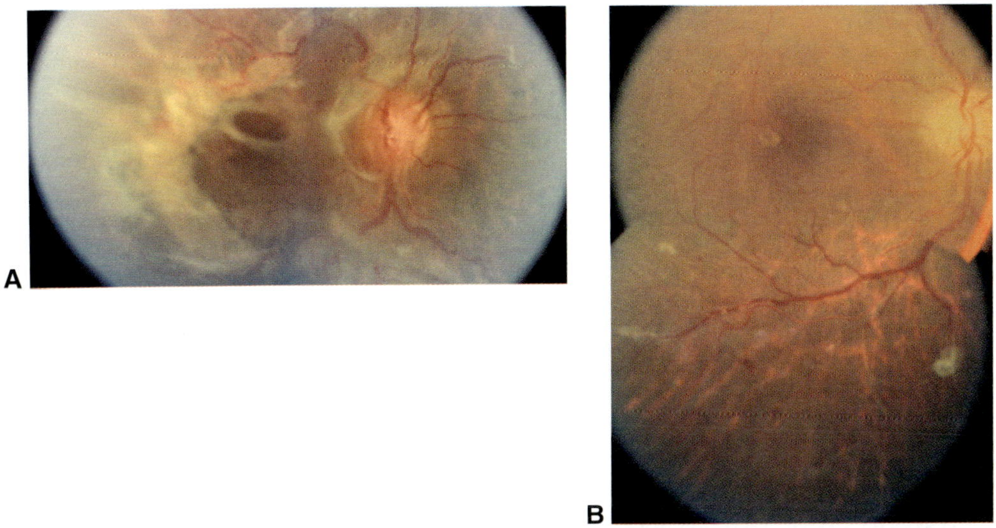

Figure 19-6 Diabetic tractional retinal detachment. **A,** The color fundus photograph montage shows fibrovascular proliferation and contracted posterior hyaloid along the retinal arcade vessels and over the macula, causing elevation and distortion of the retinal surface at the arcade vessels and in the temporal macula. **B,** The postoperative color fundus photograph montage shows flattened macula and vessels. *(Courtesy of Colin A. McCannel, MD.)*

After tractional membranes are removed, diathermy may be used to treat fibrovascular tufts and achieve hemostasis, and supplementary laser treatment may be used in the periphery to reduce ischemia.

Brunner S, Binder S. Surgery for proliferative diabetic retinopathy. In: Ryan SJ, Schachat AP, Wilkinson CP, Hinton DR, Sadda SR, Wiedemann P, eds. *Retina.* Vol 3. 5th ed. Philadelphia: Elsevier/Saunders; 2013:1876–1901.

Diabetic Macular Edema

Laser photocoagulation and intravitreal anti-VEGF or corticosteroid pharmacotherapy are currently the mainstays of treatment for diabetic macular edema. However, recalcitrant cases may be considered for vitrectomy with membrane peeling. In such cases, a standard pars plana vitrectomy is performed with mechanical release of a taut hyaloid, peeling of epiretinal membrane, and stripping of the internal limiting membrane as necessary.

Vitrectomy for Posterior Segment Complications of Anterior Segment Surgery

Postoperative Endophthalmitis

The clinical features of endophthalmitis after anterior segment surgery include marked intraocular inflammation, often with hypopyon, conjunctival vascular congestion, corneal edema, and eyelid edema. Symptoms often include pain and marked loss of vision.

The classification of postoperative endophthalmitis is based on the time of onset and the organisms most frequently isolated:

- acute-onset endophthalmitis (within 6 weeks of intraocular surgery): coagulase-negative *Staphylococcus* species including *S aureus, Streptococcus* species, gram-negative organisms
- chronic (delayed-onset) endophthalmitis (more than 6 weeks after surgery): *Propionibacterium acnes,* coagulase-negative *Staphylococcus* species, fungi
- bleb-associated endophthalmitis (months or years after surgery): *Streptococcus* species, *Haemophilus* species, gram-positive organisms

Management of postoperative endophthalmitis includes obtaining intraocular cultures and administering intravitreal antibiotics. An anterior chamber specimen is typically obtained by using a 30-gauge needle on a tuberculin syringe. A vitreous specimen can be obtained either by needle tap or by using a vitrectomy instrument. A needle tap of the vitreous is typically accomplished using a 25-gauge, 1-inch needle on a 3-mL syringe (to provide greater vacuum) introduced through the pars plana and directed toward the midvitreous cavity. Vitreous specimens are more likely to yield a positive culture result than are simultaneously obtained aqueous specimens.

Acute-onset postoperative endophthalmitis

The use of vitrectomy for acute postoperative endophthalmitis is guided by the results of the Endophthalmitis Vitrectomy Study (EVS; Clinical Trial 19-1). In the EVS, patients

CLINICAL TRIAL 19-1

Endophthalmitis Vitrectomy Study (EVS)

Objective: Evaluate the role of pars plana vitrectomy and intravenous antibiotics in management of postoperative bacterial endophthalmitis.

Participants: Patients with clinical signs and symptoms of bacterial endophthalmitis in an eye after cataract surgery or lens implantation with onset of infection within 6 weeks of surgery.

Randomization: Patients were randomly assigned to immediate pars plana vitrectomy or to immediate tap and inject. Patients were randomly assigned to receive systemic antibiotics or no systemic antibiotics and evaluated at regular intervals after treatment.

Outcome measures: Standardized visual acuity testing and media clarity.

Outcomes:

1. No difference in final visual acuity or media clarity whether or not systemic antibiotics (amikacin/ceftazidime) were employed.
2. No difference in outcomes between the 3-port pars plana vitrectomy group and the immediate tap/biopsy group for patients with better than light perception visual acuity at the study entry examination.
3. For patients with light perception visual acuity, much better results in the immediate pars plana vitrectomy group:
   a. Three times more likely to achieve ≥20/40 (33% vs 11%)
   b. Two times more likely to achieve ≥20/100 (56% vs 30%)
   c. Less likely to incur <5/200 (20% vs 47%)

Clinical impact: Study completed in 1995. Revolutionized treatment of post–cataract surgery endophthalmitis by making it an office procedure of tap and inject for most eyes.

were randomly assigned to undergo either vitrectomy or vitreous tap/biopsy. Both groups received intravitreal and subconjunctival antibiotics (vancomycin and amikacin). The EVS concluded that vitrectomy surgery was indicated in patients with acute-onset (within 6 weeks of cataract extraction) postoperative endophthalmitis with light perception vision (Fig 19-7). Patients with hand motions visual acuity or better had equivalent outcomes in both treatment groups.

Ceftazidime has largely replaced amikacin in clinical practice because of concerns of potential aminoglycoside toxicity. Intravitreal dexamethasone may reduce posttreatment inflammation, but its role in endophthalmitis management remains controversial.

Endophthalmitis Vitrectomy Study Group. Results of the Endophthalmitis Vitrectomy Study. A randomized trial of immediate vitrectomy and of intravenous antibiotics for the treatment of postoperative bacterial endophthalmitis. *Arch Ophthalmol.* 1995;113(12): 1479–1496.

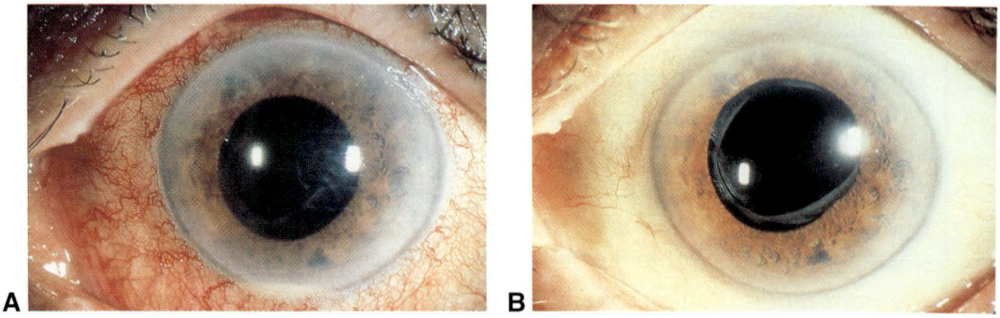

Figure 19-7 Acute-onset endophthalmitis. **A,** Patient with marked epibulbar hyperemia, iritis, hypopyon, and endophthalmitis 5 days after cataract surgery. **B,** After needle tap of vitreous and injection of intravitreal antibiotics, inflammation resolved and visual acuity improved to 20/30. *(Courtesy of Harry W. Flynn, Jr, MD.)*

Chronic (delayed-onset) endophthalmitis

Chronic endophthalmitis has a progressive or indolent course over months or years. Endophthalmitis caused by *P acnes* characteristically induces a peripheral white plaque within the capsular bag and an associated chronic granulomatous inflammation. Treatment by injection of antibiotics into the capsular bag or vitreous cavity usually does not eliminate the infection. A preferred approach is pars plana vitrectomy, partial capsulectomy with selective removal of intracapsular white plaque, and injection of intravitreal vancomycin, 1 mg, adjacent to or inside the capsular bag. If the condition recurs after vitrectomy and subtotal capsulectomy, removal of the entire capsular bag, with removal or exchange of the intraocular lens (IOL), should be considered (Fig 19-8).

Clark WL, Kaiser PK, Flynn HW Jr, Belfort A, Miller D, Meisler DM. Treatment strategies and visual acuity outcomes in chronic postoperative *Propionibacterium acnes* endophthalmitis. *Ophthalmology.* 1999;106(9):1665–1670.

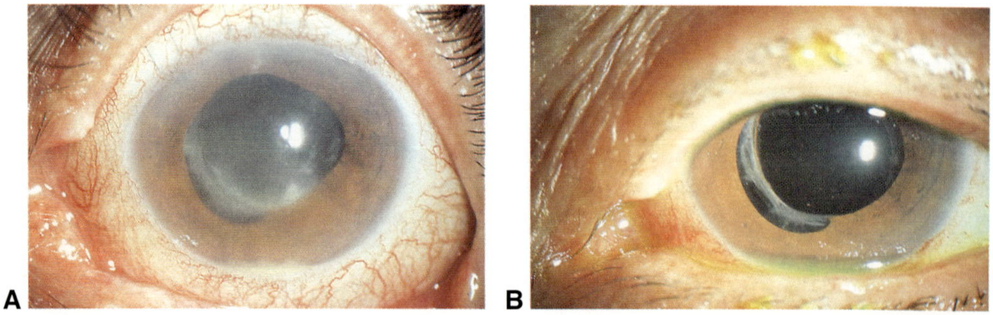

Figure 19-8 Chronic (delayed-onset) postoperative endophthalmitis. **A,** Endophthalmitis in a patient with progressive intraocular inflammation 3 months after cataract surgery. **B,** Same patient after pars plana vitrectomy, capsulectomy, and injection of intravitreal antibiotics. Culture results confirmed diagnosis of *Propionibacterium acnes* endophthalmitis. *(Courtesy of Harry W. Flynn, Jr, MD.)*

Endophthalmitis associated with conjunctival filtering blebs

Except for the additional sign of a purulent bleb, the clinical features of conjunctival filtering bleb–associated endophthalmitis are similar to those of acute-onset postoperative endophthalmitis. These features include conjunctival vascular congestion and marked intraocular inflammation, often with hypopyon (occurring months or years after glaucoma filtering surgery). The initial infection may involve the bleb only *(blebitis),* without anterior chamber or vitreous involvement. Blebitis without endophthalmitis can be treated with frequent applications of topical and subconjunctival antibiotics and close follow-up. However, when blebitis progresses to bleb-associated endophthalmitis, patients are treated by intravitreal antibiotics with or without vitrectomy. The recommended intravitreal antibiotics are similar to those used in acute-onset postoperative endophthalmitis. However, the most common causative organisms in bleb-associated endophthalmitis (eg, *Streptococcus* or *Haemophilus* spp) are more virulent than the most frequently encountered organisms in endophthalmitis that occurs after other intraocular surgeries (such as cataract surgery). Even with prompt treatment, the visual outcomes in bleb-associated endophthalmitis are generally worse than for acute-onset endophthalmitis after cataract surgery (Fig 19-9).

Greenfield DS. Dysfunctional glaucoma filtration blebs. *Focal Points: Clinical Modules for Ophthalmologists.* San Francisco: American Academy of Ophthalmology; 2002, module 4.

Retained Lens Fragments After Phacoemulsification

The incidence of posteriorly displaced, or retained, lens fragments ranges from 0.3%–1.1% in reported series. Retained lens fragments may cause severe intraocular inflammation and secondary glaucoma. Nuclear fragments usually continue to cause chronic intraocular inflammation, whereas cortical remnants usually spontaneously reabsorb (Table 19-1).

Indications for vitrectomy include secondary glaucoma, lens-induced uveitis, and the presence of large nuclear fragments. In the 4 largest reported series, 52% of patients with retained lens fragments had an IOP of at least 30 mm Hg before vitrectomy. Removal of

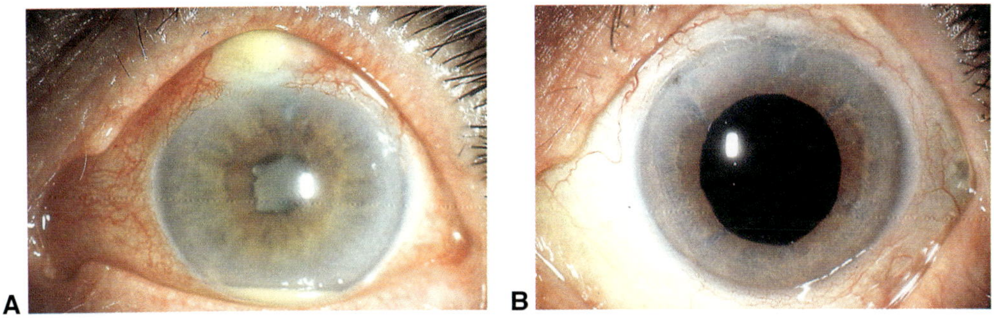

Figure 19-9 Bleb-associated endophthalmitis. **A,** Patient with endophthalmitis who had sudden onset of decreased vision, redness, and pain 2 years after glaucoma filtering surgery. **B,** Same patient after treatment with pars plana vitrectomy and injection of intravitreal antibiotics. *(Courtesy of Harry W. Flynn, Jr, MD.)*

Table 19-1 General Recommendations for Management of Retained Lens Fragments

For the anterior segment surgeon
Attempt retrieval of displaced lens fragments only if fragments are readily accessible.
Perform anterior vitrectomy as necessary to avoid vitreous prolapse into the wound.
Insert an intraocular lens if possible.
Close the cataract wound with interrupted sutures.
Prescribe topical medications as needed.
Refer the patient to a vitreoretinal consultant.
For the vitreoretinal surgeon
Observe eyes with minimal inflammation and/or a small lens fragment.
Continue topical medications as needed.
Schedule vitrectomy
if inflammation or IOP is not controlled.
if a nuclear fragment is present.
Delay vitrectomy if necessary to allow clearing of corneal edema.
Perform maximal core vitrectomy before phacofragmentation.
Start with low fragmentation power (5%–10%) for more efficient removal of the nucleus.
Prepare for secondary intraocular lens insertion if necessary.
Examine the retinal periphery for retinal tears or retinal detachment.

Modified with permission from Flynn HW Jr, Smiddy WE, Vilar NF. Management of retained lens fragments after cataract surgery. In: Saer JB, ed. *Vitreo-Retinal and Uveitis Update: Proceedings of the New Orleans Academy of Ophthalmology Symposium.* The Hague, Netherlands: Kugler; 1998:149, 150.

the lens fragments reduced this incidence by 50% or more in these series. The preferred approach is pars plana vitrectomy with or without use of a fragmatome to remove harder pieces of the lens nucleus (Video 19-4). Following lens fragment removal, the retinal periphery should be examined for the presence of retinal tears or retinal detachment in these patients.

VIDEO 19-4 Vitrectomy for removal of retained lens fragment (00:44).
Courtesy of Colin A. McCannel, MD.
Scan the QR code or access the video at www.aao.org/bcscvideo_section12.

Reported series with long-term follow-up have found that retinal detachment occurs in about 15% of eyes with retained lens fragments. Aggressive attempts to retrieve posterior lens fragments using a limbal approach are sometimes complicated by retinal detachments caused by giant retinal tears. Giant retinal tears are more commonly found 180° away from the incision used for cataract surgery.

Aaberg TM Jr, Rubsamen PE, Flynn HW Jr, Chang S, Mieler WF, Smiddy WE. Giant retinal tear as a complication of attempted removal of intravitreal lens fragments during cataract surgery. *Am J Ophthalmol.* 1997;124(2):222–226.

Modi YS, Epstein A, Smiddy WE, Murray TG, Feuer W, Flynn HW Jr. Retained lens fragments after cataract surgery: outcomes of same-day versus later pars plana vitrectomy. *Am J Ophthalmol.* 2013;156(3):454–459.

Vanner EA, Stewart MW. Vitrectomy timing for retained lens fragments after surgery for age-related cataracts: a systematic review and meta-analysis. *Am J Ophthalmol.* 2011;152(3): 345–357.

Posteriorly Dislocated Intraocular Lenses

Posterior chamber intraocular lenses (PCIOLs) may become dislocated despite seemingly satisfactory capsular support at the time of the initial surgery. Factors to consider when placing a sulcus-fixated IOL include the presence of zonular dehiscence, total amount of anterior capsular support (eg, >180°), size of the eye, and haptic-to-haptic diameter of the IOL. Foldable IOLs have a 12.5–13.0-mm haptic-to-haptic length. This length is frequently smaller than the sulcus-to-sulcus diameter into which these haptics must fit and may contribute to postoperative subluxation or dislocation of the IOL. Dislocation of a flexible IOL may also follow Nd:YAG laser capsulotomy performed soon after cataract surgery. Late dislocation of the IOL (from several days to decades after surgery) is less common but may occur as a result of trauma or spontaneous loss of zonular support in eyes with pseudoexfoliation syndrome. The options for treatment in such cases include observation only, surgical repositioning, IOL exchange, or IOL removal.

Vitrectomy for posteriorly dislocated IOLs involves removing all vitreous adhesions to the IOL in order to minimize vitreous traction to the retina when the lens is manipulated back into the anterior chamber. The IOL may be placed into the ciliary sulcus provided there is adequate support. If capsular support is inadequate, the IOL may be fixated by suturing the haptics to the iris *(iris fixation)* or sclera *(scleral fixation)* or by placing the haptics into intrascleral tunnels *(intrascleral fixation).* Alternatively, the PCIOL can be removed through a limbal incision and exchanged for an anterior chamber IOL (ACIOL; Video 19-5).

VIDEO 19-5 Vitrectomy for retrieval of posteriorly dislocated IOL (02:36).
Courtesy of Colin A McCannel, MD.
Scan the QR code or access the video at www.aao.org/bcscvideo_section12.

Smiddy WE, Flynn HW Jr. Managing retained lens fragments and dislocated posterior chamber IOLs after cataract surgery. *Focal Points: Clinical Modules for Ophthalmologists.* San Francisco: American Academy of Ophthalmology; 1996, module 7.

Cystoid Macular Edema

Cystoid macular edema (CME) that develops after anterior segment surgery usually resolves spontaneously. Treatment with corticosteroid and nonsteroidal anti-inflammatory eye drops is the first-line approach for patients with persistent CME. Periocular or intravitreal corticosteroids may be used in recalcitrant cases. Oral acetazolamide may also be useful in select cases. Pars plana vitrectomy with removal of obvious vitreous adhesions to anterior segment structures may promote resolution of CME and improve visual acuity in select cases (Fig 19-10). An IOL may require repositioning, exchange, or removal if it is deemed to irritate the iris by chafing or capture.

Suprachoroidal Hemorrhage

Suprachoroidal hemorrhage may occur during or after any form of intraocular surgery, particularly glaucoma surgery, in which large shifts in IOP are commonplace. By definition, such hemorrhages accumulate in the supraciliary and suprachoroidal space, a

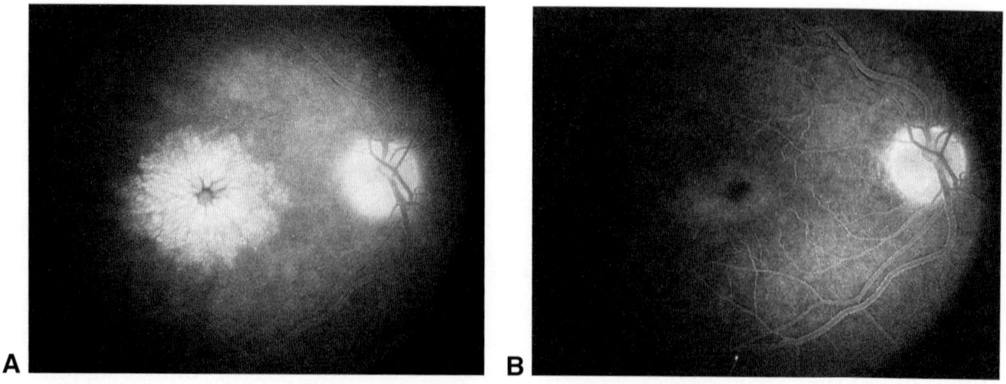

Figure 19-10 Pseudophakic cystoid macular edema (CME). **A,** Fundus photograph of patient with nonresolving CME, vitreous strands to cataract wound, and dislocated intraocular lens (IOL). **B,** Same patient after pars plana vitrectomy, removal of vitreous strands, repositioning of IOL, and periocular administration of corticosteroids. CME has markedly improved. *(Courtesy of Harry W. Flynn, Jr, MD.)*

potential space between the sclera and uvea that is modified by uveal adhesions and entries of vessels. Hemorrhages may be limited or massive and involve 1–4 quadrants. When retinal surfaces touch one another, dictated by scleral spur and the entries of the short posterior ciliary vessels and nerves, the choroidal hemorrhage is termed *appositional,* or "kissing." These hemorrhages may be further classified as nonexpulsive or expulsive; the expulsive type involves extrusion of intraocular contents. Reported risk factors for suprachoroidal hemorrhage include

- advanced age
- glaucoma
- myopia
- aphakia
- arteriosclerotic cardiovascular disease
- hypertension
- Sturge-Weber–associated choroidal hemangiomas
- intraoperative tachycardia

Transient hypotony is a common feature of all incisional ocular surgery and in a small percentage of patients may be associated with suprachoroidal hemorrhage from rupture of the long or short posterior ciliary arteries.

Surgical management strategies are controversial. Most authors recommend immediate closure of ocular surgical incisions and removal of vitreous incarceration in the wound, if possible; the primary goal is to prevent or limit expulsion. Successful intraoperative drainage of a suprachoroidal hemorrhage is rare, however, as the blood coagulates rapidly. Most surgeons recommend observation of suprachoroidal hemorrhages for 7–14 days to allow some degree of liquefaction of the hemorrhage. Determining the timing of secondary surgical intervention is aided by B-scan ultrasound, through evaluation of echographic features of clot liquefaction. Indications for surgical drainage include recalcitrant pain, increased IOP, retinal detachment, and appositional choroidal detachments associated with ciliary body rotation and angle closure. Furthermore, prolonged IOP elevation in the presence of anterior chamber hemorrhage (hyphema) increases the risk of corneal blood staining and is an indication for surgical intervention.

Surgical management of suprachoroidal hemorrhage involves placement of an anterior chamber infusion line to maintain IOP (Fig 19-11, Video 19-6). A full-thickness sclerotomy is then placed subjacent to the site of maximum accumulation of blood. After drainage of suprachoroidal blood, pars plana vitrectomy may be performed. Appositional and closed-funnel suprachoroidal hemorrhage, prolonged elevation of IOP, and retinal detachment all portend a poor visual prognosis.

VIDEO 19-6 Drainage of suprachoroidal hemorrhage (03:25).
Courtesy of Koen A. van Overdam, MD.
Scan the QR code or access the video at www.aao.org/bcscvideo_section12.

Scott IU, Flynn HW Jr, Schiffman J, Smiddy WE, Murray TG, Ehlies F. Visual acuity outcomes among patients with appositional suprachoroidal hemorrhage. *Ophthalmology.* 1997;104(12): 2039–2046.

Needle Penetration of the Globe

Factors predisposing patients to needle penetration of the globe include

- axial high myopia
- posterior staphyloma
- previous scleral buckling surgery
- poor patient cooperation at the time of the injection
- inexperience of surgeon

Management options vary with the severity of the intraocular damage. Often, blood obscures and surrounds the retinal penetration site, making laser treatment difficult. Observation or transscleral cryotherapy may be considered in such cases. When retinal detachment is associated, early vitrectomy with or without scleral buckling is often recommended. Posterior pole damage from needle extension into the macula or optic nerve is associated with a very poor visual prognosis (Fig 19-12).

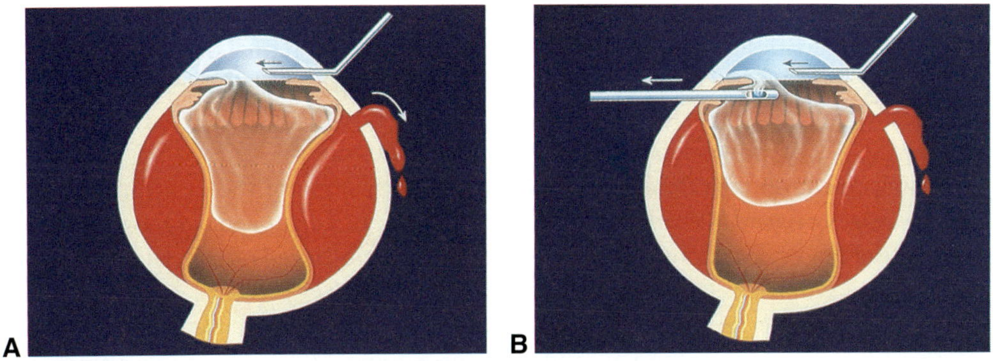

A B

Figure 19-11 Suprachoroidal hemorrhage. **A,** Schematic shows anterior infusion and simultaneous drainage of suprachoroidal hemorrhage through pars plana sclerotomy. **B,** Schematic shows pars plana vitrectomy to remove vitreous prolapse as drainage of suprachoroidal hemorrhage continues. *(Courtesy of Harry W. Flynn, Jr, MD.)*

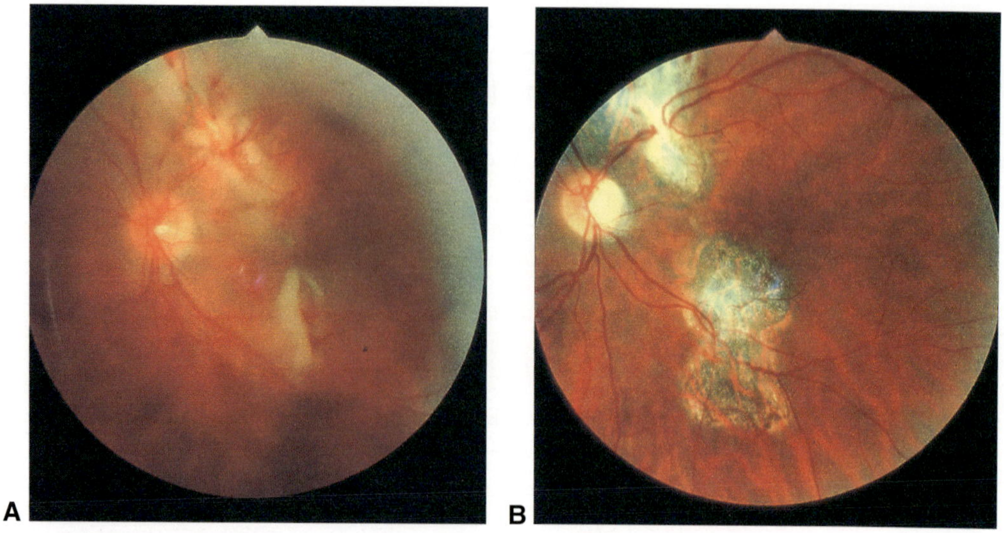

Figure 19-12 Color fundus photographs of needle penetration of the globe. **A,** Needle penetration of the globe has caused multiple retinal breaks, including damage to the macula. **B,** After retinal detachment occurred, treatment consisted of vitrectomy, fluid–gas exchange, and endolaser photocoagulation of retinal breaks. Retinal reattachment was achieved, but the visual acuity remained very poor. *(Courtesy of Harry W. Flynn, Jr, MD.)*

Rhegmatogenous Retinal Detachment Surgery

Rhegmatogenous retinal detachment occurs when a retinal break (or multiple breaks) allows ingress of fluid from the vitreous cavity into the subretinal space. Breaks can be atrophic, often associated with lattice degeneration, or they may be tractional tears, related to vitreous traction on the retina and posterior vitreous detachment (PVD). The risk of rhegmatogenous retinal detachment (RRD) in otherwise normal eyes is approximately 5 new cases in 100,000 persons per year; lifetime risk is approximately 1 in 300 persons. The most important risk factors are high myopia, family history of retinal detachment, and fellow eye retinal detachment. Pseudophakia is also an important risk factor; the reported incidence after cataract surgery is less than 1% but increases over time (Fig 19-13). Patient characteristics that increase the risk of pseudophakic retinal detachment include younger age at the time of cataract extraction, male sex, and longer axial length. A surgical complication such as posterior capsular rupture with vitreous loss has been estimated to increase the risk of retinal detachment by as much as 20-fold.

Management options for RRD include *laser demarcation* of the detachment, *pneumatic retinopexy, scleral buckling procedure,* and *vitrectomy with or without scleral buckling.* Observation can be considered for selected patients with localized retinal detachment and no associated symptoms (subclinical retinal detachment).

Selection of the treatment approach among the modalities available for retinal detachment is surgeon-dependent and remains a topic of debate among retinal surgeons. The precise configuration of the detachment, the location of the breaks, and the

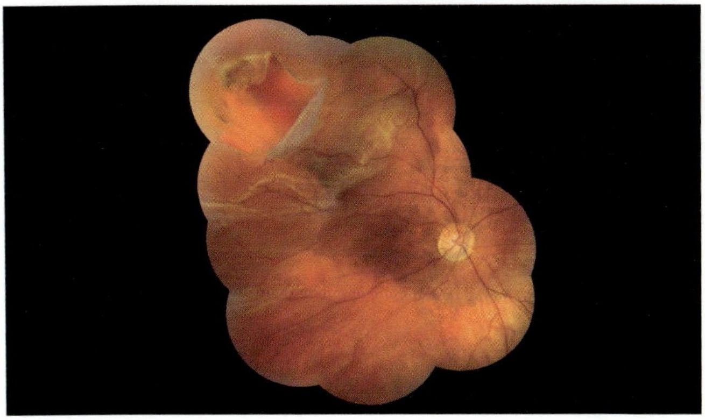

Figure 19-13 Color fundus photograph montage of a patient with symptomatic retinal detachment from a large superotemporal break after cataract surgery. *(Courtesy of Nancy M. Holekamp, MD.)*

phakic status of the eye are all considered carefully before the method of treatment is determined.

Campo RV, Sipperley JO, Sneed SR, et al. Pars plana vitrectomy without scleral buckle for pseudophakic retinal detachments. *Ophthalmology.* 1999;106(9):1811–1816.

Clark A, Morlet N, Ng JQ, Preen DB, Semmens JB. Risk for retinal detachment after phacoemulsification: a whole-population study of cataract surgery outcomes. *Arch Ophthalmol.* 2012;130(7):882–888.

Powell SK, Olson RJ. Incidence of retinal detachment after cataract surgery and neodymium: YAG laser capsulotomy. *J Cataract Refract Surg.* 1995;21(2):132–135.

Tuft SJ, Minassian D, Sullivan P. Risk factors for retinal detachment after cataract surgery: a case-control study. *Ophthalmology.* 2006;113(4):650–656.

Techniques for Surgical Repair of Retinal Detachments

Three surgical techniques have been described for eyes with primary uncomplicated rhegmatogenous retinal detachment: *pneumatic retinopexy, scleral buckling,* and *primary vitrectomy with or without scleral buckling.* These procedures all share the common goals of identifying and treating all causative retinal breaks while providing support of such breaks through external and internal tamponade as needed.

Kreissig I, ed. *Primary Retinal Detachment: Options for Repair.* Berlin: Springer-Verlag; 2005.

Pneumatic retinopexy

The goal of pneumatic retinopexy is to close the retinal breaks using an intraocular gas bubble for a sufficient time to allow the subretinal fluid to reabsorb and a chorioretinal adhesion to form around the causative break(s). The classic indications for pneumatic retinopexy include

- confidence that all retinal breaks have been identified
- retinal breaks that are confined to the superior 8 clock-hours
- a single retinal break or multiple breaks within 1–2 clock-hours

- the absence of proliferative vitreoretinopathy (PVR) grade C or D
- a cooperative patient who can maintain proper positioning
- clear media

With direct pneumatic occlusion of the causative retinal breaks in acute detachments, subretinal fluid is often completely reabsorbed within 6–8 hours.

The procedure can be performed with transconjunctival cryopexy to the causative retinal breaks; alternatively, laser retinopexy may be performed after retinal apposition. A variety of intraocular gases (eg, air, SF_6, C_3F_8) have been used for tamponade, and a concomitant anterior chamber paracentesis is generally required to normalize the elevated IOP that results from the gas injection. The patient must maintain a predetermined head posture to place the breaks in the least dependent position (Fig 19-14).

A prospective, multicenter, randomized clinical trial comparing pneumatic retinopexy with scleral buckling demonstrated successful retinal reattachment in 73% of patients who underwent pneumatic retinopexy and in 82% of those who received scleral buckle procedures—a difference that was not statistically significant. Complications from pneumatic retinopexy include subretinal gas migration, anterior chamber gas migration, endophthalmitis, cataract, and recurrent retinal detachment from the formation of new retinal breaks.

Gilca M, Duval R, Goodyear E, Olivier S, Cordahi G. Factors associated with outcomes of pneumatic retinopexy for rhegmatogenous retinal detachments: a retrospective review of 422 cases. *Retina.* 2014;34(4):693–699.

Tornambe PE, Hilton GF. Pneumatic retinopexy. A multicenter randomized controlled clinical trial comparing pneumatic retinopexy with scleral buckling. The Retinal Detachment Study Group. *Ophthalmology.* 1989;96(6):772–784.

Scleral buckling

The goal of scleral buckling is to close retinal breaks through external scleral indentation. Transscleral cryopexy is used to create a permanent adhesion between the retina and RPE at the sites of retinal breaks. The buckling material is then carefully positioned to support the causative breaks by scleral imbrication.

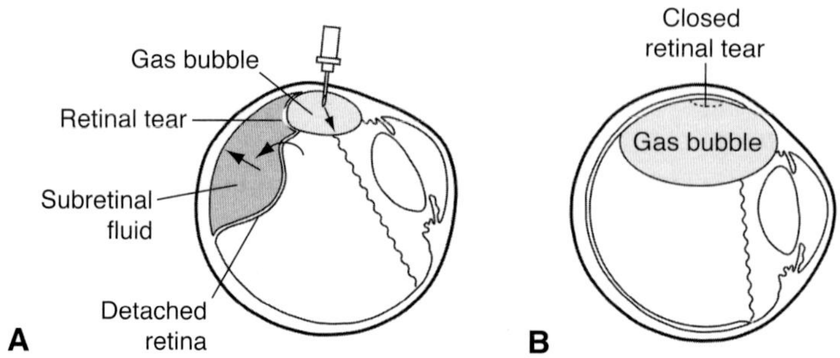

Figure 19-14 Pneumatic retinopexy. **A,** Schematic showing a small, expansile gas bubble being injected into the vitreous cavity. **B,** The bubble enlarges. The patient is positioned so the gas bubble occludes the retinal break, allowing for resorption of subretinal fluid. *(Illustration by Dave Yates.)*

The choice of scleral buckling technique (eg, encircling, segmental, or radial placement of the sponge) takes into account the number and position of the retinal breaks, the size of the eye, individual surgeon preference and training, and associated vitreoretinal findings (eg, lattice degeneration, vitreoretinal traction, and aphakia) (Fig 19-15, Video 19-7).

VIDEO 19-7 Scleral buckle for rhegmatogenous retinal detachment (05:25).
Courtesy of Colin A. McCannel, MD.
Scan the QR code or access the video at www.aao.org/bcscvideo_section12.

An increase in the IOP related to compression from the buckling effect may indicate the need for external drainage of the subretinal fluid, anterior chamber paracentesis, or

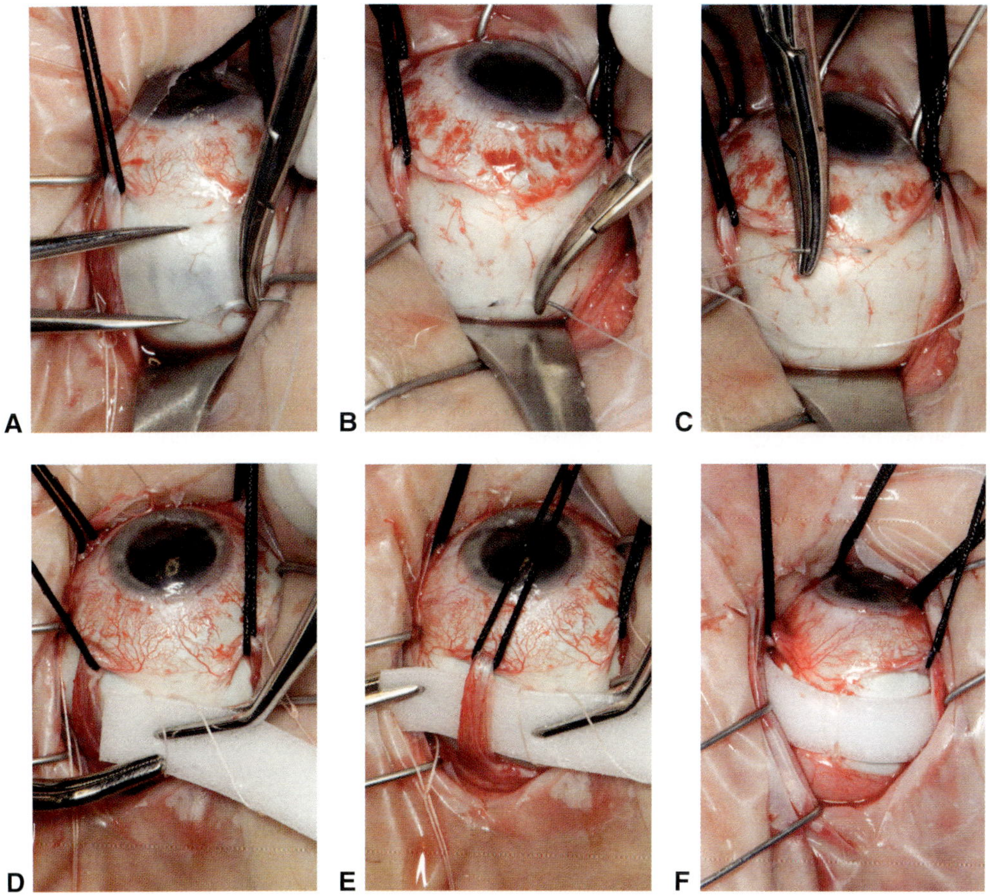

Figure 19-15 Scleral buckle procedure. The conjunctiva is opened and the rectus muscles isolated and tagged with a "0" silk suture. **A,** Intraoperative color photograph shows the eye rotated so the sclera is exposed. Using calipers, the surgeon measures and marks the location for the anterior and posterior scleral pass for the radial mattress suture. **B, C,** The posterior scleral suture pass is accomplished. **D, E,** The encircling element, a 506 sponge, is passed, using Nugent forceps, under the suture and rectus muscle. **F,** The scleral buckle is fully installed, and the tied-up radial mattress suture, with the knot rotated posteriorly, is shown. *(Courtesy of Colin A. McCannel, MD.)*

both. Chronic viscous subretinal fluid, "fish-mouthing" of large retinal breaks, and bullous retinal detachments may necessitate treatment with intraocular gas tamponade, drainage, or both. Complications of scleral buckling include induced myopia, anterior ocular ischemia, diplopia, ptosis, orbital cellulitis, subretinal hemorrhage from drainage, and retinal incarceration at the drainage site.

Primary vitrectomy

Traction on focal areas of adhesion of the vitreous to the peripheral retina (frequently at the posterior vitreous base insertion) may cause retinal breaks and allow for the subsequent migration of intraocular fluid into the subretinal space, leading to retinal detachment. Consequently, the goals of primary vitrectomy are to remove cortical vitreous adherent to retinal breaks, directly drain the subretinal fluid, tamponade the breaks (using air, gas, or silicone oil), and create chorioretinal adhesions around each retinal break with endolaser photocoagulation or cryopexy.

In general, the standard 3-port vitrectomy technique is used, employing 20-, 23-, 25-, or 27-gauge instruments. At the discretion of the surgeon, vitrectomy can be combined with a scleral buckle procedure. During vitrectomy, a complete posterior vitreous separation is ensured, and the peripheral cortical vitreous is carefully shaved toward the vitreous base to relieve traction on the retinal breaks (Fig 19-16, Video 19-8). To drain the subretinal fluid and achieve intraoperative retinal reattachment, the surgeon can use either an intentional drainage retinotomy or perfluorocarbon liquid technique. If PVR is present, it may be necessary to peel the epiretinal (and, less commonly, subretinal) membranes to facilitate the retinal reattachment. For extensive PVR, a relaxing retinotomy or retinectomy may be required. Once the retina is flattened, chorioretinal laser photocoagulation or cryopexy can be applied. Postoperative tamponade is generally provided by intraocular air or nonexpansile (isovolemic) concentrations of SF_6 or C_3F_8 gas, although complex cases may require the use of silicone oil. Complications of vitrectomy for retinal detachment include postvitrectomy nuclear sclerosis (in phakic eyes), glaucoma, PVR, and retinal redetachment.

VIDEO 19-8 Vitrectomy for rhegmatogenous retinal detachment (03:32).
Courtesy of Colin A. McCannel, MD.
Scan the QR code or access the video at www.aao.org/bcscvideo_section12.

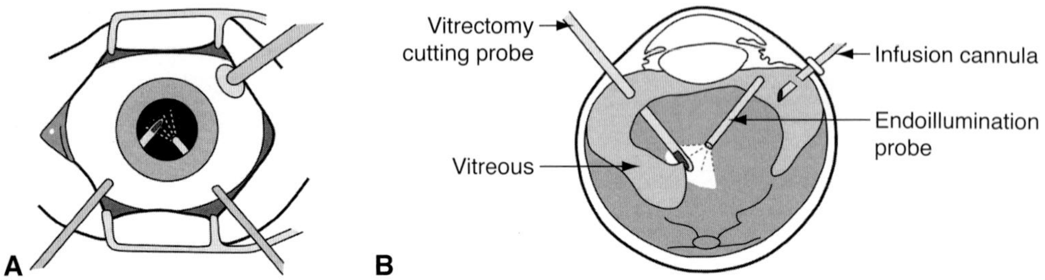

Figure 19-16 Vitrectomy. **A,** Schematic of surgeon's view of a 20-gauge, 3-port pars plana vitrectomy. **B,** A cross-sectional view of a vitrectomy, showing an infusion cannula, endoillumination probe, and vitrectomy cutting probe. *(Illustration by Dave Yates.)*

Complex retinal detachment includes giant retinal tears, recurrent retinal detachment, vitreous hemorrhage, and PVR. Pars plana vitrectomy techniques are necessary to address the common features of PVR, including proliferative membranes, retinal folds, and media opacities (see also Chapter 15). In the past, controversy surrounded the use of long-acting gas versus silicone oil in retinal tamponade for eyes with complex retinal detachment caused by advanced grades of PVR; this issue was addressed in the Silicone Study. This prospective, multicenter, randomized study concluded that tamponade with SF_6 was inferior to long-term tamponade with either C_3F_8 or silicone oil. Differences in outcomes from the use of C_3F_8 and silicone oil were statistically insignificant. A lower rate of hypotony was noted in patients treated with silicone oil than in those treated with C_3F_8.

Vitrectomy with silicone oil or sulfur hexafluoride gas in eyes with severe proliferative vitreoretinopathy: results of a randomized clinical trial. Silicone Study report 1. *Arch Ophthalmol.* 1992;110(6):770–779.

Vitrectomy with silicone oil or perfluoropropane gas in eyes with severe proliferative vitreoretinopathy: results of a randomized clinical trial. Silicone Study report 2. *Arch Ophthalmol.* 1992;110(6):780–792.

Outcomes Following Retinal Reattachment Surgery

Anatomical reattachment

The overall rate of anatomical reattachment with current techniques is 80%–90% for the primary surgery. The exact rate depends on technique and preoperative ocular findings. Subsequent reattachment surgeries have success rates in the 70% range. However, rates for final reattachment, even if multiple procedures are required, are in the 90%–100% range. Retinal detachments caused by dialyses or small holes or that are associated with demarcation lines have a better prognosis. Aphakic and pseudophakic eyes have a slightly less favorable prognosis. Detachments caused by giant tears or associated with PVR, uveitis, choroidal detachments, or posterior breaks secondary to trauma have the worst prognosis for anatomical reattachment.

Sullivan P. Techniques of scleral buckling. In: Ryan SJ, Schachat AP, Wilkinson CP, Hinton DR, Sadda SR, Wiedemann P, eds. *Retina.* Vol 3. 5th ed. Philadelphia: Elsevier/Saunders; 2013:1669–1695.

Postoperative visual acuity

The status of the macula—whether it was detached and for how long—is the primary presurgical determinant of postoperative visual acuity. If the macula was not detached ("macula-on" retinal detachment) and the retinal detachment is successfully repaired, restoration of preoperative visual acuity is usually expected. However, 10%–15% of these eyes do not return to the preoperative visual acuity.

If the macula was detached preoperatively ("macula-off" retinal detachment), damage to—or degeneration of—photoreceptors may prevent good postoperative visual acuity. Only approximately one-third to one-half of eyes with a detached macula recover visual acuity to the level of 20/50 or better. Among patients with a macular detachment of less than 1 week's duration, 75% will obtain a final visual acuity of 20/70 or better, as opposed to 50% with a macular detachment of 1–8 weeks' duration.

Other than photoreceptor damage from the detachment, factors associated with visual acuity deterioration or incomplete recovery following successful retinal reattachment surgery include irregular astigmatism, cataract progression, persistent subfoveal fluid, macular edema, or macular pucker. Intraoperative complications such as hemorrhage and preexisting ocular pathology may also limit visual recovery.

Complications of Pars Plana Vitrectomy

Nuclear sclerotic cataract is the most common complication of vitrectomy. Within 3–6 months following vitrectomy, as many as 90% of phakic eyes in patients older than 50 years may develop visually significant nuclear sclerotic cataract. Vitrectomy may also increase the long-term risk of open-angle glaucoma. Both cataract progression and glaucoma are speculated to be the result of increased oxygen tension in the eye after vitrectomy, which in turn results in oxidative damage to the lens and trabecular meshwork, respectively.

Other complications of pars plana vitrectomy include retinal tears and detachment, retention of subretinal perfluorocarbon liquid (when utilized), retinal and vitreous incarceration, endophthalmitis, and recurrent vitreous hemorrhage. Endophthalmitis after vitrectomy is rare (approximately 1 in 2000 cases) but is more common in patients with diabetes mellitus and in eyes with retained intraocular foreign bodies. Table 19-2 lists the most common complications of pars plana vitrectomy.

Banker AS, Freeman WR, Kim JW, Munguia D, Azen SP. Vision-threatening complications of surgery for full-thickness macular holes. Vitrectomy for Macular Hole Study Group. *Ophthalmology.* 1997;104(9):1442–1453.

Chang S. LXII Edward Jackson lecture: open angle glaucoma after vitrectomy. *Am J Ophthalmol.* 2006;141(6):1033–1043.

Cherfan GM, Michels RG, de Bustros S, Enger C, Glaser BM. Nuclear sclerotic cataract after vitrectomy for idiopathic epiretinal membranes causing macular pucker. *Am J Ophthalmol.* 1991;111(4):434–438.

Table 19-2 Complications of Pars Plana Vitrectomy

Complications commonly associated with pars plana vitrectomy
Postoperative nuclear sclerotic cataract
Long-term risk of open-angle glaucoma
Intraoperative or postoperative retinal break
Intraoperative or postoperative retinal detachment
Intraoperative cataract
Postoperative vitreous hemorrhage
Postoperative massive fibrin exudation
Postoperative anterior segment neovascularization
Endophthalmitis
Complications associated with silicone oil
Glaucoma
Band keratopathy
Corneal decompensation

Intravitreal Injections

Intravitreal injections are the fastest-growing procedure in ophthalmology and in medicine in general (Fig 19-17, Video 19-9). The most common indications include age-related macular degeneration, diabetic retinopathy, and venous occlusive disease–associated macular edema. The majority of injections are of anti-angiogenic agents (eg, bevacizumab, ranibizumab, and aflibercept). Other intravitreal medications used include steroid preparations, antimicrobials, and many medications used in clinical trials that will likely be approved in the coming years. The number of injections performed in the United States, estimated from Medicare procedure codes, increased from fewer than 3000 per year in 1999 to more than 2.3 million in 2012. This number is continuing to increase given the aging population, new medications available, and expanding indications.

VIDEO 19-9 Intravitreal injection of pharmacologic agent (03:11).
Courtesy of Stephen J. Kim, MD.
Scan the QR code or access the video at www.aao.org/bcscvideo_section12.

Endophthalmitis remains the most feared complication after intravitreal injection; the reported incidence ranges from 0.02% to 0.2%. Despite the possibility of respiratory organisms causing endophthalmitis (via contamination from respiratory droplets), the most common source of infection is presumed to be the patient's own conjunctiva or eyelids. Therefore, potential mechanisms of infection include direct inoculation of ocular surface bacteria into the vitreous or subsequent entry through a wound track.

Strict aseptic technique, including managing the eyelid to prevent contamination from the margin and lashes, is advocated. Despite the absence of direct evidence, there is consensus that the application of povidone-iodine, 5%, to the ocular surface for at least 60–90 seconds prior to injection is beneficial. In contrast, antibiotic use before or after injections is becoming increasingly controversial and is no longer recommended in routine situations, particularly given that repeat topical antibiotic application has been shown to select for resistant ocular flora. Multiple studies have reported that *Streptococcus viridans*, a common component of oral flora, is a more frequent cause of endophthalmitis following intravitreal injections than after other intraocular procedures, presumably from contamination by respiratory droplets. Consequently, attention should be paid to efforts that reduce the risk of respiratory-droplet contamination such as avoiding extraneous talking

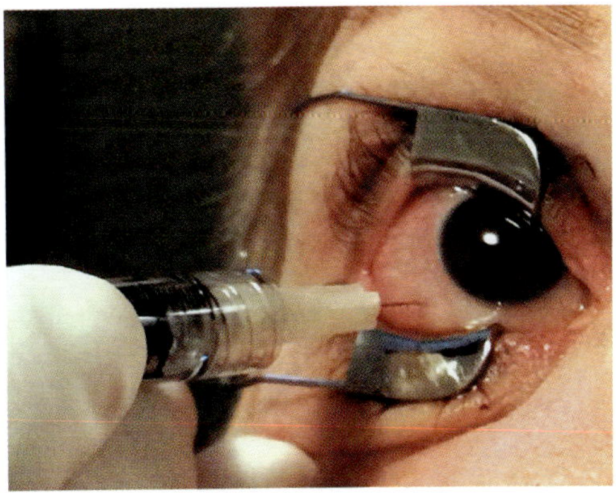

Figure 19-17 Intravitreal injection. The ocular surface was anesthetized with subconjunctival injection of lidocaine, 2%, in the inferotemporal quadrant. An eyelid speculum was inserted, and povidone-iodine, 5%, applied to the ocular surface. After 2 minutes, povidone-iodine was reapplied over the injection site and—after proper hand placement and no talking—the injection was made approximately 4 mm from the limbus. *(Courtesy of Stephen J. Kim, MD.)*

between the patient and provider and the use of a face mask during the procedure. In addition, excessive manipulation of the eyelid margin should be avoided to limit expression of bacteria-laden secretions from the meibomian glands, and aggressive treatment of blepharitis should be considered for patients with severe disease prior to intravitreal injection.

Commonly used methods for anesthesia administration before intravitreal injections include pledgets or cotton-tip applicators soaked with anesthetic and held against the site of injection, application of topical (including viscous) formulations of anesthetic, and subconjunctival lidocaine injection. There is no consensus regarding the optimal method of anesthesia for patient comfort and reduced risk of infection.

Recent outbreaks of endophthalmitis from contaminated bevacizumab have prompted periodic review of compounding pharmacy practices and accreditation status in order to minimize the risk of future outbreaks. To minimize patient risk when bilateral injections are performed, many practitioners have adopted a workflow in which different lot numbers of compounded medications are used for each eye.

Kim SJ, Chomsky AS, Sternberg P Jr. Reducing the risk of endophthalmitis after intravitreous injection. *JAMA Ophthalmol.* 2013;131(5):674–675.

Kim SJ, Toma HS. Antimicrobial resistance and ophthalmic antibiotics: 1-year results of a longitudinal controlled study of patients undergoing intravitreal injections. *Arch Ophthalmol.* 2011;129(9):1180–1188.

McCannel CA. Meta-analysis of endophthalmitis after intravitreal injection of anti-vascular endothelial growth factor agents: causative organisms and possible prevention strategies. *Retina.* 2011;31(4):654–661.

Basic Texts

Retina and Vitreous

Agarwal A. *Gass' Atlas of Macular Diseases.* 5th ed. Philadelphia: Elsevier/Saunders; 2012.

Albert DM, Miller JW, Azar DT, Blodi BA, eds. *Albert & Jakobiec's Principles and Practice of Ophthalmology.* 3rd ed. Philadelphia: Elsevier/Saunders; 2008.

Alfaro DV III, Liggett PE, eds. *Vitreoretinal Surgery of the Injured Eye.* Philadelphia: Lippincott Williams & Wilkins; 1998.

Brinton DA, Wilkinson CP. *Retinal Detachment: Principles and Practice.* 3rd ed. New York: Oxford University Press; 2009.

Duker JS, Waheed NK, Goldman DR. *Handbook of Retinal OCT.* Philadelphia: Elsevier/Saunders; 2014.

Gupta AK, Aggarwal VK, Goel N, Nayak BK. *Handbook of Clinical Trials in Ophthalmology.* New Delhi, India: Jaypee Brothers Medical Publishers; 2014.

Hartnett ME. *Pediatric Retina.* 2nd ed. Philadelphia: Lippincott Williams & Wilkins; 2014.

Ho AC, Regillo CD, eds. *Age-related Macular Degeneration Diagnosis and Treatment.* New York: Springer; 2011.

Peyman GA, Meffert SA, Conway MD, eds. *Vitreoretinal Surgical Techniques.* 2nd ed. London: Informa Healthcare; 2007.

Rizzo S, Patelli F, Chow DR, eds. *Vitreo-retinal Surgery: Progress III.* New York: Springer; 2010. *Essentials in Ophthalmology.*

Ryan SJ, Schachat AP, Wilkinson CP, Hinton DR, Sadda SR, Wiedemann P, eds. *Retina.* 5th ed. Philadelphia: Elsevier/Saunders; 2013.

Saxena S, Meyer CH, Ohji M, Akduman L, eds. *Vitreoretinal Surgery.* New Delhi, India: Jaypee Brothers Medical Publishers; 2012.

Tasman WS, Jaeger EA, eds. *Duane's Ophthalmology on DVD-ROM.* Philadelphia: Lippincott Williams & Wilkins; 2013.

Wilkinson CP, Rice TA. *Michels Retinal Detachment.* 2nd ed. St Louis: Mosby–Mosby Year Book; 1997.

Yannuzzi LA. *The Retinal Atlas.* Philadelphia: Elsevier/Saunders; 2010.

Related Academy Materials

The Academy is dedicated to providing a wealth of high-quality clinical education resources for ophthalmologists.

Print Publications and Electronic Products

For a complete listing of Academy products related to topics covered in this BCSC Section, visit our online store at http://store.aao.org/clinical-education/topic/retina-vitreous.html. Or call Customer Service at 866-561-8558 (toll free, US only) or +1 415-561-8540, Monday through Friday, between 8:00 AM and 5:00 PM (PST).

Online Resources

Visit the Ophthalmic News and Education (ONE®) Network at www.aao.org/clinical-education to find relevant videos, online courses, journal articles, practice guidelines, self-assessment quizzes, images, and more. The ONE Network is a free Academy-member benefit.

Access free, trusted articles and content with the Academy's collaborative online encyclopedia, EyeWiki, at www.aao.org/eyewiki.

Requesting Continuing Medical Education Credit

The American Academy of Ophthalmology is accredited by the Accreditation Council for Continuing Medical Education to provide continuing medical education for physicians.

The American Academy of Ophthalmology designates this enduring material for a maximum of 15 *AMA PRA Category 1 Credits*™. Physicians should claim only the credit commensurate with the extent of their participation in the activity.

The American Medical Association requires that all learners participating in activities involving enduring materials complete a formal assessment before claiming continuing medical education (CME) credit. To assess your achievement in this activity and ensure that a specified level of knowledge has been reached, a posttest for this Section of the Basic and Clinical Science Course is provided online. A minimum score of 80% must be obtained to pass the test and claim CME credit.

To take the posttest and request CME credit online:

1. Go to www.aao.org/cme-central and log in.
2. Click on "Claim CME Credit and View My CME Transcript" and then "Report AAO Credits."
3. Select the appropriate Academy activity. You will be directed to the posttest.
4. Once you have passed the test with a score of 80% or higher, you will be directed to your transcript. *If you are not an Academy member, you will be able to print out a certificate of participation once you have passed the test.*

CME expiration date: June 1, 2018. *AMA PRA Category 1 Credits*™ may be claimed only once between June 1, 2015, and the expiration date.

For assistance, contact the Academy's Customer Service department at 866-561-8558 (US only) or +1 415-561-8540 between 8:00 AM and 5:00 PM (PST), Monday through Friday, or send an e-mail to customer_service@aao.org.

Study Questions

Please note that these questions are *not* part of your CME reporting process. They are provided here for your own educational use and identification of any professional practice gaps. The required CME posttest is available online (see "Requesting CME Credit"). Following the questions are a blank answer sheet and answers with discussions. Although a concerted effort has been made to avoid ambiguity and redundancy in these questions, the authors recognize that differences of opinion may occur regarding the "best" answer. The discussions are provided to demonstrate the rationale used to derive the answer. They may also be helpful in confirming that your approach to the problem was correct or, if necessary, in fixing the principle in your memory. The Section 12 faculty thanks the Self-Assessment Committee for reviewing the self-assessment questions.

1. What is a posterior extension of the pars plana epithelium to the retinal side of the ora serrata?
   a. enclosed ora bay
   b. meridional complex
   c. dentate process
   d. peripheral retinal excavation

2. What adjacent tissue layer undergoes atrophy in conjunction with retinal pigment epithelium (RPE) atrophy?
   a. full-thickness retina
   b. full-thickness choroid
   c. choriocapillaris
   d. no adjacent atrophy; RPE usually atrophies in isolation

3. What diagnostic imaging test is quantitative for the detection of retinal thickening in diabetic macular edema?
   a. slit-lamp biomicroscopy with contact lens
   b. fluorescein angiography
   c. B-scan ultrasound
   d. optical coherence tomography

4. What represents appropriate management of a patient who has just undergone fluorescein angiography?
   a. administer aspirin
   b. observe the patient for signs of delayed adverse reactions
   c. advise the patient to avoid sunlight for 5 days after the procedure
   d. order a urine culture and sensitivity testing for urine color change

5. The activity measured in the pattern electroretinogram is generated mainly in which retinal cells?
   a. ganglion cells
   b. bipolar cells
   c. photoreceptors
   d. amacrine cells

6. What effect does demyelinating optic neuritis with recovered visual acuity have on pattern-reversal visual evoked potential (VEP) testing?
   a. delayed pattern-reversal VEP
   b. inverted pattern-reversal VEP
   c. enhanced pattern-reversal VEP
   d. reversed pattern-reversal VEP

7. What clinical finding is considered a risk factor for the development of neovascular age-related macular degeneration?
   a. multiple small drusen in 1 eye
   b. multiple small drusen in both eyes
   c. absence of pigment clumping
   d. large drusen with pigment clumping

8. Which eyes are at greatest risk for the development of an RPE tear after anti–vascular endothelial growth factor (anti-VEGF) therapy?
   a. eyes with a fibrovascular pigment epithelial detachment (PED) > 600 μm in height
   b. eyes with a large classic choroidal neovascularization (CNV)
   c. eyes with a serous PED > 600 μm in height
   d. eyes with type 2 neovascularization

9. For a patient with proliferative diabetic retinopathy and a diabetic midperipheral tractional retinal detachment, what complication is of primary concern in the initial application of panretinal photocoagulation?
   a. rhegmatogenous retinal detachment
   b. cortical cataract
   c. retinal neovascularization
   d. tractional macular detachment

10. In patients with diabetic macular edema, what is the best management strategy before considering cataract surgery?
    a. advise the patient to avoid surgery because disease progression is inevitable
    b. consider pretreating the patient with an anti-VEGF agent
    c. administer panretinal photocoagulation first
    d. plan for use of a small capsulorrhexis to avoid development of rubeosis

11. What is a characteristic clinical sequela of hypertensive choroidopathy?
    a. sub–internal limiting membrane hemorrhages
    b. linear streaks of hyperpigmentation
    c. retinal neovascularization
    d. cystoid macular edema

12. A patient who experiences an acute subarachnoid hemorrhage is found to have loss of vision and vitreous hemorrhage. What is the pathophysiologic process that has been implicated in this condition?
    a. granulocyte aggregation
    b. leukoembolization
    c. acute rise in intraocular venous pressure
    d. fat embolization

13. What condition can be associated with retinal capillary hemangioblastomas?
    a. choroidal hemangioma
    b. pheochromocytoma
    c. retinal arterial macroaneurysm
    d. astrocytoma

14. A patient incurs an acute compression injury to the thorax and experiences sudden loss of vision in both eyes. Each eye exhibits large cotton-wool spots, hemorrhages, and retinal edema. What factor would explain the relationship between the compression injury and the retinal findings?
    a. acute rise in intraocular venous pressure
    b. acute rise in systolic blood pressure
    c. compression of the central retinal vein
    d. complement activation

15. What is an accepted guideline for ophthalmoscopic screening for retinopathy of prematurity (ROP)?
    a. Screening should be performed on all premature neonates with a gestational age of 32 weeks or more.
    b. Screening should be repeated every 4 weeks on neonates who demonstrate ROP on initial examination.
    c. Screening should be performed on all premature neonates with a birth weight of 1500 g or less, with a gestational age of 30 weeks or less before hospital discharge, or who have reached 4–6 weeks of age.
    d. Screening should be performed on all premature neonates with a birth weight less than 3000 g.

16. What feature in high-risk neonates is a risk factor for ROP?
    a. fever
    b. paternal age
    c. history of blood transfusion
    d. light exposure

17. In a patient diagnosed with central serous chorioretinopathy, what finding may initiate reconsideration of the diagnosis?
    a. retinal pigment epithelial detachment
    b. serous retinal detachment
    c. large drusen
    d. pigment clumping

18. What is the most consistent diagnostic feature of circumscribed choroidal hemangiomas?
    a. association with serous detachments
    b. echographic reflectivity
    c. color of the lesion
    d. late-phase hypofluorescence on indocyanine green angiography

19. What is an important risk factor for ocular toxoplasmosis?
    a. consumption of undercooked meat
    b. exposure to ticks
    c. exposure to mosquitoes
    d. living in the Ohio River Valley

20. What is a clinical feature of the multiple evanescent white dot syndrome?
    a. RPE scarring
    b. gray-white, poorly demarcated, patchy, outer-retinal lesions
    c. severe vitreous cellular reaction
    d. gray granular pigmentation of the fovea

21. What finding in Vogt-Koyanagi-Harada disease suggests chronicity?
    a. serous retinal detachment
    b. optic disc hyperemia/edema
    c. choroidal thickening on spectral-domain optical coherence tomography (SD-OCT)
    d. choroidal depigmentation, or "sunset glow" fundus

22. A 78-year-old white man underwent uncomplicated cataract surgery 5 years before developing moderately severe panuveitis in the operated eye. What feature of this patient's presentation is most inconsistent with the diagnosis of sympathetic ophthalmia?
    a. patient's advanced age and relatively weakened immune status
    b. patient's race
    c. unilaterality
    d. time from surgery to the onset of uveitis

23. A 40-year-old black man presents with an active focal retinochoroiditis with an adjacent retinochoroidal scar. The patient recalls no prior episodes of uveitis. What is the most likely diagnosis?
    a. newly acquired toxoplasmosis (first episode)
    b. acquired toxoplasmosis reactivation
    c. congenital ocular toxoplasmosis reactivation
    d. cytomegalovirus retinitis

24. Which of the following statements regarding congenital stationary night blindness (CSNB) is true?
    a. The "complete" form of CSNB is a consequence of rod photoreceptor dysfunction.
    b. Patients with the "incomplete" form of CSNB have normal cone electroretinogram (ERG) responses.
    c. Complete X-linked stationary night blindness affects the on-bipolar cell pathway in all retinal photoreceptor types.
    d. Complete X-linked stationary night blindness is caused by mutations in *CACNA1F*.

25. A mutation of which gene in which cell type results in nonprogressive dysfunction in patients with nyctalopia and white dots?
    a. *RDH5* gene mutation in retinal photoreceptors
    b. *RDH5* gene mutation in retinal pigmented epithelium
    c. *RLBP1* gene mutation in retinal photoreceptors
    d. *ABCA4* gene mutation in retinal pigmented epithelium

26. What is a clinical finding in rod monochromacy?
    a. autosomal dominant pattern of inheritance
    b. strabismus
    c. better visual acuity in rod monochromacy than in S-cone monochromacy
    d. normal rod function shown on electroretinogram in complete achromatopsia

27. What disorder is most typically associated with a negative ERG waveform?
    a. Leber congenital amaurosis
    b. retinitis pigmentosa (RP)
    c. X-linked retinoschisis
    d. achromatopsia

28. Cystoid macular edema most commonly complicates which of the following inherited ocular disorders?
    a. Stargardt disease
    b. Best disease
    c. pattern dystrophy
    d. retinitis pigmentosa

29. What syndrome associated with RP is classified as a retinal ciliopathy involving mutations that affect the cilia of multiple organ systems, including cilia present in photoreceptor outer segments and the inner ear?
    a. Bardet-Biedl syndrome
    b. Refsum disease
    c. Zellweger syndrome
    d. Batten disease

30. What paraneoplastic retinal degeneration is associated with antirecoverin antibodies?
    a. melanoma-associated retinopathy
    b. bilateral diffuse uveal melanocytic proliferation
    c. cancer-associated retinopathy
    d. acute exudative paraneoplastic vitelliform maculopathy

31. What metabolic disorder causes a cherry-red spot?
    a. Hurler syndrome
    b. Tay-Sachs disease
    c. Gaucher disease
    d. Hunter syndrome

32. The systemic use of which drug can be complicated by pigmentary retinopathy?
    a. docetaxel
    b. paclitaxel
    c. niacin
    d. thioridazine

33. Intake of which compound(s) can cause inner segment ellipsoid disruption apparent on SD-OCT imaging?
    a. alkyl nitrite ("poppers") inhalation
    b. kola nut ingestion
    c. canthaxanthine ingestion
    d. talc injection

34. What is characteristic of retinal detachments following ocular blunt trauma in young eyes?
    a. Retinal detachments are almost always identified shortly after the trauma.
    b. Retinal detachments in this setting typically progress rapidly.
    c. Retinal detachments in this setting have a delayed presentation.
    d. Retinal detachments in this setting are typically bullous.

35. What peripheral retinal lesion is *least* likely to be associated with retinal tear or detachment?
    a. lattice degeneration
    b. meridional folds
    c. paving-stone degeneration
    d. zonular traction tufts

36. What is a risk factor for retinal detachment following cataract surgery?
    a. hyperopia
    b. younger age
    c. female sex
    d. systemic hypertension

37. What is a characteristic finding in eyes with persistent fetal vasculature?
    a. microphthalmos
    b. intraocular calcification
    c. retinal telangiectasia
    d. peripheral granuloma

38. What is a feature of Wagner disease with optically empty vitreous?
    a. systemic hypertension
    b. lens subluxation
    c. aortic regurgitation
    d. myopia

39. What is a characteristic of familial exudative vitreoretinopathy?
    a. premature birth
    b. esotropia
    c. failure of the temporal retina to vascularize
    d. history of supplemental oxygen

40. What imaging test is contraindicated in the initial evaluation of ocular trauma?
    a. plain film X-ray
    b. computed tomography of the eye and orbit
    c. magnetic resonance imaging
    d. ocular ultrasound

41. What is a characteristic feature of choroidal rupture?
    a. rarely results in subretinal hemorrhage
    b. typically radiates from the optic disc
    c. typically occurs concentric to the optic disc
    d. occurs only anterior to the equator

42. What metal is most toxic as an intraocular foreign body?
    a. aluminum
    b. zinc
    c. iron
    d. copper

43. What color wavelength is readily absorbed by macular xanthophyll?
    a. blue
    b. red
    c. green
    d. yellow

44. Photodynamic therapy is approved by the US Food and Drug Administration (FDA) for which indication?
    a. subfoveal CNV secondary to pathologic myopia
    b. subfoveal CNV secondary to posterior uveitis
    c. central serous retinopathy
    d. choroidal hemangioma

45. What is a potential advantage of subthreshold (barely visible to invisible) laser treatment over conventional laser treatment?
    a. effect is long lasting and retreatment is not required
    b. has the potential to reduce the number and size of scotomas
    c. easier means for titrating and determining the extent of treatment
    d. does not require wide pupillary dilation

46. What finding is a classic indication for pneumatic retinopexy?
    a. retinal break in any location
    b. single retinal break
    c. multiple retinal breaks spanning 3–6 clock-hours
    d. absence of proliferative vitreoretinopathy grade A or B

47. What complication can occur after retrobulbar anesthesia?
    a. acute angle-closure glaucoma
    b. respiratory depression
    c. malignant hyperthermia
    d. isolated branch retinal vein occlusion

48. What ocular characteristic affects success rate with respect to resolution of vitreomacular traction syndrome and closure of macular holes using ocriplasmin?
    a. area of vitreomacular adhesion
    b. axial length
    c. duration of symptoms
    d. lens status (phakic versus intraocular lens)

Answer Sheet for Section 12 Study Questions

Question	Answer	Question	Answer
1	a b c d	25	a b c d
2	a b c d	26	a b c d
3	a b c d	27	a b c d
4	a b c d	28	a b c d
5	a b c d	29	a b c d
6	a b c d	30	a b c d
7	a b c d	31	a b c d
8	a b c d	32	a b c d
9	a b c d	33	a b c d
10	a b c d	34	a b c d
11	a b c d	35	a b c d
12	a b c d	36	a b c d
13	a b c d	37	a b c d
14	a b c d	38	a b c d
15	a b c d	39	a b c d
16	a b c d	40	a b c d
17	a b c d	41	a b c d
18	a b c d	42	a b c d
19	a b c d	43	a b c d
20	a b c d	44	a b c d
21	a b c d	45	a b c d
22	a b c d	46	a b c d
23	a b c d	47	a b c d
24	a b c d	48	a b c d

Answers

1. **a.** A dentate process is an anterior extension of retinal tissue that separates adjacent ora bays in pars plana and is aligned with but does not reach a minor ciliary process. A meridional complex is a hyperplastic dentate process that extends across the entire length of the pars plana and merges with a ciliary process. A peripheral retinal excavation is a small, oval retinal depression posterior to the ora and is often aligned with a meridional fold or complex. It is excavated because of hypoplasia of inner retinal layers, similar to lattice degeneration.
2. **c.** Atrophy of the retinal pigment epithelium (RPE) results in adjacent outer segment and choriocapillaris atrophy. These 3 layers are interdependent on one another. The remaining retinal and outer choroidal layers are not affected by RPE loss.
3. **d.** Diabetic macular edema (DME) can be detected by slit-lamp biomicroscopy with contact lens or optical coherence tomography (OCT), but only OCT provides measurements of the thickness of the retina. Fluorescein angiography reveals leakage, which may or may not correspond to thickening. The resolution of B-scan ultrasound is generally too low to reliably detect any increase in macular thickness.
4. **b.** Most patients tolerate fluorescein angiography well without adverse effects or sequelae. Simple observation of the patient for several minutes after completion of the test is sufficient to detect an allergic reaction. Diphenhydramine, not aspirin, is most commonly used if mild signs of allergy appear. Avoidance of sunlight is not necessary because, unlike for verteporfin, no increased sun sensitivity results from fluorescein administration. A color change in the urine is expected as the dye exits the body and does not suggest an infection.
5. **a.** The pattern electroretinogram (PERG) shows the response of the central retina to a contrast stimulus. It is mostly generated in relation to the retinal ganglion cells. The (full-field) ERG is not affected in patients with dysfunction confined to the macula. Patients with generalized retinal dysfunction, and thus with abnormal results on full-field ERGs, have an abnormal PERG only if the macula is involved.
6. **a.** Optic nerve disease often results in peak-time delay in the pattern-reversal visual evoked potential (VEP). The predominant abnormality in nonarteritic anterior ischemic optic neuropathy is amplitude reduction rather than peak-time delay. Delayed pattern-reversal VEPs are frequently present in macular dysfunction. Demyelinating optic neuritis is almost invariably associated with continuing peak-time delay even after recovery of visual acuity. Compared with pattern-reversal VEPs, pattern-appearance VEPs are relatively insensitive to the presence of nystagmus.
7. **d.** According to the Age-Related Eye Disease Study (AREDS), stage 2 (multiple small or few intermediate drusen in 1 or both eyes) of the dry form of age-related macular degeneration (AMD) had a very low incidence of progression to neovascular AMD, whereas stage 3 (a few large drusen or multiple intermediate drusen) and stage 4 (geographic atrophy) eyes had high incidences of progression to neovascular AMD after 5 years (18% for stage 3, and 40% for stage 4). Pigment clumping was considered an additional risk factor according to AREDS.
8. **a.** Following anti–vascular endothelial growth factor (anti-VEGF) therapy, both a pigment epithelial detachment greater than 600 μm in height and the presence of type 1 choroidal neovascularization (CNV), as evidenced by a fibrovascular component, increase

the risk of an RPE tear. The mechanism may relate to contraction along the undersurface of the RPE monolayer as a result of the treatment.

9. **a.** In the midperiphery, the retina is considerably thinner than in the posterior pole. Panretinal photocoagulation (PRP) may lead to some degree of contraction of fibrovascular proliferative tissue as it involutes. The contraction can exert sufficient traction to cause a retinal tear, which in turn can cause a retinal detachment. Retinal tears from PRP treatment are rare in the posterior pole because of the thicker retina in that location. Although a cortical cataract could develop if there is pigment on the lens that absorbs the laser light, this complication is both rare and not the primary concern. By definition, in proliferative diabetic retinopathy, retinal neovascularization is already present. The tractional detachment is described to be in the periphery, not the macula. As such, tractional macular detachment is not a primary concern but should always be kept in mind as a possibility.

10. **b.** It is advisable to treat any preexisting DME prior to cataract surgery in an attempt to minimize or prevent worsening as a result of the surgical procedure. In patients with DME, anti-VEGF agents are excellent treatment options and may help reduce the risk of worsening the macular edema. Progression of diabetic retinopathy or DME is not inevitable if managed appropriately and aggressively. PRP can sometimes worsen DME in the short run but may help reduce DME in the long run. A small capsulorrhexis would have no expected impact in preventing worsening of DME.

11. **b.** In hypertensive choroidopathy, lobular nonperfusion of the choriocapillaris may occur, resulting in Elschnig spots (hyperpigmented spots surrounded by margins of hypopigmentation) or Siegrist streaks (linear configurations of hyperpigmentation following the meridional course of choroidal arteries). Sub–internal limiting membrane hemorrhages, retinal neovascularization, and cystoid macular edema (CME) are characteristic sequelae of hypertensive retinopathy, not hypertensive choroidopathy.

12. **c.** The clinical presentation is consistent with Terson syndrome, which is caused by abrupt intracranial hemorrhage. The mechanism is suspected to be that the hemorrhage causes an acute rise in the intraocular venous pressure, resulting in a rupture of peripapillary and retinal vessels. Granulocyte aggregation, leukoembolization, and fat embolization are not thought to be causative or contributory factors in Terson syndrome. They are, however, thought to play roles in the pathogenesis of Purtscher retinopathy and Purtscherlike retinopathy.

13. **b.** Von Hippel–Lindau disease is characterized by retinal capillary hemangioblastomas in association with angiomatous lesions of the central nervous system and cysts and tumors in the viscera. Manifestations include cerebellar hemangioblastoma, pancreatic cysts, renal cell carcinoma, and pheochromocytoma. Diffuse choroidal hemangioma is associated with Sturge-Weber syndrome, whereas circumscribed choroidal hemangiomas have no systemic disease or syndrome association. Retinal astrocytic hamartomas, or retinal astrocytomas, are benign lesions and may be associated with tuberous sclerosis or neurofibromatosis type 1. On the other hand, central nervous system astrocytomas can be malignant tumors. Retinal arterial macroaneurysms are associated with hypertension and atherosclerotic disease.

14. **d.** Purtscher retinopathy typically follows acute compression injuries to the thorax or head. It is thought to be a result of injury-induced complement activation, which causes granulocyte aggregation and leukoembolization. This process in turn occludes small arterioles such as those found in the peripapillary retina.

15. **c.** Several risk factors have been associated with the development of retinopathy of prematurity (ROP) in premature neonates, including low birth weight, low gestational age, oxygen therapy, apnea, sepsis, and others. Premature infants with a birth weight of 1500 g or less, of gestational age of 30 weeks or less, or who require supplemental oxygen are particularly at risk of developing ROP. Initial examination of the peripheral retina by indirect ophthalmoscopy in these neonates is recommended before hospital discharge, or by 4–6 weeks of postnatal age (or within the 31st to 33rd week of postconceptional or postmenstrual age, whichever is later). Retinal examinations are repeated every 1–2 weeks until the retina becomes fully vascularized or ROP is noted. If ROP develops, weekly examinations should be performed to watch for possible progression to threshold disease.
16. **c.** Premature babies that have been septic, have required a blood transfusion, and have poor postnatal weight gain have been shown in several studies to be at higher risk of developing ROP. Light exposure, paternal age, and fever (without sepsis) have not been shown to increase the risk of ROP development.
17. **c.** Central serous chorioretinopathy (CSR) is characterized by the presence of retinal pigment epithelial detachments, serous retinal detachments, and macular and/or inferior peripheral pigmentary changes. Large drusen are not a feature of CSR and should suggest an alternate or concurrent diagnosis of AMD-related macular degeneration.
18. **b.** Circumscribed choroidal hemangiomas are among the rarest intraocular tumors. In Sturge-Weber disease, choroidal hemangiomas may be diffuse and typically have a tomato ketchup appearance. For circumscribed choroidal hemangiomas, the color may vary from white to tomato ketchup red, depending on the overlying RPE. On indocyanine green angiography, persistent diffuse hyperfluorescence may be apparent in the late phase. Serous retinal detachments may be associated with choroidal hemangiomas, but they are usually less severe than those that occur with malignant melanoma of the choroid. Echography of circumscribed choroidal hemangiomas usually demonstrates a highly reflective mass with uniform, high internal spikes; this feature is the most consistent finding.
19. **a.** Consumption of undercooked or raw meat or of substances contaminated with cat feces are risk factors for ocular toxoplasmosis. Exposure to ticks increases the risk of Lyme disease, whereas exposure to mosquitoes increases the risk of acquiring various infectious disease–causing organisms (eg, the parasites that cause malaria or the West Nile virus). The Ohio River Valley is endemic for the ocular histoplasmosis syndrome.
20. **b.** Multiple evanescent white dot syndrome is characterized by the presence of multiple, small gray-white dots at the level of the deep retina/RPE in the posterior pole. Foveal granularity, when present, appears as tiny yellow-orange dots. Mild vitritis may or may not be present but is not severe when present. RPE scarring is not a feature, as the condition typically resolves spontaneously over 2–6 weeks.
21. **d.** Serous retinal detachment, optic disc hyperemia, and choroidal thickening are all signs of the acute uveitic phase of Vogt-Koyanagi-Harada disease. Choroidal depigmentation, or "sunset glow" fundus, is a sign of recurrent/chronic disease and occurs late in the course of the condition.
22. **c.** Sympathetic ophthalmia is always bilateral. Bilaterality may be difficult or impossible to document if the inciting eye is phthisical or has been removed. Sympathetic ophthalmia may occur in any race at any age and at any time following eye surgery or trauma.

23. **b.** The vast majority of ocular toxoplasmosis is acquired. The presence of a retinochoroidal scar is strong support for prior infection, meaning that this particular episode is not primary and that infection could have occurred either at or long after birth. The absence of an adjacent or nearby retinochoroidal scar together with a positive serum test result for anti-*Toxoplasma gondii* IgM antibody would constitute strong supportive evidence for an acutely acquired infection. Cytomegalovirus retinitis is rare and is typically observed in severely immunosuppressed individuals.

24. **c.** Complete X-linked congenital stationary night blindness (CSNB) is caused by mutations in the *NYX* gene and affects the on-bipolar cell pathways in rods and all cone systems. Incomplete X-linked CSNB is a result of mutations in the *CACNA1F* gene; it involves both on- and off-bipolar cell cone pathways and causes very abnormal cone-system ERG responses. Although the rod-specific ERG (dim-flash, dark-adapted 0.01) is abnormal in CSNB, the presence of a normal a-wave in response to a bright flash under scotopic conditions confirms normal photoreceptor phototransduction.

25. **b.** Fundus albipunctatus is caused by a mutation in the gene *RDH5*. *RDH5* encodes 11-*cis*-retinol dehydrogenase, a microsomal enzyme in the RPE that converts 11-*cis*-retinol into 11-*cis*-retinal and is therefore involved in the regeneration of rhodopsin. Patients with mutations in this gene have very delayed rhodopsin regeneration, and although levels eventually normalize, the process may take many hours in the dark. Mutations in the gene *RLBP1* result in retinitis punctata albescens. *ABCA4* is a gene that, depending upon the exact mutation, may cause fundus flavimaculatus, cone–rod dystrophy, retinitis pigmentosa (RP), or AMD, among others.

26. **d.** Complete achromatopsia, or rod monochromacy, has an autosomal recessive inheritance pattern. Patients usually present with early-onset nystagmus not strabismus. Electroretinography typically shows normal rod function but undetectable cone function. Visual acuity in S-cone monochromacy, in which there are functioning S cones, is usually better than that in rod monochromacy.

27. **c.** A negative ERG waveform refers to a preserved a-wave and a selectively reduced b-wave; it can be present in several clinical diseases including CSNB, X-linked retinoschisis, paraneoplastic retinopathy, and central retinal artery occlusion.

28. **d.** Among the conditions listed, RP is the most common condition complicated by CME; it has been reported to occur in approximately 10%–20% of RP patients. Although CNV can complicate Stargardt disease, Best disease, and pattern dystrophies, CME is rarely reported in these disorders. Acetazolamide has been shown to reduce CME in patients with RP.

29. **a.** In addition to Bardet-Biedl syndrome, other syndromic forms of RP associated with retinal and systemic ciliary dysfunction include Usher, Alström, Senior-Løken, Joubert, and Jeune syndromes. Patients with these forms often have hearing loss and renal disease in addition to RP.

30. **c.** Antirecoverin antibodies may be found in the serum of patients with cancer-associated retinopathy (CAR) and are highly suggestive of the presence of a systemic malignancy, such as small cell carcinoma of the lung. In some cases, these systemic malignancies may not be clinically detectable for some time after the onset of vision loss. Other antiretinal antibodies that can be present in patients with retinal degeneration include antienolase and antitransducin antibodies; because they are less specific, their presence supports a diagnosis of CAR less strongly. In such cases, *autoimmune retinopathy* is the preferred diagnostic terminology.

31. **b.** The most common cause of a cherry-red spot from metabolic disorder is Tay-Sachs disease. Other metabolic syndromes, such as Niemann-Pick disease, may also cause cherry-red spots. Hunter and Hurler syndromes cause a pigmentary retinopathy, whereas Gaucher disease causes white preretinal opacities that are well visualized with OCT imaging.

32. **d.** The taxanes (docetaxel, paclitaxel) and niacin may induce a microcystic form of macular edema that is detected on SD-OCT and does not leak on fluorescein angiography. The phenothiazine thioridazine can cause a severe pigmentary retinopathy that can develop within a few weeks or months of high-dose utilization. Toxicity is rare with thioridazine doses of less than 800 mg/day.

33. **a.** Alkyl nitrite ("poppers") inhalation has been associated with central disruption of the inner segment ellipsoid layer on spectral-domain optical coherence tomography (SD-OCT) analysis, sometimes referred to as *poppers maculopathy.* Ingestion of kola nuts or canthaxanthine or injection of talc may cause a crystalline maculopathy.

34. **c.** Retinal detachments following trauma in young patients typically have a delayed presentation. The delay results from the fact that the vitreous is still formed (ie, not syneretic), which has 3 effects: (1) the formed vitreous prevents fluid movement under the retina by acting like a cork on the break, (2) the vitreous prevents the retina from assuming a bullous shape, and (3) the progression is slow as the vitreous slowly liquefies over time.

35. **c.** Lattice degeneration is among the peripheral retinal lesions most associated with increased risk of retinal detachment. Meridional folds may develop a tear at the posterior edge of the fold, and zonular traction tufts are a cause of small retinal flap tears, often seen following cataract surgery. Paving-stone degeneration is not associated with increased retinal detachment risk, as it does not affect the vitreoretinal interface.

36. **b.** Risk factors for the development of retinal detachment following cataract surgery are male sex, younger age, myopia, increased axial length, and posterior capsular tear. Hyperopia is not considered a risk factor for retinal detachment.

37. **a.** In anterior persistent fetal vasculature (previously known as *hyperplastic primary vitreous*), the hyaloid artery remains, and a white vascularized fibrous membrane or mass is present behind the lens. Associated findings include microphthalmos, a shallow anterior chamber, and elongated ciliary processes that are visible around the small lens.

38. **d.** Wagner disease is characterized by an optically empty vitreous, myopia, strabismus, and cataract but no associated systemic findings.

39. **c.** Familial exudative vitreoretinopathy (FEVR) is characterized by failure of the temporal retina to vascularize. Although it is phenotypically similar to ROP, patients are born full term and have normal respiratory status. Differentiation of FEVR from ROP is also aided by the family history and a careful examination of all family members.

40. **c.** All of the listed tests are helpful in evaluating ocular trauma, particularly to assess for the presence or absence of an intraocular foreign body. Plain films, although still useful, may not allow visualization of small metallic or nonradiopaque foreign bodies. Similarly, computed tomography is very helpful but may not allow visualization of nonradiopaque foreign bodies. Ocular ultrasound must be performed with great caution, particularly when the eye is open, as compression of the eye can lead to extrusion of intraocular content. Magnetic resonance imaging (MRI) can be performed only after the presence of a ferromagnetic intraocular foreign body has been excluded and should therefore be avoided in the initial assessment. MRI offers the advantage of providing visualization of even nonradiopaque material such as wood.

41. **c.** When the eye is compressed along its anterior–posterior axis, tears may occur in the Bruch membrane, which has little elasticity, as well as in the overlying RPE and fibrous tissue investing the choriocapillaris. Adjacent subretinal hemorrhage is common. Choroidal ruptures occur typically in the periphery and concentric to the optic disc. There is no effective treatment for choroidal rupture.

42. **d.** Pure copper is especially toxic to the retina, and prompt removal is required. Copper causes acute chalcosis, which manifests as severe inflammation and may lead to loss of the eye. If copper is alloyed with another metal so that the material has a final copper content of less than 85% (eg, brass, bronze), chronic chalcosis may occur. Iron is also very toxic and can cause siderosis and vision loss. Zinc and aluminum tend to cause minimal inflammation and may become encapsulated. However, any very large foreign body may incite inflammation and thereby cause anterior and posterior proliferative vitreoretinopathy.

43. **a.** Macular xanthophyll readily absorbs blue but minimally absorbs yellow, red, and infrared wavelengths. Therefore, the blue wavelength should be avoided during laser photocoagulation (especially in the macula) in order to minimize thermal macular retinal damage.

44. **a.** Photodynamic therapy (PDT) is approved by the US Food and Drug Administration (FDA) for the treatment of certain types of subfoveal CNV in AMD and of subfoveal CNV secondary to ocular histoplasmosis syndrome and myopia. PDT has generally fallen out of favor for the management of CNV because more effective treatments have become available. PDT is currently the most successful treatment for CSR and circumscribed choroidal hemangiomas; however, its use is off-label for these indications.

45. **b.** Compared with conventional macular photocoagulation, delivery systems that apply subthreshold (barely visible to invisible) laser spots have the potential to reduce the number and size of scotomas. The shorter laser-energy pulses result in less or no thermal damage. However, titrating the amount of treatment is rendered difficult by the lack of visible feedback.

46. **b.** The classic indications for pneumatic retinopexy include confidence that all retinal breaks have been identified, retinal breaks that are confined to the superior 8 clock-hours, a single retinal break, multiple breaks within 1–2 clock-hours, the absence of proliferative vitreoretinopathy grade C or D, a cooperative patient who can maintain proper positioning, and clear media.

47. **b.** Reported complications of retrobulbar anesthesia include brainstem suppression with subsequent respiratory arrest. Combined central retinal artery and vein occlusion has been reported, but isolated branch retinal vein occlusion has not. Both malignant hyperthermia and acute angle-closure glaucoma are not known complications of retrobulbar anesthesia.

48. **a.** The area of vitreomacular adhesion (VMA) is an important predictor of successful resolution of vitreomacular traction using ocriplasmin. VMA resolved in 33.6% of eyes in which the size of adhesions was 1500 μm or smaller on OCT but in only 10.3% of adhesions larger than 1500 μm.

Index

(*f* = figure; *t* = table)